Digital Technologies in Craniomaxillofacial Surgery

Alex M. Greenberg
Editor

Digital Technologies in Craniomaxillofacial Surgery

Springer

Editor
Alex M. Greenberg
Columbia University
New York, NY, USA

ISBN 978-1-4939-1531-6 ISBN 978-1-4939-1532-3 (eBook)
https://doi.org/10.1007/978-1-4939-1532-3

Library of Congress Control Number: 2017913738

Printed on acid-free paper

This Springer imprint is published by the registered company Springer Science+Business Media, LLC part of Springer Nature.
The registered company address is: 233 Spring Street, New York, NY 10013, U.S.A.

Preface

It is with great pleasure that I present this first comprehensive book on the subject of digital technologies in Craniomaxillofacial Surgery. With the development of CT scanning and advanced imaging, 3D visualization of the facial bones and soft tissues has evolved to now include the virtual planning of surgical procedures and intraoperative navigation. These technologies can allow surgeons to preplan procedures to ensure precise surgical results. Rather than using the surgeon's 3D perception to imagine bone cuts, fitting of osteotomy segments, and grafts, these tools allow preoperative enactment and template design. 3D stereolithographic and rapid printed models can be used for osteotomy design, anatomically accurate implant fabrication, and communication with the surgical team. In this new textbook, we are able to review many of the latest advances in 3D modeling, software for virtual surgical planning (VSP), navigation, surgical cutting and drill templates, surgical occlusal splints, cranioplasty, radiation therapy, and custom facial and cranial implants. These innovative technologies allow for improved cost savings, time savings, improved outcomes, and the development of new surgical techniques.

I am indebted to my many colleagues from the many disciplines of Oral and Maxillofacial Surgery, Plastic and Reconstructive Surgery, Otolaryngology/Head and Neck Surgery, Neurosurgery, and Oral and Maxillofacial Radiology, as well as the 3D printing industry who have contributed to this work.

New York, NY, USA   Alex M. Greenberg

Contents

Contributors

Oleh M. Antonyshyn, MD, FRCSC Division of Plastic Surgery, Sunnybrook Health Sciences Centre, University of Toronto, Toronto, ON, Canada

Christopher Beaudreau, BS 3D Systems, Littleton, CO, USA

Joshua B. Bederson, MD Department of Neurosurgery, The Mount Sinai Hospital, Icahn School of Medicine at Mount Sinai, New York, NY, USA

Gido Bittermann, DMD, MD, Dr Department of Craniomaxillofacial Surgery, University of Freiburg, Freiburg, Germany

Vincent Carrao, DDS, MD Division of Oral and Maxillofacial Surgery, The Mount Sinai Hospital, Icahn School of Medicine at Mount Sinai, New York, NY, USA

Andrew M. Christensen, BS Division of Medical Physics, University of Ottawa, Ottawa, ON, Canada

Anthony B. Costa, PhD Department of Neurosurgery, The Mount Sinai Hospital, Icahn School of Medicine at Mount Sinai, New York, NY, USA

Glenn Edwards, BES, BArch Calavera Surgical Design, Toronto, ON, Canada

Nils-Claudius Gellrich, MD, DDS, Prof Dr Department of Oral & Craniomaxillofacial Surgery, Hannover Medical School, Hannover, Germany

Satish Govindaraj, MD Department of Otolaryngology, The Mount Sinai Hospital, Icahn School of Medicine at Mount Sinai, New York, NY, USA

Gerald T. Grant, DMD, MS, FACP Oral Health and Rehabilitation, University of Louisville School of Dentistry, Louisville, KY, USA

Alex M. Greenberg, DDS Division of Oral and Maxillofacial Surgery, Columbia University College of Dental Medicine, New York, NY, USA

The New York Presbyterian Hospital, New York, NY, USA

The Mount Sinai Hospital, New York, NY, USA

Samer Elia Haber, MD Plastic and Maxillofacial Surgery Department, Hôtel Dieu de France Hospital, Beirut, Lebanon

Hugo St. Hilaire, DDS, MD, FACS Division of Plastic & Reconstructive Surgery, Department of Surgery, Louisiana State University, New Orleans, LA, USA

Benjamin Johnson, BS 3D Systems, Littleton, CO, USA

Sarah M. Kidwai, MD Department of Otolaryngology, The Mount Sinai Hospital, Icahn School of Medicine at Mount Sinai, New York, NY, USA

James G. Mainprize, PhD Department of Physical Sciences, Sunnybrook Research Institute, Toronto, ON, Canada

James Leighton Mayo, MD Aesthetic and Reconstructive Surgery Institute, Orlando Health-University of Florida Cancer Center of Orlando, Orlando, FL, USA

Marc C. Metzger, DMD, MD, PhD, Prof Dr Department of Maxillofacial and Oral Surgery, University of Freiburg, Freiburg, Germany

Arjun K. Parasher, MD Department of Otolaryngology, The Mount Sinai Hospital, Icahn School of Medicine at Mount Sinai, New York, NY, USA

Anup Patel, MD, MBA Yale Plastic Surgery, New Haven, CT, USA

Majeed Rana, MD, DDS, PD Dr Department of Oral & Craniomaxillofacial Surgery, Hannover Medical School, Hanover, Germany

Michael Rensberger, MS 3D Systems, Littleton, CO, USA

Kyle J. Riley, BA Icahn School of Medicine at Mount Sinai, New York, NY, USA

Rainer Schmelzeisen, MD, DDS, PhD, FRCS, Prof Dr Department of Maxillofacial and Oral Surgery, University of Freiburg, Freiburg, Germany

Raj Shrivastava, MD Department of Neurosurgery, The Mount Sinai Hospital, Icahn School of Medicine at Mount Sinai, New York, NY, USA

Derek M. Steinbacher, DMD, MD, FACS Craniomaxillofacial Surgery, Yale University School of Medicine, New Haven, CT, USA

Leslie H. Sultan, DDS Department of Surgery, Broward Health Medical Center, Fort Lauderdale, FL, USA

Mohammad Tofigh, DDS, MD Private Practive, Oral and Maxillofacial Surgery, New York, NY, USA

Katherine Weimer, BS, MS 3D Systems, Littleton, CO, USA

Samuel J. Zeichner, DMD, MA, MS(Hyg) Division of Oral and Maxillofacial Radiology, Columbia University College of Dental Medicine, New York, NY, USA

University of Basel Faculty of Medicine, Department of Clinical Morphology, Biomedical Engineering/Hightech Research Center, Allschwil, Switzerland

Introduction to *Digital Technologies in Craniomaxillofacial Surgery*

1

Alex M. Greenberg

The purpose of this textbook is to review digital technologies in craniomaxillofacial surgery that have become important new tools for surgeons. As a result of improvements in digital imaging technology and the software programs that are able to utilize their data, a wide variety of applications have been developed [1, 2]. These applications include the use of virtual surgical planning (VSP) for the design and intraoperative implementation of surgical procedures involving orthognathic surgery, resection and immediate reconstruction of tumors, distraction osteogenesis, cranioplasty, cosmetic facial implants, dental implant placement, and facial fractures. Stereolithographic and rapid printing allows the fabrication of highly accurate 3D models and surgical templates to support these various craniomaxillofacial surgical procedures (Fig. 1.1). Primary to all of these applications have been advances in CT scanning specifically cone beam CT (CBCT), which has become widely available as an outpatient office scanning procedure [3]. CBCT has a significantly lower radiation exposure [3] and provides high levels of 3D imaging at a reduced cost. For the first time, 3D imaging has become available in an office setting with CBCT software applications that provide surgeons with powerful diagnostic and treatment tools (Figs. 1.1, 1.2, 1.3, and 1.4). Data from CBCT can be uploaded to various vendors for use with virtual surgical planning (VSP).

Stereolithographic model fabrication, rapid manufacturing, and rapid printing allow the implementation of VSP or other planning methods by the production of accurate anatomic models, cutting and drilling guides (Fig. 1.5) [4], prefabrication of bone plates, occlusal splints [5], and other surgical hardware. Orthognathic surgical procedures that required 6–8 h of planning utilizing hand drawn tracings of cephalometric x-rays, the production of mounted dental casts, the cutting of plaster models, and hand fabrication of occlusal splints are now replaced with highly accurate and timesaving virtual surgical planning and rapid printed cutting guides and occlusal templates (Fig. 1.6) [6]. Distraction osteogenesis can also be planned and performed utilizing VSP with cutting and drill guides for the creation of osteotomies and the placement of hardware. Stereolithographic models can be sterilized and used in surgery for various applications. Stereolithographic models can also be utilized to practice osteotomy cuts and design bone cutting procedures (Figs. 1.7–1.15). Stereolithographic models can also be utilized for the custom fabrication of patient-specific implants for facial cosmetic surgery utilizing solid silicone or PTFE (Figs. 1.16–1.24) [7]. The precision placement of dental implants utilizing software planning with surgical drill guides fabricated by rapid printing allows flapless placement with control of implant trajectory and depth (Figs. 1.25–1.32) [3, 8]. Immediate temporization through laboratory or CADCAM milling in coordination with dental implant software planning can allow for teeth in a day procedures. Cranioplasty procedures with mesh and methylmethacrylate are now replaced by 3D modeling using VSP to create patient-specific cranial and craniofacial implants [9]. Cranial implants made with PEEK can be CNC milled, or titanium mesh fabricated by titanium implants can be fabricated using selective laser melting (SLM), electron beam melting (EBM), and direct metal sintering (DMLS) [2].

Navigation has proven to be a valuable new tool for the management of complex head and neck tumor surgery, craniofacial surgery, endoscopic sinus surgery, and orthographic surgery to ensure the correct resection of margins, repositioning of segments, and immediate reconstruction with complex bone grafts in 3D real-time space [10–15]. Complex surgery for facial transplantation, war injury-related facial reconstruction, cancer ablation, and immediate reconstruction can benefit from intraoperative

A.M. Greenberg (✉)
Division of Oral and Maxillofacial Surgery, Columbia University College of Dental Medicine, 18 East 48th Street Suite 1702, New York, NY 10017, USA
e-mail: nycimplant@aol.com

A.M. Greenberg (ed.), *Digital Technologies in Craniomaxillofacial Surgery*, https://doi.org/10.1007/978-1-4939-1532-3_1

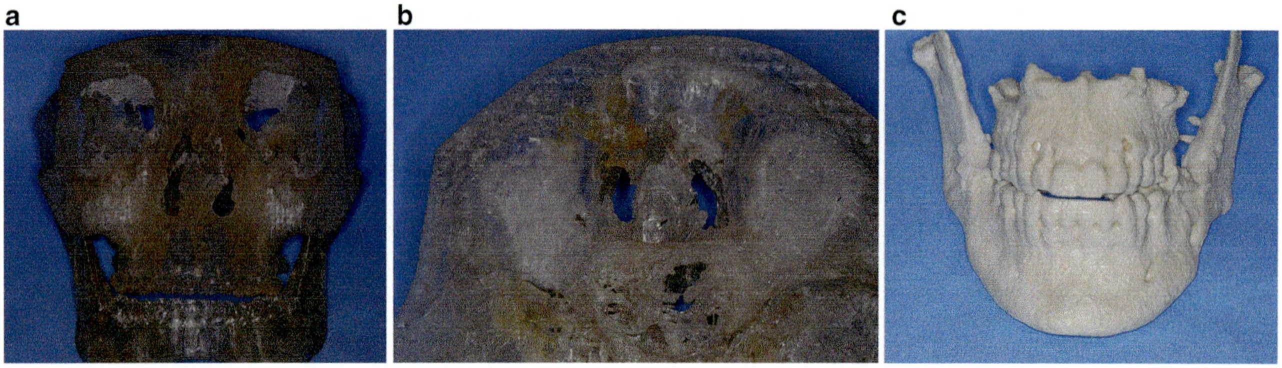

Fig. 1.1 Stereolithographic model of skull with meningocele anterior cranial base and hypertelorism with nasal deformity and skeletal Class III malocclusion Figs. (**a**) and (**b**). (**a**) Frontal view. (**b**) Superior view. (**c**) 3D printed maxilla and mandible

Fig. 1.2 CBCT axial view of mandible

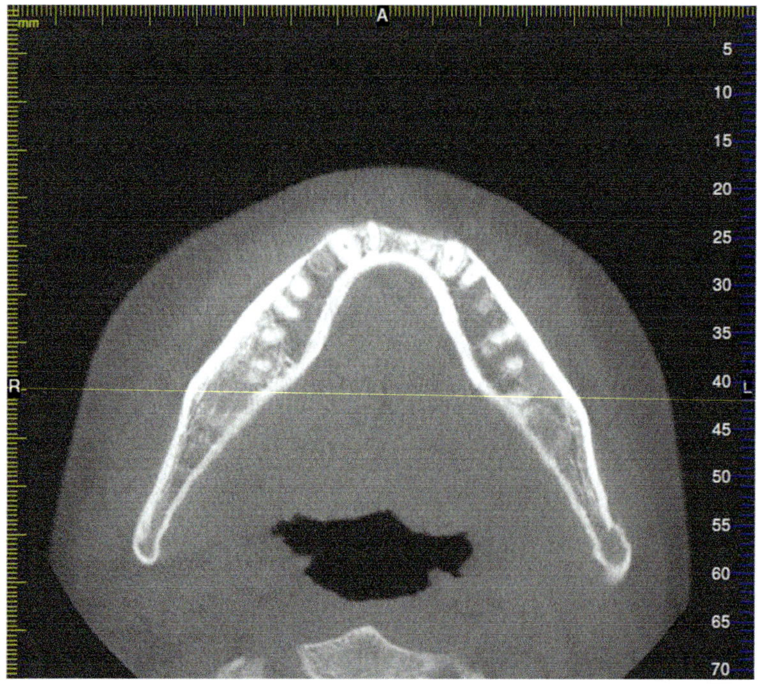

cutting guide utilization. Head and neck tumor surgery can be preoperatively precisely digitally planned for both the resection and immediate reconstruction with microvascular osteomyocutaneous grafts with dental implant planning as a single procedure with rapid printed or milled bone cutting guides, drill guides, and occlusal splints (Figs. 1.33–1.43) [16]. New frontiers in facial transplantation also benefit from preoperative digital planning and the use of cutting guides (Figs. 1.44–1.50) [17]. Digital planning for radiation therapy for head and neck tumors with improved accuracy for preoperative, intraoperative, and postoperative beam orientation and more precise field of exposure is a new area of interest.

Digital technologies are just at the beginning of providing surgeons with important tools to allow more accurate, precise surgical procedures with the advantage of improved patient outcomes. The savings of time allows surgeons to care for more patients in an efficient manner compared to traditional analog methods. Sharing of information through the Internet whether data transfer, sharing of images, and participation of doctors as teams improves communication and reduces misdiagnosis and errors that were acceptable in the past. Innovations can multiply more rapidly in the digital environment, and entire fields of surgery can be upended overnight by breakthrough techniques that can be practiced virtually before implementation in the operating room.

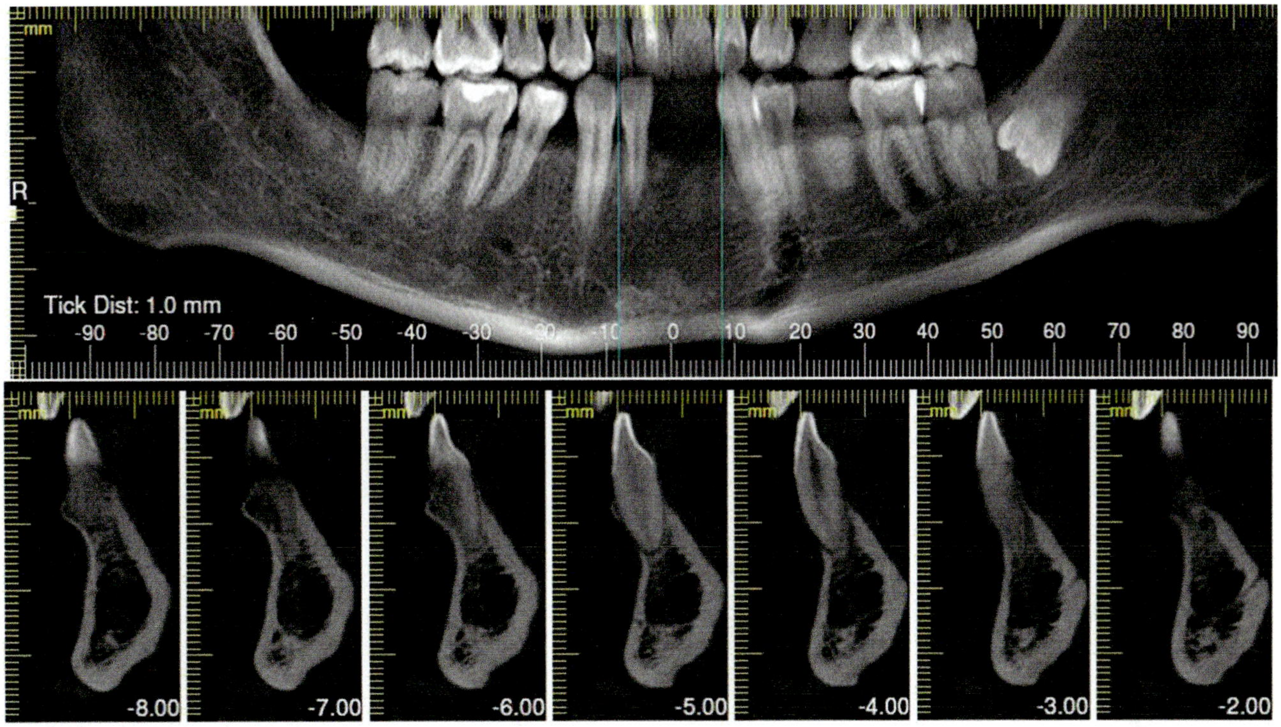

Fig. 1.3 CBCT panoramic and sagittal oblique views of mandible

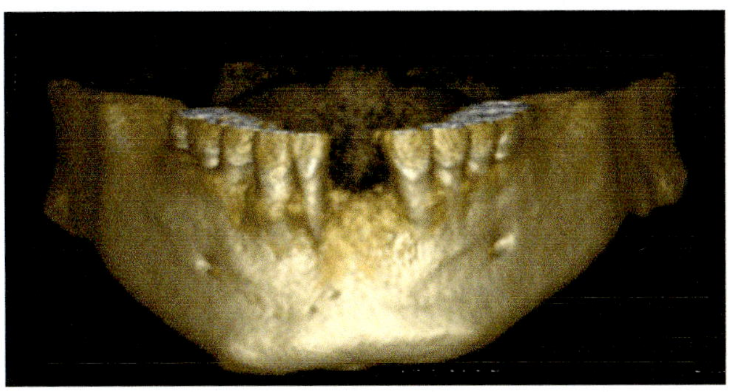

Fig. 1.4 CBCT 3D view of mandible

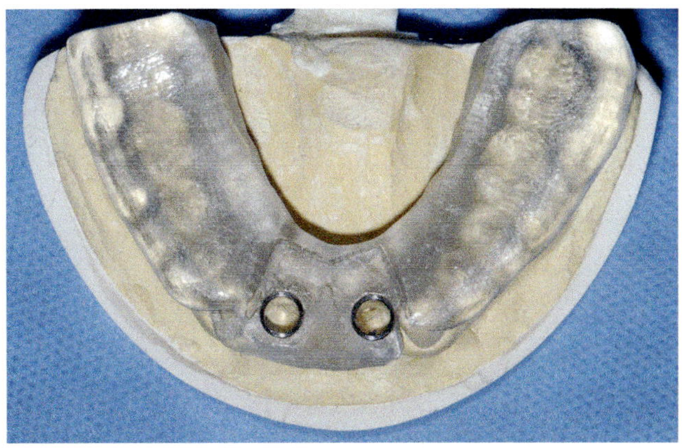

Fig. 1.5 Dental implant 3D printed surgical drill guide

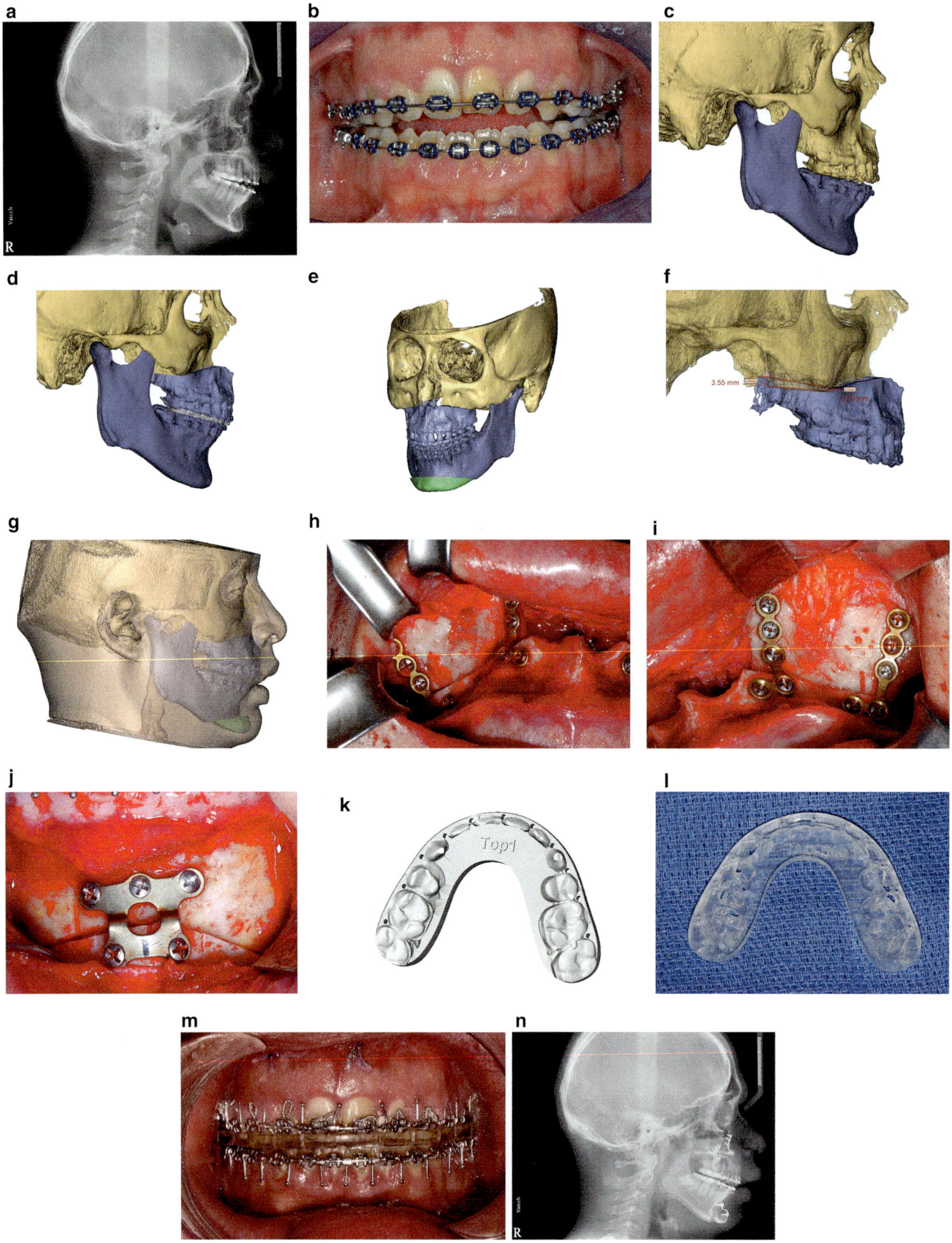

Fig. 1.6 VSP for orthognathic surgery with 3D printed occlusal splint. (**a**) *Lateral* cephalometric radiograph of Class II skeletal malocclusion with retrogenia. (**b**) *Frontal* occlusal view of Class II skeletal malocclusion with anterior open bite and presurgical orthodontic appliance. (**c**) *Right lateral* VSP 3D presurgical image of skull and Class II skeletal malocclusion with anterior open bite (Materialise, Plymouth, MI, and DuPuy Synthes Craniomaxillofacial, Paoli, PA, USA). (**d**) VSP 3D image of right lateral view of LeFort I osteotomy

Figures 1.7–15 Patient had prior bilateral zygomatic arch osteotomies for narrowing of facial width, and desired additional facial width narrowing. Stereolithographic model obtained for diagnosis and planning of bilateral zygomatic arch osteotomies with medial repositioning and reduction osteoplasties of the zygomatic bodies and posterior zygomatic arches.

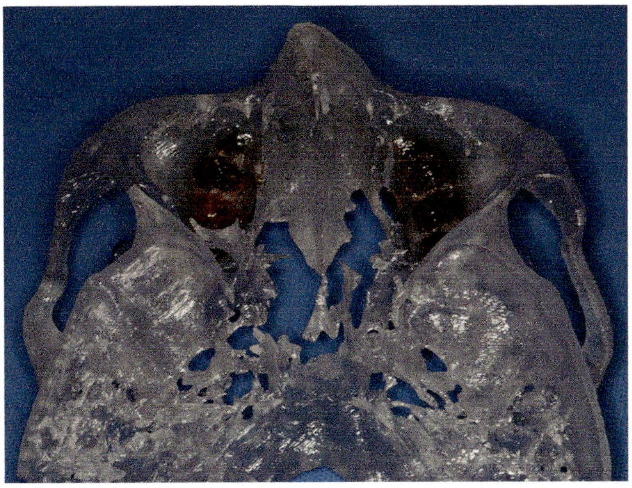

Fig. 1.7 Stereolithographic skull model superior view with bilateral zygomatic arch deformities from prior medial repositioning osteotomies

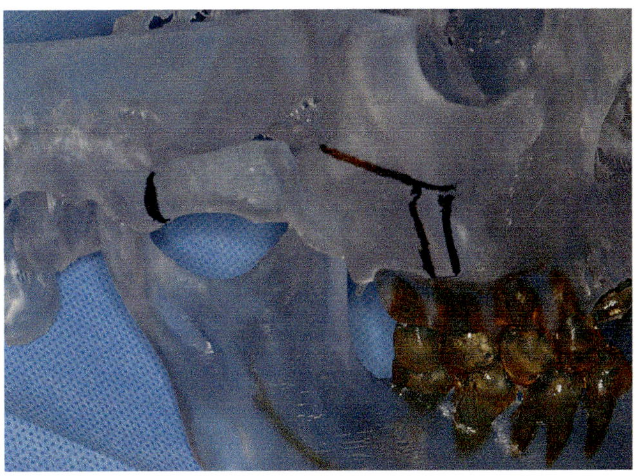

Fig. 1.8 Stereolithographic skull model *right lateral* view with *right* zygomatic arch deformity with planned revision osteotomy for medial repositioning

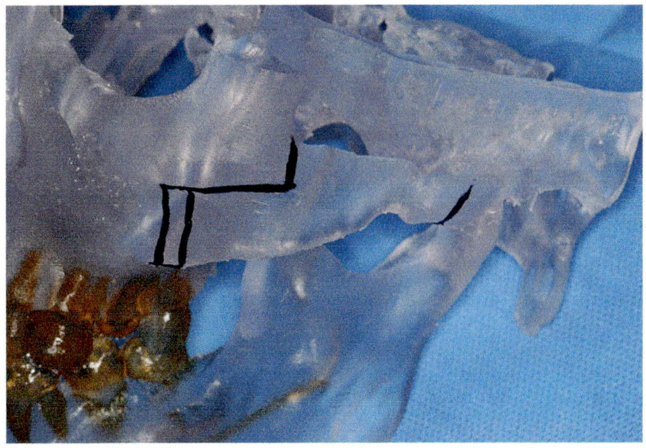

Fig. 1.9 Stereolithographic skull model *left lateral view* with *left* zygomatic arch deformity with planned revision osteotomy for medial repositioning

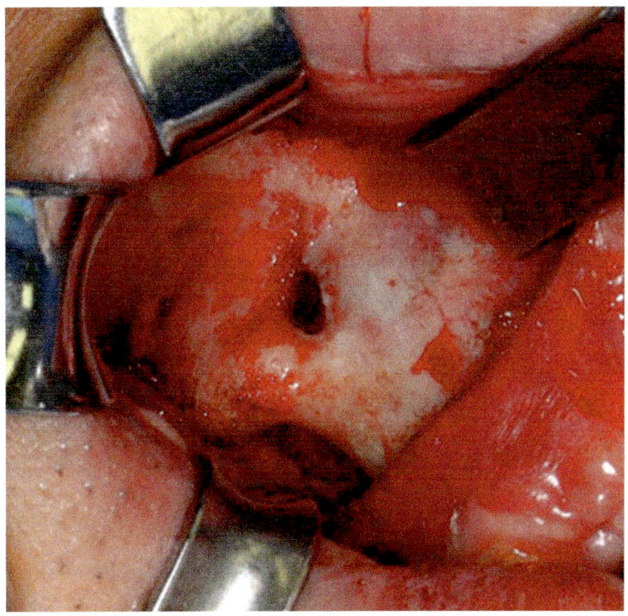

Fig. 1.10 Intraoperative *right* zygomatic region initial exposure via buccal incision

Fig. 1.6 (continued) with virtual occlusal splint. (Materialise, Plymouth, MI, USA and DuPuy Synthes Craniomaxillofacial, Paoli, PA, USA). (**e**) VSP 3D image of left 3/4 view of planned LeFort I osteotomy with virtual occlusal template and anterior horizontal mandibular osteotomy correction (Materialise, Plymouth, MI, USA and DuPuy Synthes Craniomaxillofacial, Paoli, PA, USA). (**f**) VSP 3D image close-up of *right lateral view* of LeFort I osteotomy with planning for maxillary wedge ostectomy and a posterior differential impaction and advancement (Materialise, Plymouth, MI, USA and DuPuy Synthes Craniomaxillofacial, Paoli, PA, USA). (**g**) VSP *right lateral* 3D skin and bone view of LeFort I osteotomy and anterior horizontal mandibular osteotomy correction (Materialise, Plymouth, MI, USA and DuPuy Synthes Craniomaxillofacial, Paoli, PA, USA). (**h**) Intraoperative view of *right side* of LeFort I osteotomy with miniplate fixation (DuPuy Synthes Craniomaxillofacial, Paoli, PA, USA). (**i**) Intraoperative view of *left side* of LeFort I osteotomy with miniplate fixation (DuPuy Synthes Craniomaxillofacial, Paoli, PA, USA). (**j**) Intraoperative view of genioplasty with chin plate fixation (DuPuy Synthes Craniomaxillofacial, Paoli, PA, USA). (**k**) VSP virtual occlusal splint (Materialise, Plymouth, MI, USA and DuPuy Synthes Craniomaxillofacial, Paoli, PA, USA). (**l**) VSP 3D printed occlusal splint (Materialise, Plymouth, MI, USA and DuPuy Synthes Craniomaxillofacial, Paoli, PA, USA). (**m**) Postoperative occlusal splint in place, note precise fit of occlusion. (**n**) Postoperative *right lateral* cephalometric radiograph

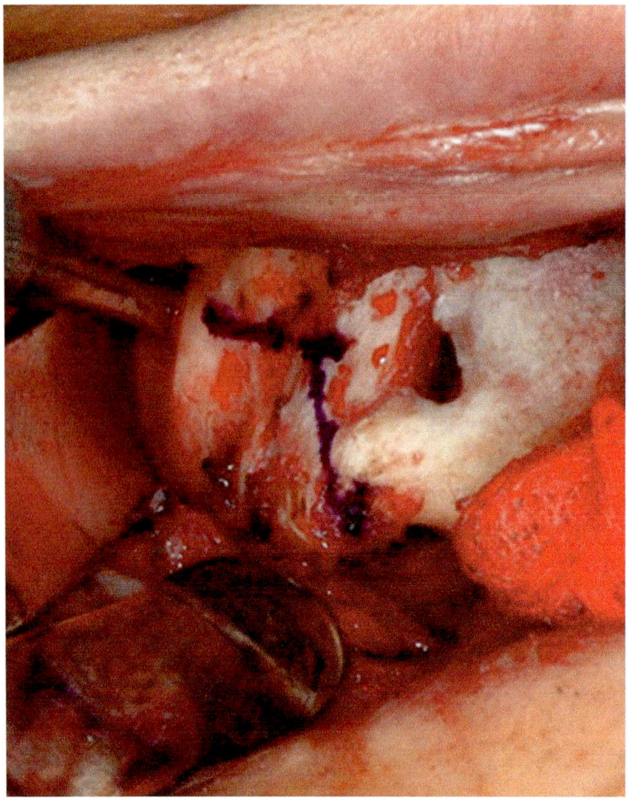

Fig. 1.11 Intraoperative *right* zygomatic body and arch revision osteotomy for medial repositioning outlined

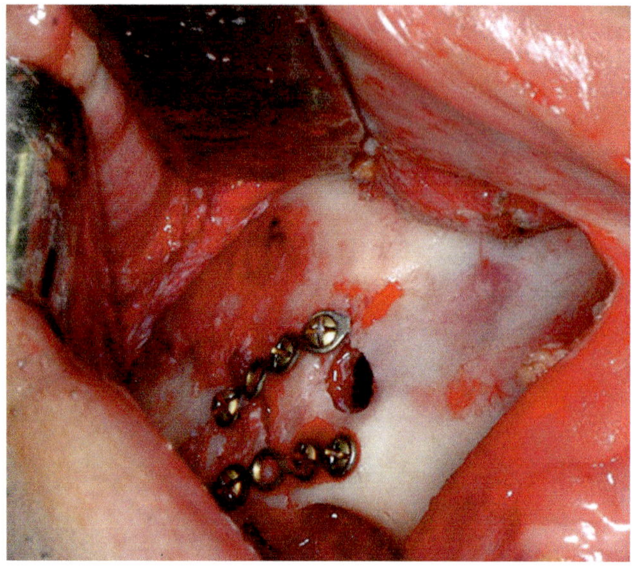

Fig. 1.13 Intraoperative *right* zygomatic body and arch osteotomy medially repositioned following osteoplasty zygomatic body reduction and internal fixation (DuPuy Synthes Craniomaxillofacial, Paoli, PA, USA)

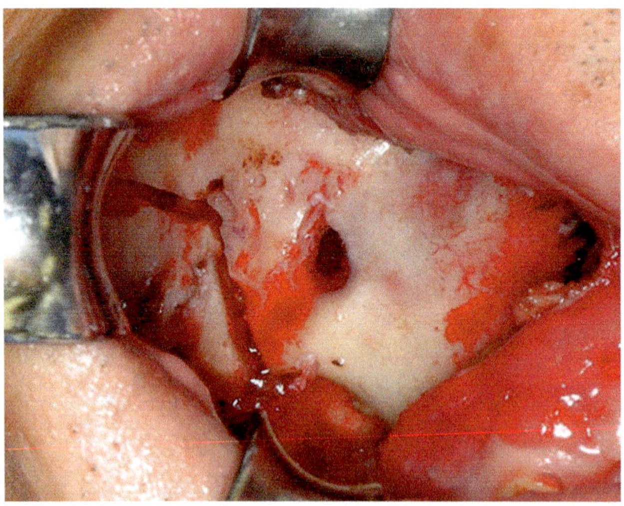

Fig. 1.12 Intraoperative *right* zygomatic body and arch osteotomy for medial repositioning completed as planned

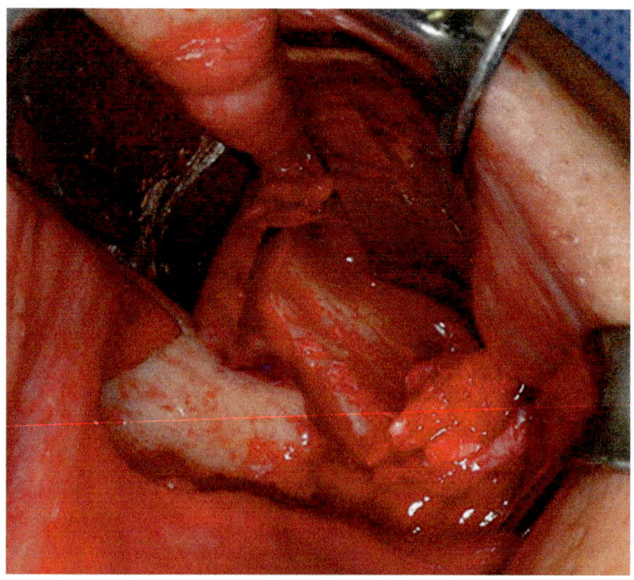

Fig. 1.14 Intraoperative *left* zygomatic body and arch osteotomy for medial repositioning completed as planned

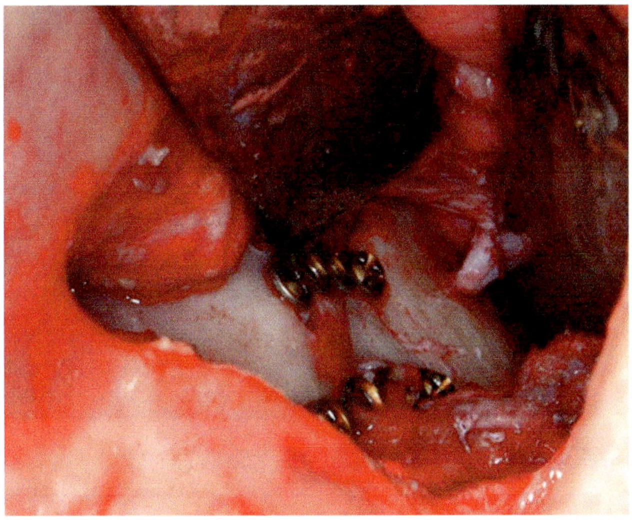

Fig. 1.15 Intraoperative *left* zygomatic body and arch osteotomy medially repositioned following zygomatic body reduction osteoplasty and internal fixation (DuPuy Synthes Craniomaxillofacial, Paoli, PA)

Figures 1.16–24 the patient desired improved contours at the geniomandibular notches and additional chin augmentation. Submental ptosis would also be improved by the chin implant. A custom solid silicone chin implant was designed, fabricated, and inserted.

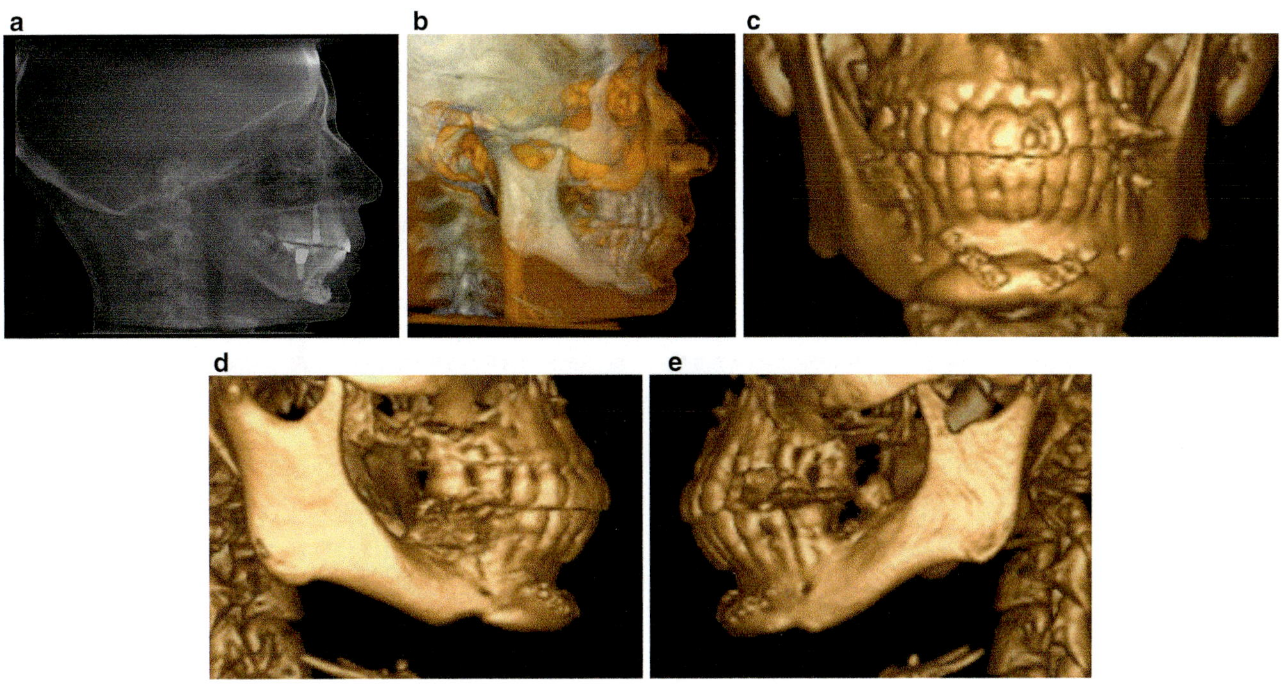

Fig. 1.16 CBCT views of chin 10 years following anterior mandibular horizontal osteotomy with retained hardware and prominent geniomandibular notches. (**a**) Right *lateral* cephalometric view. (**b**) 3D skin and bone transparent right *lateral* view. (**c**) 3D *frontal* view. (**d**) 3D right *lateral* view. (**e**) 3D left *lateral* view

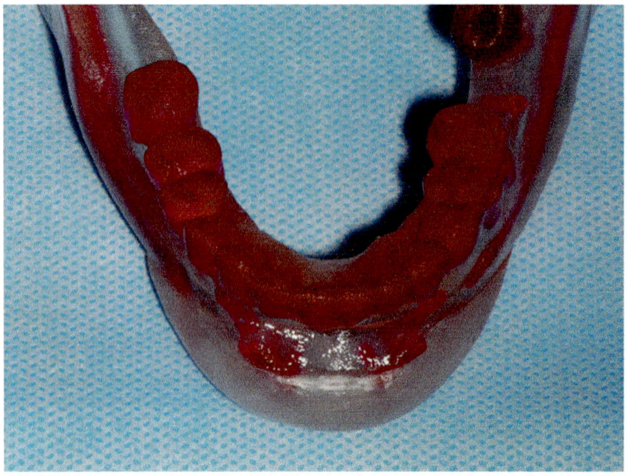

Fig. 1.17 Stereolithographic model superior view of custom chin implant waxup

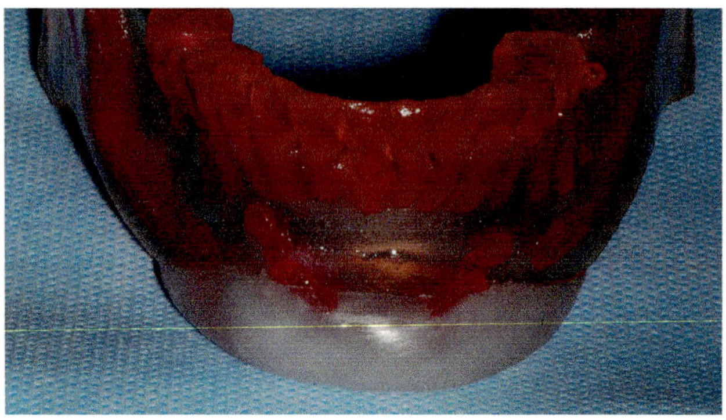

Fig. 1.18 Stereolithographic model *anterior* view of custom chin implant waxup

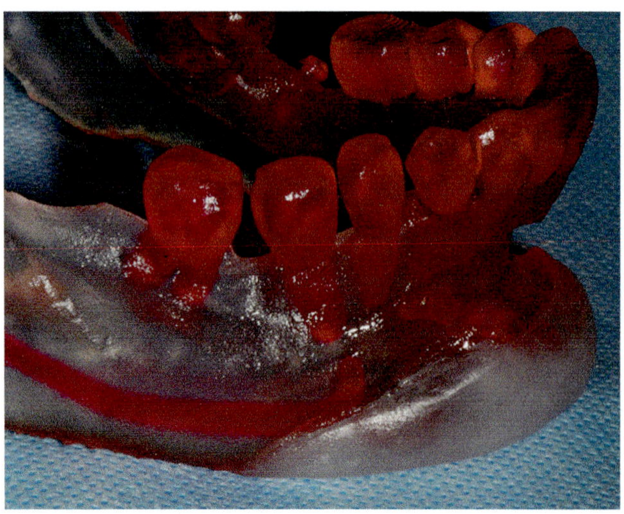

Fig. 1.19 Stereolithographic model *right lateral view* of custom chin implant waxup

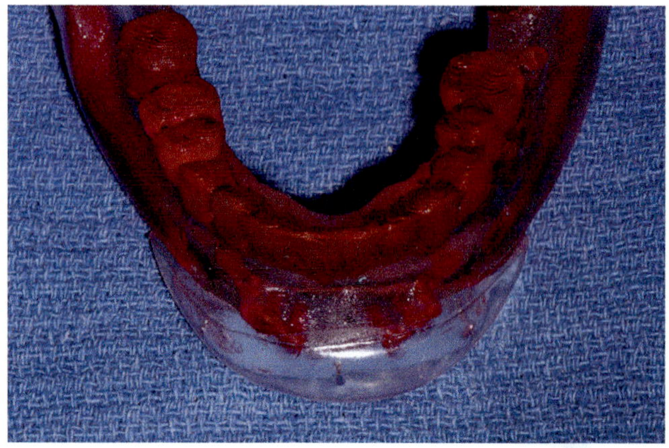

Fig. 1.20 Stereolithographic model superior view of custom chin solid silicone implant fitted to 3D model (Implantech, Ventura, CA, USA)

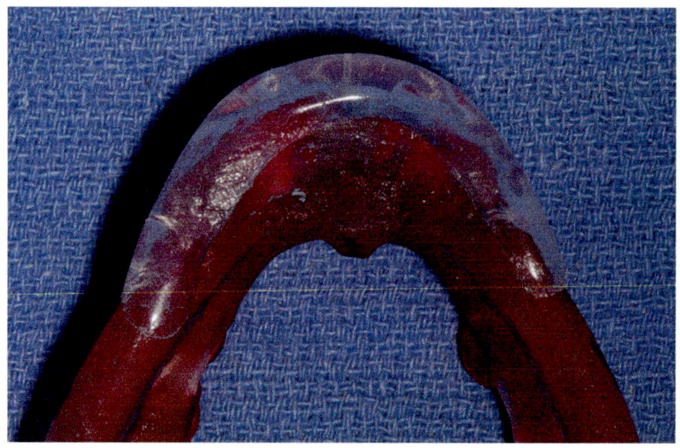

Fig. 1.21 Stereolithographic model inferior view of custom chin solid silicone implant fitted to 3D model (Implantech, Ventura, CA, USA)

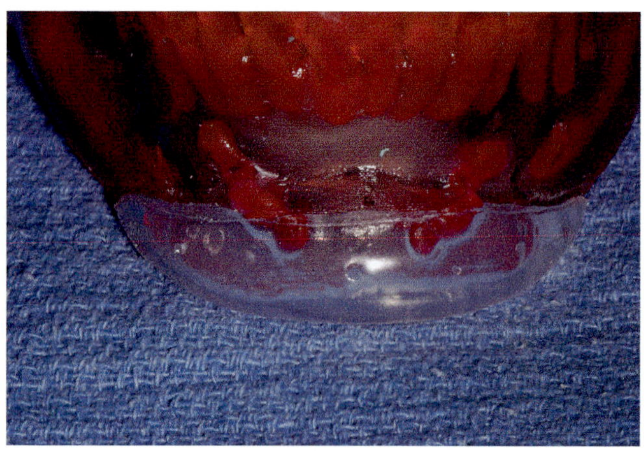

Fig. 1.22 Stereolithographic model *anterior* view of custom chin solid silicone implant fitted to 3D model (Implantech, Ventura, CA, USA)

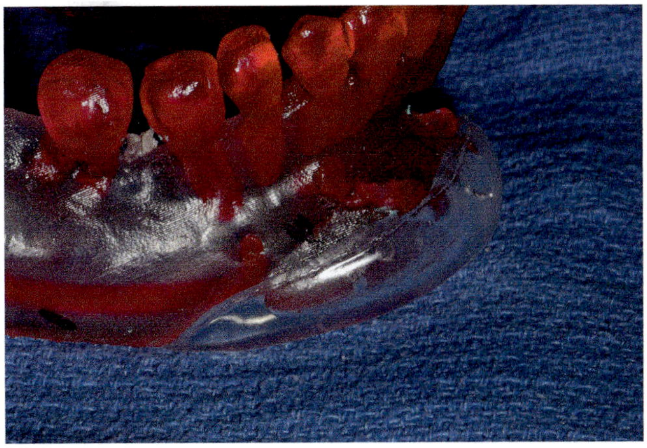

Fig. 1.23 Stereolithographic model *right lateral view* of custom chin solid silicone implant fitted to 3D model (Implantech, Ventura, CA, USA)

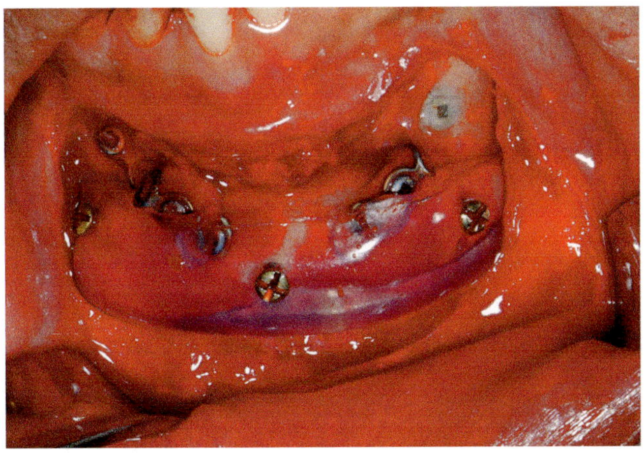

Fig. 1.24 *Intraoperative* view of buccal vestibular incision with custom chin solid silicone implant placement (Implantech, Ventura, CA, USA) and three screws for fixation (DuPuy Synthes Craniomaxillofacial, Paoli, PA, USA)

Figures 1.25–32 Patient with osteosarcoma of the right maxillary region underwent right hemimaxillectomy with immediate fibular osteomyocutaneous graft and later digital planning with 3D printed surgical guide for the precise placement of dental implants for an implant supported fixed prosthesis.

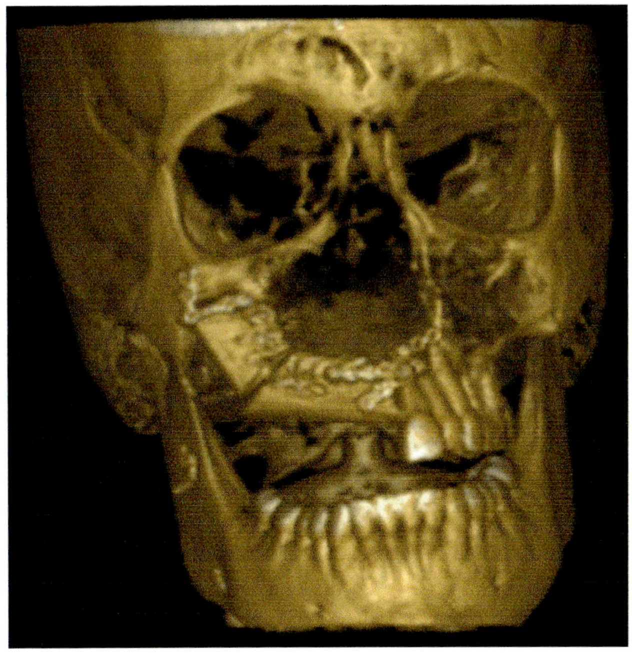

Fig. 1.25 CBCT *frontal* 3D view of *right* hemimaxillectomy with immediate fibular bone graft reconstruction for the management of osteosarcoma

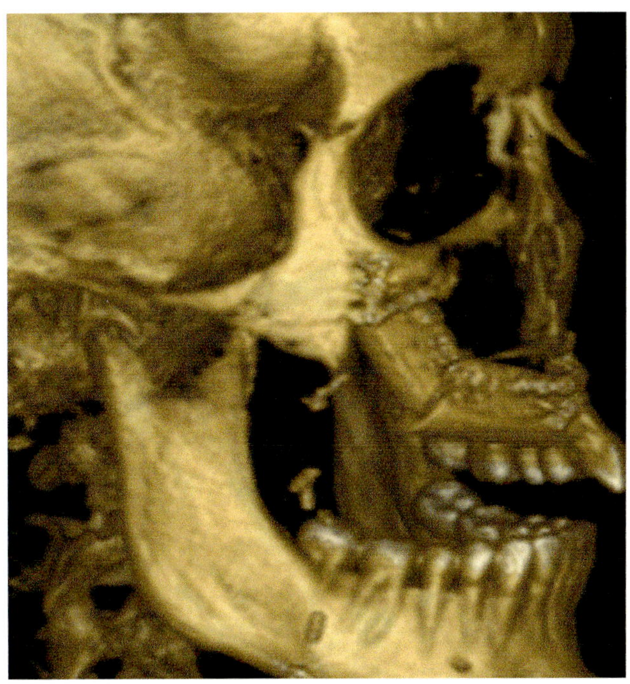

Fig. 1.26 CBCT *right lateral* 3D view of *right* hemimaxillectomy with immediate fibular bone graft reconstruction for the management of osteosarcoma

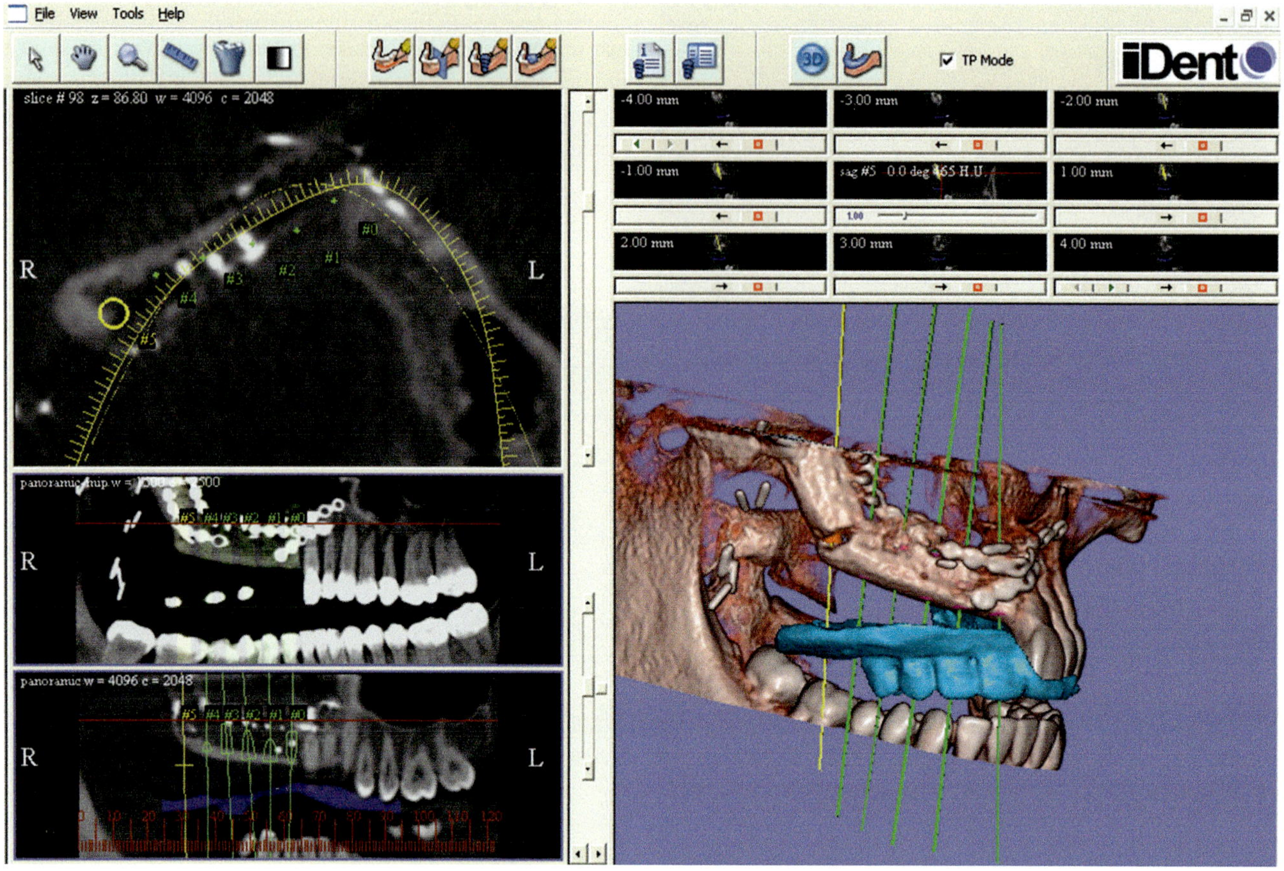

Fig. 1.27 Treatment planning window for dental implant placement into *right* fibular bone graft reconstruction following *right* hemimaxillectomy with immediate fibular bone graft reconstruction for osteosarcoma (ImplantMaster, iDent Imaging, Inc., NY, NY, USA)

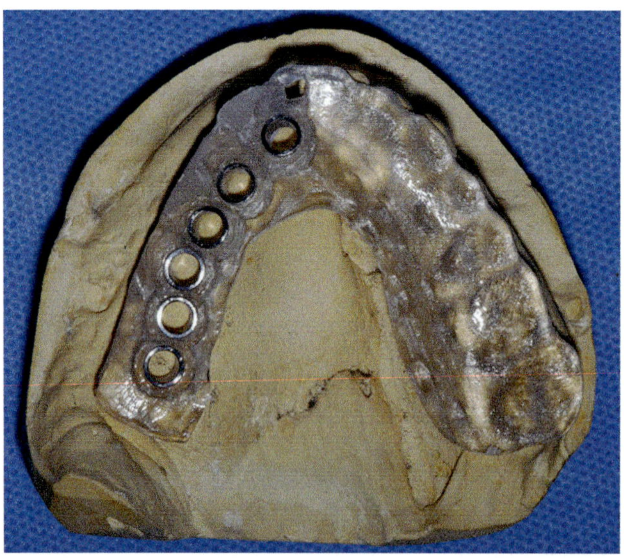

Fig. 1.28 Surgical drill guide produced by rapid printing (Ident Imaging, Inc., NY, NY, USA)

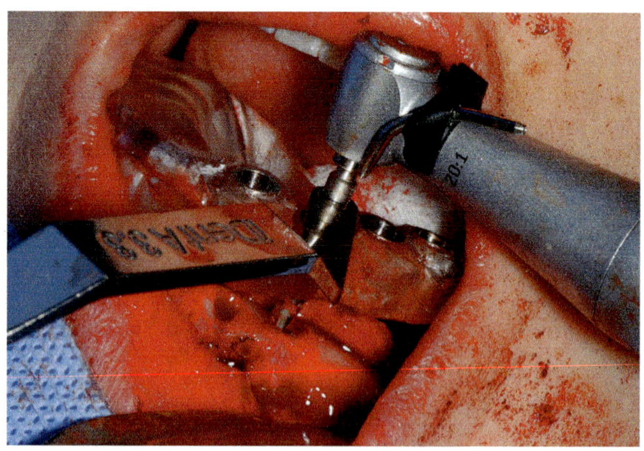

Fig. 1.29 Intraoperative view of surgical drill guide with hand tool and drill for dental implant osteotomy creation (Ident Imaging, NY, NY, USA)

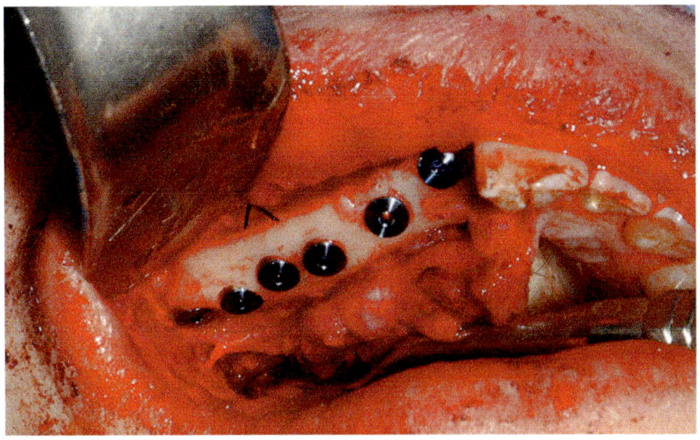

Fig. 1.30 Intraoperative view of dental implant placement in *right* maxillary fibular bone graft reconstruction following *right* hemimaxillectomy (Zimmer Biomet 3i, Palm Beach Gardens, FL, USA)

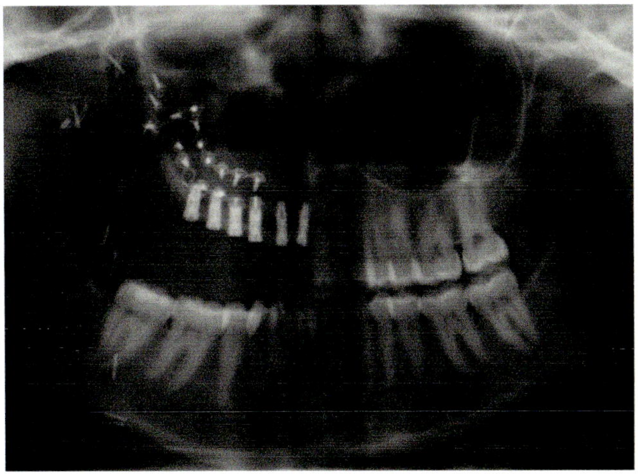

Fig. 1.31 Postoperative panoramic radiograph with six dental implants placed

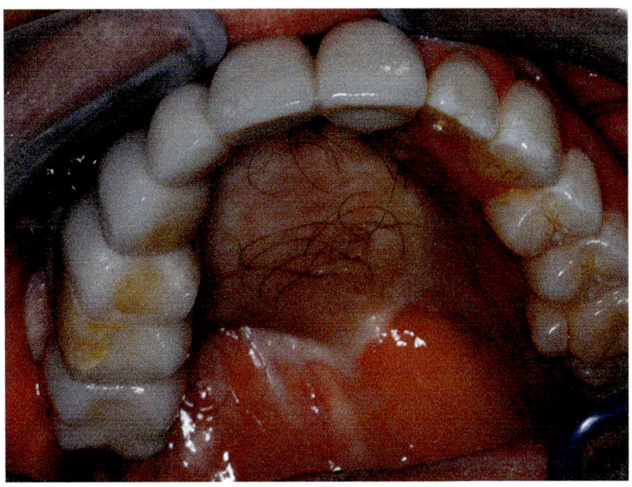

Fig. 1.32 Postoperative intraoral frontal occlusal view of final implant-supported prosthesis

Figures 1.33–43 Digital 3D planning for resection of left mandibular tumor with immediate fibular osteomyocutaneous flap reconstruction and custom prebent bone plate, with simultaneous dental implant placement (Materialise, Plymouth, MI, USA and DuPuy Synthes Craniomaxillofacial, Paoli, PA, USA) (Case courtesy Hugo St. Hilaire, MD, DDS, Department of Plastic Surgery, Louisiana State University, New Orleans, LA).

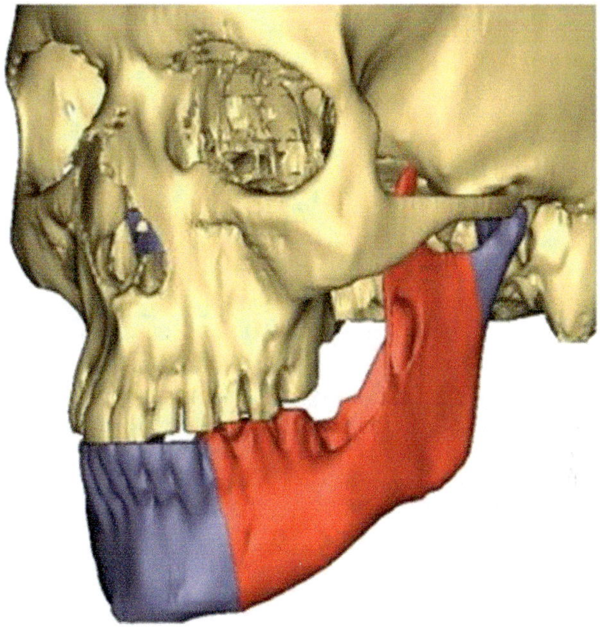

Fig. 1.33 Digital 3D planning for resection of *left* mandibular tumor (Materialise, MI, and DuPuy Synthes Craniomaxillofacial, Paoli, PA, USA) (Case courtesy Hugo St. Hilaire, MD, DDS, Department of Plastic Surgery, Louisiana State University, New Orleans, LA)

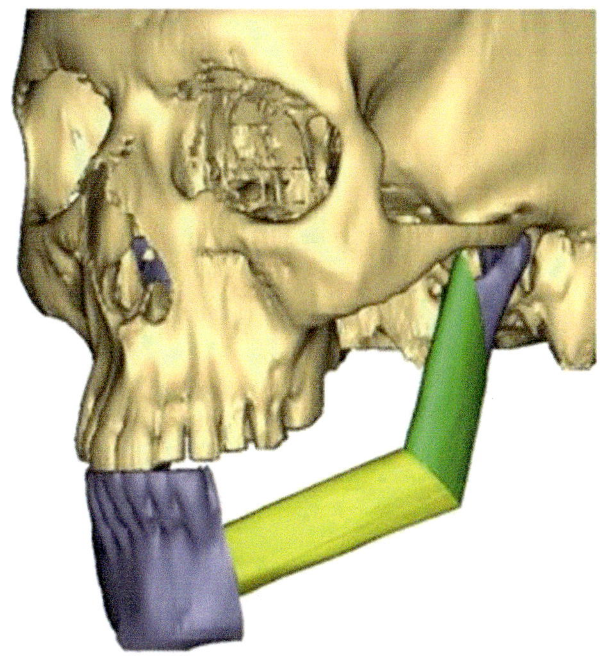

Fig. 1.34 Digital 3D planning for resection of *left* mandibular tumor with immediate fibular osteomyocutaneous flap reconstruction (Materialise, MI, and DuPuy Synthes Craniomaxillofacial, Paoli, PA, USA) (Case courtesy Hugo St. Hilaire, MD, DDS, Department of Plastic Surgery, Louisiana State University, New Orleans, LA)

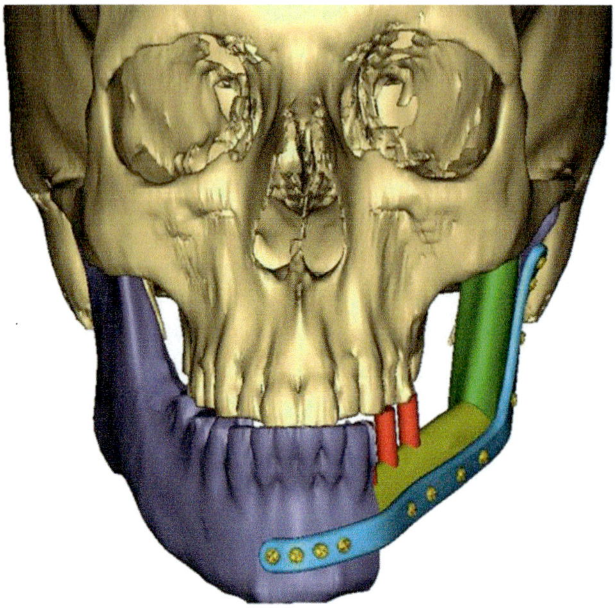

Fig. 1.35 Digital 3D planning for resection of *left* mandibular tumor with immediate fibular osteomyocutaneous flap reconstruction and custom prebent bone plate with simultaneous dental implant placement frontal view (Materialise, Plymouth, MI, USA and DuPuy Synthes Craniomaxillofacial, Paoli, PA, USA) (Case courtesy Hugo St. Hilaire, MD, DDS, Department of Plastic Surgery, Louisiana State University, New Orleans, LA)

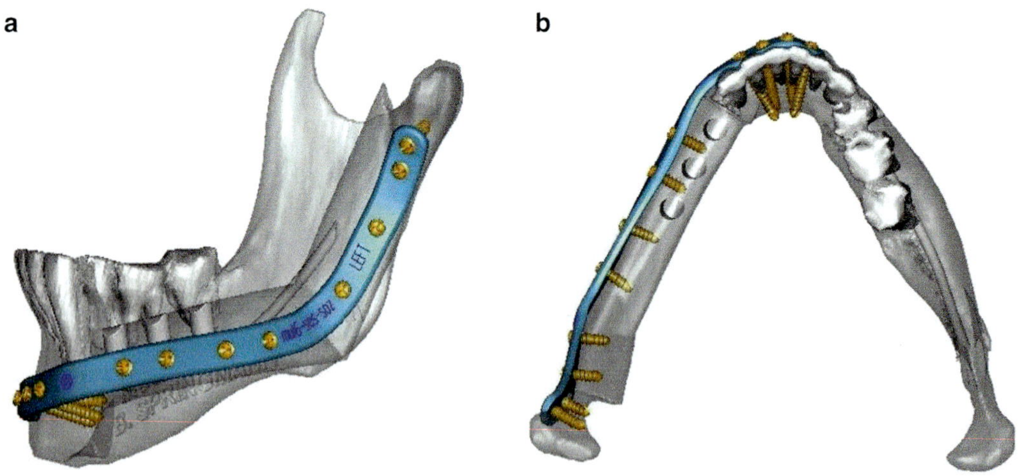

Fig. 1.36 Digital 3D planning for resection of *left* mandibular tumor with immediate fibular osteomyocutaneous flap reconstruction and custom prebent bone plate and simultaneous dental implant placement (**a**)*left lateral view*, and (**b**)*superior view* (Materialise, Plymouth, MI, USA and DuPuy Synthes Craniomaxillofacial, Paoli, PA, USA) (Case courtesy Hugo St. Hilaire, MD, DDS, Department of Plastic Surgery, Louisiana State University, New Orleans, LA)

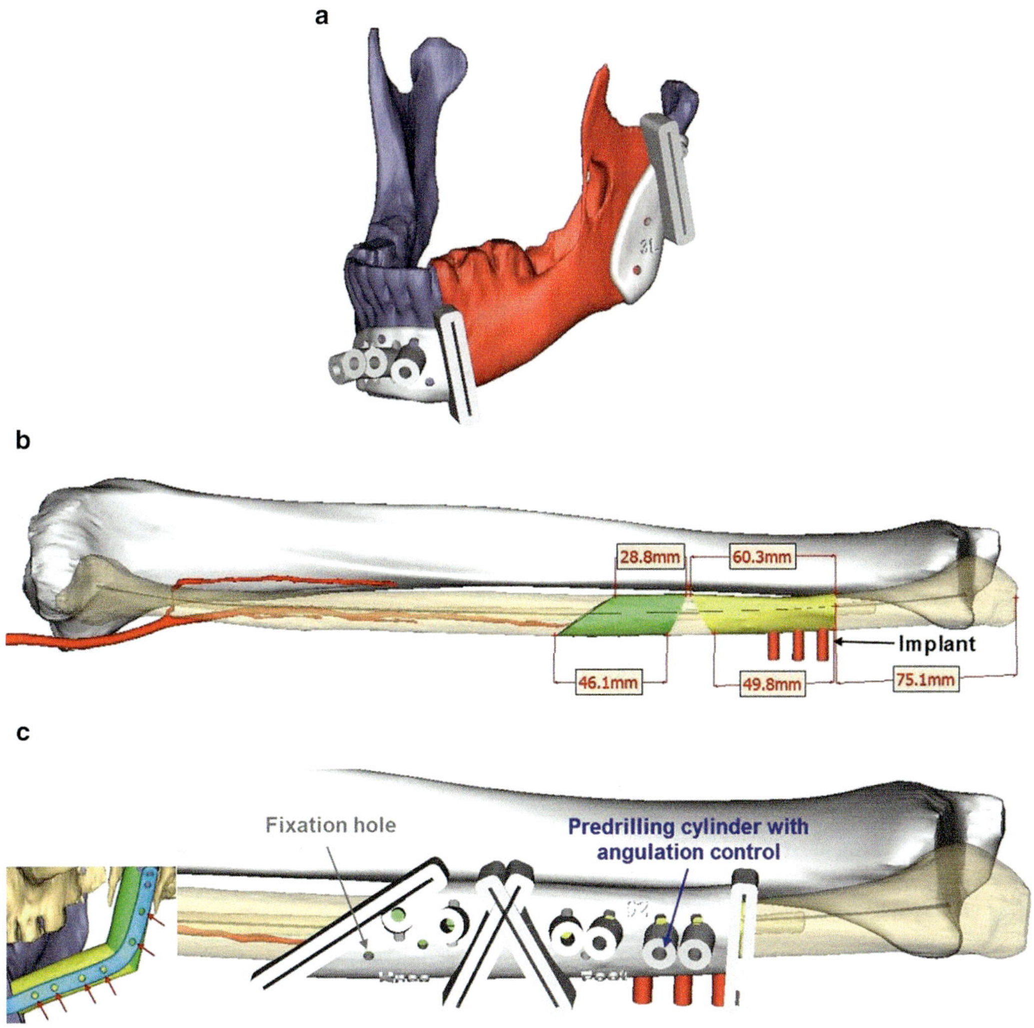

Fig. 1.37 Digital 3D planning for resection of *left* mandibular tumor with combination surgical cutting guides and drill guides for bone plate placement for immediate fibular osteomyocutaneous flap reconstruction. (**a**) Mandibular *left* symphysis and *left* subcondylar cutting/drill guides. (**b**) *Right* fibular bone segment plan. (**c**) *Right* fibular bone cutting and drill guide (Materialise, Plymouth, MI, USA and DuPuy Synthes Craniomaxillofacial, Paoli, PA, USA) (Case courtesy Hugo St. Hilaire, MD, DDS, Department of Plastic Surgery, Louisiana State University, New Orleans, LA)

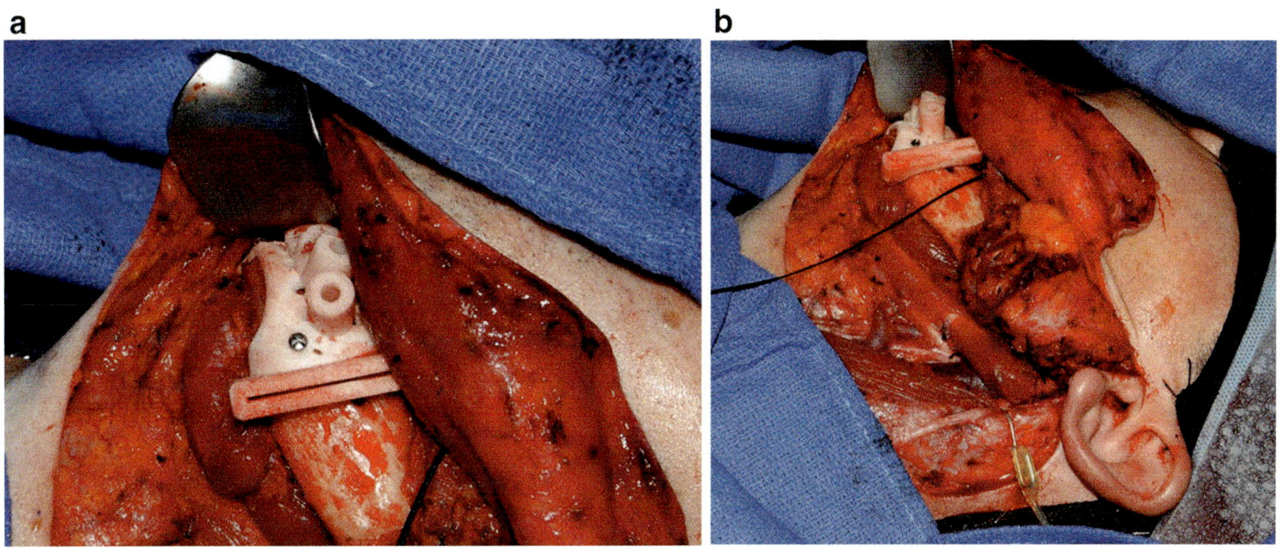

Fig. 1.38 Intraoperative view of *left* mandibular tumor with *left* anterior mandibular combination cutting guide and drill guide. (**a**) Closeup view. (**b**) Full mandibular view (Materialise, Plymouth, MI, USA and DuPuy Synthes Craniomaxillofacial, Paoli, PA, USA) (Case courtesy Hugo St. Hilaire, MD, DDS, Department of Plastic Surgery, Louisiana State University, New Orleans, LA)

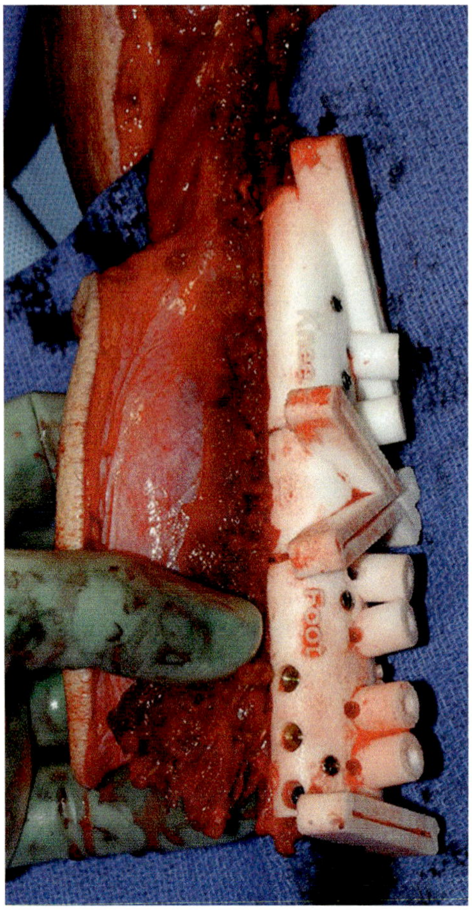

Fig. 1.39 Intraoperative view of *right* fibular osteomyocutaneous graft with combination surgical cutting guide and drill guide for bone plate placement (Materialise, Plymouth, MI, USA and DuPuy Synthes Craniomaxillofacial, Paoli, PA, USA) (Case courtesy Hugo St. Hilaire, MD, DDS, Department of Plastic Surgery, Louisiana State University, New Orleans, LA)

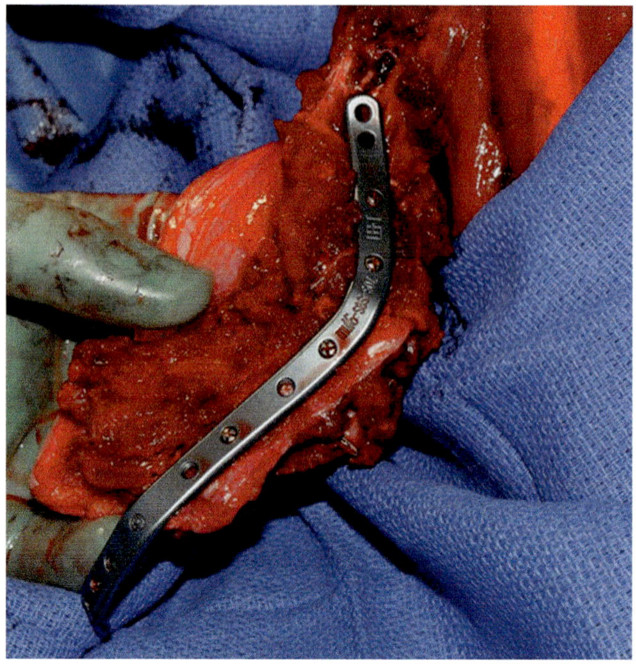

Fig. 1.40 Intraoperative view of *right* fibular osteomyocutaneous graft after segmentation with custom prebent bone plate placement following the use of a combination surgical cutting guide and drill guide (Materialise, Plymouth, MI, USA and DuPuy Synthes Craniomaxillofacial, Paoli, PA, USA) (Case courtesy Hugo St. Hilaire, MD, DDS, Department of Plastic Surgery, Louisiana State University, New Orleans, LA)

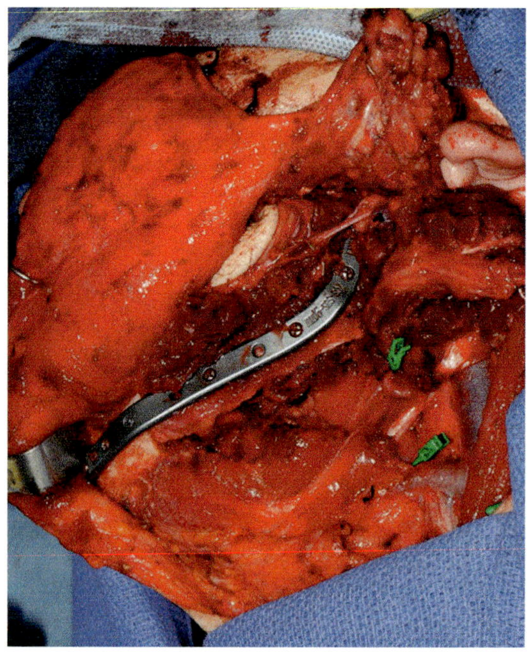

Fig. 1.41 Intraoperative view of *right* fibular osteomyocutaneous graft after segmentation with custom prebent bone plate placement following the use of a combination surgical cutting guide and drill guide and inset into the left posterior mandible partial mandibulectomy defect post-resection of tumor with fixation of the symphysis and body segments (Materialise, Plymouth, MI, USA and DuPuy Synthes Craniomaxillofacial, Paoli, PA, USA) (Case courtesy Hugo St. Hilaire, MD, DDS, Department of Plastic Surgery, Louisiana State University, New Orleans, LA)

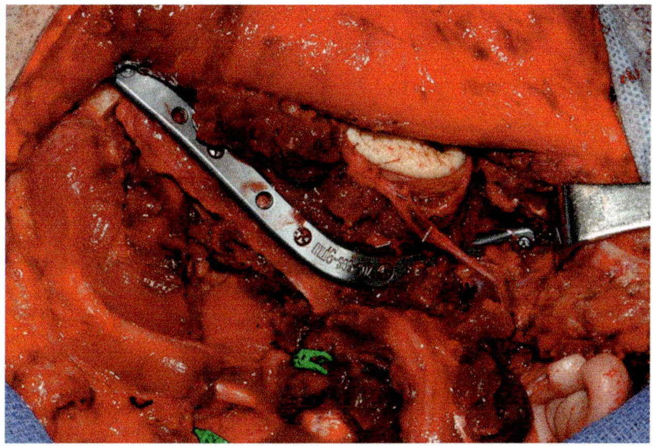

Fig. 1.42 Intraoperative view of *right* fibular osteomyocutaneous graft after segmentation with custom prebent bone plate placement following the use of a combination surgical cutting guide and drill guide and inset into the left posterior mandible partial mandibulectomy defect post-resection of tumor with fixation of the condylar segment (Materialise, Plymouth, MI, USA and DuPuy Synthes Craniomaxillofacial, Paoli, PA, USA) (Case courtesy Hugo St. Hilaire, MD, DDS, Department of Plastic Surgery, Louisiana State University, New Orleans, LA)

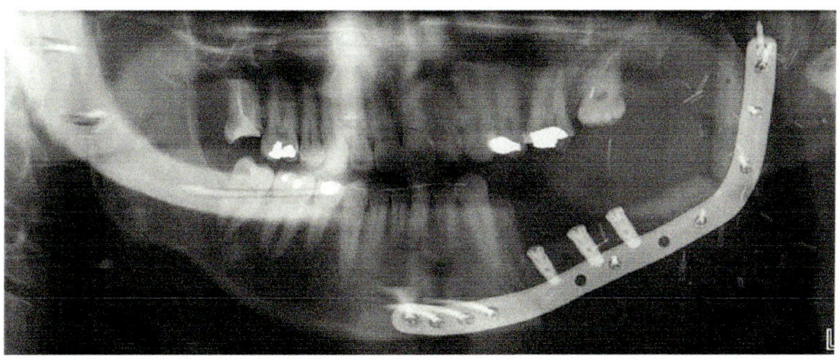

Fig. 1.43 Postoperative panoramic radiograph demonstrates the *right* fibular osteomyocutaneous graft reconstruction of the *left* mandibular defect following resection of tumor with custom prebent bone plate and dental implant placement following the use of a combination surgical cutting guide and drill guide (Materialise, Plymouth, MI, USA and DuPuy Synthes Craniomaxillofacial, Paoli, PA, USA) (Case courtesy Hugo St. Hilaire, MD, DDS, Department of Plastic Surgery, Louisiana State University, New Orleans, LA)

Figures 1.44–50; Total face, eyelids, ears, scalp, and skeletal subunit transplant: a reconstructive solution for the full face and total scalp burn using 3D digital planning and rapid printed cutting guides.(3D Systems Healthcare, Littleton, CO, USA), (Case courtesy Eduardo D. Rodriguez, MD, DDS, Department of Plastic and Reconstructive Surgery, New York University, New York, NY).

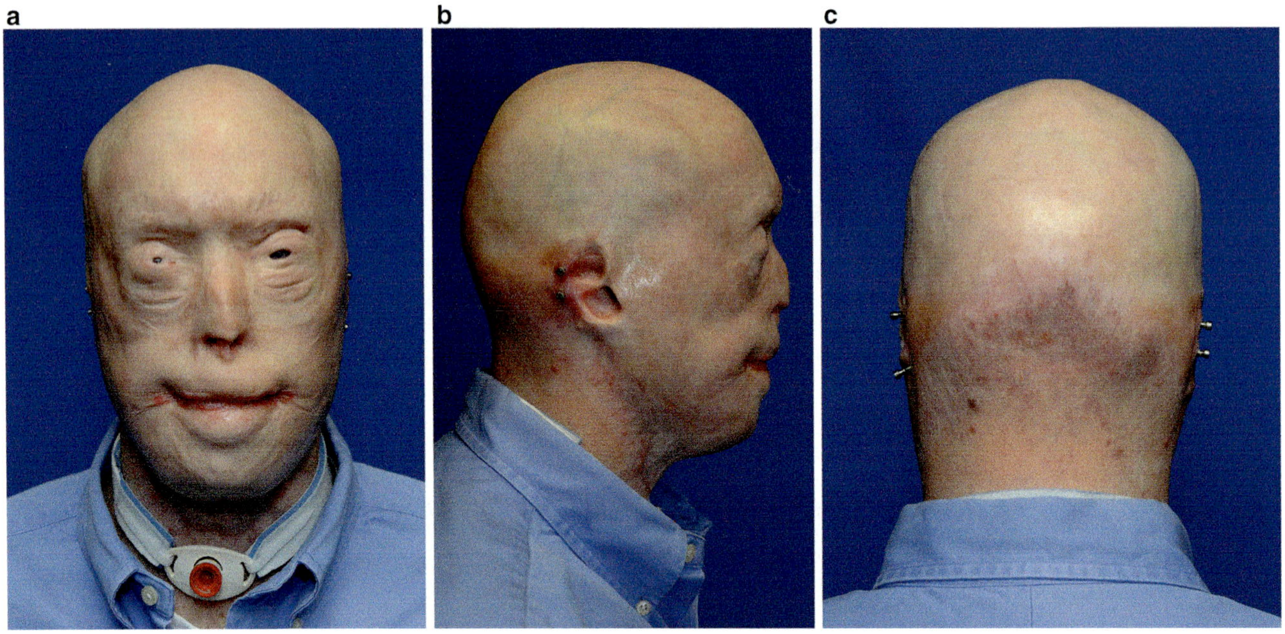

Fig. 1.44 Preoperative patient with total face, eyelids, ears, and scalp severe burn injuries. Note implants for retention of auricular prostheses. (**a**) Frontal view. (**b**) Right lateral. (**c**) Posterior (Printed with permission and copyrights retained by Eduardo D. Rodriguez, MD, DDS, Department of Plastic and Reconstructive Surgery, New York University, New York, NY; Source: Total face, eyelids, ears, scalp, and skeletal subunit transplant: a reconstructive solution for the full face and total scalp burn. Plastic and Reconstructive Surgery. 138(1):205–219, July 2016) (3D Systems Healthcare, Littleton, CO, USA)

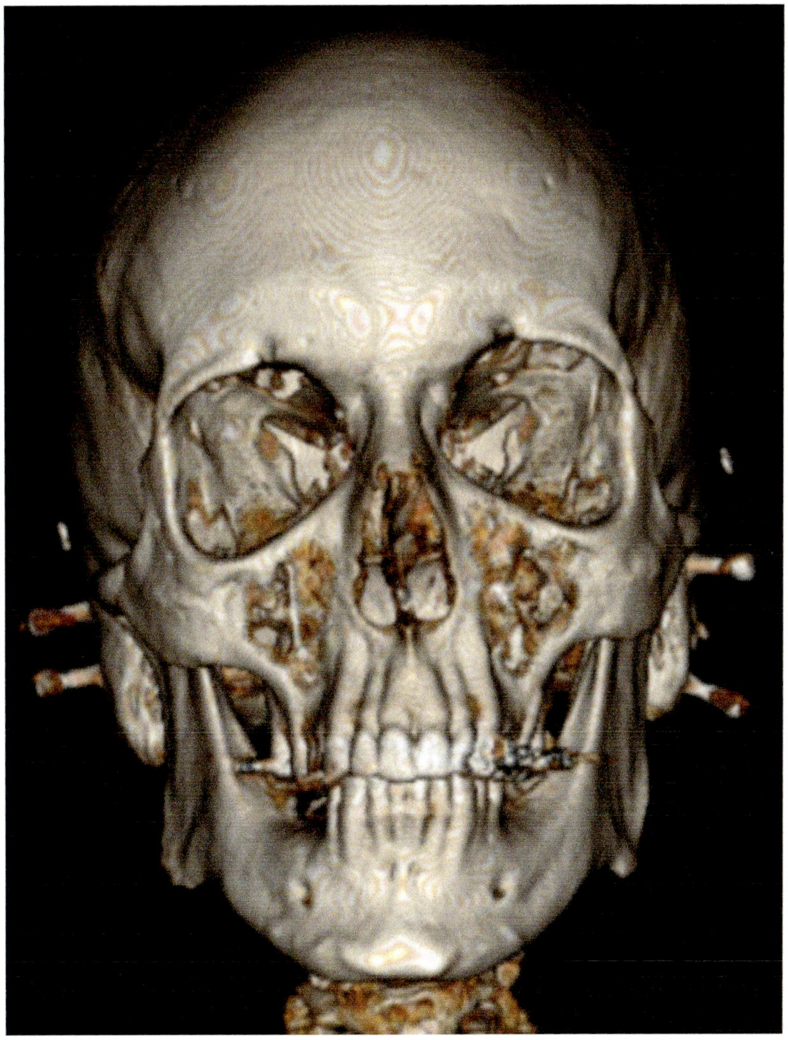

Fig. 1.45 Preoperative 3D CT scan of recipient. (Printed with permission and copyrights retained by Eduardo D. Rodriguez, MD, DDS, Department of Plastic and Reconstructive Surgery, New York University, New York, NY; Source: Total face, eyelids, ears, scalp, and skeletal subunit transplant: a reconstructive solution for the full face and total scalp burn. Plastic and Reconstructive Surgery. 138(1):205–219, July 2016)

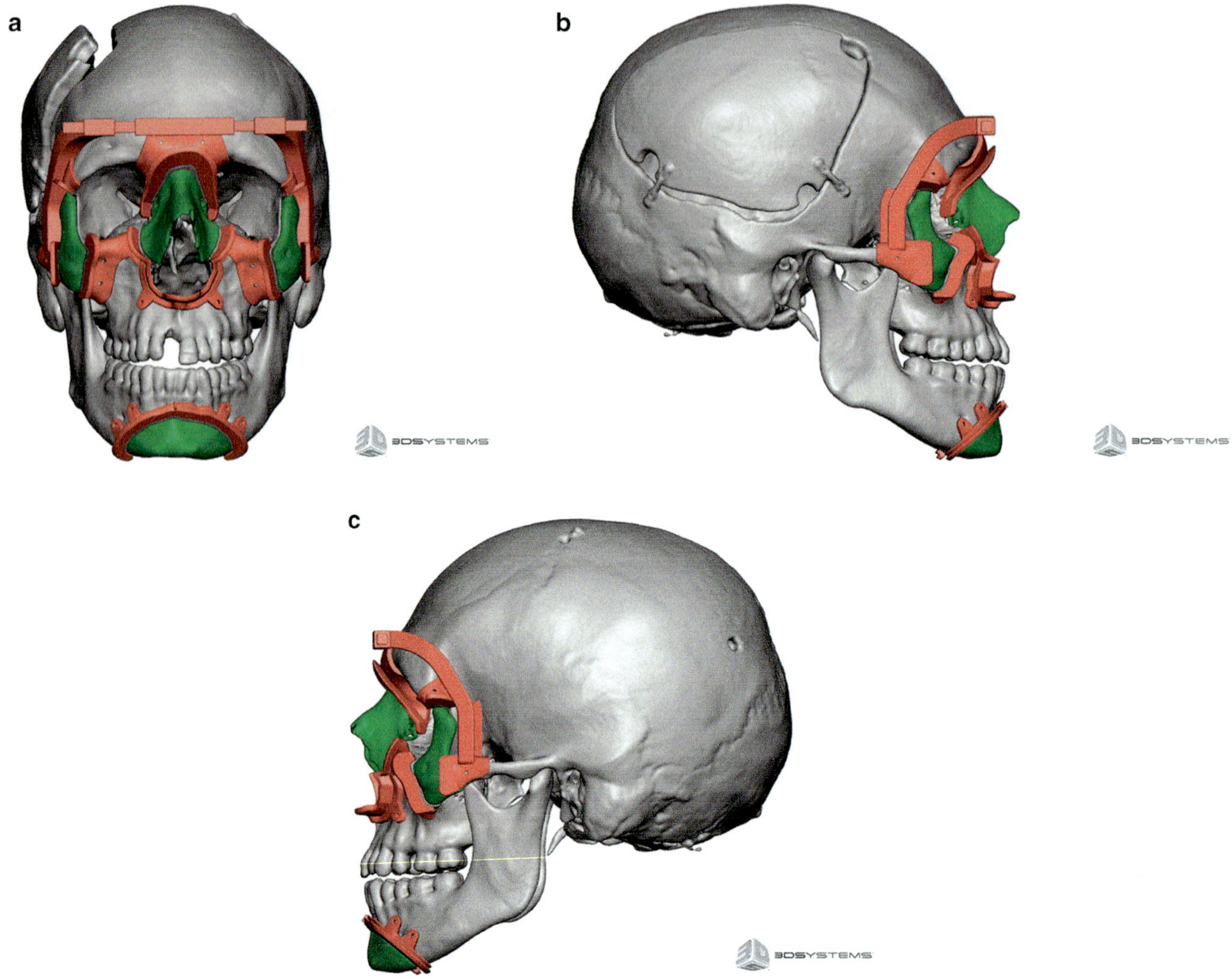

Fig. 1.46 Virtually designed cutting guides for the donor skeleton (*red*). Virtually planned nasal and genial skeletal segments to be removed (*green*) and orbitozygomatic regions to be augmented (*green*). (**a**) Frontal view. (**b**) Right lateral view. (**c**) Left lateral view (Printed with permission and copyrights retained by Eduardo D. Rodriguez, MD, DDS, Department of Plastic and Reconstructive Surgery, New York University, New York, NY; Source: Total face, eyelids, ears, scalp, and skeletal subunit transplant: a reconstructive solution for the full face and total scalp burn. Plastic and Reconstructive Surgery. 138(1):205–219, July 2016). (3D Systems Healthcare, Littleton, CO, USA)

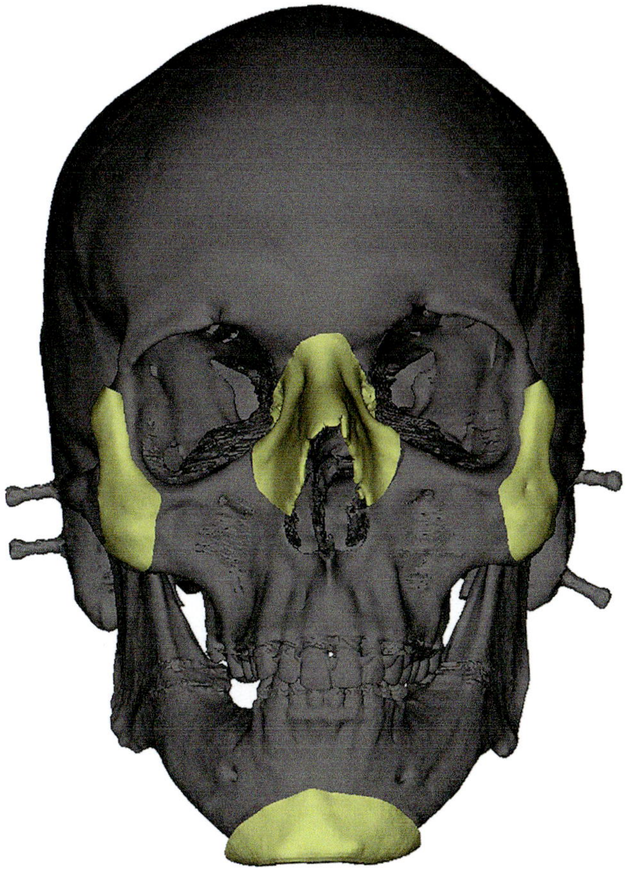

Fig. 1.47 Virtual plan of nasal, orbitozygomatic, and genial regions to be augmented on recipient 3D facial skeleton (Printed with permission and copyrights retained by Eduardo D. Rodriguez, MD, DDS, Department of Plastic and Reconstructive Surgery, New York University, New York, NY; Source: Total face, eyelids, ears, scalp, and skeletal subunit transplant: a reconstructive solution for the full face and total scalp burn. Plastic and Reconstructive Surgery. 138(1):205–219, July 2016). (3D Systems Healthcare, Littleton, CO, USA)

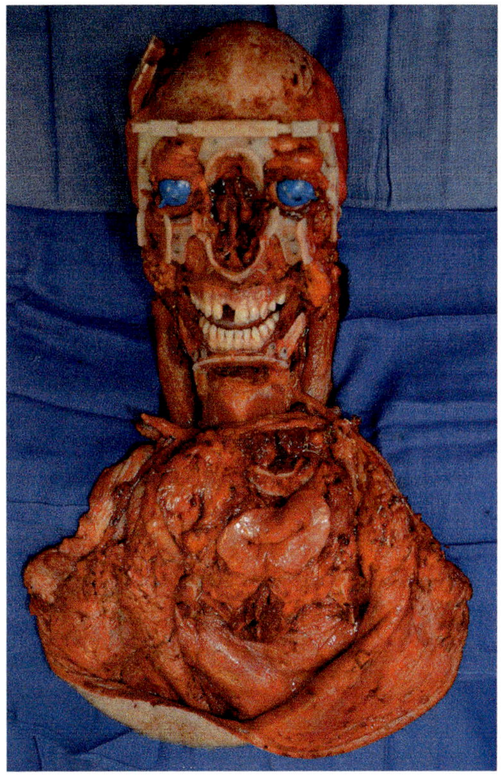

Fig. 1.48 Donor allograft following completion of the facial procurement but before the division of the vascular pedicles with cutting guides for the donor skeleton for the planned nasal, orbitozygomatic, and genial skeletal segments to be removed for recipient augmentation (Printed with permission and copyrights retained by Eduardo D. Rodriguez, MD, DDS, Department of Plastic and Reconstructive Surgery, New York University, New York, NY; Source: Total face, eyelids, ears, scalp, and skeletal subunit transplant: a reconstructive solution for the full face and total scalp burn. Plastic and Reconstructive Surgery. 138(1):205–219, July 2016). (3D Systems Healthcare, Littleton, CO, USA)

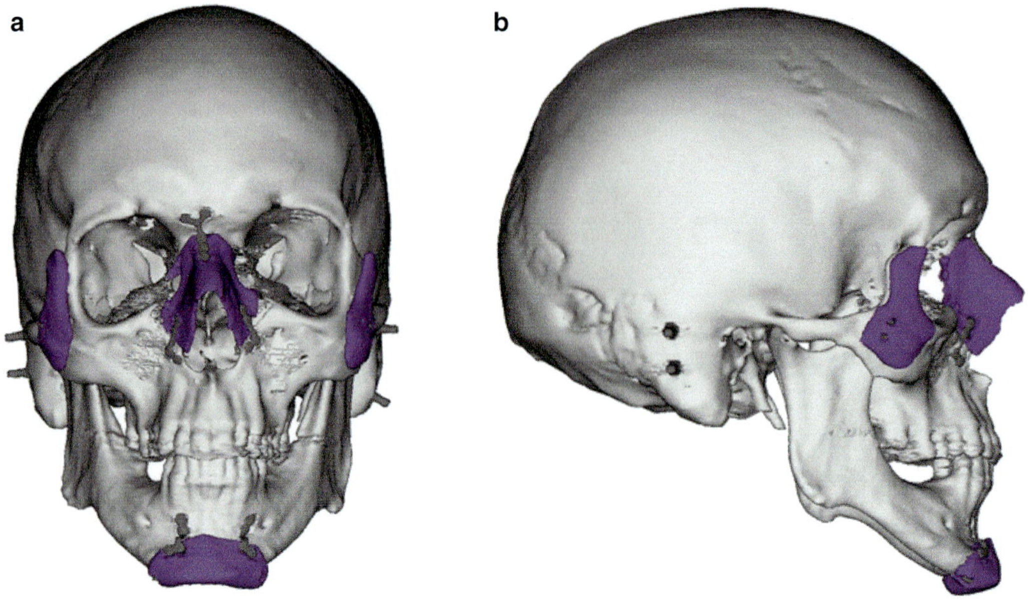

Fig. 1.49 Postoperative 3D CT facial skeleton of recipient following precise harvest of donor bone segments with cutting guides from the donor skeleton for the augmentation of the recipient with nasal, orbito-zygomatic, and genial skeletal segments of the recipient in association with the transplantation of the facial soft tissue flap. (**a**) Frontal view. (**b**) Right lateral view (Printed with permission and copyrights retained by Eduardo D. Rodriguez, MD, DDS, Department of Plastic and Reconstructive Surgery, New York University, New York, NY; Source: Total face, eyelids, ears, scalp, and skeletal subunit transplant: a reconstructive solution for the full face and total scalp burn. Plastic and Reconstructive Surgery. 138(1):205–219, July 2016). (3D Systems Healthcare, Littleton, CO, USA)

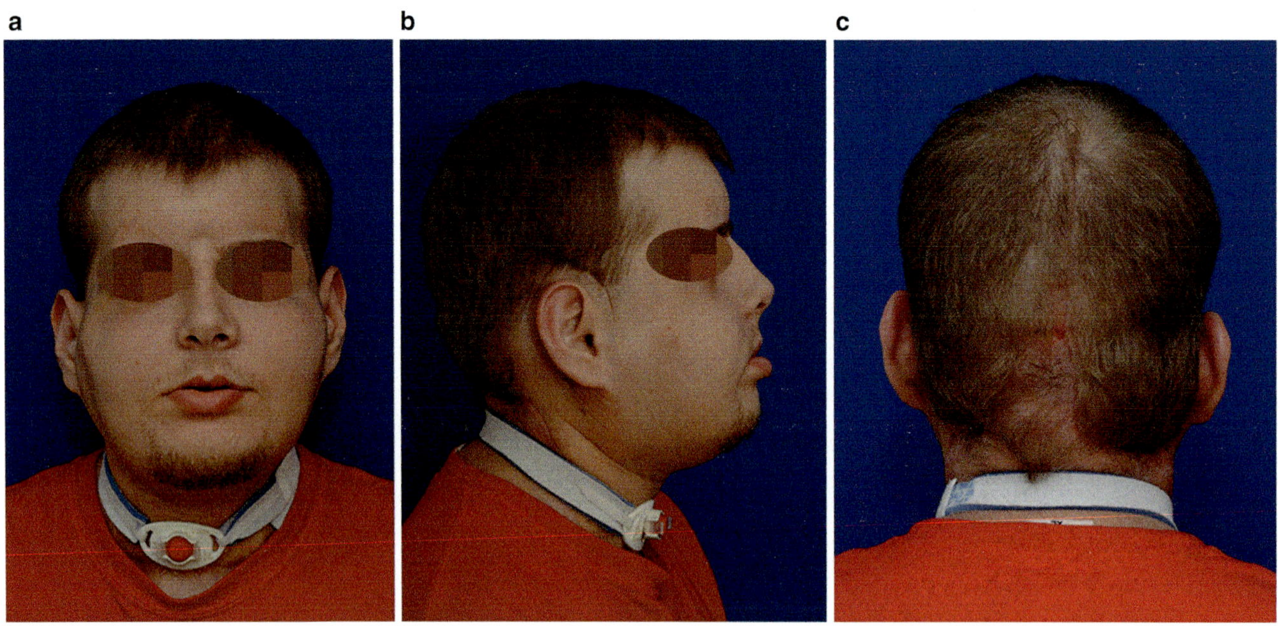

Fig. 1.50 Postoperative view of recipient following facial transplantation. (**a**) Frontal. (**b**) Right lateral. (**c**) Posterior (Printed with permission and copyrights retained by Eduardo D. Rodriguez, MD, DDS, Department of Plastic and Reconstructive Surgery, New York University, New York, NY; Source: Total face, eyelids, ears, scalp, and skeletal subunit transplant: a reconstructive solution for the full face and total scalp burn. Plastic and Reconstructive Surgery. 138(1):205–219, July 2016)

References

1. Wang JC, Nagy L, Demke JC. Image-guided surgery and craniofacial applications: mastering the unseen. Maxillofac Plast Reconstr Surg. 2015 Nov 21;37(1):43.
2. Mehra P, Miner J, D'Innocenzo R, Nadershah M. Use of 3-d stereolithographic models in oral and maxillofacial surgery. J Maxillofac Oral Surg. 2011 Mar;10(1):6–13.
3. Greenberg AM. Digital technologies for dental implant treatment planning and guided surgery. Oral Maxillofac Surg Clin North Am. 2015 May;27(2):319–40.
4. Schepers RH, Kraeima J, Vissink A, Lahoda LU, Roodenburg JL, Reintsema H, Raghoebar GM, Witjes MJ. Accuracy of secondary maxillofacial reconstruction with prefabricated fibula grafts using 3D planning and guided reconstruction. J Craniomaxillofac Surg. 2016 Apr;44(4):392–9.
5. Polley JW, Figueroa AA. Orthognathic positioning system: intraoperative system to transfer virtual surgical plan to operating field during orthognathic surgery. J Oral Maxillofac Surg. 2013 May;71(5):911–20.
6. Zinser MJ, Sailer HF, Ritter L, Braumann B, Maegele M, Zöller JE. A paradigm shift in orthognathic surgery? A comparison of navigation, computer-aided designed/computer-aided manufactured splints, and "classic" intermaxillary splints to surgical transfer of virtual orthognathic planning. J Oral Maxillofac Surg. 2013 Dec;71(12):2151.e1–21.
7. Binder WJ. Custom-designed facial implants. Facial Plast Surg Clin North Am. 2008 Feb;16(1):133–46.
8. Vercruyssen M, Jacobs R, Van Assche N, van Steenberghe D. The use of CT scan based planning for oral rehabilitation by means of implants and its transfer to the surgical field: a critical review on accuracy. J Oral Rehabil. 2008 Jun;35(6):454–74.
9. Gerbino G, Zavattero E, Zenga F, Bianchi FA, Garzino-Demo P, Berrone S. Primary and secondary reconstruction of complex craniofacial defects using polyetheretherketone custom-made implants. J Craniomaxillofac Surg. 2015 Oct;43(8):1356–63.
10. Andrews BT, Thurston TE, Tanna N, Broer PN, Levine JP, Kumar A, Bradley JP. A multicenter experience with image-guided surgical navigation: broadening clinical indications in complex craniomaxillofacial surgery. J Craniofac Surg. 2015 Jun;26(4):1136–9.
11. Zavattero E, Viterbo S, Gerbino G, Ramieri G. Navigation-aided endoscopic sinus surgery. J Craniofac Surg. 2015 Jan;26(1):326–7.
12. Bolzoni Villaret A, Battaglia P, Tschabitscher M, Mattavelli D, Turri-Zanoni M, Castelnuovo P, Nicolai P. A 3-dimensional transnasal endoscopic journey through the paranasal sinuses and adjacent skull base: a practical and surgery-oriented perspective. Neurosurgery. 2014 Mar;10(Suppl 1):116–20; discussion 120.
13. Lobo B, Heng A, Barkhoudarian G, Griffiths CF, Kelly DF. The expanding role of the endonasal endoscopic approach in pituitary and skull base surgery: a 2014 perspective. Surg Neurol Int. 2015 May 20;6:82.
14. Dehdashti AR, Ganna A, Witterick I, Gentili F. Expanded endoscopic endonasal approach for anterior cranial base and suprasellar lesions: indications and limitations. Neurosurgery. 2009 Apr;64(4):677–87; discussion 687–9.
15. van Nunen DP, Janssen LE, Stubenitsky BM, Han KS, Muradin MS. Stereolithographic skull models in the surgical planning of fronto-supraorbital bar advancement for non-syndromic trigonocephaly. J Craniomaxillofac Surg. 2014 Sep;42(6):959–65.
16. Mazzoni S, Marchetti C, Sgarzani R, Cipriani R, Scotti R, Ciocca L. Prosthetically guided maxillofacial surgery: evaluation of the accuracy of a surgical guide and custom-made bone plate in oncology patients after mandibular reconstruction. Plast Reconstr Surg. 2013 Jun;131(6):1376–85.
17. Sosin M, Ceradini D, Levine J, Hazen A, Staffenberg D, Saadeh P, Flores R, Sweeney N, Bernstein GL, Rodriguez E. Total face, eyelids, ears, scalp, and skeletal subunit transplant: a reconstructive solution for the full face and total scalp burn. Plast Reconstr Surg. July 2016;138(1):205–19.

The Digital Thread for Personalized Craniomaxillofacial Surgery

2

Andrew M. Christensen, Katherine Weimer, Christopher Beaudreau, Michael Rensberger, and Benjamin Johnson

Introduction: The Digital Thread

Digital technologies are impacting healthcare in every possible way. Their impact on treatment can be seen across the specialty of craniomaxillofacial (CMF) surgery, from dental implant technology, to personalized implants, and virtual surgical planning for reconstructive surgeries. Digital medical imaging has made a broad impact on patient care throughout the body, but perhaps nowhere more visible than in the specialties involving care of the CMF area. As three-dimensional volumetric imaging has become standard of care for treating patients with CMF trauma, disease, and deformities, digital technologies utilizing these medical images have been rapidly evolving to meet the increased demand. With a digital "3D patient" at their fingertips, surgeons are eager to find new ways to diagnose, treatment plan, and execute surgery.

Digital medical imaging technologies are a basis for the personalization of surgery, by applying surgical procedures to the individual patient before surgery. An example might be surgical planning for the placement of dental fixtures or surgical planning of orthognathic surgery; both guided by tactile guides which transfer the surgical plan to the patient. Most of these techniques rely on medical imaging to drive the digital workflow, which in general terms includes the following major steps: (1) medical imaging, (2) medical image processing, (3) virtual surgical planning, (4) haptic design, (5) 3D printing, (6) surgical rehearsal, and finally (7) the surgery. This workflow, referred to as a "digital thread" (Fig. 2.1), becomes very important to leveraging tools in ways to deliver accurate, time efficient, and powerful treatment methodologies. The digital thread is a series of interconnected technologies which create a clinical workflow for a given surgical application.

The earliest uses of 3D technology involved 3D printed anatomical models of bone, used for hands-on visualization, diagnosis, and treatment planning [1, 2] (Fig. 2.2). Anatomical models when used for preoperative planning were shown to reduce surgical time and enhance overall treatment of many reconstructive maxillofacial procedures [3]. The next stage of the technology involved customization of implants for the CMF area, which has become commonplace. Implant applications such as custom cranioplasty [4], custom total temporomandibular joint replacement [5], custom facial implants [6], and obvious areas like fully edentulous reconstruction by dental implants are all areas known to CMF surgeons which use digital technology. In the last 5 years, the technology has continued to evolve into driving personalized surgery for bony and soft tissue reconstruction. This is done using virtual tools (i.e., software) translated to the operating room by output of models, guides, templates, and implants using 3D printing. This new area is known as virtual surgical planning (VSP) and is finding application in numerous areas across the anatomical spectrum, ranging from CMF surgery to orthopedic surgery. Thousands of patient surgeries per year are now being impacted by VSP technology for "everyday" procedures ranging from total knee arthroplasty to bimaxillary orthognathic surgery (Fig. 2.3).

3D printing can be defined as the translation of a CAD (computer-aided design) software file into the physical world using technology known as additive manufacturing, a group of technologies which lay down successive axially oriented layers of material to create a physical object (Figs. 2.4 and 2.23). Traditional manufacturing techniques like machining, milling, injection molding, and forging are all suited toward large runs of the same part. 3D printing is agnostic to the complexity or number of parts in a single run. This benefits customized part production because 3D printing can produce 20 individual parts just as easily as it can produce 20 parts which are identical. Many different techniques now exist

A.M. Christensen (✉)
Division of Medical Physics, University of Ottawa, Ottawa, ON, Canada
e-mail: biomdlr@me.com

K. Weimer • C. Beaudreau • M. Rensberger • B. Johnson
3D Systems, 5381 South Alkire Circle, Littleton 80127, CO, USA
e-mail: denver.healthcare@3dsystems.com

A.M. Greenberg (ed.), *Digital Technologies in Craniomaxillofacial Surgery*, https://doi.org/10.1007/978-1-4939-1532-3_2

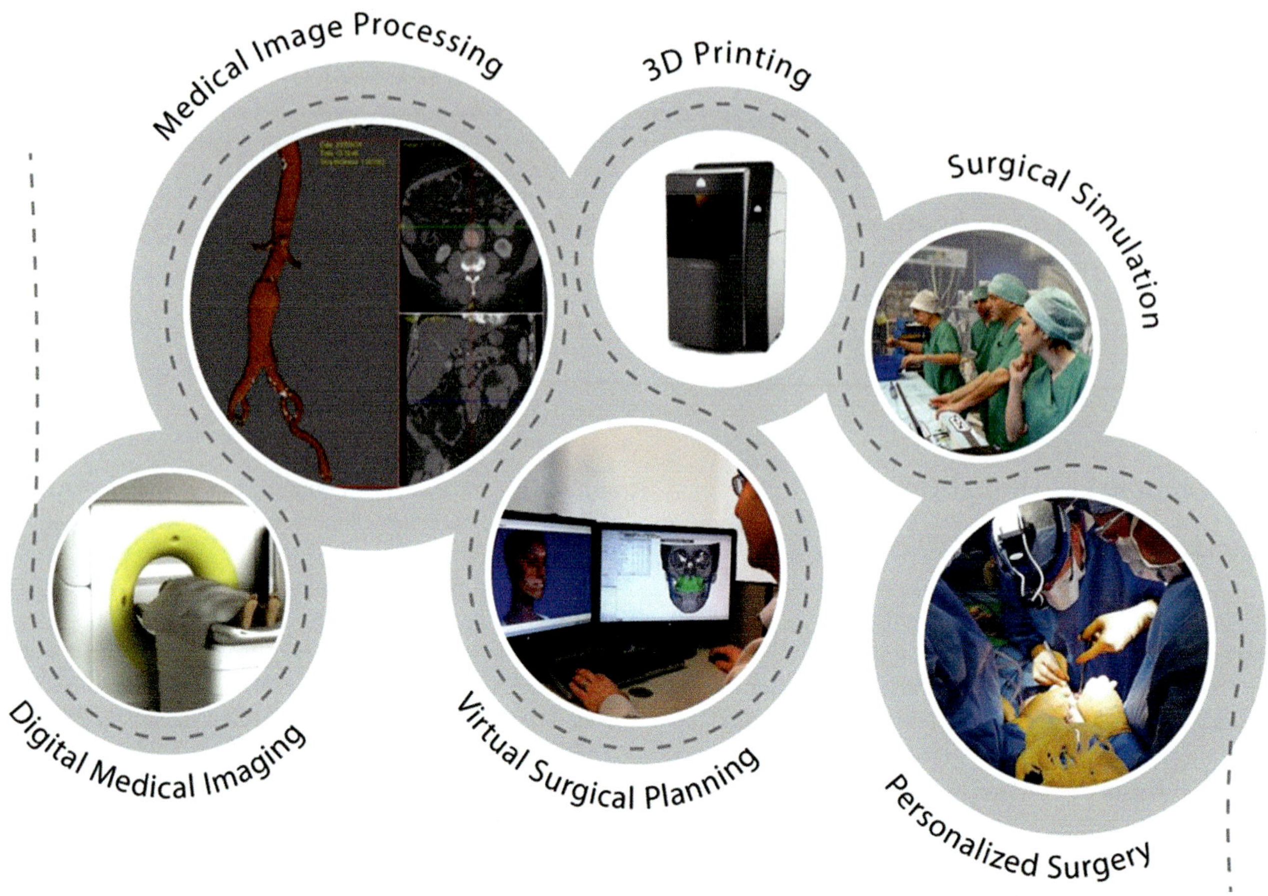

Fig. 2.1 The digital thread for personalized surgery includes major steps for using medical image data to drive patient treatment using 3D printing-centric technology (Courtesy 3D Systems Healthcare, Rock Hill, SC, USA)

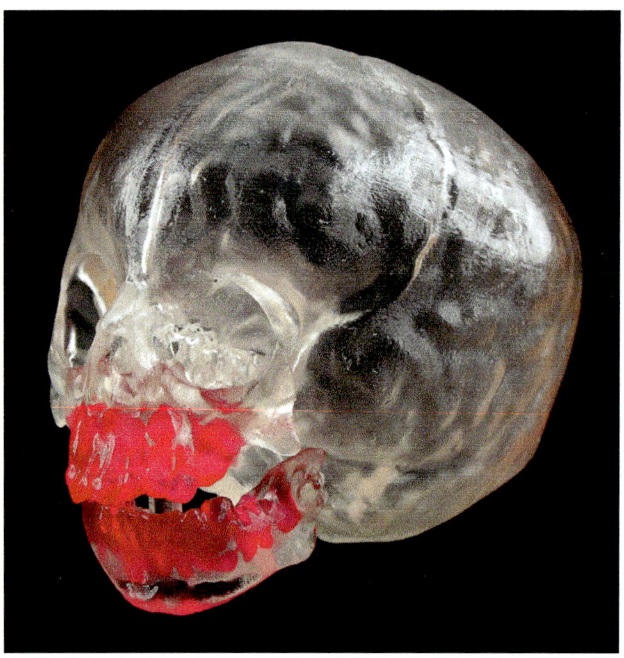

Fig. 2.2 Stereolithography (SLA) model of an infant cranium showing selective coloration (*in red*) of tooth structures (Courtesy 3D Systems Healthcare, Rock Hill, SC, USA)

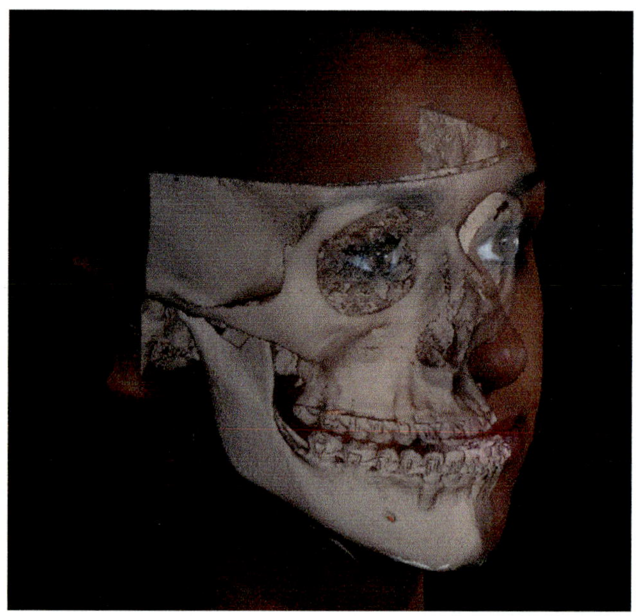

Fig. 2.3 A computer rendering of a composite model showing a "digital patient" with overlay of soft tissue coloring by either photograph or stereophotogrammetry in preparation for virtual surgical planning of orthognathic surgery (Courtesy 3D Systems Healthcare, Rock Hill, SC, USA)

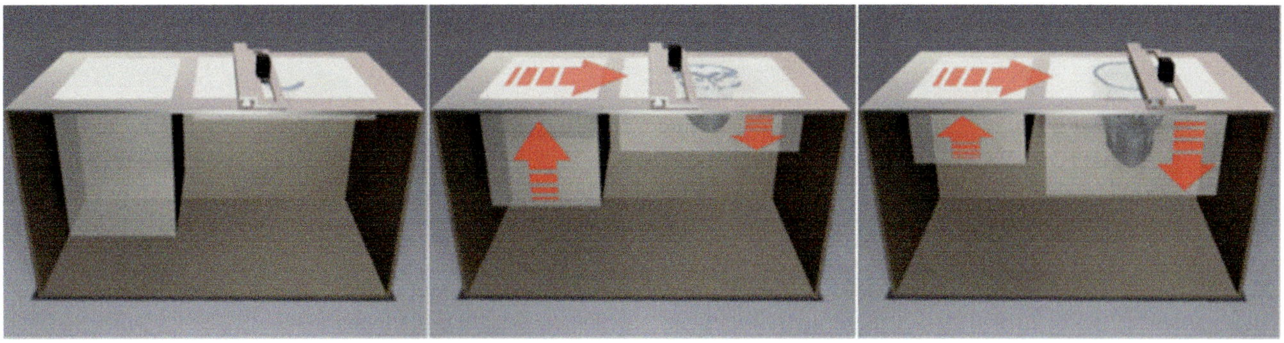

Fig. 2.4 Schematic of the ColorJet printing (CJP) 3D printing process showing a model being created in successive, axial layers (Courtesy 3D Systems Healthcare, Rock Hill, SC, USA)

under the umbrella of 3D printing, and many of them have application to healthcare one way or another through different materials, colors, material properties, or accuracy levels.

Medical Imaging and Image Processing

Medical Imaging Background

Imaging modalities utilized in the diagnosis and surgical treatment of CMF cases are varied. As has been mentioned, what traditionally included CT and MRI now commonly includes CBCT, laser scanning, intraoral scanning, and sometimes even photogrammetry. The collection of morphometrically accurate data for anatomical features of a patient forms the basis for personalized surgical intervention. It is therefore critically important that proper protocols are both established and followed when collecting medical imaging data to ensure necessary information is obtained without the need for costly and harmful repeat procedures.

Computed tomography is typically used for imaging of dense tissues such as bone. A smooth, but not soft, reconstruction kernel is well suited for image processing. Sharp algorithms, however, are associated with increased noise that make segmentation more difficult. Magnetic resonance imaging (MRI) used for soft tissues such as brain and tumors is a technique not often associated with CMF surgical planning. T1- and T2-weighted acquisitions do not resolve structures with low proton densities like bone, making identification of these anatomies difficult. The ability to image patients without ionizing radiation is attractive though, and developments in MRI acquisition techniques like "Black Bone MRI" protocols could pave the way for more widespread use [7, 8].

Medical Imaging Considerations

Medical, multi-detector CT (MDCT) scanners found in the hospital setting typically have excellent contrast resolution and good spatial resolution with slice spacing from 0.625 to 1.25 mm and pixel sizes less than 0.5 mm. Studies at this resolution with contiguous scanning are ideal for the digital CMF workflow (Fig. 2.5). Imaging data of any type with slice spacing over 2.5 mm risks compromising accuracy of the 3D generated patient model; over the last 10 years, CBCT imaging systems with flat panel detectors have gained acceptance for head and neck imaging. The CBCT modality is characterized by excellent spatial resolution at reduced patient dose, but with the expense of increased scatter and noise [9] (Fig. 2.6). High spatial resolution studies over a large of field of view create an immense amount of data, and it is our experience that studies smaller than 0.4 mm voxels can become cumbersome to process because of the large amount of computation required to handle the data. In some select instances (perhaps evaluation of individual teeth or arches), a smaller voxel size may be necessary but should be paired with a smaller field of view to better manage the computational limitations. There are many factors outside of spatial resolution that can affect the quality of the medical imaging data. Before any type of medical imaging data is used for personalized surgery, it should be evaluated for suitable use. Although some artifacts are common across all

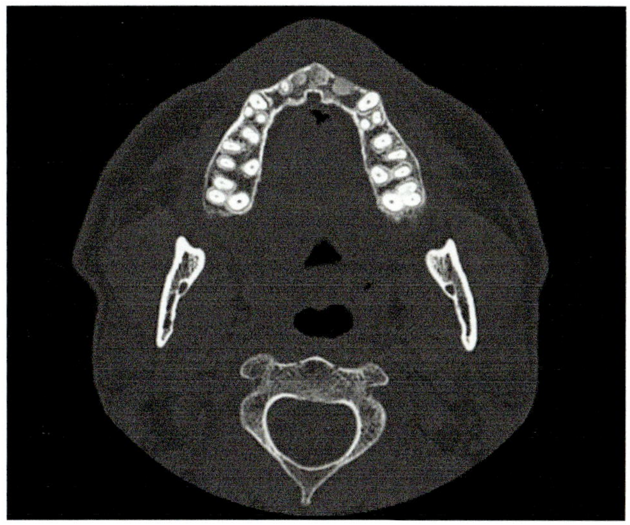

Fig. 2.5 Example axial image of medical computed tomography (CT) scan showing good delineation between hard and soft tissue (Courtesy 3D Systems Healthcare, Rock Hill, SC, USA)

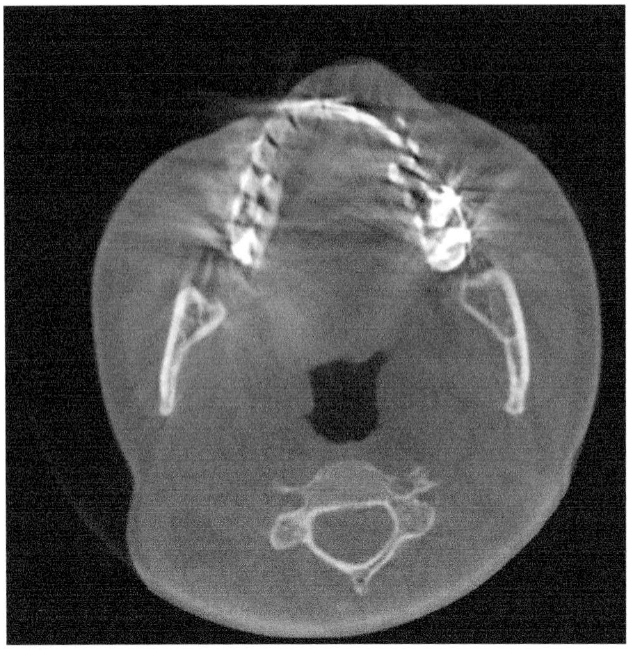

Fig. 2.6 Example axial image of cone beam CT (CBCT) scan showing lower contrast to noise ratio and less discretion between hard and soft tissues (Courtesy 3D Systems Healthcare, Rock Hill, SC, USA)

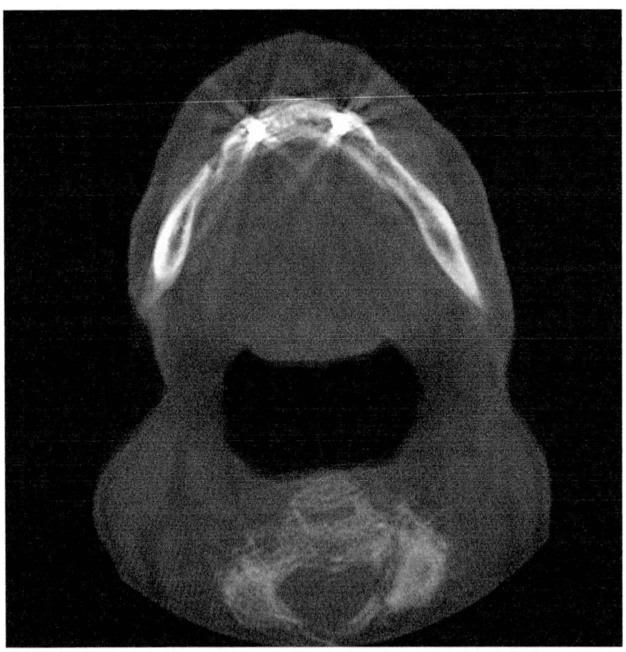

Fig. 2.7 Example axial image of cone beam CT (CBCT) scan showing motion artifact; note the blurry "double" images shown in anterior and spinal areas (Courtesy 3D Systems Healthcare, Rock Hill, SC, USA)

medical imaging platforms, the list below focuses on artifacts and issues common to CT and CBCT modalities used for CMF imaging:

1. Patient Motion. Perhaps the most prevalent study artifact is patient motion occurring during image acquisition. Patient movement results in streaks, blurry images, and double contours not suitable for treatment planning [10] (Fig. 2.7). Causes of patient movement are varied from a noncompliant subject to involuntary movements such as breathing. Children are a key demographic for craniomaxillofacial surgery, and it can be difficult for a child to sit still in a CBCT scanner for the 10–30 s required for image acquisition. Additionally, patients may present with physical impairments that make it difficult to remain without motion during the image scanning process.
2. Metal Artifact. X-rays passing through dense metallic materials are attenuated and scattered, resulting in streak artifacts in the image reconstruction (Fig. 2.8). Metal artifact reduces the quality of the images and makes accurate image processing more difficult. Plates and screws from a previous surgery, braces from orthodontic treatment, amalgam fillings for dental caries, dental restorations and implants, and even bullet fragments from gunshot wounds are all potential sources of metal artifact.
3. Field of View. For treatment of CMF deformities, it is imperative that the entire region of interest is captured in the scan. As simple as this seems, mistakes in patient imaging oftentimes necessitate a rescan. A more common occurrence of insufficient field of view occurs in CBCT scanners seen in oral surgery, dental, and orthodontic offices. Many of these scanners are dual purpose for dental-specific applications and are also expected to capture sufficient anatomy for more expanded oral surgery operations in the maxilla, mandible, and cranium. Often, limited field of view CBCT scanners are unsuccessfully

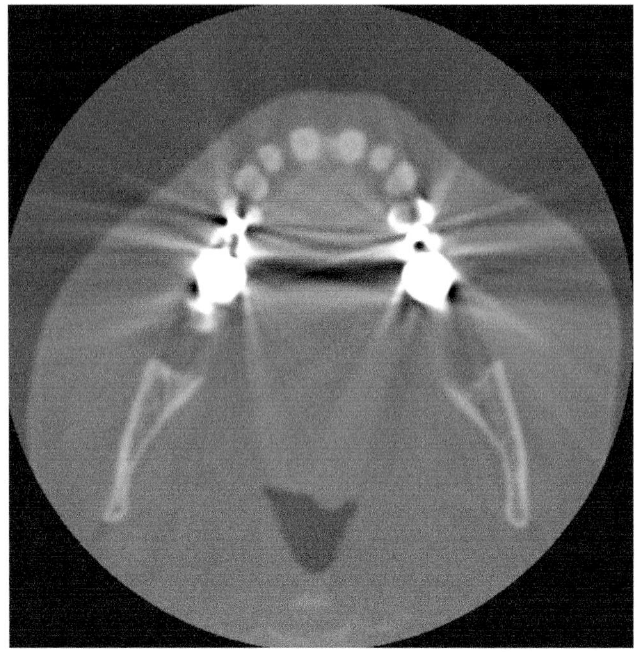

Fig. 2.8 Example axial image of medical computed tomography (CT) scan showing extreme metallic artifact in the area of the dentition (Courtesy 3D Systems Healthcare, Rock Hill, SC, USA)

used for capturing midface and cranium bony anatomy. Software solutions used to obviate this issue include aligning and then stitching of multiple scan volumes together to create a single volume. If done correctly, this does work in limited applications, but it creates a risk of inaccuracy that could follow all the way to the operating room.

4. Age of Scan. Especially relevant in the growing child, the date of image acquisition can have an effect on the accuracy of the data once in the three-dimensional environment. For example, an infant requiring mandibular distraction for airway constraints will have drastically different imaging studies at 1 week of age and at 6 months of age due to growth of the child. The age of the scan is also critical in patients who are undergoing orthodontic treatment. If the patient's teeth have moved after the imaging was conducted, the accuracy of the final tools used in surgery will be compromised. Scan date issues are also common in trauma and cranial vault reconstruction. Determining if a scan is still current enough to not affect the representation of the anatomy is not trivial and should be discussed with the medical team before use in personalized surgery.
5. Calibration and Maintenance of Imaging Equipment. Any equipment used as a medical device for clinical application requires scheduled maintenance and calibration to repeatedly produce accurate results. In-office CBCT equipment is particularly susceptible to lapses in upkeep and calibration, resulting in detrimental effects to imaging quality. As we begin to rely more heavily on medical imaging data for the basis of complicated and aggressive designs in personalized surgery, it is the obligation of the clinicians using this technology to understand where the risks lie.

Medical Image Processing

Processing of medical image data into 3D representations of patient anatomy involves segmenting out structures of interest from the 2D image stack based on the radiodensity of each pixel. Anatomical structures such as teeth, bone, nerve canals, implants, tumors, and skin surfaces can be assigned to a grouping of pixels and then interpolated between slices to create a 3D volumetric representation. Medical image processing can be performed using automated or manual segmentation techniques, and there are advantages and disadvantages to both.

It is almost certain that the future of personalized surgery will require advancements in automatic segmentation of medical imaging data. In automated segmentation, the user (or automated computer) would decide the most appropriate technical parameters of selection and apply those parameters to the region of interest (ROI) of the data. Algorithms for automated segmentation are typically based either on gray value features of the image or on previously segmented structures that can be used for comparison [11]. Advantages are in the time saving aspect and lack of subjective decisions being made by the technical liaison segmenting the anatomy. Disadvantages occur when the image data falls outside the scope of automation and the algorithm fails to converge on a correctly segmented anatomical structure. Based on the previously stated list of risks and artifacts when acquiring medical imaging data, automation of medical imaging data in craniomaxillofacial surgery is not currently common.

Manual segmentation is laborious and operator dependent but is currently considered the "gold standard" of image processing [12]. The manual segmentation process is particularly suited to CMF cases with CBCT imaging, metal artifact, and patients presenting with uncommon anatomy as a result of trauma, disease, or deformity.

Manual segmentation requires a slice by slice intervention with the data to digitally label the pixels associated with a region of interest based on gray levels. Additional tools such as eroding, region growing, extruding, adding, and subtracting are used as needed to create an accurate segmentation. Manual segmentations require expert knowledge of anatomy and imaging data to produce robust digital files appropriate for use. Any errors introduced at this step in the process propagate downstream and produce deleterious effects in the accuracy of surgical planning.

The last step in medical image processing is to create CAD files of desired anatomies that can be used universally on many software platforms for further design work. Successfully segmented and interpolated image data will result in a volume rendering of the anatomy. In a volume rendering, there are no actual surfaces (or meshes) that can be cut, reshaped, moved, or used as a design basis. The volumes must be converted into a surface file prior to manipulation of the structures. Conversion to a surface file involves wrapping a mesh around the selected volume of data by fitting points on the volume and connecting the points to create a triangulated surface mesh. These elements wrap around the contour of the shape desired in a sheet-like fashion to form a geometric surface file of the area of interest. This type of geometric file can be imported into other software programs and is suitable to be digitally manipulated.

Alternative Medical Imaging Techniques

An interesting area of newer data acquisition formats in CMF surgeries is the use of laser surface scanning and stereophotogrammetry. Laser surface scanning is noninvasive and uses light and camera technology to generate a three-dimensional mapping of a surface. It does this by capturing points on the scanned object and then creates a surface from those points. This type of technology is prevalent in digital intraoral scanning and can obviate the need for traditional impressions and dental casts. Stereophotogrammetry is a system that uses multiple cameras with known locations and the scanned object as an additional point in space. With these multiple known points in space, the triangulation method can be used to record a three-dimensional location of the object in space. The result is a surface file with color and texture of the object being scanned. This type of scanning is most common for taking nonintrusive color and texture scans of the face, impressions, teeth, or plaster models of the teeth (Fig. 2.26).

Virtual Surgical Planning

Introduction

Virtual surgical planning (VSP) is quickly becoming the standard of care in CMF surgery, especially in applications where osteotomies are performed [13–26]. This includes but is not limited to orthognathic surgery, fibula free flap reconstruction of the maxilla or mandible, trauma reconstruction, distraction osteogenesis, and even cranial vault reconstruction. This does not mean that soft tissue and vascular surgery are out of touch with VSP; they are just at this moment less impacted by VSP.

Virtual surgical planning is at its basis the idea of taking digital anatomy of a patient and using it to drive surgical treatment through surgical planning in a digital environment paired with 3D printed guides, templates, and models meant to carry the plan from the computer to the operating room. This method often takes software and engineering skills to manipulate the data in an accurate and time-effective manner. Although the clinician may be quite capable of this task, they usually do not have the required software, time, or honed skills to do this in a cost or time-effective way [27, 28]. As such, a service center with a technical liaison is often used to aid in the virtual surgical planning process. The clinician can interact with the service center via synchronous collaboration (webmeeting) platforms such as GoToMeeting® (Citrix Systems, Fort Lauderdale, FL). This allows the clinician to focus on making the clinical and surgical decisions without getting lost in the technical software processes involved with creating an accurate digital surgical plan. During a webmeeting, the keyboard and mouse control can be given to the clinician to make the screen sharing process even more efficient. Multiple parties from the medical team can join the webmeeting, and the geographic location is obviated. All that is needed is a computer, tablet, or smartphone with an Internet connection.

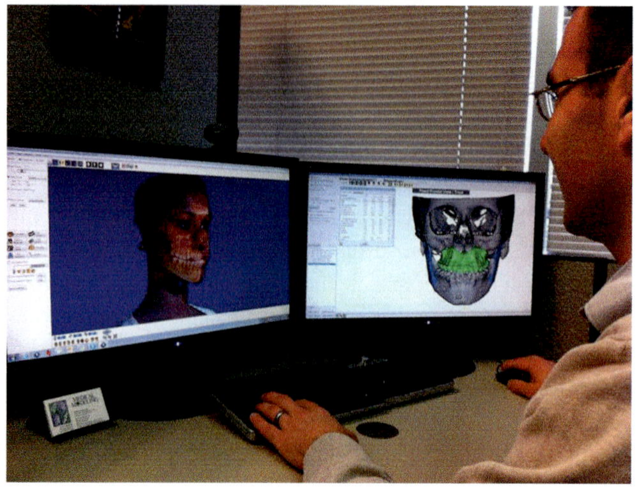

Fig. 2.9 Collaborative webmeetings allow for synchronous discussion between surgeon and engineer while viewing the patient image on screen (Courtesy 3D Systems Healthcare, Rock Hill, SC, USA)

Toolbox

During the webmeeting with the technical liaison (typically a biomedical engineer) and the clinician, various aspects of the surgical operation can be simulated (Fig. 2.9). Although more realistic surgical simulation will be touched on later, it is important to know that the common reference to virtual surgical planning is not intended to be a true surgical rehearsal. The simulation of the operation is simplified into common CAD tasks that will allow for manipulation of the patient's anatomy into a simulated final surgical outcome. Any virtual surgical plan is a combination of one of the following data manipulations:

1. Anatomic osteotomies: Using cutting planes and subtraction techniques, a virtual cutting path can be applied to the patient's anatomy. This cutting path can vary in thickness and shape to simulate both straight-line or curved osteotomies. Likewise drill holes for pins or screws can also be simulated (Fig. 2.10).
2. Reshape Anatomy: Bony reconstructive surgery does not always fall in the category of a straight-line osteotomy or drill hole. Many times an irregular osteotomy, reshaping using a burr or other surgical tools is used. Although this is more difficult to simulate, it is possible to mimic this surgical action using force-feedback (haptic) technology by the digital designer. Much like the surgeon burrs or carves the bony anatomy to desired shape; this can be simulated as well digitally (Fig. 2.11).
3. Repositioning Anatomy: Using various point tracking and measurement tools, anatomic osteotomies can be repositioned digitally to reach the surgeon's desired simu-

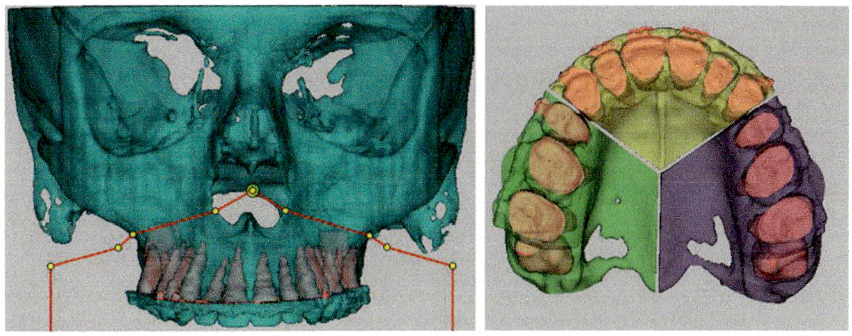

Fig. 2.10 Virtual osteotomies are performed which separate the bones of the computer model much like during the actual procedure. Note the different colored maxillary segments and teeth following virtual osteotomy (Courtesy 3D Systems Healthcare, Rock Hill, SC, USA)

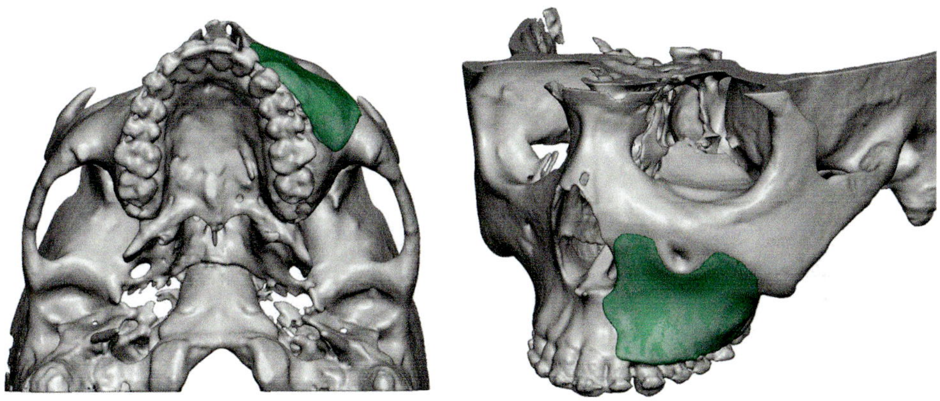

Fig. 2.11 Adding material to the anatomy or digitally burring down anatomy can be performed in a virtual environment, as here in *green* augmenting the left malar area (Courtesy 3D Systems Healthcare, Rock Hill, SC, USA)

lated final position. For orthognathic surgery, this would be implemented by correcting midline asymmetries until desired facial proportions are met. For a trauma case, this would translate to repositioning the bony segments back to their original location. For a reconstruction case, this could mean repositioning malposed anatomy or misaligned condyles back to their original state. In all instances of repositioning, the surgeon and/or technical liaison have the ability to do fine or gross movements on the anatomy (Fig. 2.12).

4. Targeting Anatomically Correct Results: The methods previously described (osteotomies, reshaping, and repositioning) can be assisted by real-time comparison to anatomically correct references. This can be achieved in several fashions, but two methods are used most commonly:

(a) Mirroring Data: When patient anatomy is available that has been unaffected by a defect or deformity, this region can be mirrored across the midsagittal plane and overlaid against the affected anatomy. This provides a patient-specific reference dataset in order to optimize the digital plan [29] (Fig. 2.13).

(b) Normative Data: When patient anatomy unaffected by a defect or deformity is unavailable, for example, in a panfacial traumatic injury, normative data can be utilized to optimize the digital plan. Studies have been performed to generate statistically "normal" cephalometric datasets based on different age ranges and genders. These datasets can then be transformed into digital surface models that can be overlaid on the existing patient anatomy for reference [30–33] (Fig. 2.14).

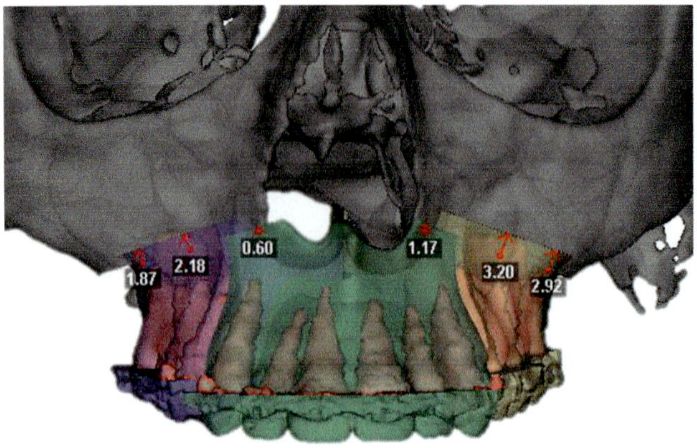

Fig. 2.12 Bony gaps and overlaps can be measured with precision during the virtual planning session. Note the bony overlaps here caused by impaction of the multipiece maxillary segment (Courtesy 3D Systems Healthcare, Rock Hill, SC, USA)

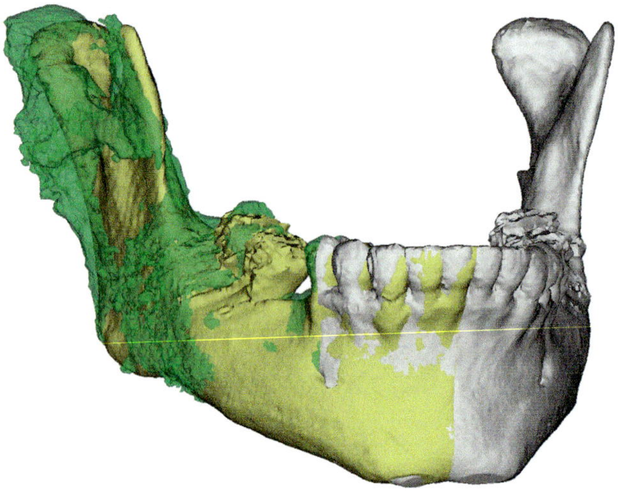

Fig. 2.13 Contralateral anatomy can be used for guidance if the pathologic anatomy is limited to a single side. Here the patient's unaffected left ramus is used in a mirrored fashion (*in yellow*) to ascertain how much deformity has occurred on the right (Courtesy 3D Systems Healthcare, Rock Hill, SC, USA)

5. Soft Tissue Simulation: The use of predictive soft tissue simulation analyses is becoming more prevalent in CMF surgery. Specifically in orthognathic surgical planning, the clinician has the ability to see what a "predicted" soft tissue outcome may look like for his or her patient. Many of these soft tissue algorithms are not validated, but are becoming more interesting for patient education and teaching purposes. It is an obvious next step to validate these three-dimensional soft tissue simulations in order to plan the desired soft tissue changes and determine what bony anatomy repositioning is required to achieve the soft tissue target.
6. Measurements: Measurements or cephalometric landmarks and analysis are often used to make critical surgical planning decisions. Although this can commonly be overlooked as a valuable planning tool, it is critical in the success of an accurate plan. Two-dimensional and three-dimensional measurements in the form of points, lines, planes, and angles are used to create many types of measurements. For example, at any time you can measure the thickness of the bone at the osteotomy site and the depth of the inferior alveolar nerve at various points of the mandible, create a perpendicular plane to establish the midsagittal plane of a patient, and also create a ratio of cephalometric points that allow for proper facial form (Fig. 2.15). It is frequently of interest to know how far a certain landmark has moved from its original position. This is also possible and very easy to do in the digital environment. Without these digital tools, it would be nearly impossible to quantify this type of request using traditional treatment planning methods.

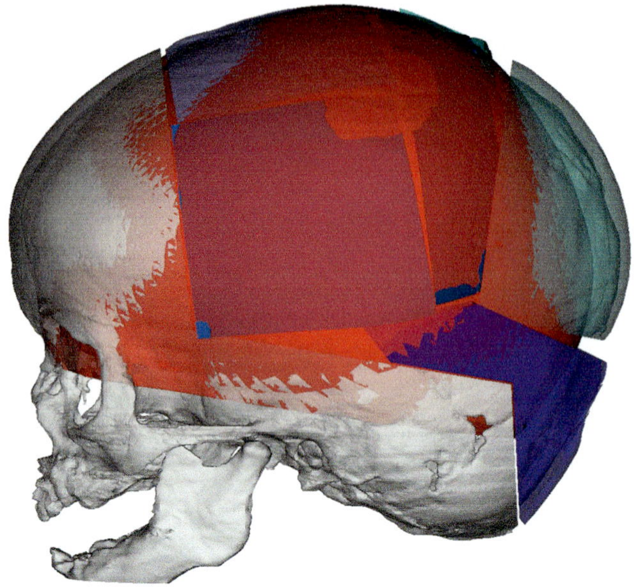

Fig. 2.14 Age-matched normative data can be used during a planning session to determine correct scale. Note the *red* normative dataset superimposed on the postoperative view following simulation of a cranial vault reconstruction (Courtesy 3D Systems Healthcare, Rock Hill, SC, USA)

Virtual surgical planning can be applied to a wide range of craniomaxillofacial surgeries [13]. Depending on whether a clinician is using a service center or doing the virtual surgical planning on his or her own, the digital process to manipulate the meshed anatomy into a final surgical plan can take 30 min to several hours depending on the complexity of the case. Once the surgical planning process is complete, the simulated final meshed surface files are exported for design of custom models, surgical guides, and templates that are used to transfer the virtual plan to surgical environment in

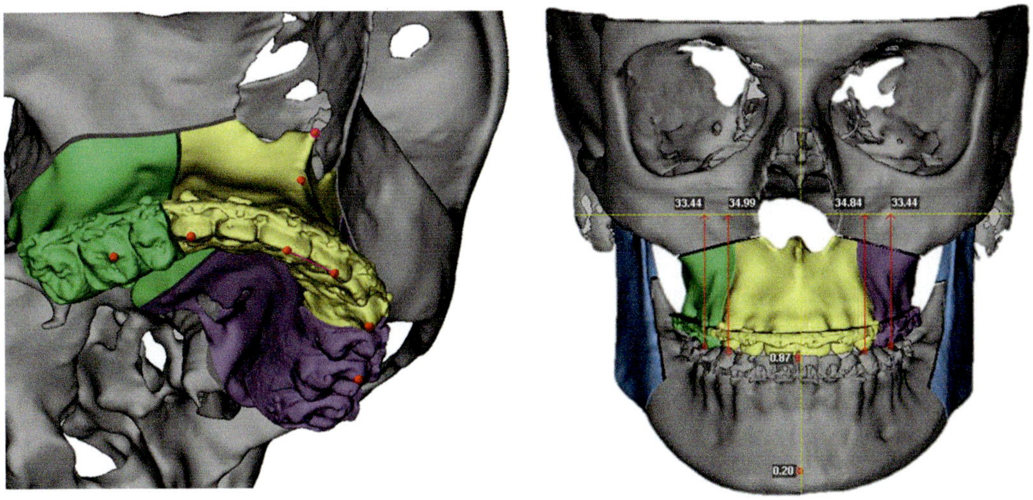

Fig. 2.15 Bony landmarks can be used to determine symmetry and overall balance when planning for orthognathic surgery (Courtesy 3D Systems Healthcare, Rock Hill, SC, USA)

the operating room. One can even use the simulated surgical planning data to design a custom implant specifically for that particular patient and that particular surgical plan.

Risks of surgical planning are not completely obviated. One of the common pitfalls discussed is that in many instances such a detailed presurgical plan does not allow for any (or much) intraoperative decision-making to take place when it references the presurgical plan. It also can prohibit the surgeon's ability to change the surgical plan based on intraoperative findings. There are also added costs to surgical planning that may not have been accrued otherwise, though these may be offset or even overcome by time saved in the operating room and/or the elimination of traditional methods of presurgical planning [16, 27]. Lastly, it has been discussed that presurgical planning and reliance on digital technologies can take the "art" out of surgery. Where technology can impact patient care in a beneficial way, it must proceed and most would argue that the benefits outweigh the drawbacks, including reducing certain aspects of the artistry of surgery.

Design

Introduction

Virtual surgical planning is constrained to simple image visualization and measurements if one is not able to transfer the surgical plan to the operating room using physical means. Utilizing CAD and computer-aided manufacturing (CAM) tools is a typical way to create patient-specific models, surgical guides, and templates to transfer the surgical plan to the operating room [33] (Figs. 2.16 and 2.17). Most of the design tools used in the field of medical devices today are developed for an engineer or designer to use, rather than a surgeon or clinician. There is currently a push to transfer these perceptual digital design tools to the surgeon's desktop. To do so, a change in mind-set must take place on behalf of both the teams creating the design tools as well as the surgeons who should be using them. The design tools must be made available more cost-effectively, become more intuitive to use, and be time effective to truly reach the surgeon's desktop on a large scale.

In addition to using traditional setup of a designer postured at a computer using a mouse, true perceptual design can take place using tools that give the designer force feedback and actual sensation of touching the object they are digitally designing. This form of perceptual design uses a haptic device (Fig. 2.18). The haptic device replaces the traditional mouse strokes with those of a physical sense of touch on the model much like you would do while sculpting clay. This type of perceptual design software, such as Geomagic® Freeform® (3D Systems, Rock Hill, SC), provides the designer (or surgeon) with a sense of touch that is missing in other design platforms. Unfortunately this sense of touch and feel when designing in a virtual clay environment cannot yet be translated through webmeeting interaction, but these types of perceptual design tools are becoming less expensive and will continue to become more accessible to the surgeon's desktop.

To translate the VSP to the operating room, a clinical transfer from the digital world to the physical world must take place, typically using 3D printing technologies. There are many strategies for making this transfer. Each of these is decided by both the type of VSP that was performed and the preferences of the clinician. Transfer to the operating room

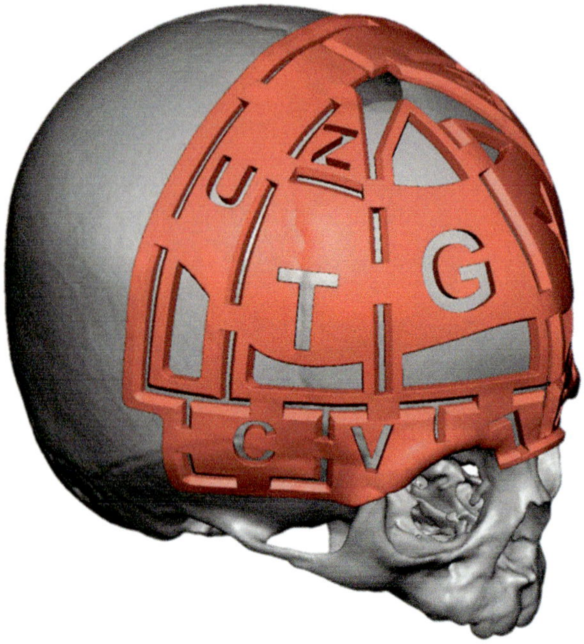

Fig. 2.16 3D printed templates like this one for craniosynostosis repair are able to accurately translate the surgical plan from the computer to the operating room (Courtesy 3D Systems Healthcare, Rock Hill, SC, USA)

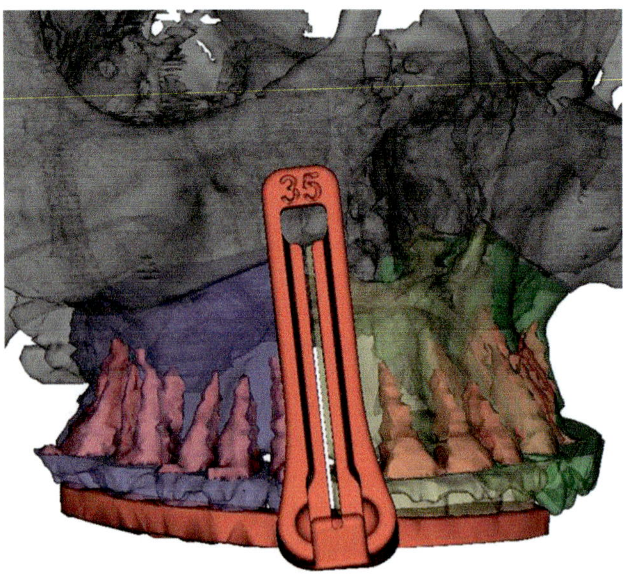

Fig. 2.17 A 3D printed surgical guide which fits the occlusal surface of the maxilla will guide an interdental osteotomy (Courtesy 3D Systems Healthcare, Rock Hill, SC, USA)

can take place by creating bone-borne templates to guide osteotomies, templates to guide position of bone, an advanced technique of predictive hole placement to guide the positioning of implants or secondary positioning guides, and templates to reshape the bone [22, 34] (Fig. 2.19).

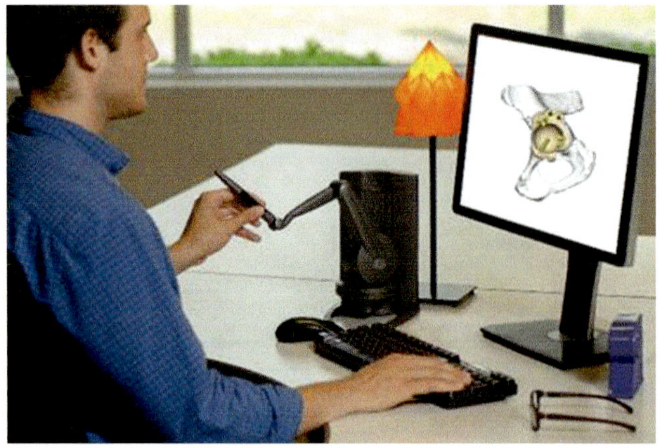

Fig. 2.18 An engineer may use a haptic feedback device combined with powerful CAD software to allow for "feeling" the patient's anatomy or guide/implant designs in a very tactile way (Courtesy 3D Systems Healthcare, Rock Hill, SC, USA)

Clinical Transfer Using Guides/Implants

Digital osteotomies can be transferred to the patient in a practical way by designing a bone-borne guide. A bone-borne osteotomy guide is specifically designed to fit in one – and only one – location on the patient's anatomy. This bone-borne portion allows the guide to fit lock-in-key with the anatomy, thus forcing the guide and subsequent osteotomy into the digitally planned position (Fig. 2.20). When the guide is positioned on the patient's anatomy as designed, the surgeon can perform the osteotomy with confidence that it is in the same position as discussed during the VSP meeting.

Perhaps the most useful type of guide to transfer the VSP to the operating room is a positioning guide [35]. The simple idea behind this type of guide is to transfer the existing bony location to the new virtually planned final position. To reposition bony anatomy, a number of techniques can be used. Using the unique three-dimensional shape of the patient's anatomy can allow for positioning guides to be created to reference one landmark to another. This technique is commonly seen in creation of intermediate and final occlusal splints for orthognathic surgery. This technique can also be used to reference a piece of moving anatomy to one that is stationary or unaltered (Fig. 2.21).

A concept called "predictive hole placement" can be used [23, 34, 36]. This process relates pre-osteotomy and pre-movement reference marks to a secondary positioning guide that aligns with those same marks. To further explain, before any osteotomies or burring is performed, the "future" position of the positioning guide holes is marked on the bony anatomy. The osteotomies can then be performed, and the

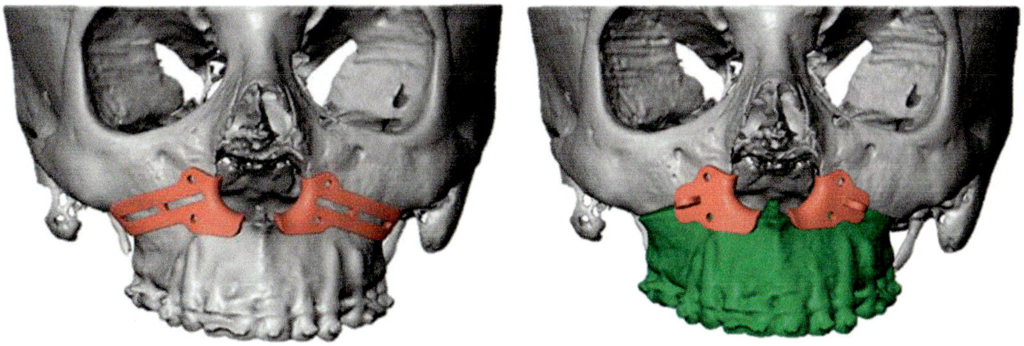

Fig. 2.19 Guides like these accurately transfer information from the computer to the patient using a technique called predictive hole placement. The technique relies on predrilling holes from a first surgical guide which match up with holes in a second surgical guide (Courtesy 3D Systems Healthcare, Rock Hill, SC, USA)

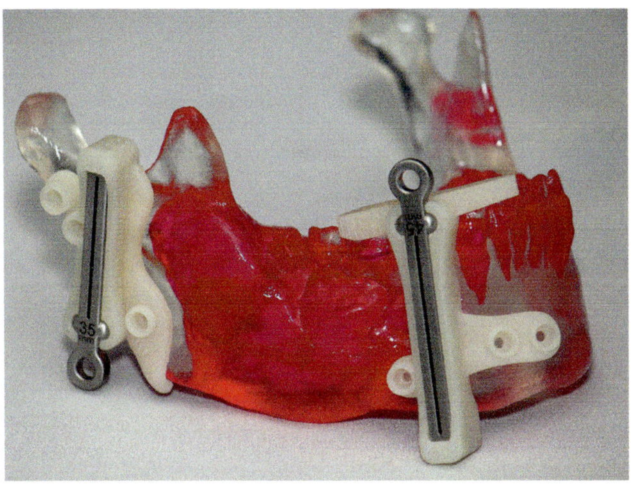

Fig. 2.20 Surgical guides are meant to "key" onto one and only one area of the patient's anatomy to accurately transfer a surgical plan to surgery. In this case an osteotomy will be guided using a bone-borne guide which fits tightly against the patient's mandibular angle (Courtesy 3D Systems Healthcare, Rock Hill, SC, USA)

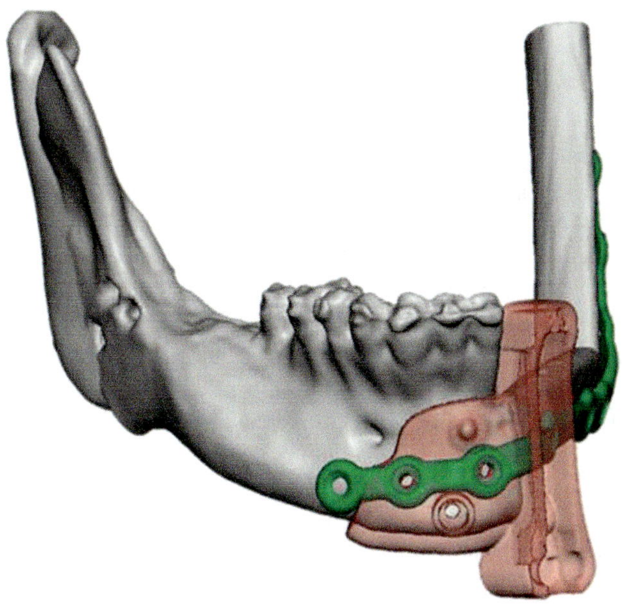

Fig. 2.21 For pre-bent or customized fixation plates, the concept of predictive hole placement can be very useful. Note here that two holes in the *green* plate intersect with the same holes in the *red* surgical guide (Courtesy 3D Systems Healthcare, Rock Hill, SC, USA)

positioning guide can be inserted and aligned to the predrilled holes. Where the predrilled holes line up with the positioning guide, the final position of the anatomy has been achieved.

A more clever way to reposition bony anatomy in CMF surgery is to use the customized implant as a positioning guide [23]. By using the predictive hole placement concept as previously described, the custom implant itself can take the place of the secondary positioning device. The workflow is as follows:

1. The first surgical guide is placed on the patient, and reference holes that match the future position of the implant are marked or drilled on the patient's anatomy.
2. Next, the guide is removed, and the planned osteotomies and general movements are performed.
3. The personalized (or off-the-shelf) implant is placed on the patient's anatomy. The implant is aligned appropriately to the predrilled holes and fixed to the patient's anatomy. The implant and relative bony anatomy will now be positioned as intended in the VSP.

If a surgeon is reshaping bone, either in the form of a graft or simply burring the anatomy down, various design techniques can be used to transfer these operations to the operating room. The graft site is somewhat irrelevant, as the virtually planned or perfected piece of bone can be transferred to the operating room by way of a bone graft template.

This is essentially a plastic representation of the ideal piece of bone that the surgeon will need to replicate in the operating room. If reshaping a graft, instead of guessing at how much bone to harvest or what shape that graft should be, a template could be designed that exactly replicates the shape of the void to be filled. An advanced form of this guide would be a burr guide that would aid the surgeon in burring down bone (e.g., on a fibrous dysplasia case) until the desired perfected shape is reached. These burring/graft template guides can be simple in design but can save several minutes of valuable OR time. It can also work to minimize morbidity at the graft donor site as the surgeons are able to more precisely gather only the graft they need.

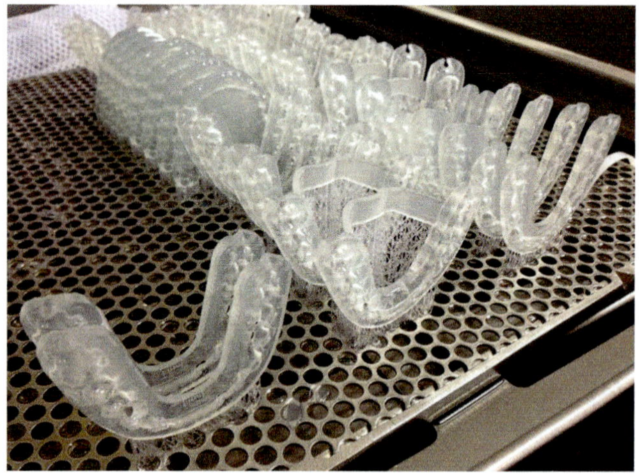

Fig. 2.22 Orthognathic splints for intermediate or final occlusal positioning can be generated using the stereolithography (SLA) 3D printing technique in either opaque or clear resins (Courtesy 3D Systems Healthcare, Rock Hill, SC, USA)

3D Printing Technologies

Background (Figures 2.22 and 2.23)

3D printing was invented when a scientist named Chuck Hull created a physical part out of resin in 1983 in a process later coined "stereolithography" [58]. Following this groundbreaking work, many additional techniques were developed which are all classified as "3D printing." Different processes use different methods to deposit different materials, but all of these concepts have one major thing in common: they are all creating parts in an additive fashion. Additive manufacturing has been used to describe the way that 3D printing works, the concept being that layers of material are deposited sequentially on top of each other until a 3D object is formed. In a similar fashion to a CT scan, the 3D printer lays down horizontal cross sections of material which are fused to the layer below either by light, chemical reaction, or heat. Although the concept of 3D printing is over 30 years old, there is more interest than ever in this technology which keeps developing and finding new applications.

In its application to CMF surgery, 3D printing's first application was to print anatomical models for use of preoperative surgical planning. This form of printing was purely for visualization and hands-on surgical planning [1, 2]. Next came customized implants aided by 3D printing models, templates, or even two part molds [37, 38]. Since then custom surgical guides and templates are being 3D printed from VSP prior to surgery creating a category of printing for surgery. 3D printing in implantable metals is now becoming more common, with applications for implants in the spine, hip, knee, and others. These metallic implants meet the same standards as their traditionally manufactured counterparts. Bioprinting of scaffolds or living tissues remains the next frontier for 3D printing, with researchers working on applications ranging from bone and skin to organs like the heart and liver [39].

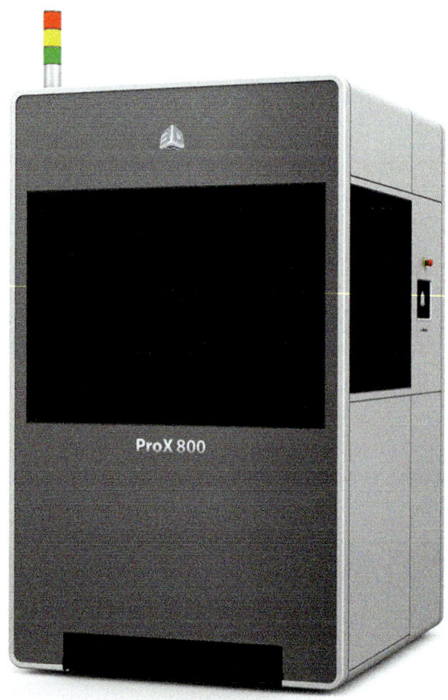

Fig. 2.23 Example of a 3D stereolithographic printer. The stereolithography (SLA) process was the first 3D printing process invented back in the 1980s and is still widely used today. Opaque or translucent resins are cured by an ultraviolet laser in sequential layers to form a 3D object (Courtesy 3D Systems Healthcare, Rock Hill, SC, USA)

Processes/Materials

The most common types of 3D printing technology seen in CMF surgery are as follows:

1. *SLA – Stereolithography*. Stereolithography is a technique using an ultraviolet laser to cure successive layers

of photopolymer. This technique renders translucent or opaque models which can also include selective coloration (Fig. 2.24). Parts produced using the SLA technique can also be produced in a biocompatible polymer suitable for cleaning and sterilization prior to use in the sterile field.

2. *SLS – Selective Laser Sintering*. Selective laser sintering is a technique which uses a fiber laser to melt plastic powder layer by layer, typically using nylon materials. The resultant models are very durable, can be biocompatible, and are typically opaque. These models are suited for surgical tool applications (Fig. 2.25).
3. *MJP – MultiJet Printing*. MultiJet printing technology uses ink-jetting to deposit photopolymer materials which are cured using UV lights layer by layer. A benefit of this technology is the ability to jet out multiple materials at once, for instance, black and white, to create color differentiation. MJP can also jet out rigid or flexible materials and even combinations of materials to create a wider palette of colors or durometers of flexibility.
4. *CJP – ColorJet Printing*. ColorJet printing is a technique whereby a liquid is jetted onto the surface of a powder bed, "gluing" successive layers of composite plaster or plastic powder together. Multiple print heads or combination color print heads can be used to print parts in full color (Fig. 2.26).
5. *PJP – Plastic Jet Printing*. Plastic jet printing technology relies on a filament plastic material, typically PLA (polylactic acid) or ABS (acrylonitrile butadiene styrene), which is fed through a heated extrusion nozzle and deposited onto a platform. These models are typically fairly rough and used typically for low-resolution printing applications.
6. *DMP – Direct Metal Printing*. Direct metal printing refers to a group of techniques which melt successive layers of metal powder using a laser energy source. Typical metals used in DMP include titanium, titanium alloy, cobalt-chrome alloy, and stainless steel. Applications range from creation of surgical instruments to off-the-shelf and personalized long-term implants for many areas of reconstructive surgery (Fig. 2.27).

Although some of the previously mentioned types of 3D printing have a greater footprint in CMF surgery, they are all somewhat irrelevant unless we understand the types of materials that each machine can utilize for printing. It is also relevant to understand how these materials can be used in the clinical/surgical setting. Figure 2.28 illustrates different aspects of each technology in their application.

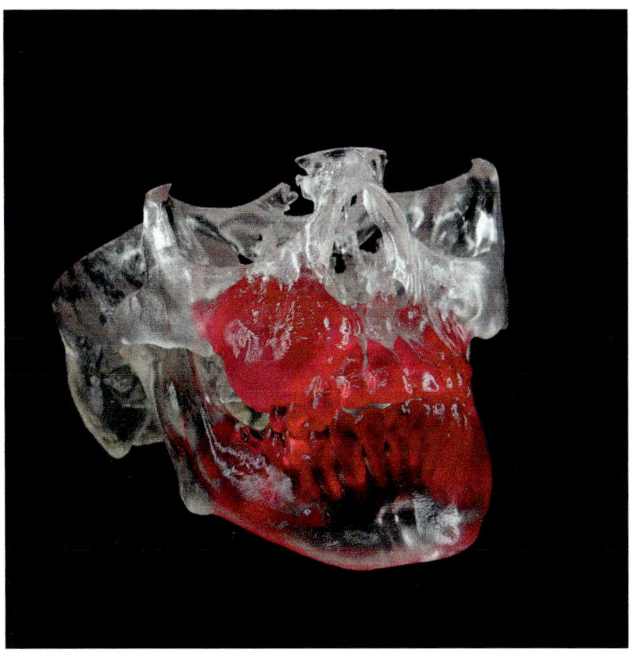

Fig. 2.24 A translucent stereolithography (SLA) 3D printing model showing selective coloration of a mass in the right maxilla, in combination with tooth roots (Courtesy 3D Systems Healthcare, Rock Hill, SC, USA)

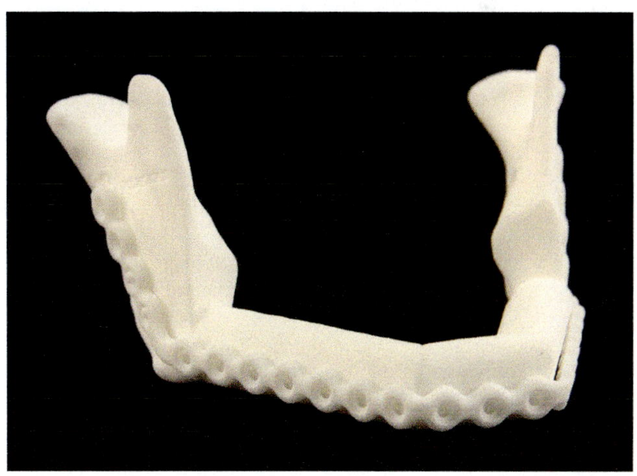

Fig. 2.25 The selective laser sintering (SLS) 3D printing technique relies on a fiber laser to melt nylon powder, forming an object layer by layer. Here SLS parts are used in preparation for a mandibular reconstruction surgery (Courtesy 3D Systems Healthcare, Rock Hill, SC, USA)

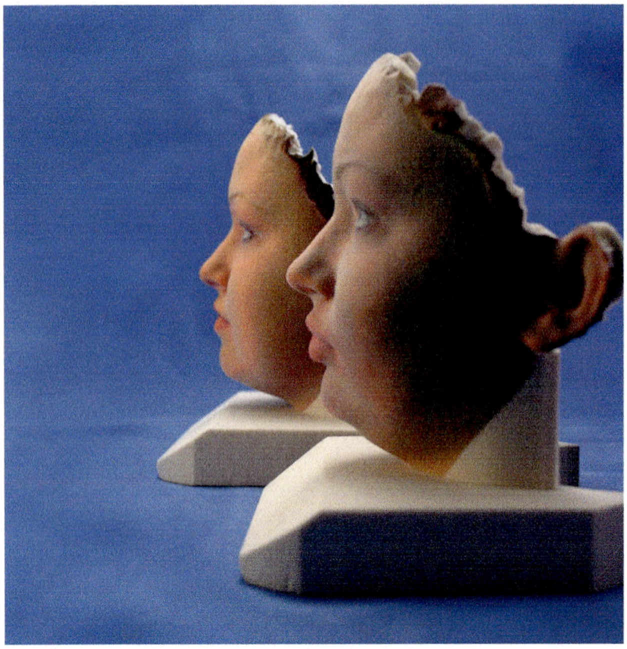

Fig. 2.26 ColorJet printing (CJP) typically uses either composite plaster or plastic powder which is held together by liquid which is ink-jetted onto its surface, forming an object layer by layer. In this case the photograph shows side-by-side comparison of pre- and postsurgery photogrammetry dataset output by CJP; notice the chin movement (Courtesy 3D Systems Healthcare, Rock Hill, SC, USA)

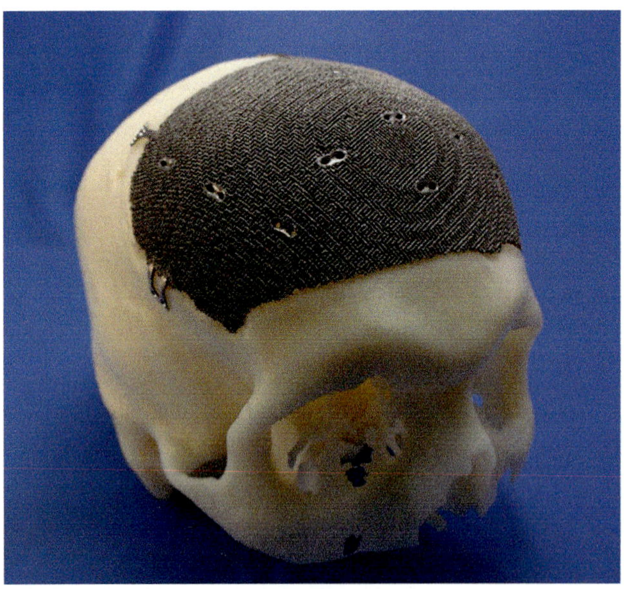

Fig. 2.27 A porous titanium alloy cranioplasty implant created using direct metal printing (DMP) technology allows for integration of solid and porous sections in one part (Courtesy 3D Systems Healthcare, Rock Hill, SC, USA)

Application to Craniomaxillofacial Surgery

Orthognathic Surgery (Figure 2.29)

Orthognathic surgery, also known as corrective jaw surgery, is a procedure in which the jaws are osteotomized and repositioned in a way that increases facial symmetry and aesthetics, optimizes respiratory function, and provides a functional occlusion. Traditional presurgical preparation techniques for orthognathic surgery are time intensive and technically challenging, in fact more than many other types of CMF surgery. Virtual surgical planning has not changed this fact, but has largely shifted this preparation from the clinician to a service center in order to optimize efficiency [27, 40].

Traditional preparation for orthognathic surgery includes patient evaluation, cephalometric tracing, physical model surgery, and surgical splint generation. This is a meticulous process that can take anywhere from 1 to 5 h depending on the complexity of the case and experience level of the clinician. Virtual surgical planning, whether completed by the clinician or through a service center, has increased the efficiency and accuracy of this process dramatically [26, 28, 40]. The steps and inputs required for digital treatment planning of orthognathic surgery are outlined as follows.

Data Collection

As with traditional planning for orthognathic surgery, and more so than most other virtually planned procedures, the virtual surgical planning process for orthognathic surgery requires extensive data collection and compilation in order to fully and accurately treatment plan. Beyond just a CT or CBCT scan of the patient as a foundation for the planning, additional imagery of the patient's occlusal anatomy, 2D and/or 3D color imagery of the patient's facial features, and data records of the patient's natural head position are also collected at the time of the initial patient visit. It is important to consider when and how this data is collected in order to maximize the accuracy of the process. As many of these types of patients are active in the orthodontic process, it is important that these records are collected as close to the surgical procedure as is reasonable and in a similar timeframe as a whole. Any additional occlusal adjustment or movement between when the records for virtual surgical planning are taken and the time of surgery can affect the accuracy of the transfer of the plan to the surgical environment. For instance, if the patient's CBCT scan is acquired 3 weeks prior to surgery, the patient's occlusal impressions should be done within a few days of this if not at the same appointment in order to ensure the multiple datasets match each other. At

Fig. 2.28 Table illustrating different 3D printing processes and different material/use characteristics (Courtesy 3D Systems Healthcare, Rock Hill, SC, USA)

3D Printing Process	Visualization Models		Surgical Models	Surgical Guides	Implants
	Color	Monochromatic			
SLA	Yes	Yes	Yes	Yes	No
SLS	No	Yes	Yes	Yes	No – nylon Yes – materials like PEEK/PEKK
MJP	Yes	Yes	Yes	No	No
CJP	Yes	Yes	No	No	No
PJP	Yes	Yes	Yes, limited	No	No
DMP	No	No	No	No	Yes – titanium,

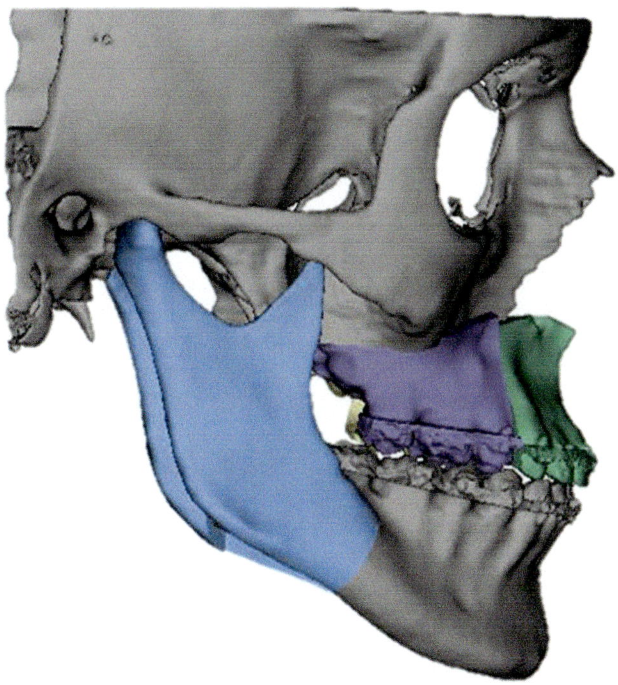

Fig. 2.29 Orthognathic surgical planning has been performed on this two jaw case; note setback of the mandible by BSSO and advancement of the maxilla using a multipiece LeFort I (Courtesy 3D Systems Healthcare, Rock Hill, SC, USA)

this point the collaborating clinicians should ensure that the patient will not have any further dental movement.

The dental artifact present in the medical imaging data from the patient scan creates the need for additional techniques to be performed to capture accurate dental anatomy. Most commonly an impression is taken of the patient's occlusal anatomy at the clinical evaluation, and physical stone models are poured and sent to a service center. These physical models are then digitized using laser surface imaging technology. While this analog to digital method is most common, it has its drawbacks such as the time and material needed to create the analog representation of the dental anatomy, but also the process of acquiring the impression is technique sensitive and can induce inaccuracies to the overall process. New technologies are becoming more readily available in which optical or laser surface imagery of the occlusal anatomy can be obtained directly without the need for analog production. Over time this method will likely replace more traditional methods as the need for digital and accurate patient records increases.

Another piece of important data to be considered during the data collection process is the idea termed NHP (natural head position or neutral head posture) [41, 42, 43]. This is the idea that we should virtually treat patients from a position that is natural rather than the position in which they were scanned during the CT or CBCT scanning process. There is much debate regarding what the exact definition of this position is, but ultimately it falls to the clinician's preference. Multiple techniques exist to record this position during the patient evaluation ranging from simple digital photos of the patient to the use of transducer technology to record the pitch, roll, and yaw of the head and to transposing horizontal and vertical planes onto the face using a series of self-leveling lasers and radiopaque fiducial devices. Similar to the definition of NHP itself, there is some debate regarding the optimal technique to record head position, which again falls mostly to surgeon's preference at this point in time.

Data Preparation

Once the above series of data is collected, it is then compiled and prepared for the virtual surgical treatment plan. As previously described, the CT or CBCT imaging data is segmented in order to extract the surface representation of the bony anatomy, the soft tissue or facial anatomy, the dental root anatomy, and the inferior alveolar nerve information. After the additional information of the occlusal surface anatomy is digitized, it is then overlaid against surface anatomy of the bone in order to create a composite model, joining accurate surfaces of the bone and the much higher-resolution occlusal anatomy from the occlusal scans [44]. The two-dimensional or three-dimensional color facial imagery is also overlaid on the facial surface anatomy from the CT or CBCT scan in order to provide additional detail and appreciation of the patient's features. Lastly the now digital patient's anatomy is oriented from the as scanned position to a position that better reflects the patient's daily natural head position.

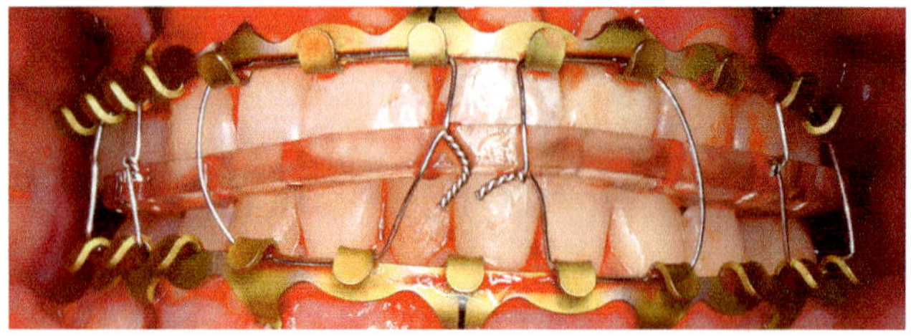

Fig. 2.30 Once virtual surgical planning has been completed, a splint is digitally designed and manufactured. Note that this represents the final surgical splint (Courtesy 3D Systems Healthcare, Rock Hill, SC, USA)

Treatment Planning

Once the digital patient has been created, the clinician is ready to treatment plan the simulated surgical procedure either on his/her own or with the assistance of a service center. The patient's anatomy, both bony and soft tissue, is evaluated using a series of cephalometric landmarks and measurements. Through digital osteotomies and repositioning the bony anatomy, these landmarks are transposed, and measurements are adjusted to achieve a target based on historically developed normal facial measurements that are established to optimize facial symmetry and aesthetics, while maintaining or increasing respiratory function and maximizing a functional occlusion. Soft tissue or facial simulated outcomes are also beneficial during the treatment planning phase.

Transfer of the Plan

Now that the optimal plan for the patient is established virtually, it must be transferred in some fashion to the operating environment. This is done with the combination CAD/CAM produced physical guides ranging from surgical occlusal splints (Fig. 2.30) to more complex bone-borne osteotomy and repositioning devices, along with a detailed case summary overviewing the plan determined during the online treatment planning session [36, 45]. This two-dimensional report outlines the movement of all bony anatomy quantitatively as well as qualitatively, indicating the steps of the surgical process as well as areas of concern that may come into play during the procedure such as bony interferences that would need to be reduced.

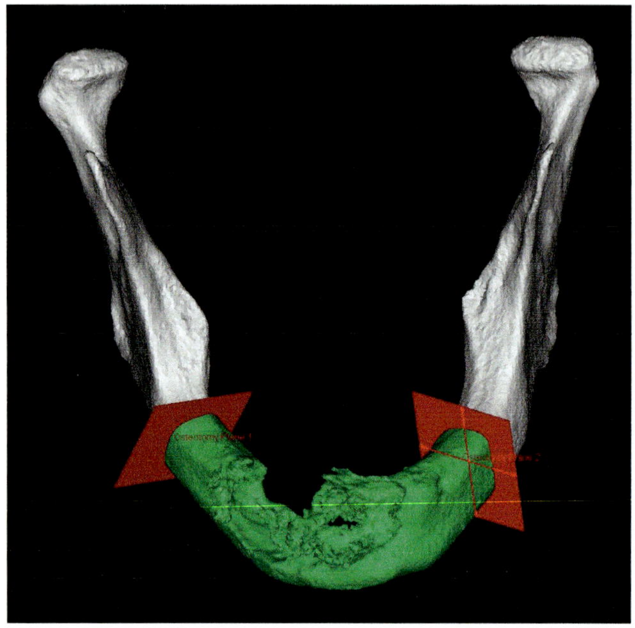

Fig. 2.31 Anterior mandible will be resected in this case and digital osteotomy lines (shown in *red*) align with the surgeon's planned osteotomies (Courtesy 3D Systems Healthcare, Rock Hill, SC, USA)

Fibula Free Flap Reconstruction

Generally speaking, CMF reconstruction with free tissue transfer requires a multidisciplinary and team approach in the operating room. Commonly there is a team of surgeons working on the resection, while another team prepares the fibula free flap for transfer. It is not uncommon for surgical teams to include any combination of oral and maxillofacial, plastic and reconstructive, ENT, and prosthodontic specialists. The planning session allows for all of these surgeons to be present and ensure that all important clinical details are considered. Other stakeholders (e.g., rigid fixation vendor and/or dental lab if appropriate) can also join the planning session, to advise on the appropriate application of their products for a given case [15, 46].

The surgical planning webmeeting begins with evaluation of patient anatomy, history, and diagnosis. The first important goal is to accurately define the anticipated surgical defect (Fig. 2.31). Plans for resection can be simulated, reviewed, and confirmed against the axial/coronal/sagittal CT slices as well as the 3D model. If the patient presents with existing defects and/or malpositioning of anatomy, the position of any mobile bone fragments can be corrected to achieve more ideal anatomical contour.

Once the resection defect is defined, focus shifts to design of the bony free flap that will be used for reconstruction (Fig. 2.32). Often, the patient's preoperative anatomy will

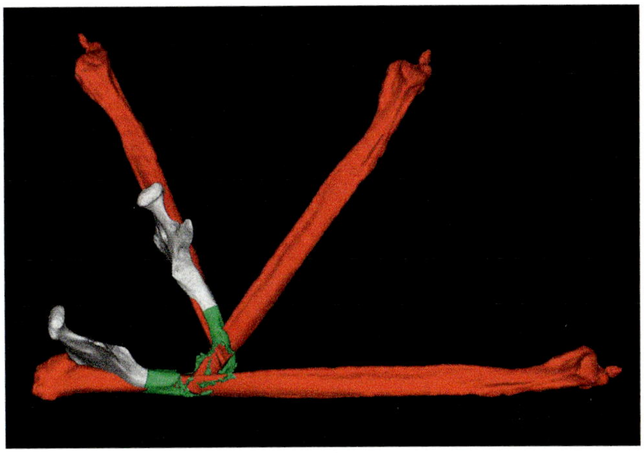

Fig. 2.32 Importing autogenous tissue, in this case a free flap from the fibula, aids in creating an accurate depiction of the surgery to be performed. In this example, precise osteotomies between host and graft can be optimized for a better fit (Courtesy 3D Systems Healthcare, Rock Hill, SC, USA)

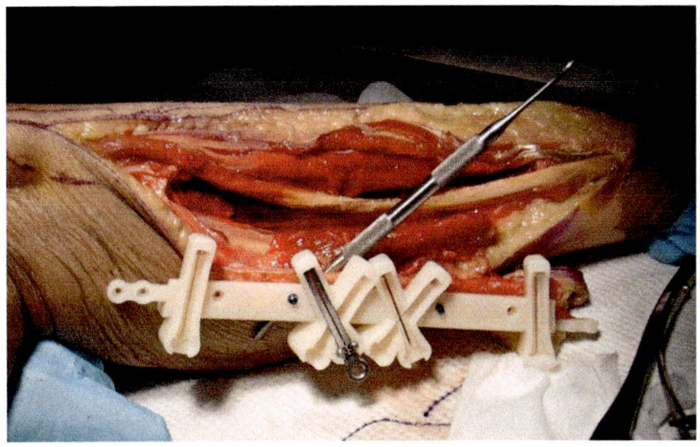

Fig. 2.33 The clinical transfer for a fibula free flap reconstruction case involves a bony "miter box" which allows for creation of closing wedge osteotomies in the fibula (Courtesy 3D Systems Healthcare, Rock Hill, SC, USA)

serve as a good reference for the size and shape of the reconstruction. However, some pathologies tend to expand or distort native anatomy. A history of previous resection or traumatic injury can also reduce the suitability of native anatomy to serve as a good reference. In these situations, unaffected anatomy can be mirrored from the contralateral side, or normative datasets can be imported for comparison [28]. It is important to know which fibula will be used as a donor site, as well as which blood vessels in the recipient site will be used for anastomosis. As a rule, cutting guides that will be produced for clinical transfer of the virtual surgical plan to the operating room will work only for a single, specific plan. Clearly, it is critical to consider all clinical implications of a particular flap design. Measurements can be made during planning to ensure that minimum size is maintained for each segment of fibula, and bony contact can be optimized by adjusting the geometry of planned cuts [16].

Planning can also include the primary placement of immediate osseointegrated dental implants into the fibula reconstruction. It is also possible to design a CAD/CAM immediate provisional dental prosthesis. This cutting-edge "jaw-in-a-day" technique allows for a patient to undergo resection, reconstruction, and dental rehabilitation in a single surgical stage – a process that traditionally takes multiple operations over the course of several months [23]. This added level of complexity requires specialized, advanced guides to be designed and a very close collaboration between the surgeons, the surgical planning service center, the rigid fixation vendor, and the dental lab that will produce the prosthesis. It has been shown that the use of VSP can reduce operative time, while increasing case complexity and improving rates of dental rehabilitation [13].

After the surgical plan is finalized, closing discussion will surround guide designs. Surgical access, special clinical requirements (if applicable), manufacturing requirements, and surgeon preference should all be considered to optimize guide design [28]. Custom, patient-specific hardware can be made to match the surgical plan, or a bending template can be provided for use in pre-bending a stock reconstruction plate.

Physical models, guides, and templates are 3D printed to transfer the digital plan into the operating room. Bone-borne cutting guides are produced to guide the resection cuts, and a fibula cutting guide is made, which acts as a plan-specific "miter box" for use on the fibula bone (Fig. 2.33). Fibula guides can also incorporate special features to guide the placement of endosseous dental implants in preplanned locations. These patient-specific guides and templates are manufactured via stereolithography, using sterilizable and biocompatible resins. Cutting slots in the plastic guides are specially designed to integrate with stainless steel slot inserts. By acting as an intermediate between the saw blade and the plastic guide, these metal inserts act to reduce or eliminate the scatter of plastic dust into an open surgical site. They also help to more tightly control the path of the saw blade during use.

It has been shown that operative and ischemic times can be shortened with the use of VSP and that overall case complexity is generally increased. A recent study performed at NYU also showed that patients whose fibula free flap reconstructions were planned using VSP have ultimately received full dental rehabilitation at unprecedented rates [13].

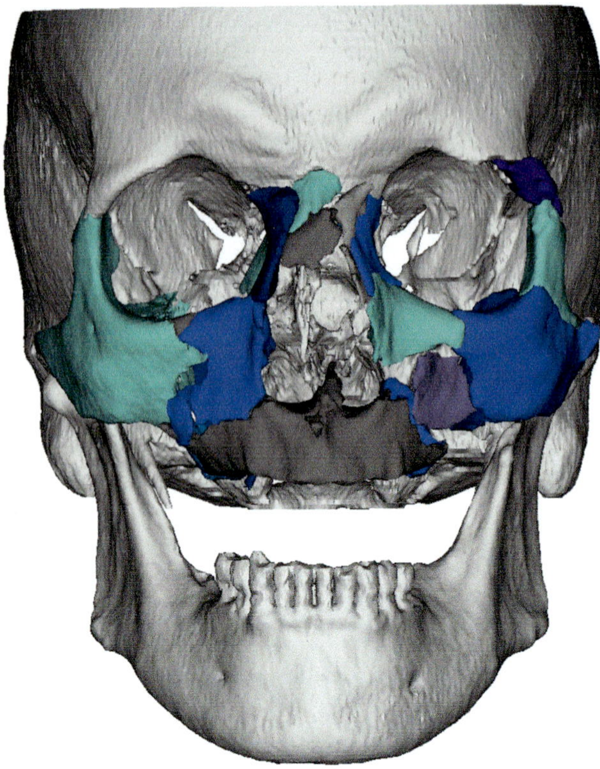

Fig. 2.34 For post-traumatic reconstruction, multiple bony fragments can be reduced into a more anatomical position before guiding this reduction using 3D printed templates (Courtesy 3D Systems Healthcare, Rock Hill, SC, USA)

Trauma

VSP can be used to assist with either primary or secondary facial trauma reconstruction. For primary management of traumatic injuries, data processing of a patient's CT can take additional time. This time is spent segmenting individual bony segments in what are often complex, comminuted facial fractures. During planning, these individual segments are repositioned to achieve fracture reduction and reconstruct pre-injury contour (Fig. 2.34). Once again, mirrored or normative anatomy can serve as an excellent reference during planning.

Anatomical models of the simulated postoperative anatomy can be produced and used for pre-contouring plates for use at the time of surgery. Existing bony defects (common for blowout fractures of the orbital floor) can also be patched with perfected anatomy for use in pre-bending implants. For defects where bone grafting is anticipated, templates of these perfected regions can be produced to help with harvesting and shaping bone grafts intraoperatively. Additionally, positioning guides can be designed to temporarily hold bony fragments in their reduced position while plates are applied [35].

Stereotactic navigation can be a helpful tool to give real-time intraoperative feedback and confirmation of bony positioning, akin to an intraoperative "GPS." To facilitate this, the new positions of reduced bony fragments can be back-converted into modified DICOM images. This dataset can then be loaded into the navigation system and registered to patient anatomy. It has been shown that the use of VSP and intraoperative navigation aids in predictably reestablishing normal orbital volume and malar projection, leading to a more favorable position of the globe and facial symmetry [21].

Distraction Osteogenesis

As with orthognathic surgery, distraction osteogenesis is performed in order to achieve facial symmetry and aesthetics, increase respiratory function, and maximize occlusal function depending on the specific needs of the patient. However, unlike orthognathic surgery, the bony anatomy does not undergo osteotomies and repositioning, but rather cut and slowly guided into the correct position using a series of distractor devices. This process of slowly guiding the bone to the optimal position allows for continuous bony growth.

One of the more challenging aspects of this type of procedure is to determine the placement of the distractor device in order to apply the correct vector of bony growth. Utilizing VSP allows the clinician to import the exact device they plan on using overlaid on the patient's unique anatomy. At this point the vector of distraction can be planned in order to optimize the final bony position with the device orientated appropriately. While this visualization is important, the process is not complete until that position is transferred effectively to the operating room environment. Using CAD/CAM produced patient-specific surgical tools that reference not only the patient's unique bony anatomy, the osteotomy site, and drill hole locations but also the footprint of the specific distractor device (Fig. 2.35), the clinician can replicate intraoperatively the exact position that the distractor device was orientated virtually [18, 47].

TMJ Reconstruction

Treatment of temporomandibular joint disorders utilizing total joint replacement is a complex procedure for a variety of reasons. Oftentimes the anatomy is altered from its normal and can be difficult to visualize and anticipate surgically. Also the procedure has limited visible access and is in close proximity to several key anatomical structures including the middle cranial fossa, middle ear, multiple facial nerve branches, and the internal carotid artery. Visualization of these landmarks prior to the surgical procedure using patient-

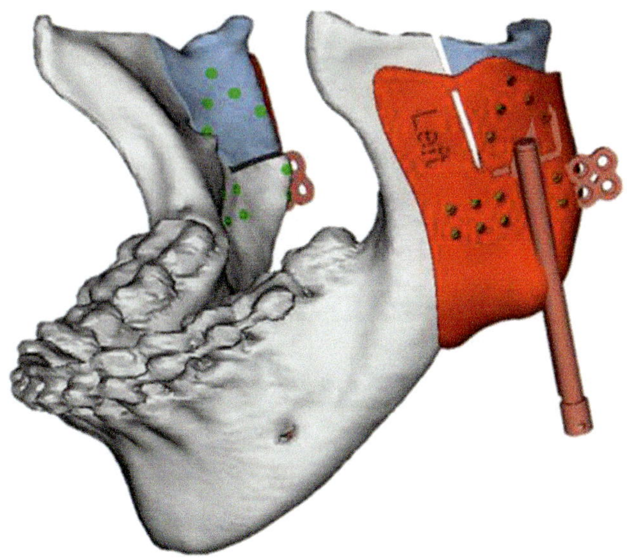

Fig. 2.35 Surgical guides for distraction osteogenesis often contain both information on an osteotomy (shown as a vertical line on this particular guide) as well as screw hole placement for positioning guidance of the distractor (Courtesy 3D Systems Healthcare, Rock Hill, SC, USA)

specific imagery may improve surgical outcomes as well as safety during the procedure [48, 49]. In addition to the complexities associated with the surgical procedure itself, it can be challenging to select the appropriately sized stock prosthesis or create a patient-specific designed custom prosthesis. The use of virtual surgical planning can assist not only with visualization, but also with the selection or development of a total joint replacement, both in off-the-shelf and personalized form [48, 49].

Stock Alloplastic TMJ System

When a stock alloplastic TMJ system is used for total joint reconstruction, it may be difficult to appropriately select and position the correct prosthesis for a given patient. Traditionally the clinician has a series of tools that he would use to measure or gauge the appropriate-sized joint intraoperatively. With the use of VSP, the appropriately sized joint can be preselected and overlaid against the patient's anatomy. With the joint in place, any needed bony resections can also be planned to remove ankylosis and any interferences with the prosthesis components. After the appropriate joint is selected and placed, patient-specific surgical tools can be developed using CAD/CAM technology that will guide necessary resections as well as the placement of the prosthesis in order to mimic the virtual surgical plan [48].

Patient-Specific TMJ Replacement Solution

Utilizing patient-specific imaging data to create a fully custom joint reconstruction is a process that has evolved dramatically over the last several years. There are a few commonly used solutions for this process that range from a fully digital CAD/CAM prosthesis to a combination of digital and analog methods to generate a custom fitting prosthesis. These common methods can be utilized in conjunction with virtual surgical planning to guide not only the design of the prosthesis but also any bony resections and the placement of the joint reconstruction itself [3, 49].

Custom Implants

VSP technology can also be leveraged to produce patient-specific implants. Simulated postoperative anatomy can be used in the CAD/CAM production of varying types of implants, ranging from titanium reconstruction plates and meshes to custom silicone implants for aesthetic applications and everything between.

Customized reconstruction plates can be produced with CAD/CAM to match a virtual surgical plan. In this application, resection guides can also incorporate predictive hole placement which corresponds to screw hole locations in the final plate design, with bone depth maps provided to aid in screw length selection intraoperatively. Custom crib meshes can be designed to follow idealized anatomical contours, which can be packed with bone graft and/or other biological materials at the time of surgery.

Full thickness calvarial implants can be produced for either primary or staged reconstruction following ablative or post-traumatic craniotomies [50]. If a single-stage resection and reconstruction is needed, guides can be produced to help create a defect that should fit ideally with the customized implant. Onlay implants can also be produced in PEEK, PMMA, and porous polyethylene materials for various applications, all designed using CT-based planning.

Patients seeking aesthetic CMF augmentation also find a solution with virtual surgical planning. Custom implants can be designed digitally according to surgeon and/or patient specifications (Fig. 2.36). Templates of these implants can then be produced with 3D printers and used to create master patterns for traditional mold-based production of a customized silicone onlay.

Other Applications

Craniosynostosis

Craniosynostosis is a congenital disorder whereby one or more sutures in an infant's skull fuse prematurely. This can lead to an abnormal head shape and occasionally to increased intracranial pressure and/or neurodevelopmental impairment [27]. One technique for correcting this disorder involves cutting and reshaping the bones of the calvarium to achieve a more normal head shape. This surgical correction commonly takes place between 6 and 12 months of age.

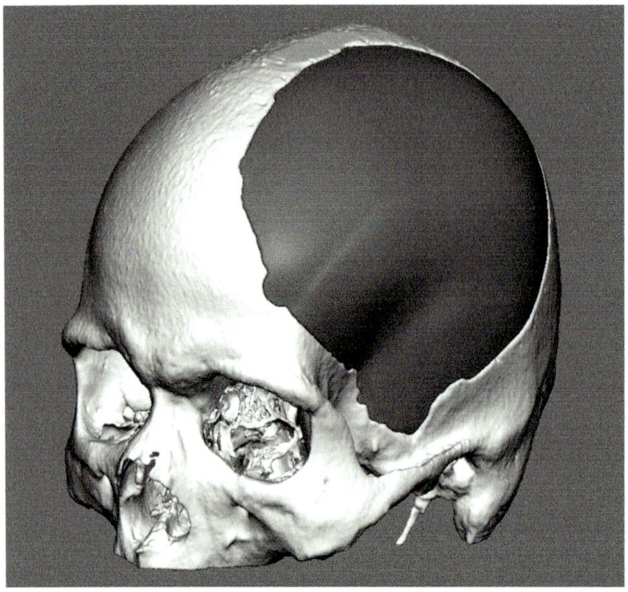

Fig. 2.36 Personalized implants like this cranioplasty plate can be designed using the patient's data as input (Courtesy 3D Systems Healthcare, Rock Hill, SC, USA)

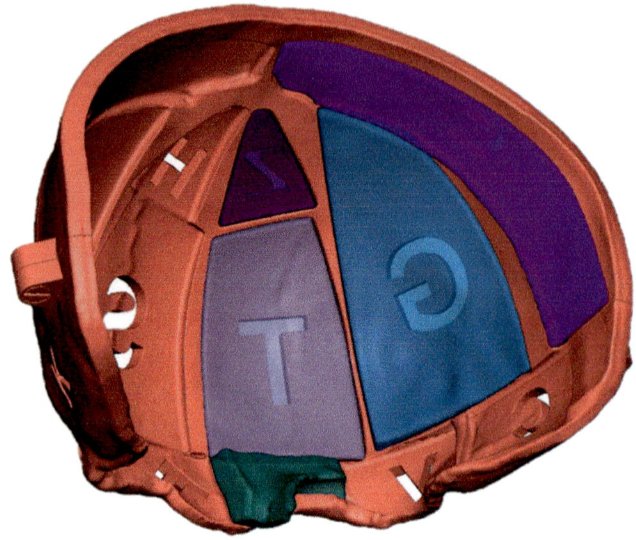

Fig. 2.37 For cranial reconstruction, one might use a series of templates both to section the bony segments and later to position them in a new array. This guide is the second positioning guide for a cranial vault reconstruction (Courtesy 3D Systems Healthcare, Rock Hill, SC, USA)

In using VSP for craniosynostosis correction, a recent craniomaxillofacial CT scan is required. Due to the rapid pace of growth during infancy, large changes in size and shape can occur in relatively little time. This prohibits a large delay between scan acquisition and surgical correction using CT-based guides. Age-matched normative datasets have been developed for patients from 8 to 12 months of age [51], which prove to be a powerful reference tool during virtual surgical planning [47].

Collaboration and cooperation between neurosurgical and craniofacial specialists is a must for these complex reconstructions. Once again, all parties can be present during the initial planning meeting in order to ensure that the surgical plan is acceptable for all involved. Planned osteotomy sites can be verified against planar CT slices to confirm safe distances from underlying intracranial anatomy such as the sagittal and transverse dural venous sinuses [47].

For clinical transfer, a series of marking and positioning guides are used (Figs. 2.16 and 2.37). After exposure of the calvarium, bone-borne marking guides are placed and used to mark out all of the planned osteotomies along with orientation characters. The neurosurgical team will generally perform the osteotomies which define the outer borders of the overall craniotomy, removing the affected calvarium as intact as possible. This pre-marked subtotal calvarium is then cut and reshaped on a back table, following the pre-marked cutting paths. Commonly, bone flaps are moved, rotated, and reoriented in a complex way in order to achieve the final desired shape. To help facilitate these movements, the previously marked registration characters are used in conjunction with matching features in a set of positioning guides. These guides reinforce appropriate positioning of these bony flaps prior to fixation. One common technique involves inserting all bony flaps into a bowl-shaped set of positioning guides before plating on the deep/intracranial surface of the reshaped segments. The guides can then be removed leaving a neocalvarium that can be replaced and fixated onto the skull base to cover the cranial defect. Fixation is generally performed using resorbable plating systems in these young children [27, 33, 47].

Facial Allotransplantation

Facial allotransplantation (i.e., face transplant) is one of the most difficult and advanced microsurgical operations that exist. Only considered in extreme cases, the risks are tremendous. Many times the patients who are candidates for a face transplant operation have both soft and hard tissue defects, particularly if their disfigurement is due to traumatic injury. One of the many important factors for these long and arduous operations is making sure that the donor anatomy is shaped to fit directly with a properly prepared recipient site. VSP has a clear application to transplantation cases where a bony component is required [52].

It is, of course, likely that there will be ample time to get a high-quality CT scan of the recipient to use with VSP. It usually takes many months of preparation and regulatory and ethics approvals before a patient can officially be listed on the transplant list and await a suitable donor. This window allows for guides to be designed and manufactured for use in establishing a planned bony defect at the time of surgery. These guides can be on standby and ready to sterilize and take to surgery within a moment's notice.

Guides can also be created to help harvest donor bone with the appropriate size and shape to fit into the recipient's surgically created defect(s) (Figs. 1.44–1.50). Bone-borne guides, of course, would require a donor CT scan, which can be its own challenge under the time constraints that generally surround organ donors. These recipient guides would require expediting the data processing, guide design, manufacturing, and shipping operations as much as possible [53].

Microtia Reconstruction

Patients suffering from microtia (underdeveloped or missing ear structures) or traumatic ear injuries can also be helped using VSP. A popular technique for creating an ear for these patients involves carving a series of structures out of autogenous rib cartilage and then stacking these segments together and covering them with a soft tissue flap. This method avoids the increased infection risk associated with implanting prosthetic ears but is a more technically challenging surgery to perform.

If a patient has a full ear on the unaffected side, this ear can be measured or captured with imaging such as a CT or MRI scan or optical or laser surface capture. Custom guides and templates can then be created at the appropriate dimensions to help the surgeon to size and shape the cartilage intraoperatively to achieve the ideal result (Figs. 2.38 and 2.39). A guide is also created which helps to hold the separate cartilage structures stacked together in the correct shape. This guide is designed with relief features to allow the surgeon to suture and/or wire the structures together permanently, all while they are being supported and held in the appropriate configuration. The completed complex can then be implanted.

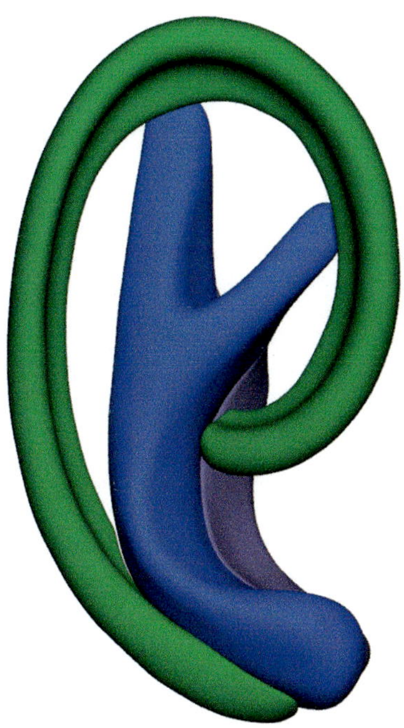

Fig. 2.38 Templates can serve as guides for harvesting of autogenous tissue, here for costochondral rib cartilage for auricular reconstruction (Courtesy 3D Systems Healthcare, Rock Hill, SC, USA)

Postoperative Analysis

Postoperative CT/CBCT scans are often acquired for patients who received CMF surgery. If a preoperative imaging data also exists, a comparison can be drawn between the two datasets. This can be particularly interesting if preoperative VSP was performed, so that the actual surgical results can be compared with the virtual surgical plan. Analysis of volume, shape, and cephalometric or anatomical landmark measurements can be performed (Fig. 2.40). There are several published studies that have evaluated postoperative results compared to virtual surgical plans for orthognathic surgery and fibula free flap reconstruction. These can be helpful tools for evaluating accuracy of VSP, and all have shown promising results [13, 14, 20, 54].

Summary

Digital technologies have indeed made a major impact on patient treatment in the area of craniomaxillofacial reconstruction. Looking back over the last 15 years at the progression is interesting, starting with (1) anatomical modeling, leading to (2) personalization of implants and finally onto (3) personalization and guidance of surgical procedures. This progression from simple surgeries to more complex surgeries continues to push forward, with digital technologies now poised to break ground in surgeries ranging from full-face transplants to concomitant mandibular prosthetic reconstructions following tumor reconstruction [55–57].

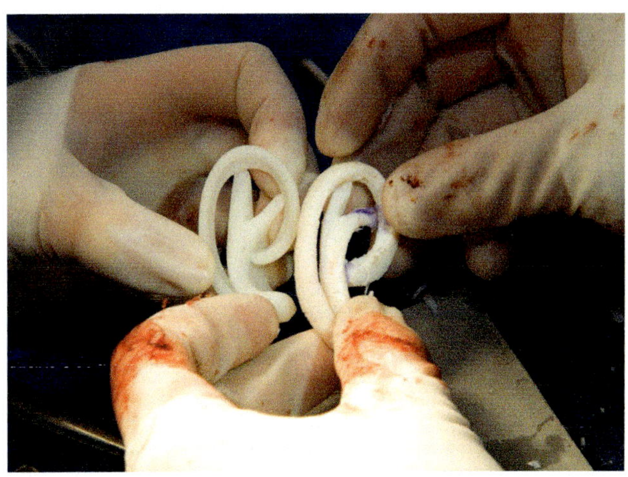

Fig. 2.39 During surgery the template is compared to the harvested graft (Courtesy 3D Systems Healthcare, Rock Hill, SC, USA)

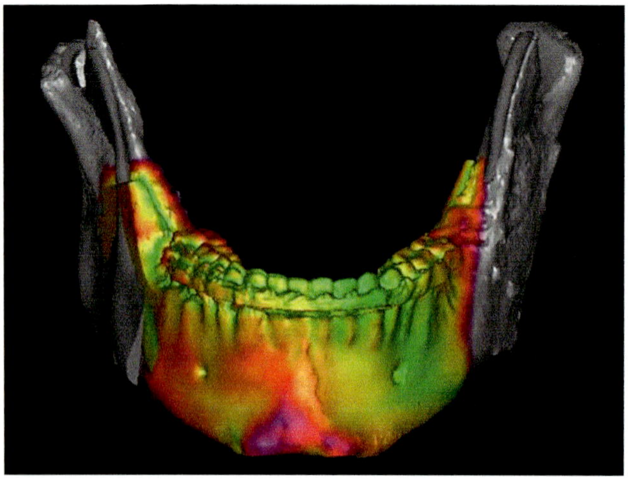

Fig. 2.40 Color-mapping overlays such as this can be used to qualitatively compare two objects. The color scale would represent relative differences between the two objects; in this case a preoperative plan is compared with actual postsurgical outcome (Courtesy 3D Systems Healthcare, Rock Hill, SC, USA)

Software technology has enabled some of the advancements, but the biggest key has been the creation of individual digital threads. These optimized workflows for guiding different surgical techniques are enabling surgical efficiency and, more importantly, optimizing patient care. Because a digital surgical plan exists, there is for the first time an objective measure for surgical outcomes. This measure can not only help with training of the next generation but also establishes a baseline for comparison between surgeons, centers, and geographic locations. The concept of highly realistic surgical simulation combined with more and more precise guidance in surgery are continuing to push the limits of CMF surgery. New applications for digital planning and the use of 3D printing tools will come about based on advancements in 3D printing processes, materials, and design techniques. In the future one can imagine that most major reconstructive surgical procedures will be powered by personalization and integrated digital technologies.

References

1. Mankovich N, Cheeseman A, Soker N. The display of three-dimensional anatomy with stereolithographic models. J Digit Imaging. 1990;3:200.
2. Stoker N, Mankovich N, Valentino D. Stereolithographic models for surgical planning. J Oral Maxillofac Surg. 1992;50:466.
3. Erickson D, Chance D, Schmitt S, et al. An opinion survey of reported benefits from the use of stereolithographic models. J Oral and Maxillofac Surg. 1999;57:1040.
4. Eppley B. Craniofacial reconstruction with computer-generated HTR patient-matched implants: use in primary bony tumor excision. J Craniofac Surg. 2002;13(5):650–7.
5. Wolford L. Temporomandibular joint reconstruction of the complex patient with Techmedica custom-made total joint prosthesis. J Oral Maxillofac Surg. 1994;52(1):2–10.
6. Binder W, Kaye A. Reconstruction of posttraumatic congenital facial deformities with three-dimensional computer-assisted custom-designed implants. Plast Reconstr Surg. 1994;94:775.
7. Eley K, McIntyre A, Watt-Smith S, Golding S. "black bone" MRI: a partial flip angle technique for radiation reduction in craniofacial imaging. Br J Radiol. 2012;1011:272–8.
8. Eley K, McIntyre A, Watt-Smith S, Golding S. "black bone" MRI: a partial flip angle technique for radiation reduction in craniofacial imaging. Br J Radiol. 2012;1013:659.
9. Miracle A, Mukherj S. Conebeam CT of the head and neck, part 1: physical principles. Am J Neuroradiol. 2009;30(6):1088–95.
10. Schulze R, Heil U, Gross D, Bruellmann D, Dranischnikow E, Schwanecke U, Schoemer E. Artefacts in CBCT: a review. Dentomaxillofac Radiol. 2011;40(5):265–73.
11. Sharma N, Aggarwal L. Automated medical image segmentation techniques. J Med Phys. 2010;35(1):3–14.
12. Bryan F, Xu Z, Asman A, Allen W, Reich D, Landman B. Self-assessed performance improves statistical fusion of image labels. J Med Phys. 2014;41(3):031903.
13. Avraham T, Franco P, Brecht L, Ceradini D, Saadeh P, Hirsch D, Levine J. Functional outcomes of virtually planned free fibula flap reconstruction of the mandible. Plastic Reconstruct Surg. 2014;134:628e.
14. Xia J, Sheychenko L, Gateno J, Teichgraeber J, Taylor T, Lasky R, English J, Kau C, Mcgrory K. Outcome of computer–aided surgical simulation in the treatment of patients with craniomaxillofacial deformities. J Oral Maxillofac Surg. 2011;69(7):2014–24.
15. Markiewicz M, Bell R. The use of 3D imaging tools in facial plastic surgery. Facial Plast Surg Clin North Am. 2011;19:655–82.
16. Roser S, Ramachandra S, Blair H, Grist W, Carlson G, Christensen A, Weimer K, Steed M. The accuracy of virtual surgical planning in free fibula mandibular reconstruction: comparison of planned and final results. J Oral Maxillofac Surg. 2010;68:2824–32.
17. Antony A, Chen W, Kolokythas A, Weimer K, Cohen M. Use of virtual surgery and stereolithography-guided osteotomy for mandibular reconstruction with the free fibula. Plast Reconstr Surg. 2011;128(5):1080–4.
18. Haddock N, Monaco C, Weimer K, Hirsch D, Levine J, Saddeh P. Increasing bony contact and overlap with computer-designed offset cuts in free fibula mandible reconstruction. J Craniofac Surg. 2012;23:1592–5.
19. Broe P, Tanna N, Franco P, Thanik V, Levine S, Garfein E, Saadeh P, Ceradini D, Hirsch D, Levine J. Ten-year evolution utilizing computer-assisted reconstruction for giant ameloblastoma. J Reconstr Microsurg. 2013;29:173–80.
20. Doscher M, Garfein E, Bent J, Tepper O. Neonatal mandibular distraction osteogenesis: converting virtual surgical planning into an operative reality. Int J Pediatr Otorhinolaryngol. 2014;78:381–4.
21. Saad A, Winters R, Wise M, Dupin C, Hilaire HS. Virtual surgical planning in complex composite maxillofacial reconstruction. Plast Reconstr Surg. 2013;132(3):626–33.
22. Foley B, Thayer Q, Honeybrook A, McKenna S, Press S. Mandibular reconstruction using computer-aided design and computer-aided manufacturing: an analysis of surgical results. J Oral Maxillofac Surg. 2013;71:e111–9.
23. Markiewicz M, Bell R. Modern concepts in computer-assisted craniomaxillofacial reconstruction. Curr Opin Otolaryngol Head Neck Surgery. 2011;19:295–301.
24. Patel A, Levine J, Brecht L, Saadeh P, Hirsch D. Digital technologies in mandibular pathology and reconstruction. Atlas Oral Maxillofac Surg Clin North Am. 2012;131:95–106.

25. Levine J, Soo Bae J, Soares M, Brecht L, Saadeh P, Cerandini D, Hirsch D. Jaw in a day: total maxillofacial reconstruction using digital technology. Plast Reconstr Surg. 2013;131:1383.
26. Gelesko S, Markiewicz M, Weimer K, Bell R. Computer-aided orthognathic surgery. Atlas Oral Maxillofac Surg Clin North Am. 2012;20:107–18.
27. Mardini S, Alsubaie S, Cayci C, Chim H, Wetjen N. Three-dimensional preoperative virtual planning and template use for surgical correction of craniosynostosis. J Plas Reconst Asthetic Surg. 2014;67(3):336–43.
28. Hsu S, Gateno J, Bell R, Hirsch D, Markiewicz M, Teichgraeber J, Xia J. Accuracy of a computer-aided surgical simulation protocol for orthognathic surgery: a prospective multicenter study. J Oral Maxillofac Surg. 2013;71:128–42.
29. Xia J, Phillips C, Gateno J, Teichgraeber J, Christensen A, Gliddon M, Lemoine J, Liebschner M. Cost-effectiveness analysis for computer-aided surgical simulation in complex cranio-maxillofacial surgery. J Oral Maxillofac Surg. 2006;64(12):1780–4.
30. Matros E, Albornoz C, Rensberger M, Weimer K, Garfein E. Computer-assisted design and computer-assisted modeling technique optimization and advantages over traditional methods of osseous flap reconstruction. J Reconstr Microsurg. 2013;29(3):173–80.
31. DeLong B, Weimer K, Press S. Development of an anthropometric skull for use in severe maxillofacial trauma reconstruction. In: AAOMS 94th Annual Meeting, San Diego, CA; 2012.
32. Lewallen J, Frederick J, Press S. Modifications of a halo-supported external fixator as an adjunct to complex maxillofacial trauma: a report of 10 cases. J Maxillofac Trauma. 2012;1:2–12.
33. Saber N, Phillips J, Looi T, Usmani Z, Burge J, Drake J, Kim P. Generation of normative pediatric skull models for use in cranial vault remodeling procedures. Childs Nerv Syst. 2012;28:405–10.
34. Burge J, Saber N, Looi T, French B, Usmani Z, Anooshiravani N, Kim P, Forrest C, Phillips J. Application of CAD/CAM prefabricated age-matched templates in cranio-orbital remodeling in craniosynostosis. J Craniofac Surg. 2011;22:1810–3.
35. Hirsch D, Garfein E, Christensen A, Weimer K, Saadeh P, Levine J. Use of computer-aided design and computer-aided manufacturing to produce orthognathically ideal surgical outcomes: a paradigm shift in head and neck reconstruction. J Oral Maxillofac Surg. 2009;67:2115–22.
36. Xia J, Gateno J, Teichgraeber J. A new paradigm for complex midface reconstruction: a reversed approach. J Oral Maxillofac Surg. 2009;67:693–703.
37. Tepper O, Sorice S, Hershman G, Saadeh P, Levine J, Hirsch D. Use of virtual 3-dimensional surgery in post-traumatic craniomaxillofacial reconstruction. J Oral Maxillofac Surg. 2011;69:733–41.
38. Polley J, Figueroa A. Orthognathic positioning system: intraoperative system to transfer virtual surgical plan to operating field during orthognathic surgery. J Oral Maxillofac Surg. 2013;71:911–20.
39. Murphy S, Atala A. 3D bioprinting of tissues and organs. Nat Biotechnol. 2014;32(8):773–85.
40. McCormick S, Drew S. Virtual model surgery for efficient planning and surgical performance. J Oral Maxillofac Surg. 2011;69:638–44.
41. Xia J, Gateno J, Teichgraeber J, Christensen A, Lasky R, Lemoine J, Liebschner M. Accuracy of a computer-aided surgical simulation (CASS) system in the treatment of complex craniomaxillofacial deformities: a pilot study. J Oral Maxillofac Surg. 2007;65(2):248–54.
42. Xia J, McGrory J, Gateno J. A new method to orient 3-dimensional computed tomography models to the natural head position: a clinical feasibility study. J Oral Maxillofac Surg. 2011;69(3):584–91.
43. Schatz E, Xia J, Gateno J. Development of a technique for recording and transferring natural head position in 3 dimensions. J Craniofac Surg. 2010;21(5):1452–5.
44. Gateno J, Xia J, Teichgraeber J, Rosen A. A new technique for the creation of a computerized composite skull model. J Oral Maxillofac Surg. 2003;61:222–7.
45. Xia J, Gateno J, Teichgraeber J. A new clinical protocol to evaluate cranio-maxillofacial deformity and to plan surgical correction. J Oral Maxillofac Surg. 2009;67(10):2093.
46. Sharaf B, Levine J, Hirsch D, Bastidas J, Schiff B, Garfein E. Importance of computer-aided design and manufacturing technology in the multidisciplinary approach to head and neck reconstruction. J Craniofac Surg. 2010;21(4):1277–80.
47. Chim H, Wetjen N, Mardini S. Virtual surgical planning in craniofacial surgery. Semin Plast Surg. 2014;28:150–8.
48. Chandran R, Keeler G, Christensen A, Weimer K, Caloss R. Application of virtual surgical planning for total joint reconstruction with a stock alloplast system. J Oral Maxillofac Surg. 2011;69:286–94.
49. Haq J, Patel N, Weimer K, Matthews S. Single stage treatment of ankylosis of the temporomandibular joint using patient-specific total joint replacement and virtual surgical planning. Br J Oral Maxillofac Surg. 2014;52:350–5.
50. Roberson D, Rosenberg W. Traumatic cranial defects reconstructed with the HTR-PMI cranioplatic implant. J Craniomaxillofac Trauma. 1997;3:8.
51. Seruya M, Borsuk D, Khalifian S, Carson B, Dalesio N, Dorafshar A. Computer-aided design and manufacturing in craniosynostosis surgery. J Craniofac Surg. 2013;24:1100–5.
52. Dorafshar A, Brazo P, Mundinger G, Mohan R, Brown E, Rodriguez E. Found in space: computer-assisted orthognathic alignment of a total face allograft in six degrees of freedom. J Oral Maxillofac Surg. 2014;72(9):1788–800.
53. Chim H, Amer H, Mardini S, Moran S. Vascularized composite allotransplantation in the realm of regenerative plastic surgery. Mayo Clin Proc. 2014;89(7):1009–20.
54. Hanasono M, Skoracki R. Computer-assisted design and rapid prototype modeling in microvascular mandible reconstruction. Laryngoscope. 2013;123:597–604.
55. Brown E, Dorafshar A, Bojovic B, et al. Total face, double jaw, and tongue transplant simulation: a cadaveric study using computer-assisted techniques. Plastic and Reconstructive Surgery. 2012;130(4):815–23.
56. Jacobs J, Dec W, Levine J, McCarthy J, Weimer KMK, Ceradini D. Best face forward: virtual modeling and custom device fabrication to optimize craniofacial vascularized composite allotransplantation. Plast Reconstr Surg. 2013;131:64.
57. Bell R. Computer planning and intraoperative navigation in craniomaxillary surgery. Atlas Oral Maxillofac Surg Clin North Am. 2010;22:135–56.
58. Hull C. Apparatus for production of three-dimensional objects by stereolithography. 3D Systems Corporation, assignee, Patent US4575330. 11 Mar 1986. Print.

Cone Beam CT

3

Samuel J. Zeichner

Introduction

In parallel with advances in digital imaging, cone beam CT (CBCT), also known as digital volumetric tomography (DVT), first emerged for investigational purposes in 1982 as an adaption of conventional fan-beam CT [1]. The original intent was as an alternative modality for angiography. Marketable scanners did not arrive until more than a decade later. That is, practical versions had to wait for advancements in flat-panel display (FPD) technologies, improved computer power, and the implementation of x-ray tubes with low-power requirements. CBCT, characterized by a conical x-ray beam and the use of 3-D reconstruction algorithms, seemed well suited for specific head and neck imaging tasks requiring high isotropic dimensions (uniform in x, y, and z planes), high spatial resolution, and low patient radiation dose. Thus, CBCT found its niche in craniomaxillofacial imaging including otorhinolaryngology and dentistry.

This chapter is not intended to be a technical compendium of the principles of cone beam CT, but rather the text describes the technology at the level of relevance for clinicians. Upon completion of this chapter, the reader will be able to:

1. Explain the concept of tomographic imaging.
2. Compare and contrast conventional multidetector CT with CBCT technologies.
3. Describe the acquisition of data in CBCT systems.
4. Understand basic image-processing methods used in CBCT.
5. List the capacities and limitations of CBCT, and understand the underlying principles as they relate to the clinical limitations.
6. Appreciate the clinical indications as well as the contraindications for the use of CBCT.

S.J. Zeichner (✉)
Division of Oral and Maxillofacial Radiology, Columbia University College of Dental Medicine,
New York, NY, USA

University of Basel Faculty of Medicine, Department of Clinical Morphology, Biomedical Engineering/Hightech Research Center, Gewerbestrasse 14–16, 4123 Allschwil, Switzerland
e-mail: sjz2110@cumc.columbia.edu; samzeichner@gmail.com

Overview of the Fundamental Principles of CT and CBCT

Tomography (from the Greek tomos—slice) is a radiographic technique wherein a given layer or plane of tissue within a body part is displayed without superimposition of adjacent structures. Thus, a tomogram represents a slice or sectional image of the body. In fact, an entire field of radiology known as sectional imaging encompasses a variety of tomographic modalities. Among these modalities are computed tomography and, its derivative, cone beam computed tomography.

Computed tomography has been available for more than four decades. CT is discussed here because it shares much technology with its later evolutionary offshoot, CBCT. Computed tomography, as introduced by its originator, Sir Godfrey Hounsfield in 1967, initially was termed computerized axial tomography or "CAT scanning." The name aptly described the process. That is, a well-collimated pencil-shaped x-ray beam translated and then rotated around a supine patient. The beam traversed the patient toward a detector located opposite the source of the x-ray photons. The photon beam was differentially attenuated within the patient. Then, the detector measured the intensity of photons striking it. Subsequently, an image could be reconstructed in the axial plane via computer algorithms—hence the term computerized *axial* tomography. By moving the patient mechanically along his/her long axis, a second rotation of the x-ray beam would produce another axial image. Continuing in this "step-and-shoot" manner, multiple contiguous images or slices could be acquired in axial planes through the anatomic area of interest. This, of course, resulted in long examination times (5 min) and relatively

A.M. Greenberg (ed.), *Digital Technologies in Craniomaxillofacial Surgery*, https://doi.org/10.1007/978-1-4939-1532-3_3

high patient radiation doses. Later generations of scanners were able to reduce acquisition time. Such scanners employed a collimated, *fan-shaped* x-ray beam that continuously rotated around the patient in a helical geometry striking *multiple* solid-state detectors (typically >1000). These mechanically complex scanners required concurrent motion of the x-ray tube and detectors and corresponding simultaneous movement of the patient couch [2]. This generation of scanners, known as multidetector helical CT (MDCT), dominated the CT market by 2005. Today, MDCT has become the first-line imaging modality for radiologists in the diagnostic workup of patients. In short, CT scanners evolved to greater sophistication and mechanical complexity in an effort to achieve shorter acquisition times and greater image resolution.

In contrast to the sophistication of conventional MDCT, CBCT represents a series of technological compromises. Unlike conventional *fan-beam multidetector* CT, cone beam CT systems use a *conical* beam of x-ray photons that passes through the patient and strikes a *single* detector. This single detector typically has the shape and dimensions of a 1 cm thick stack of A4 paper. In CBCT, there is no complex mechanical gantry. Rather, a rigid connecting arm (C-arm) connects the x-ray source and detector. The patient remains stationary at a location between the source and detector. In a CBCT apparatus, the x-ray tube and detector rotate only once around the patient. Because of the conical shape, an entire volume of anatomic interest rather than a single slice is acquired in one rotation. This results in several hundred 2-D (i.e., raw data) x-ray projections being acquired by the detector. Therefore, the acquisition time is short. The dose is relatively low, and the apparatus is smaller, less complex, and vastly less expensive to manufacture than MDCT.

Technical Background of CBCT

It is instructive to further compare and contrast CBCT with conventional MDCT. The physical principles of CBCT resemble, yet remain distinct from, conventional CT. Both modalities require (1) a moving source of x-ray photons, (2) a mechanism to position a patient within the x-ray beam with known geometry, (3) a means to detect and convert x-ray photons that have passed through a patient into a digital signal, and (4) a method to produce multidimensional images and/or to export a dataset for further evaluation. However, the particular mechanisms differ, thus accounting for the characteristic advantages and limitations of each modality. This will be addressed in detail in a subsequent section.

From a technical perspective, a CT (or CBCT) radiologic examination entails two phases: (1) data acquisition and (2) data reconstruction/evaluation. In the data acquisition phase, three technical elements come into play: the x-ray source, the gantry/couch assembly that houses the source and positions the patient, and the image receptor. The data reconstruction/evaluation phase takes place within the computer components of the CT or CBCT apparatus.

Phase 1: Data Acquisition

The x-ray source: conventional CT requires a rotating source capable of producing x-ray photons with energies as great as 160 kV. A substantial gantry is needed to support and move the heavy, intricate x-ray tube. In contrast, a typical CBCT unit uses a significantly smaller, lighter, and less heat-producing tube such as those found in dental x-ray machines. A CBCT unit employs tube voltages between 80 and 120 kV and a tube current between 0.5 and 10 mA [3].

Whereas in conventional CT examinations, a mechanical couch moves a patient along the axial plane in conjunction with serial x-ray exposures, in CBCT the patient is stationary. There is no requirement for a couch; the patient sits or stands. Only the x-ray source and detector move. Thus, a conical x-ray beam rotates around the patient with a fixed z-axis. Typically, this is accomplished by one centric revolution. (However, in some CBCT units, the field of view may be extended or modified by moving the source horizontally and applying a second rotation or by applying an eccentric rotation.) During the rotation, the x-ray beam tends to be pulsed rather than continuous. The total acquisition time ranges between 10 and 40 s. It can be appreciated that the simplified construction of CBCT, the shortened acquisition times, and the low-intensity x-ray beam result in a comparatively low-dose, low-cost tomographic x-ray examination.

The image receptor: the next part of the image acquisition process requires x-ray photons to be converted to a useful series of images. In the analog era, the image receptor was film. In the digital age, the receptor is electronic. In most MDCT scanners in use today, multiple linear arrays of detectors comprised of a radiation-sensitive element (e.g., cadmium tungstate, gadolinium oxide, or gadolinium oxysulfide) convert the absorbed x-rays to light. A silicon photodiode detects the light, and the resulting electrical current is amplified and converted into a digital signal. Subsequently, in the data reconstruction phase, the digital signals are expressed as shades of gray that form an image. This multidetector technology is both expensive and mechanically complex.

Not until the development of digital flat-panel detectors in 1992 did CBCT technology become practical [4]. A flat-panel detector is a single panel rather than an array of detectors.

FPDs may be of two varieties: direct-conversion FPDs or indirect-conversion FPDs. The first is a selenium-based technology that uses an amorphous selenium-coated thin-film-transistor (TFT) array to capture and convert x-ray energy directly into digital signals. It is a direct-conversion technology that converts x-ray beams into electric charges directly. This type of FPD does not require light-emitting materials as with CR systems, intermediate steps, or additional processes to capture and convert the incident x-ray energy (as with silicon-based systems or CCD systems). Under a bias voltage applied across the detector structure, incident x-rays directly generate electron-hole pairs in the selenium layer. Individual storage capacitors associated with each detector element collect these charges for readout by customized electronics within the array.

The second type of flat-panel sensor uses thin films of silicon integrated with arrays of photodiodes. A coating of a crystalline cesium iodide (CsI:Tl) scintillator or a rare-earth scintillator (terbium-doped gadolinium oxysulfide, Gd_2O_2S:Tb) overlays these photodiodes. When x-rays strike these scintillator layers, visible light is emitted proportional to the incident x-ray energy. Then the light photons are converted into an electric charge by the photodiode arrays. Thus, this type of indirect-conversion detector technology is a two-step process for x-ray detection, i.e., the scintillator converts the x-ray beams into visible light, and light then is converted into an electric charge by the amorphous silicon photodiodes. Dissimilar to the previously described amorphous selenium direct-conversion system, this indirect mechanism results in lower resolution images. The image is degraded because the light photons diffuse within the scintillation layer through which they travel before striking the subjacent photodiode array. Whereas, such indirect flat-panel systems are noisy, most CBCT units sold between 2005 and 2012 were manufactured with indirect FPD technology [5].

Whereas FPDs are innovative, cost-saving imaging technologies, the aforementioned systems suffer from performance limitations about which the clinician should be aware. Most notably, contrast resolution suffers because of increased x-ray scatter, light diffusion, reduced temporal resolution, and diminished dynamic range of FPDs. Further limitations arise from nonlinearity of response to radiation, lack of uniformity of response throughout the area of the detector, and bad pixels [6].

Phase 2: Data Reconstruction/Evaluation

The data reconstruction/evaluation phase takes place within the computer components of the CT or CBCT apparatus. As described above, x-ray photons passing through a patient are differentially attenuated by anatomic structures within the patient. Then, the non-attenuated x-ray photons interact in the detector component of the CT or CBCT devices to generate a digital signal proportional to the intensity of the incident photons. At this stage, a computer is needed to convert digital signals to images that can be interpreted by a clinician or to other forms of datasets that are clinically relevant.

The task of the computer system in MDCT is to convert raw data acquired in the acquisition phase to a volumetric three-dimensional representation of an anatomic region. The raw data is comprised of hundreds of individual 2-D projection frames each with over one million pixels with 12 to 16 bits of data assigned to each pixel. The processing uses computationally complex reconstruction algorithms. This process is termed simply *reconstruction*. In contrast to MDCT, cone beam CT data reconstruction is performed by a personal computer rather than a high-end workstation.

Conventional CT has evolved to use several advanced reconstruction techniques including filtered back projection, iterative techniques, and many supplemental algorithms to correct artifacts [7]. The principle reconstruction algorithm used in conventional CT (and shared in a simplified form with CBCT) is based on the filtered back projection. In this method, a large set of x-ray projections are collected from the photons striking the detectors. In a typical scanner, 800–1500 projections are collected at rotational intervals of less than 1°. Computationally, the multiple projections are "folded back" upon each other. Thus, the end results represent overlapping of all projections that were acquired from the initial scan. This mathematical process produces blur. To compensate, a computational adjustment must be made. The adjustment is known as a "filter," hence the term "filtered back projection." It should be noted that all these mathematical manipulations produce image artifacts that subsequently must be corrected by means of additional filters.

The reconstruction process for CBCT fundamentally differs from MDCT. As noted previously, a MDCT radiological examination is comprised of a collection of individual "slices" obtained by sequential rotations of the scanner around the patient. The computational task in MDCT is to stack the slices upon each other in order to display a 3-D volume. In contrast, CBCT acquires a 3-D volume in one rotation of the scanning apparatus. The computational task in CBCT is to "decompose" the volumetric data to create individual slices from the total volume acquired. That is, the process is the converse. To accomplish this, CBCT uses an extremely basic filtered back projection known as the modified Feldkamp algorithm. Similar to the reconstruction algorithms employed in MDCT, the modified Feldkamp algorithm engenders multiple imaging artifacts. Presently, manufacturers of CBCT struggle devising supplemental filters to compensate for artifacts in the context of diminished processing power inherent in CBCT workstations.

Thus, whereas the end product of CBCT and MDCT is the same, a three-dimensional representation of an anatomic region, the technical mechanisms differ. These differences underscore the limitations of CBCT technology as addressed in the next section.

Subsequent to the data reconstruction process, CBCT and MDCT workstations secondarily process the data to yield various types of image display. Depending on the capability of the software, there are many options of image construction from the 3-D volumetric dataset. Manufacturers of CBCT units supply proprietary image display software of varying capabilities. In addition, at this writing, there are no fewer than eight third-party venders producing software for imaging CBCT datasets. Most CBCT software applications display primary image reconstruction in the three anatomic planes of imaging: axial, sagittal, and coronal planes. These are known as multiplanar reconstructions. The software generally permits orientation and navigation by means of intersection lines or crosshairs in the display window. Most basic software applications allow the clinician to adjust brightness and contrast, manipulate slice thickness, and smooth, sharpen, or magnify the image.

In addition to this standard multiplanar display, venders offer task-specific manipulations of the dataset. Among these are panoramic reconstructions, cross-sectional reconstructions along a curved plane such as used in implant treatment planning, temporomandibular joint reconstructions, airway displays, three-dimensional displays, and surface renderings of various complexities.

A feature of high-end image-processing software is the ability to perform surface and volume rendering. Surface rendering can be useful to generate a drilling or surgical guide for implant placement via a rapid prototyping machine or to print out a real physical model of the rendered object for surgical treatment planning. Whereas the image manipulation known as "segmentation" is integral to medical radiological diagnosis, the diminished computational power of CBCT workstations struggle with this procedure. This is because segmentation requires the ability to find edges by thresholding gray levels. As noted previously, CBCT has poor gray-level discrimination. Thus, it remains difficult to measure airway or sinus volumes or quantify bony defects in three dimensions with CBCT.

To recapitulate, the basic principle behind computed tomography is to acquire multiple views of an object over a range of angular orientations. In a subsequent step, a computer program (an algorithm) manipulates these views to form a coherent image. Alternately, the data can be exported as a clinically useful dataset. In its simplest form, a MDCT scanner consists of an x-ray tube that emits a finely collimated, fan-shaped beam directed through a patient. After passing through the patient, the x-ray photons strike a series of scintillation detectors that measure the number of photons that exit the patient. This information produces a single, cross-sectional image (slice) of the patient. Next, the patient repositions with respect to the x-ray source/detector assembly, and the scanner acquires another cross-sectional image. Subsequently, computer software reassembles the resulting stack of many discrete, axial images into a unified whole that represents a three-dimensional patient.

Similar to other forms of digital imaging, the CT scanner's computer assigns numbers to the image. The numbers correspond to a shade of gray. These shades of gray reside in grid-like boxes on the image known as pixels (picture elements). Because each slice actually has a thickness, the boxes are really cubes in three dimensions. The cubic elements are termed voxels (volume elements).

Thus, the CT numbers represent tissue density. The more dense the body part that is imaged, the higher the CT number. Most fan-beam MDCT scanners can display more than 2000 shades of gray. In honor of its inventor, these gray shades are named Hounsfield units (HU). The power of MDCT imaging lies in this modality's ability to demonstrate subtle differences in tissue density. For example, CT can distinguish gray matter from white matter and blood from clotted blood or discern subtleties in bone density.

The principle behind CBCT, as its name implies, is a cone-shaped x-ray beam, with the x-ray source and detector rotating around a point (or field) of interest of the patient. The conical shape of the beam distinguishes this technique from MDCT. In contrast to MDCT, only one rotation or less is needed to acquire a full three-dimensional dataset. By rotating an x-ray source around a fixed point (isocenter) in the object of interest and acquiring projections from many different angles, a three-dimensional volume (typically cylindrical) can be created. The CBCT computer "decomposes" the volumetric dataset to create individual slices from the total volume acquired. Similar to MDCT, during the mathematical process, voxels are assigned individual gray levels, each having a particular gray value that represents the average density within this volume element. Cone beam CT does not have the capacity to display many shades of gray. Thus, tissue densities are poorly defined with this modality. CBCT workstations, to varying extents, can transform the volumetric dataset to task-specific image displays according to the needs of the clinician.

Limitations of CBCT

Technological advances enabled the development of CBCT and fostered its proliferation into the clinical armamentarium of craniomaxillofacial surgeons and other head and neck specialists. As stated earlier, the specific technological advances in x-ray tubes, FPDs, and computer systems represented compromises compared to existing technology [8]. Thus, three categories of CBCT limitations merit discussion here.

1. The x-ray tube compromise:

Beam geometry: the shift of the conventional, tightly collimated, fan-shaped beam in MDCT to the divergent, cone-shaped beam in CBCT generates significant scatter radiation in the imaging field. Such off-axis, low-energy scatter in the patient during image acquisition diminishes contrast. The scattered photons merely contribute noise to the image that degrades the capacity of CBCT to display subtle shades of gray. Scatter is expressed as the scatter-to-primary ratio (SPR). In large-volume CBCT systems, the SPR can be as high as 3.0 compared with approximately 0.2 in conventional MDCT systems [9]. Thus, CBCT is of little clinical utility for the assessment of soft tissue structures.

Beam quality: all CT scanners inherently produce polyenergetic x-ray beams. That is, the beam is a collection of photons having assorted energies. As this x-ray beam passes through a patient, the lower-energy photons are preferentially attenuated. The mean energy of the polyenergetic beam is now higher. This process is called beam hardening. Because CBCT uses lower kilovolt peak energies compared with MDCT, beam-hardening artifacts are more pronounced in CBCT. One type of beam-hardening artifact is known as cupping. Cupping results when the x-ray beam is differentially absorbed in metallic structures. As a result of this artifact, objects proximal to the metallic structures shrink or disappear. The region adjacent to the dense material appears black because the detector is "fooled" by the preponderance of high-energy photons striking it. Another beam quality artifact, streaks with dark bands, appears in association with dense objects in the beam. The streaks and bands obscure structures in the neighboring field of interest. Thus, CBCT is limited in clinical situations involving surgical hardware, metallic implants, or dental restorations.

2. The flat-panel display compromise: the use of FPDs introduces higher levels of noise in the resultant CBCT images than with the detectors used in MDCT. In the case of indirect FPDs, light diffuses within the thickness of the scintillation layer contributing to the noise. Additionally, with flat-panel detectors, the active area of each detector is only a portion of the entire imaging area. This portion is known as the "fill factor." With CBCT, the fill factor may be as small as 35%. Such FPDs capture fewer x-ray photons and the result is more image noise. In addition, FPDs have inherent low temporal resolution. The rotating CBCT photon beam challenges the electronics of the FPD. Signal refresh rates (known as frame rate) cannot keep up with signal acquisition. All the above factors result in image degradation.
3. The computational compromise: CBCT workstations employ diminished processing power compared to MDCT. As noted previously, scatter degrades image quality. In the high-end imaging workstations found in MDCT, the effects of scatter are compensated by means of scatter correction algorithms. The most robust algorithm is based on Monte Carlo simulation. Monte Carlo computations require significant processing power. These are not easily adaptable to the PC-based workstations used in CBCT. Nonetheless, some scatter subtraction or homogeneous processing algorithms are used in most clinical CBCT systems. As a result, there has been recent improvement in image uniformity and contrast to noise ratio. Also noted previously was the need for back-filtered projections to be supplementarily computer-processed to reduce blur. These existing supplementary algorithms are not easily adaptable to computers used for CBCT. Thus, PC workstations represent further compromise in the ability to resolve image degradation by computational means.

Capacities of CBCT

Just as the technology dictates the limitations of CBCT, the technology accentuates its strengths. For example, a cone-shaped beam is isotropic (or nearly isotropic). That is, there is no dimensional distortion of objects in all projection planes. This greatly simplifies accurate dimensional measurements such as those needed to plan dental implant procedures, to manufacture surgical devices or prostheses, or for operative navigation.

Another technological advantage of CBCT is high spatial resolution. The spatial resolution of an imaging system is its ability to discriminate objects of different attenuation at small separation distances. With CBCT, this is largely the result of its inherent isotropic data acquisition and advancing FPD technology. Spatial resolution typically is expressed in line pairs/mm (lp/mm). It should be noted that spatial resolution reflects several components of the imaging system including focal spot size, detector element size, smoothing filter, and reconstructed voxel size. Thus, CBCT manufacturers' propensity to represent spatial resolution as "minimum voxel dimension" is misleading.

Some investigators have reported that the spatial resolution of CBCT exceeds MDCT by a factor of 2–5. However, in an actual clinical environment, it is more realistic to conclude that the spatial resolution of CBCT is on a par with MDCT. Accordingly, current literature places CBCT spatial resolution at about 1 lp/mm [10, 11].

Evidence-Based Applications of CBCT

As with many new technologies, clinicians and researchers have published myriads of manuscripts describing new and novel applications for CBCT. Before reaching conclusions, one must scrutinize this extensive literature to determine what are "evidence-based" applications for cone beam CT.

In 2008, the European Commission formed a panel of experts to prepare guidelines for the appropriate application of CBCT. This project, known as SEDENTEXCT, published the guidelines in 2012 [12]. The panel reviewed more than 350 publications addressing applications of CBCT that appeared in the literature between 2000 and 2012. The conclusions of the panel are instructive and are summarized below. In brief, despite the popularity of CBCT, the SEDENTEXCT project could not establish evidence to support almost 50% of published applications for CBCT in craniomaxillofacial surgery. Whereas the evidenced-based applications for CBCT are fluid and evolving, the present consensus is:

Contraindications for CBCT:

1. CBCT *is not indicated* for caries detection and diagnosis.
2. CBCT *is not the modality of choice* for assessing bony pathosis. When it is likely that evaluation of soft tissues will be needed, then MDCT or MR is preferred to CBCT. (However small-field high-resolution CBCT may be indicated for evaluation of bony invasion of the jaws by oral carcinoma when the initial imaging modality used for diagnosis and staging does not provide satisfactory information.)
3. CBCT *is not indicated* for the localization of nonerupted teeth except when the information cannot be obtained adequately by lower-dose conventional radiography.
4. The use of CBCT to derive density measurements of bone *is not recommended.*
5. CBCT *should not be used* routinely for orthodontic diagnosis. (However, it may be justified for complex cases of skeletal abnormality, particularly those requiring combined orthodontic/surgical management.)
6. CBCT *is not indicated* for planning the placement of temporary anchorage devices in orthodontics.
7. CBCT *is not indicated* as a standard method for identification of periapical pathosis. (However, small-field, high-resolution CBCT may be indicated in selected cases when conventional radiographs give a negative finding or when there are contradictory positive clinical signs and symptoms.)
8. CBCT *is not indicated* as a standard method for demonstration of root canal anatomy. (However, small-field, high-resolution CBCT may be indicated for selected cases where conventional radiographs provide equivocal or inadequate information for treatment planning.)
9. CBCT *is not indicated* for examination of the TMJ except as an alternative to where MDCT would be used because it is a lower dose.
10. CBCT *is not indicated* as a method of imaging periodontal bone support. (However, small-field, high-resolution CBCT may be indicated in selected cases of infra-bony defects and furcational lesions where clinical and conventional radiographic examinations do not provide the information needed for management.)

Possible indications for CBCT:

1. Small-field, high-resolution CBCT *may be justifiable* for selected cases where endodontic treatment is complicated by concurrent factors such as resorption lesions, combined periodontal/endodontic lesions, and atypical pulp anatomy.
2. Small-field, high-resolution CBCT *may be indicated* for selected cases when planning surgical endodontic procedures.
3. CBCT *may be indicated* for presurgical assessment of a nonerupted tooth in selected cases where conventional radiographs fail to provide the information required.
4. Small-field, high-resolution CBCT *may be indicated* in selected cases of suspected or established inflammatory root resorption or internal resorption, where 3-D information is likely to alter the management or prognosis of the tooth.
5. For maxillofacial fracture, where cross-sectional imaging is judged to be necessary, CBCT *may be indicated* as an alternative imaging modality to MDCT but only where soft tissue detail is not required.

Indications for CBCT:

1. CBCT *is indicated* for cross-sectional imaging prior to implant placement.
2. Small-field, high-resolution CBCT *is indicated* in the assessment of dental trauma in selected cases, where conventional intraoral radiographs provide inadequate information for treatment planning.
3. CBCT *is indicated* for assessing cleft palate and is preferred to MDCT because the radiation dose is lower.
4. CBCT has been shown to be *an effective means* of providing data for the manufacture of surgical guides in implant dentistry.
5. CBCT *is indicated* where bone information is required in orthognathic surgical planning, for obtaining 3-D datasets of the craniofacial skeleton.
6. CBCT *is indicated* when conventional radiographs suggest a direct interrelationship between a mandibular third molar and the mandibular canal and when the decision to perform surgical removal has been made.

Evidence-based guidelines for other head and neck applications of CBCT have not been formulated. The literature reports the use of CBCT for paranasal sinus imaging [13, 14], airway imaging [15], and imaging of the middle ear and proximal structures [16, 17].

It is not surprising that the evidence-based indications and contraindications for the application of CBCT reflect the technological strengths and weaknesses of this modality. Specifically, tasks that require gray-level discrimination or differentiation of soft tissues are not possible with CBCT. Moreover, CBCT is limited in clinical situations involving surgical hardware, metallic implants, or dental restorations because of beam artifacts and inadequate computational power to filter artifacts. On the other hand, the evidence supports tasks that rely on high spatial resolution and accurate isotropic measurement capability. Thus, CBCT demonstrates clinical utility for surgical treatment planning, navigation, or 3-D modeling. High-resolution, small field of view CBCT exhibits utility in selected diagnostic situations in dentistry and perhaps otorhinolaryngology.

Summary

Cone beam computed tomography is a form of tomographic imaging. It is a derivative of multidetector computed tomography. CBCT is a technology characterized by compromises. As a consequence, CBCT has limited capabilities, most notably the inability to differentiate soft tissue densities and meager computational capacities of the image-processing system. The principle advantage of CBCT is its dimensional accuracy and high spatial resolution. Moreover, it is vastly less expensive and generally exhibits lower radiation dose than its forerunner, MDCT. A critical view of the literature reflects that the evidence-based applications of CBCT in craniomaxillofacial surgery are restricted.

References

1. Robb RA. The dynamic spatial reconstructor: an x-ray videofluoroscopic CT scanner for dynamic volume imaging of moving organs. IEEE Trans Med Imaging. 1982;1:22–3.
2. Kalender WA. Computed tomography. Fundamentals, system technology, image quality, applications. 2nd ed. Erlangen: Publicis Corporate Publishing; 2005.
3. Kau CH, Bozic M, English J, Lee R, Bussa H, Ellis RK. Cone-beam computed tomography of the maxillofacial region-an update. Int J Med Robot. 2009;5(4):366–80.
4. Kalender WA. Flat-detector computed tomography (FD-CT). Eur Radiol. 2007;17:2767–79.
5. Nemtoi A, Czink C, Haba D, Gahleitner A. Cone-beam CT: a current overview of devices. Dentomaxillofac Radiol. 2013;42:20120443.
6. Scarfe W, Farman A. What is cone-beam CT and how does it work? Dent Clin N Am. 2008;52:707–30.
7. van den Hoff J. Evaluation of tomographic data. In: Salzer R, editor. Biomedical Imaging: Principles and Applications. Hoboken: Wiley; 2012. Ch 2.
8. Miracle AC, Mukherji SK. Cone-beam CT of the head and neck, part 1: physical principles. AJNR Am J Neuroradiol. 2009;30(6):1088–95.
9. Sierwerdsen JH, Jafray DA. Cone beam CT with a flat-panel imager: magnitude and effects of x-ray scatter. Med Phys. 2001;28:230–1.
10. Suomalainen A, Kiljunen T, Käser Y, Peltola J, Kortesniemi M. Dosimetry and image quality of four dental cone beam computed tomography scanners compared with multislice computed tomography scanners. Dentomaxillofac Radiol. 2009;38(6):367–78.
11. Schulze RKW, Brüllmann D. Spatial resolution in CBCT machines for dental/maxillofacial applications—what do we know today? Dentomaxillofac Radiol. 2015;44(1):20140204. Review
12. European Commission. Cone beam CT for dental and maxillofacial radiology: evidence based guidelines. Radiation Protection Publication; 2012. p, 172.
13. Güldner C, Pistorius SM, Diogo I, Bien S, Sesterhenn A, Werner JA. Analysis of pneumatization and neurovascular structures of the sphenoid sinus using cone-beam tomography (CBT). Acta Radiol. 2012;53(2):214–9.
14. Prisman E, Daly MJ, Chan H, Siewerdsen JH, Vescan A, Irish JC. Real-time tracking and virtual endoscopy in cone-beam CT-guided surgery of the sinuses and skull base in a cadaver model. Int Forum Allergy Rhinol. 2011;1(1):70–7.
15. Haskell JA, McCrillis J, Haskell BS, et al. Effects of mandibular advancement device on airway dimensions assessed with cone beam computed tomography. Semin Orthod. 2009;15:132–58.
16. Peltonen LI, Aarnisalo AA, Kortesniemi MK, Suomalainen A, Jero J, Robinson S. Limited cone-beam computed tomography imaging of the middle ear: a comparison with multislice helical computed tomography. Acta Radiol. 2007;48(2):207–12.
17. Dahmani-Causse M, Marx M, Deguine O, Fraysse B, Lepage B, Escudé B. Morphologic examination of the temporal bone by cone beam computed tomography: comparison with multislice helical computed tomography. Eur Ann Otorhinolaryngol Head Neck Dis. 2011;128(5):230–5.

Craniomaxillofacial Reconstruction Based on 3D Modeling

4

Gerald T. Grant

Introduction

Current treatment planning and reconstruction of craniofacial trauma has been advanced greatly due to the increase in the use of software to convert medical image files in the form of Digital Imaging and Communications in Medicine (DICOM) to 3D reconstructions and ultimately files which can be converted for fabrication of medical models and surgical guides using additive or subtractive manufacturing technologies (Fig. 4.1). In addition, advances in photogrammetry systems allow for capture of the surface of the head and neck using camera systems that can be registered to medical images to help in the surgical planning for head and neck reconstructions [1].

Medical imaging devices such as computed tomography (CT), magnetic resonance imaging (MRI), ultrasound, and recently cone beam CT (CBCT) are used to capture the hard and soft internal structures for craniofacial imaging. Scanning systems such as white light scanners, lasers, and camera systems using photogrammetry also provide the data needed to accurately capture soft tissue surfaces for measurement and registration. All of these capture devices have file formats that are easily converted for 3D reconstructions and ultimately digital virtual surgical planning (VSP) [2].

In addition to imaging advances, software has become more accessible that allows conversion of the DICOM files to the .stl and similar file formats, more appropriate for use with 3D reconstruction and "3D printing" (Fig. 4.2). Currently, commercial software can be obtained that is designed to help with the virtual surgical manipulation to develop cutting as well as positioning guides that can be fabricated using additive manufacturing technologies (3D printing) or subtractive manufacturing technologies (milling).

The advantages of these systems is that the virtual plan can be executed by maintaining the digital file from image capture, to virtual surgical planning, and the fabrication of surgical guides. These techniques have proven to provide surgeons greater confidence in executing their plan, reducing operating times, follow-up surgical revisions, and reduced unfavorable outcomes (Fig. 4.3). In addition, they provide patient-centered care and better esthetic and functional outcomes [3–5].

Craniofacial Imaging

Computer tomography is the preferred method of imaging for head and neck reconstructions. The Hounsfield scale enables identification of soft and hard tissues by their density; this allows for segmentation of the images for reconstruction of 3D models with minimal artifact, but at the expense of radiation exposure to the patient [6]. In contrast, CBCT scanners have become more common in dental practices; their low radiation exposure provides a unique opportunity to capture hard tissue images that have been used from endodontic diagnosis to dental implant planning [7, 8]. However, although there is a low radiation exposure to the patient, CBCT is subject to severe artifact due to dental restorations (Fig. 4.4), and other metallic objects (Fig. 4.5) and lack the contrast to segment soft tissue structures for use with 3D reconstruction of structures other than bone [9]. For this reason, a standard for CBCT such as the Hounsfield scale for CT has not been developed.

Magnetic resonance imaging provides imaging of the internal soft tissue from the reaction of hydrogen atoms with a strong magnetic field. Although this spares the patient from X-ray radiation exposure, bone has a negative return and requires that the patient remain still for an extended time.

In addition to scanning to provide some description of the internal structures, surface imaging can provide valuable information as to the prediction of soft tissue placement, measurement, as well as volume estimation. These images are generally captured by using multiple camera capture systems employing photogrammetry techniques or scanning technology [10] (Fig. 4.6). The multicamera systems have

G.T. Grant (✉)
Oral Health and Rehabilitation, University of Louisville School of Dentistry, 501 South Preston Street, Louisville, KY 40202, USA
e-mail: gerald.grant@louisville.edu

A.M. Greenberg (ed.), *Digital Technologies in Craniomaxillofacial Surgery*, https://doi.org/10.1007/978-1-4939-1532-3_4

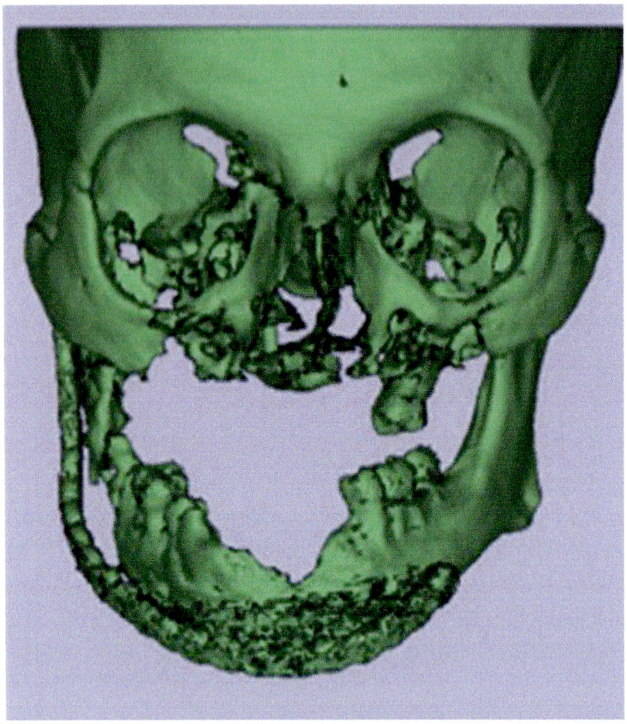

Fig. 4.1 3D model of mid-face and mandibular trauma (Mimics Innovation Suite, Materialise, Leuven, Belgium)

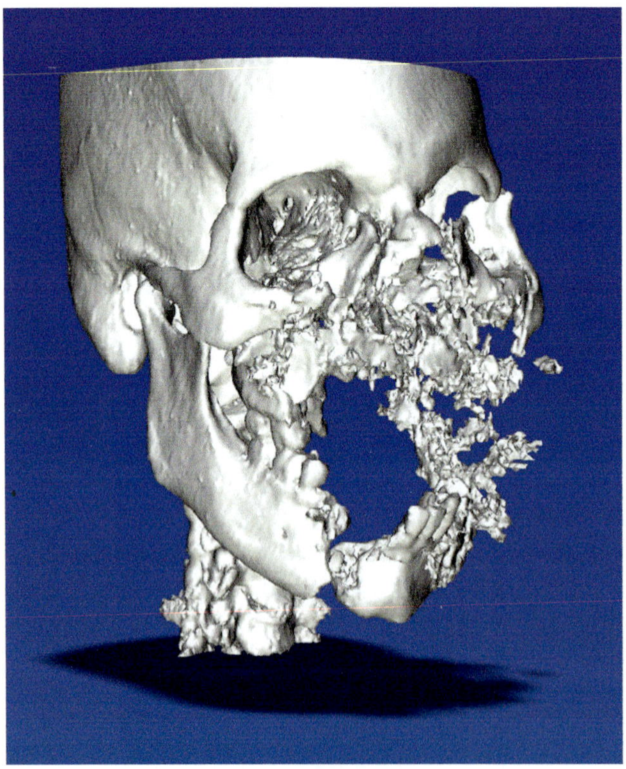

Fig. 4.2 Mid-face trauma model fabricated from a CT scan (Mimics Innovation Suite, Materialise, Leuven, Belgium)

the advantage in that image capture is very short (less than a second), and the surface to be captured is related to the number of cameras in the array. This short capture time is ideal for head and neck capture, especially in documenting soft tissue defects in children [11]. These images can be registered to CT and CBCT scans to allow for measurement of soft and hard tissues (Fig. 4.7).

Surface scanning systems using light or lasers require time to capture the image and some expertise for the operator. As a result, they are not well suited for use in reconstruction of the head and neck, but very useful in capture of the surface for tracking wound healing from burns or amputation impressions for prosthetics [12]. However, registering the surfaces can provide information on the volume changes between surfaces that could provide a means to follow swellings or wound healing.

The recent advances in intraoral scanners provide the advantage of scanning the dentition as well. These scans can be registered to CT and CBCT scans to compensate for the poor scan quality of teeth due to artifact from dental restorations and other hardware.

Since the medical images are generally stored as medical DICOM files, they can be converted to a common modeling file, generally an .stl file. The file format from dental intraoral scanners may be a direct .stl from the scanning system, but more often they are proprietary and have to be converted to an .stl. Once they are in this file format, they can be registered to each other to develop a hard and soft tissue model, providing captured data for multiple sources and providing a more accurate representation in virtual or physical model fabrication for treatment planning (Figs. 4.7 and 4.8).

Virtual Surgery

Virtual surgery is a term that is often used to describe the surgical planning from medical images using software. Software that is designed for surgical planning accepts DICOM images and converts them to a 3D format. The most common 3D format file used for radiology applications to date is Standard Tessellation Language (STL). Accurate 3D printing is based on the conversion of image data from DICOM to .stl files. However, a second relatively new file format called Additive Manufacturing File Format (AMF) supported by the American Society of Testing and Materials (ASTM) F42 committee on additive manufacturing has been designed to enable the user to incorporate such features as surface texture, color, and material properties into the 3D models. It may become widely used in the future [13]. These types of files are characterized by triangular meshes, which relate each point in space to each other to develop a 3D model (Fig. 4.9).

Images can be brought into different software packages, which allow for segmentation of the bones and soft tissue, registration of different images, and fabrication of surgical

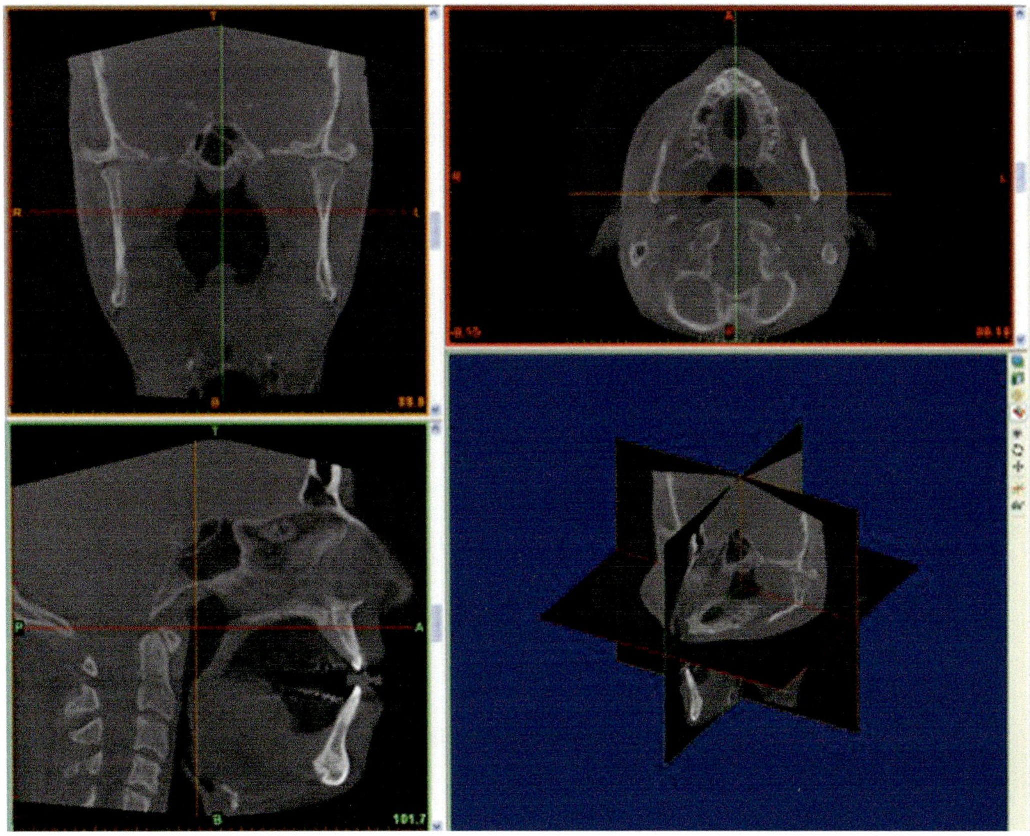

Fig. 4.3 Conversion of a CT model into modeling software, note three views and 3D reconstructions (Mimics Innovation Suite, Materialise, Leuven, Belgium)

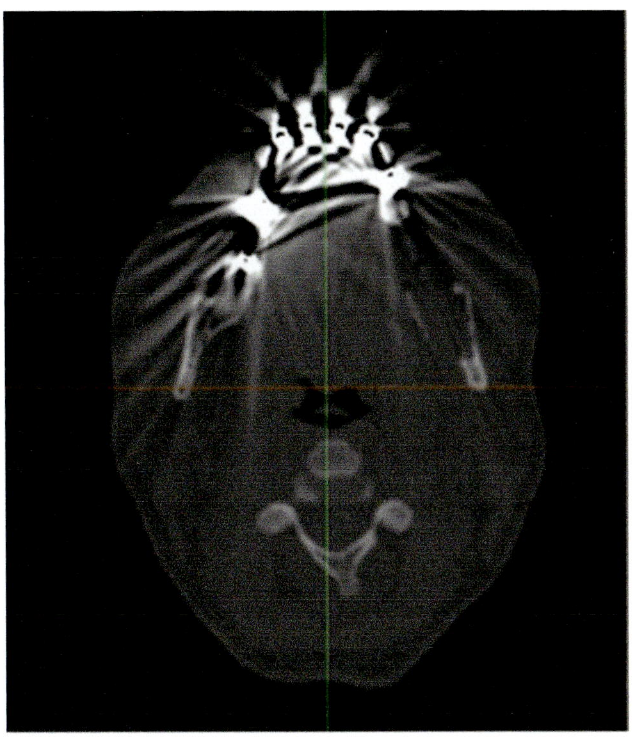

Fig. 4.4 Artifact from dental restorations is a problem especially in CBCT; the area of the artifact needs to be removed to develop models

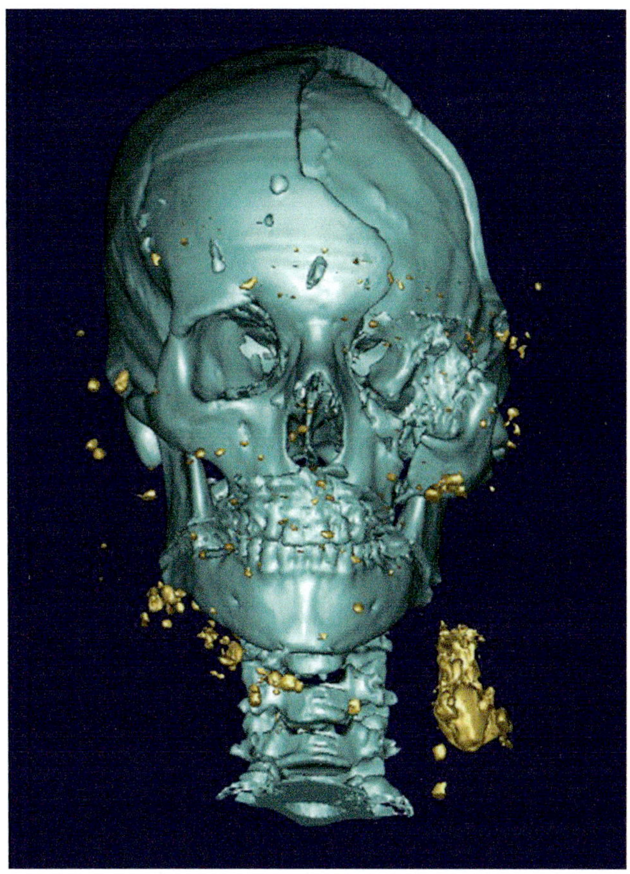

Fig. 4.5 Note bone trauma and metal fragments in the 3D rendered model from CT scan (Mimics Innovation Suite, Materialise, Leuven, Belgium)

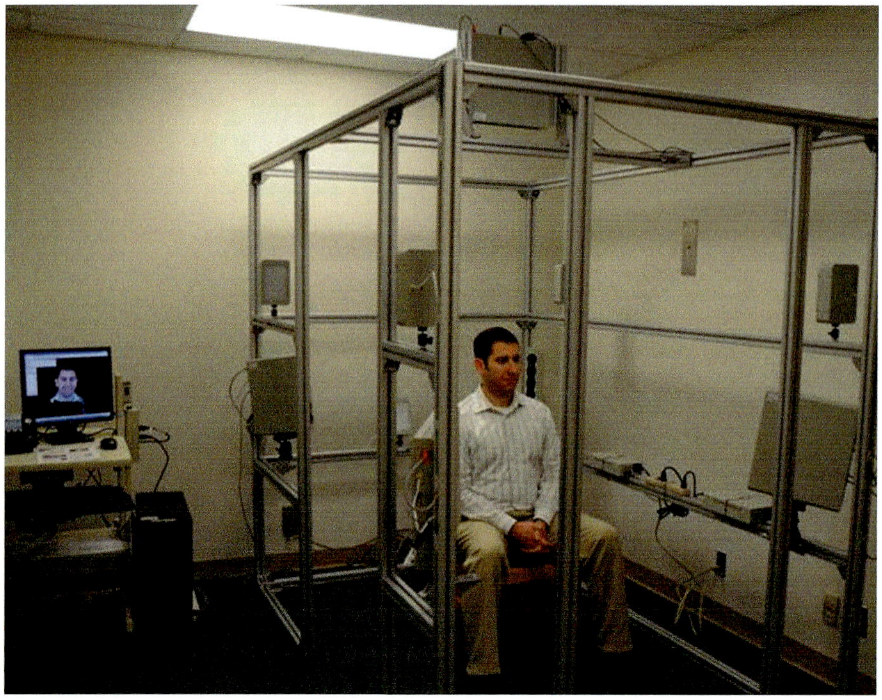

Fig. 4.6 A photogrammetry camera, five cameras can capture the entire head in 1/32 of a second (3dMD Head System, 3dMD, LLC, Atlanta, GA, USA)

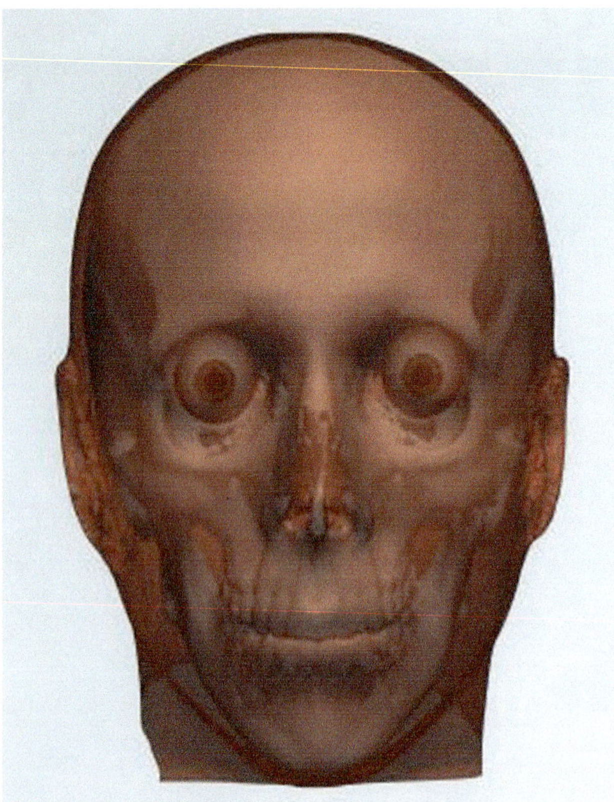

Fig. 4.7 Soft tissue and hard tissue models can be developed from CT, CBCT scans as well as registration of CT/CBCT with digital surface images (Mimics Innovation Suite, Materialise, Leuven, Belgium)

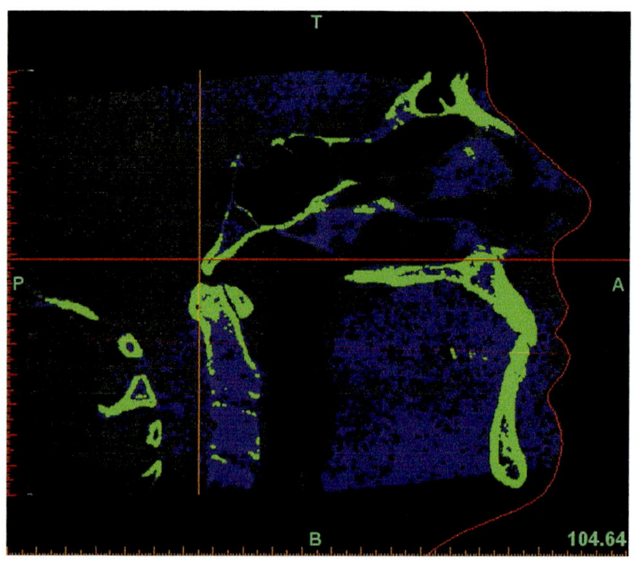

Fig. 4.8 Many of the CBCT systems have airway options (3D Vultus, 3dMD, LLC, Atlanta, GA, USA)

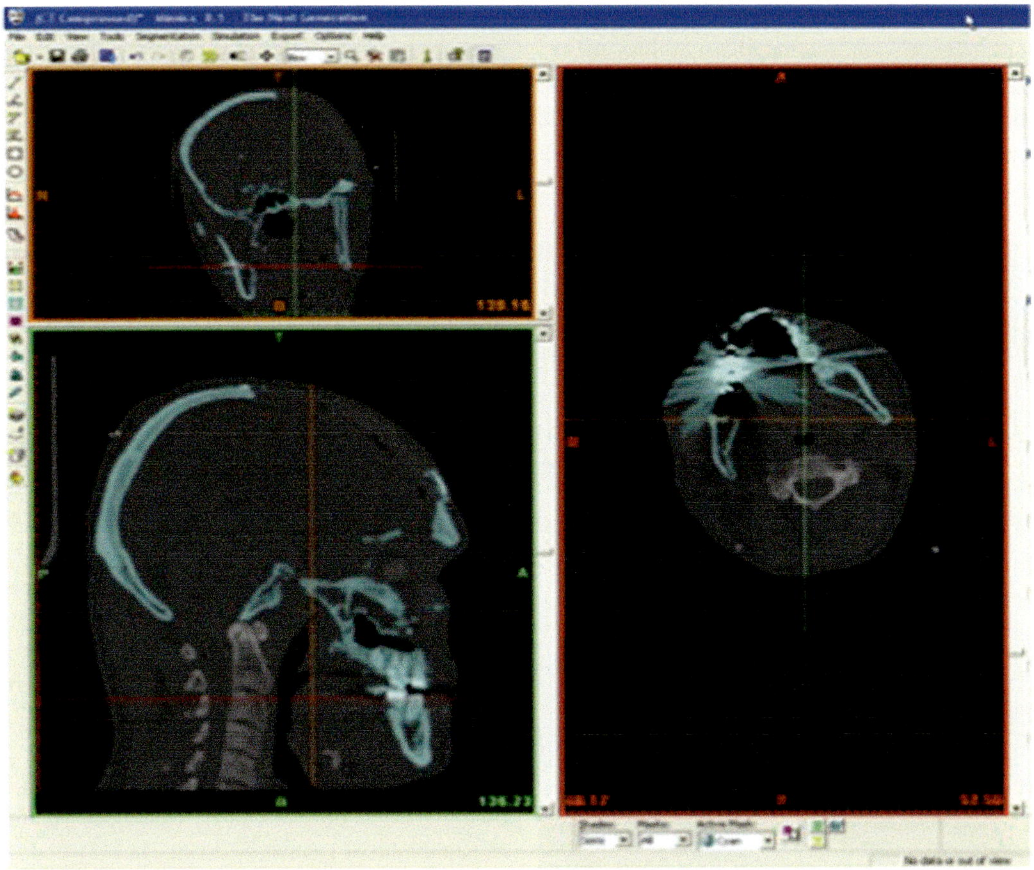

Fig. 4.9 CT scan in modeling software; note the artifact; features of the program allow to manually remove artifact to develop a model (Mimics Innovation Suite, Materialise, Leuven, Belgium)

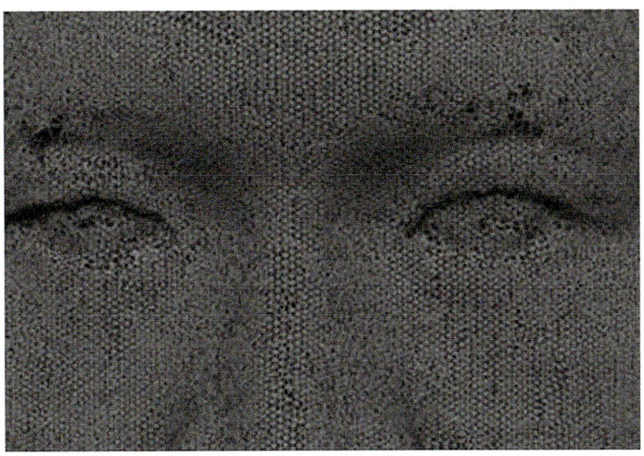

Fig. 4.10 A wire mesh is developed in the .stl formats; triangles connect each of the coordinate points. The smaller the triangles, the more accurate the measurement of the models (3D Vultus, 3dMD, LLC, Atlanta, GA, USA)

cutting guides, positioning guides, as well as design of custom reconstruction plates, grafts, and implants (Figs. 4.10–4.13).

The better-known systems are those that have been commercially available for dental implant placement. Most of these softwares are proprietary to an implant system, but more recently they have become more general in their use. In

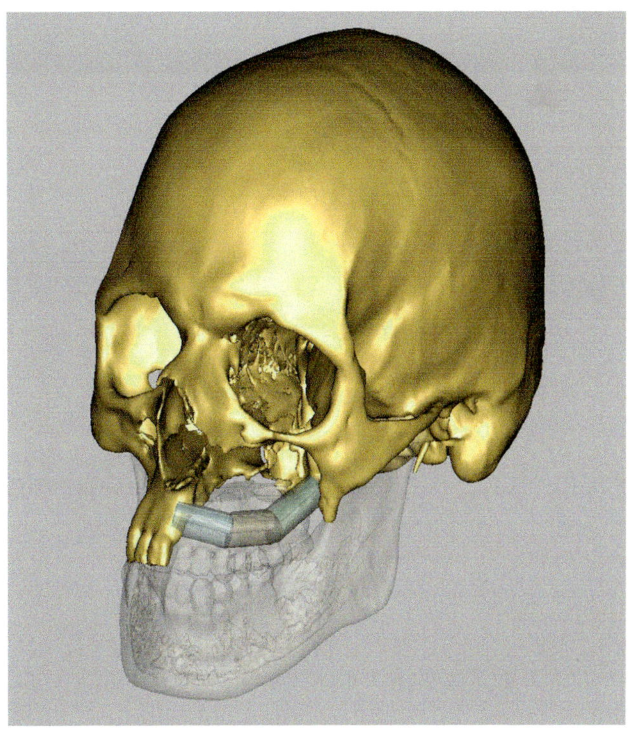

Fig. 4.11 Fibula graft designed for maxillary defect (Surgicase CMF, Materialise, Leuven, Belgium)

some instances, they have been "partnered" with a CBCT imaging system and a CAD/CAM dentistry system for the restorations as well. The restoration can be designed and the implant positioned. The product is a surgical guide and a temporary or permanent milled restoration, to provide a single- to a full-arch restoration at the time of implant placement (Figs. 4.14 and 4.15.).

Most of the virtual surgical technologies for craniofacial reconstruction use registration technology. This technique is used when there are missing anatomical segments, to restore a contour or follow the progression of a lesion or process. It involves having two scans of the same individual, a pre-trauma for a template for reconstruction and a post-trauma image, but it can also be used to track swellings and changes in morphology of anatomical structures (Figs. 4.16 and 4.17). If a pre-trauma record is not available, then scans of family members, a library, mirroring an unaffected side, or even some forensic reconstruction software can be used as a template for reconstruction [14]. Once areas of the scans where there have been no changes, such as bony landmarks (the bridge of the nose, calvarias, etc.) have been located, most software will provide a "best fit" algorithm to put the two scans together, but you often need to make small adjustments (Fig. 4.17). Once you have the images registered, missing anatomical segments can be "replaced"; changes between the two images in a given area can be measured, etc... This is a very useful tool for predicting bony reconstructions and developing surgical guides for graft harvest and placement, as well as custom reconstruction plates. Swellings and tumors can be followed over time to determine the rate of growth or shrinkage [15].

In addition to registration, some softwares offer the ability to shape and design surgical guides during the planning phase, such as replacing missing mandibular sections using a fibula flap reconstruction. Once the area is identified to be restored, the fibula can be manipulated to provide the best fit and a cutting guide is designed to provide the results planned for digital fabrication [16].

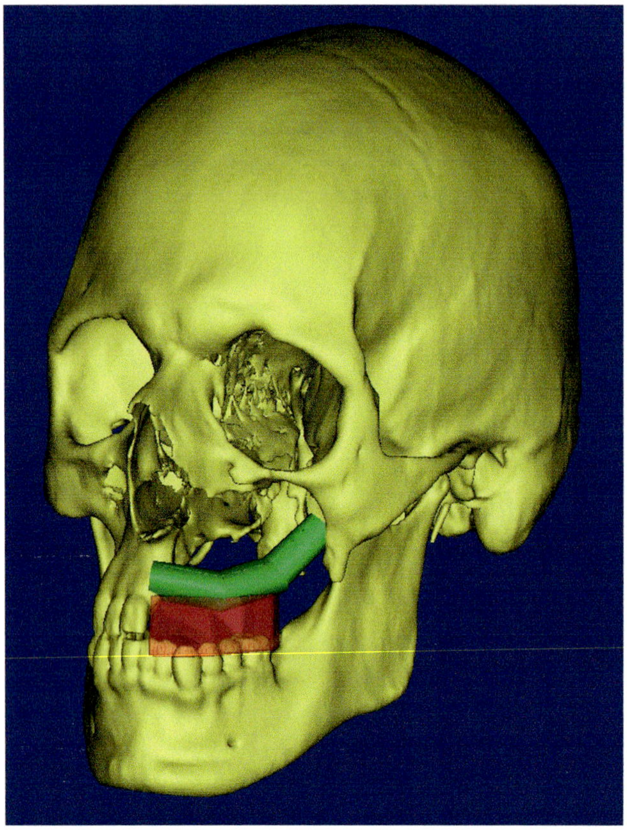

Fig. 4.12 Positioning of the teeth and associated structures registered from pre-traumatic images (Surgicase CMF, Materialise, Leuven, Belgium)

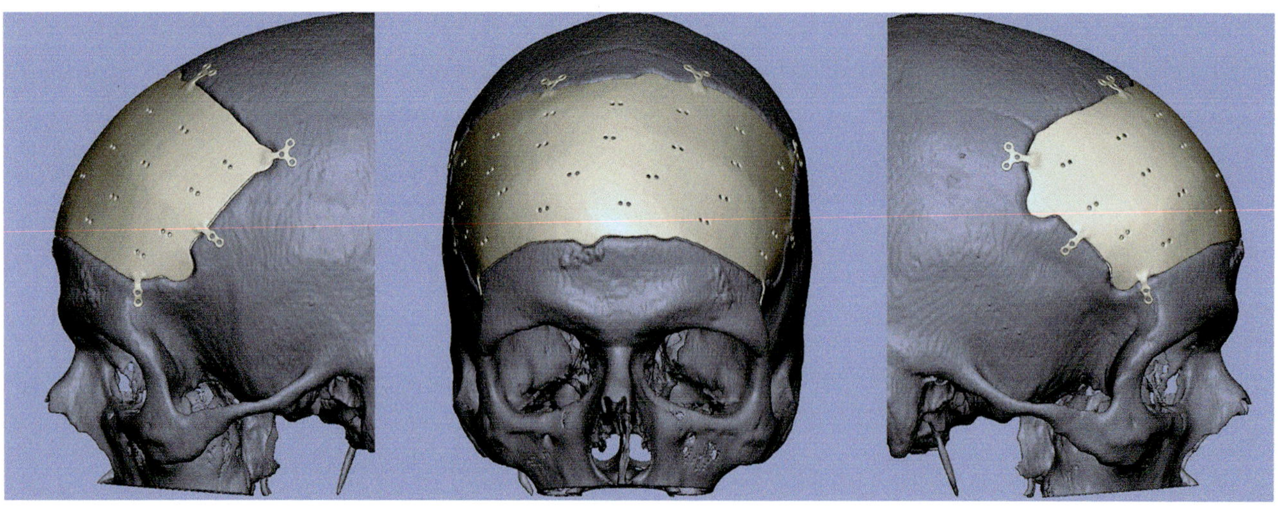

Fig. 4.13 Design for fabrication of cranial implant (Mimics Innovation Suite, Materialise, Leuven, Belgium)

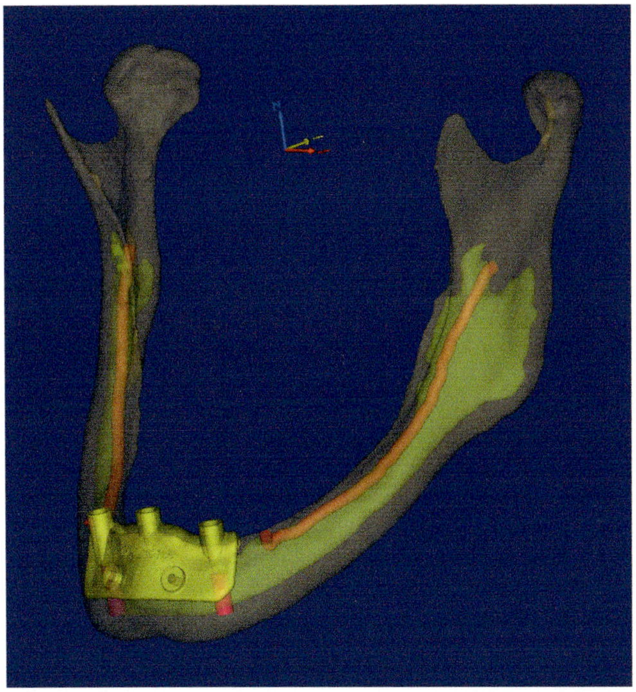

Fig. 4.14 Digital design of edentulous mandible with inferior alveolar nerve highlighted and surgical guide (Mimics Innovation Suite, Materialise, Leuven, Belgium)

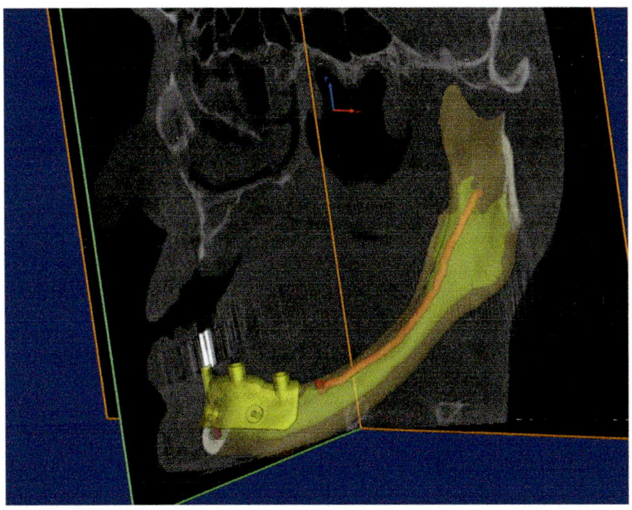

Fig. 4.15 Edentulous mandible positioned in the planes of the CT scan (Mimics Innovation Suite, Materialise, Leuven, Belgium)

Medical Models

In addition to virtual surgical planning, fabrication of medical models for presurgical planning has become very helpful in not only the planning phase, but as surgical guides for cutting, repositioning, and bending of bars, design of implants, as well as education of residents and patients (Figs. 4.18–4.22).These models are designed from medical images, generally CT or CBCT, but can be a combination of

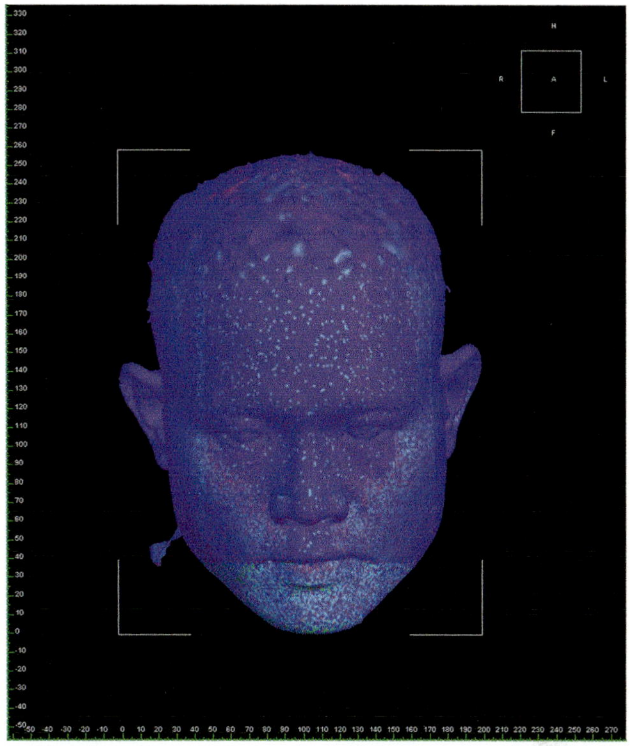

Fig. 4.16 Preliminary photogrammetry shot of patient with no swelling (3D Vultus, 3dMD, LLC, Atlanta, Georgia, USA)

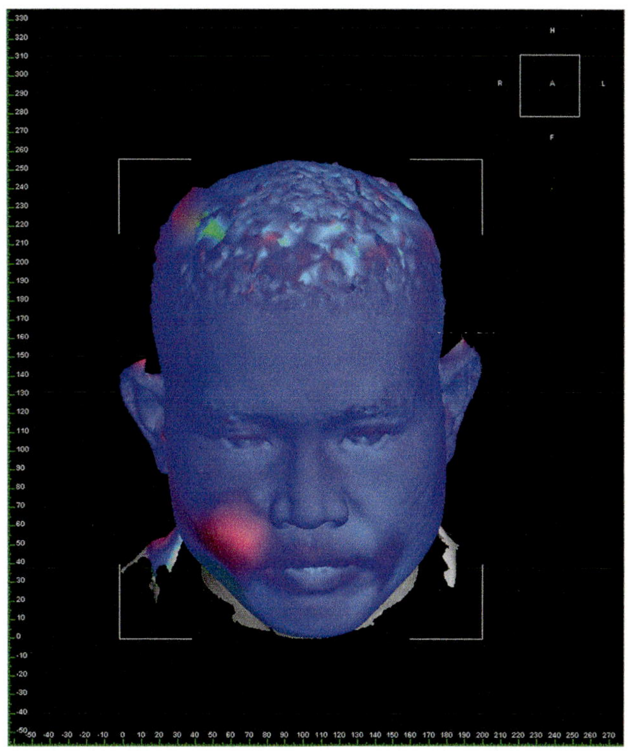

Fig. 4.17 Registration of the photogrammetry shot of patient of the original and with swelling noted on the *right* (3D Vultus, 3dMD, LLC, Atlanta, GA, USA)

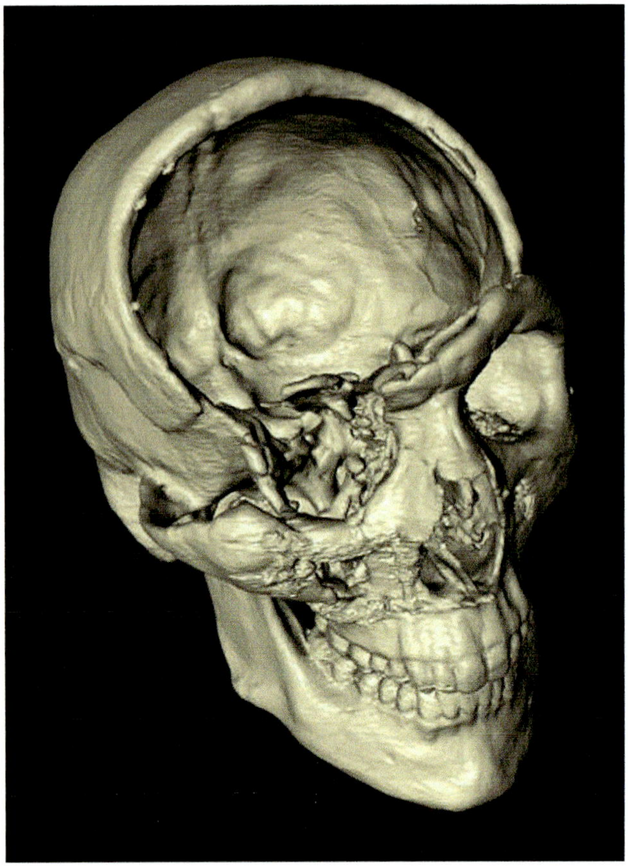

Fig. 4.18 Example of a 3D design from DICOM of a complex cranial fracture (Mimics Innovation Suite, Materialise, Leuven, Belgium)

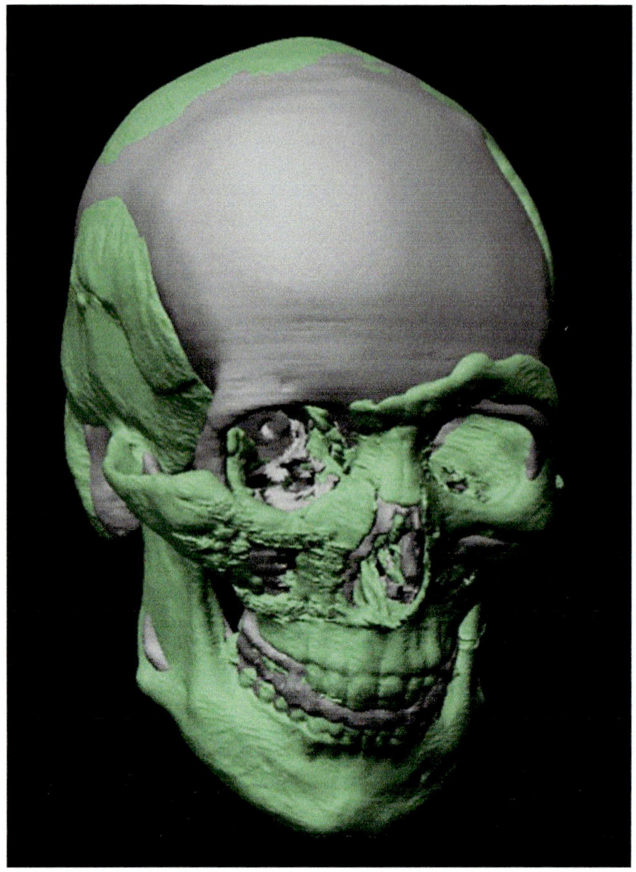

Fig. 4.19 By registering a pre-traumatic or similar skull to Fig. 4.18, the contours of the defect can be re-established to fabricate an implant and for treatment planning (Mimics Innovation Suite, Materialise, Leuven, Belgium)

many different scans as discussed previously. Models are reconstructed as an .stl file that is produced once the DICOM files have been converted through some kind of planning software. The .stl represents the 3D model that can be used for fabrication with additive or subtractive manufacturing technologies. Medical images are captured and described as "slices" in DICOM. These "slices" provide the information needed to develop a 3D model. The model captures all the required data in the scan per slice, so any internal features are maintained. The resolution of the model is relative to the size of the image slice; however, 1 mm or less is usually the maximum slice size adequate to fabricate an accurate surgical model [1]. Additive manufacturing or "3D printing" is ideal for the fabrication of anatomic models. Once a 3D model has been designed, it is once again "sliced" to provide layers to be fabricated based on the additive manufacturing technology used. The internal features are reproduced in the model and in some systems an anatomical structure can be given another color or darkened to separate the structures in the model. Subtractive techniques (milling) will only provide the surface contours from a solid block and are not well suited for medical models.

Medical models can be produced that provide a full-size or scaled model of the area in question; vessels, tumors, and hard tissues can all be produced from the medical images (Fig. 4.23). These models are an excellent guide to preplanning a reconstruction or tumor resection case. Models can be produced in clear materials with internal structures such as impacted teeth or nerves colored within the model (Fig. 4.24). Solid models from powder bed binding techniques provide models that will allow vessels, tumors, and bone all to be colored. Models can also be design to assemble and disassemble allowing a solid model to be taken apart to get to the internal structures (Fig. 4.25).

In addition to surgical models, physical models from imaging provide unique opportunities in graduate dental and medical education in helping to understand and coordinate three-dimensional structures with the images.

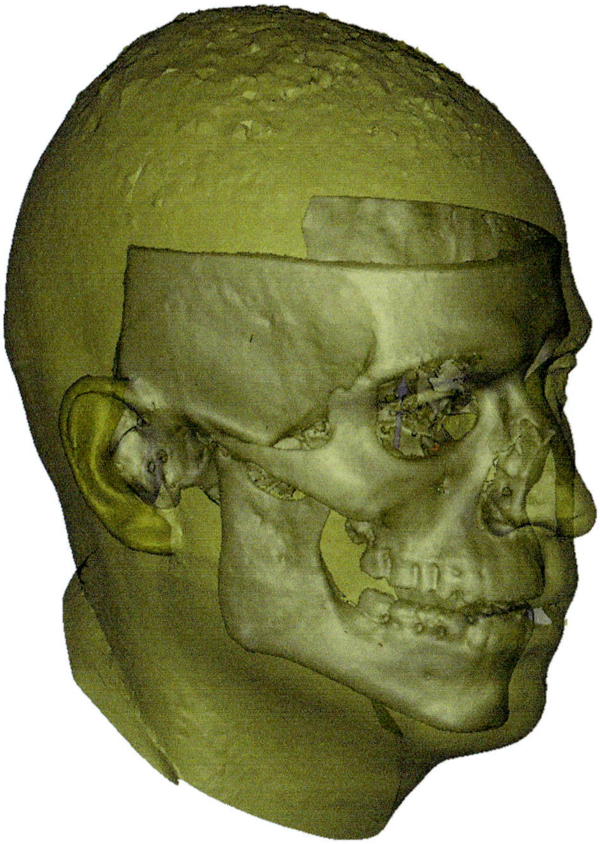

Fig. 4.20 A CBCT scan of bone and a surface 3D model of the soft tissue from photogrammetry can be registered to provide a more accurate reconstruction for treatment planning (3D Vultus, 3dMD, LLC, Atlanta, GA, USA)

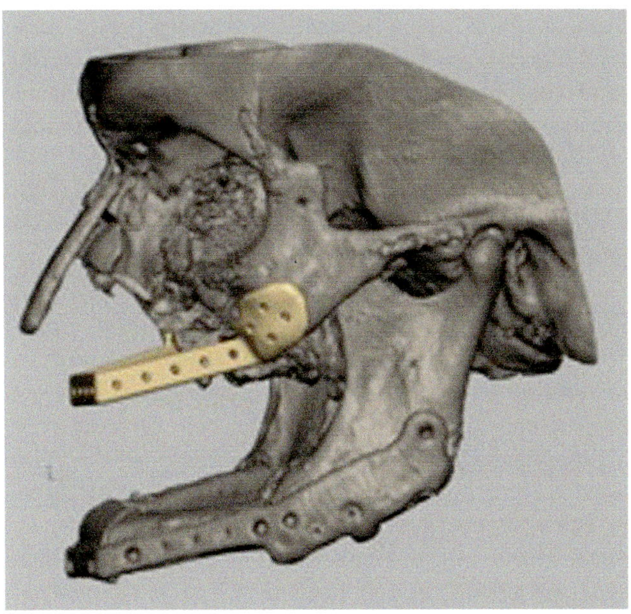

Fig. 4.21 A reconstruction custom implant support was designed to provide the projection for this complex mid-face reconstruction from a severe gunshot wound to the face left lateral 3D view (Mimics Innovation Suite, Materialise, Leuven, Belgium)

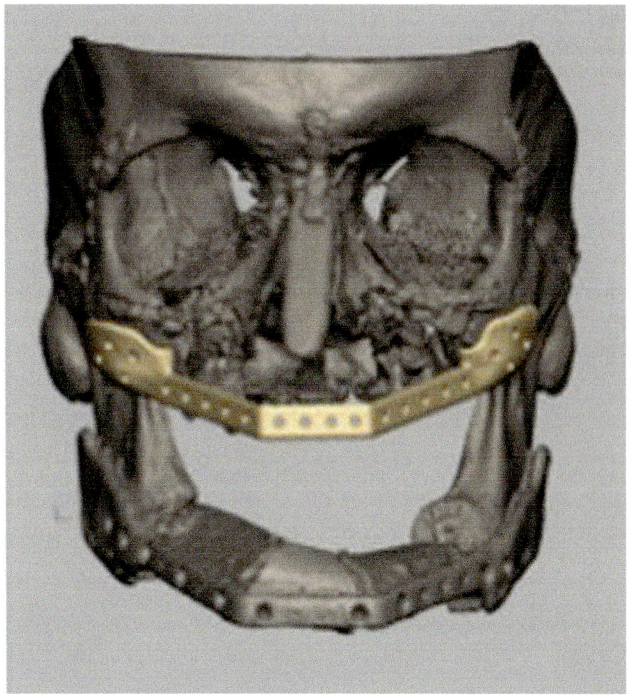

Fig. 4.22 Facial view of the same patient of Figure 4.21 (Mimics Innovation Suite, Materialise, Leuven, Belgium)

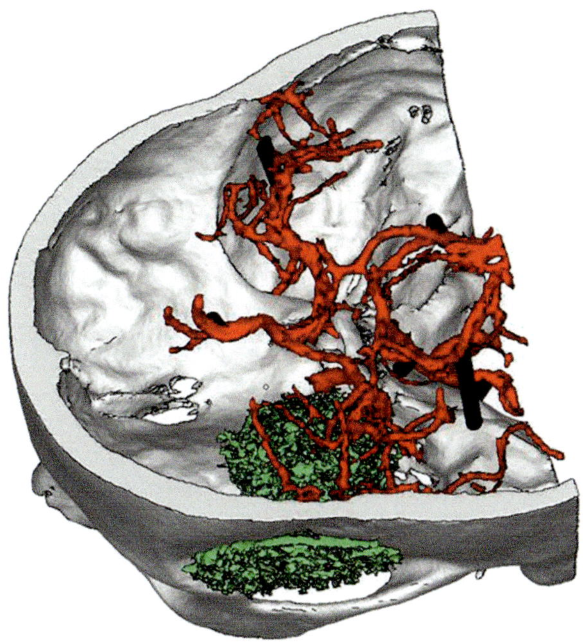

Fig. 4.23 Contrast with CT scans provides the opportunity to fabricate designs and models that separate tumors and vessels (Mimics Innovation Suite, Materialise, Leuven, Belgium)

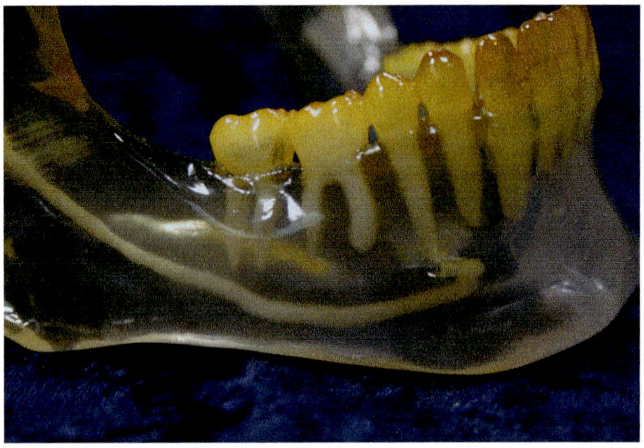

Fig. 4.24 Stereolithographic model, the teeth and the nerve can be treated to show as separate color (SLA 7000, 3D Systems Healthcare, Rock Hill, SC, USA)

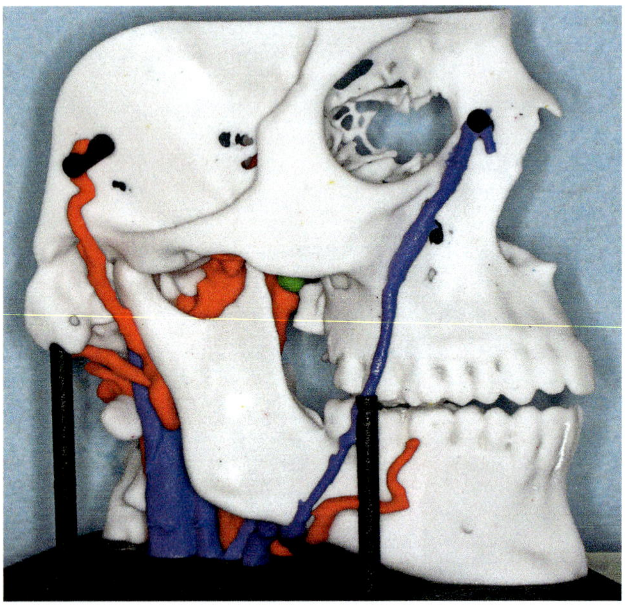

Fig. 4.25 Binder jetting techniques allow models to be printed in color, generally from a gypsum type of material, providing unprecedented information for treatment planning and in patient education (Project 660, 3d Systems Healthcare, Rock Hill, SC USA)

Face Alloplastic Transplants and Digital Technologies

Advances in facial reconstruction have recently been approached using a facial alloplastic transplantation of the missing facial structures that can take up to 30 h [17, 18]. The advantage is that not only the soft tissue but all of the structures including bone, muscle, nerves, and vasculature can be included in the graft. Over 25 patients have undergone a face transplant as of early 2014 worldwide [19]. However, most of the current maxillofacial single-jaw surgeries have suffered from some type of malocclusion [17]. In addition, the patient must commit to some type of daily antirejection treatment for the life of the graft. Recent developments in the use of image registration of donor and recipient, virtual surgical manipulation to develop the best outcome for dental occlusion, and combinations of cutting guides and guided surgical technologies have promise in addressing a lot of the issues with surgical time and difficult occlusal problems [20] (Figs. 4.26 and 4.27).

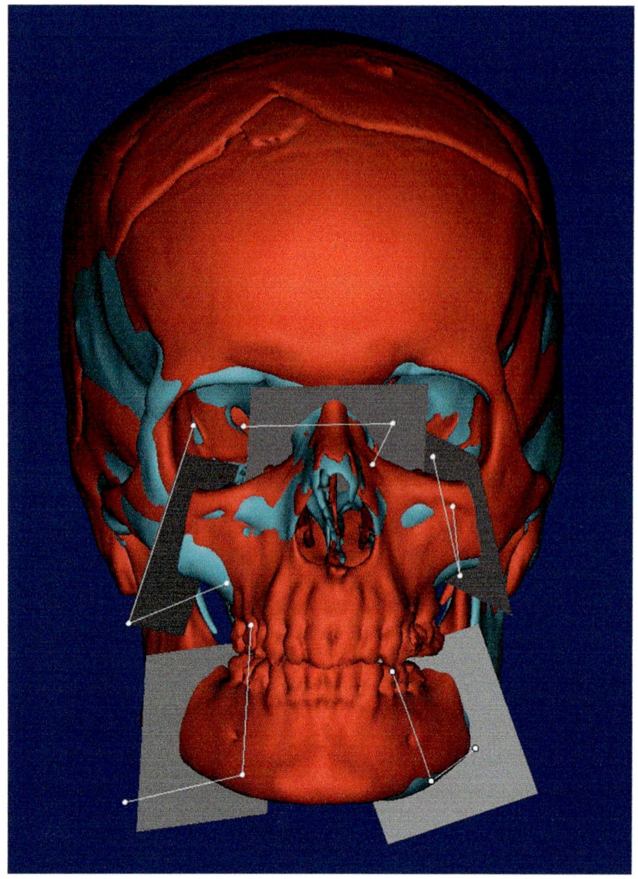

Fig. 4.26 The donor and recipient skulls can be registered to each other with cutting planes inserted for boney cuts in a face transplant (Mimics Innovation Suite, Materialise, Leuven, Belgium)

Future Expectations

Medical imaging technologies have begun to expand well past the radiographs and CT scanning; new advances in 3D digital photography, surface scanning, and ultrasound have provided images that can be developed into 3D models and in some instances the added dimension of movement. Reconstruction of medical images into 3D images of hard and soft tissues, virtual surgical manipulation of those images, and the manufacturing of surgical guides and custom devices have provided unprecedented opportunities in the reconstruction of the head and neck.

It has been reported that this technology has proven to decrease operating time and increase better outcomes for

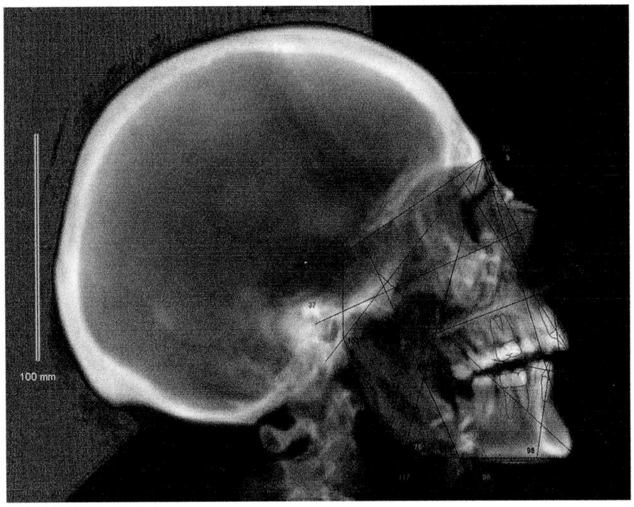

Fig. 4.27 Cephalometric calculations for a face transplant of the maxilla and anterior mandible (Dolphin Imaging, Dolphin Imaging and Management, Chatsworth, CA, USA)

patients [21]. Recently the Specialty of Radiology has embraced segmentation, 3D modeling, and the printing of medical models. In addition, working groups on the manufacturing of medical models can now be found as part of not only medical specialy groups such as the Radiology Society of North America, but in engineering such as the Society of Manufacturing Engineers.

References

1. Taft RM, Kondor S, Grant GT. Accuracy of rapid prototype models for head and neck reconstruction. J Prosthet Dent. 2011 Dec;106(6):399–408.
2. Grant GT, Liacouras PC, Kondor S. Maxillofacial trauma imaging in the trauma patient. Atlas Oral Maxillofac Surg Clin North Am. 2013 Mar;21(1):25–36.
3. Kozakiewicz M, Elgalal M, Loba P, et al. Clinical application of 3D pre-bent titanium implants for orbital floor fractures. J Craniomaxillofac Surg. 2009;37(4):229–34.
4. Cui J, Chen L, Guan X, Ye L, Wang H, Liu L. Surgical planning, three-dimensional model surgery and preshaped implants in treatment of bilateral craniomaxillofacial post-traumatic deformities. J Oral Maxillofac Surg. 2014;72(6):1138–e1-14.
5. Muller A, Krishnan KG, Uhl E, Mast G. The application of rapid prototyping techniques in cranial reconstruction and preoperative planning in neurosurgery. J Craniofac Surg. 2003;14(6):899–914.
6. Zurl B, Tiefling R, Whinkler P, Kindi P, Kapp KS. Hounsfied units variations: impact on CT density based conversion tables and their effects on dose distribution. Strahlenther Onkol. 2014 Jan;190(1):88–93.
7. Patel S, Dawood A, Ford TP, Whaites E. The potential applications of cone beam computed tomography in the management of endodontic problems. Int Endod J. 2007 Oct;40(10):818–30.
8. Jacobs R, Quirynen M. Dental cone beam computed tomography: justification for use in planning oral implant placement. Periodontol. 2014;66(1):203–13.
9. Makins SR. Artifacts interfering with interpretation of cone beam tomography images. Dent Clin N Am. 2014 Jul;58(3):485–95.
10. Maal TJ, van Loon B, Plooij JM, Rangel F, Ettema AM, Borstlap WA, Berge SJ. Registration of 3-dimenstional facial photographs for clinical use. J Oral Maxillofac Surg. 2010 Oct;68(10):2391–401.
11. Simanca E, Morris D, Zhao L, Reisberg D, Viana G. Measuring progressive soft tissue change with nasoalveolar molding using a three-dimensional system. J Craniofac Surg. 2011 Sept;22(5):1622–5.
12. Edgar D, Day R, Briffa NK, Cole J, Wood F. Volume measurements using the Polhemus FastSCAN 3D laser scanning: a novel application for burns clinical research. J Burn Care Res. 2008 Nov-Dec;29(6):994–1000.
13. Hiller J, Lipson H. STL 2.0: a proposal for a universal, multimaterial Additive Manufacturing File Format. In: Proceedings of the Solid Freeform Fabrication Symposium (SFF'09), Austin;2009. p. 266–278.
14. Parks CL, Richard AH, Monson KL. Preliminary performance assessment of computer automated facial approximations using computed tomography scans of living individuals. Forensic Sci Int. 2013;233(1-3):133–9.
15. Lindsay RW, Herberg M, Liacouras P. The use of three dimensional technology and additive manufacturing to create templates for soft-tissue reconstructions. Plast Reconstr Surg. 2012 Oct;130(4):629e–31e.
16. Antony AK, Chen WF, Kolokythas A, Weimer KA, Cohn MN. Use of virtual surgery and stereolithography-guided osteotomy for mandibular reconstruction with the free fibula. Plast Reconstr Surg. 2011 Nov;128(5):1080–4.
17. Gordon CR, Susarla S, Peacock Z, et al. Le Fort-based maxillofacial transplantation: current state-of-the-art and refined technique. J Craniofac Surg. 2012;23:81–7.
18. Siemionow M, Papay F, Alam D, et al. Near total face transplantation in severely disfigured patient in the USA. Lancet. 2009;374:203–9.
19. Singhal D, Pribaz JJ, Pomahac B. The Brigham and Women's Hospital face transplant program: a look back. Plast Reconstr Surg 2012 Jan;129(1):81e–88e.
20. Gordon CR, Murphy RJ, Coon D, Otake Y, Basafa E, Al Rakan M, Rada E, Susarla S, Swanson E, Fishman E, Santiago G, Brandacher G, Andrew Lee WP, Liacouras P, Grant G, Armand M. Preliminary development of a preliminary development of a workstation for craniomaxillofacial surgical procedures – introducing a computer-assisted planning and execution (CAPE) system. J Craniofac Surg. 2014;25(1):273–83.
21. Hsieh TY, Dedhia R, Cervenka B, Tollefson TT. 3D Printing: current use in facial plastic and reconstructive surgery. Curr Opin Otolaryngol Head Neck Surg 2017 Aug; 25(4)291–299.

Clinical Cone Beam CT and CT-Guided Dental Implant Surgery

5

Alex M. Greenberg and Leslie H. Sultan

CT scanning, rapid printing and prototyping, optical scanning, and CAD CAM milling can now be utilized in a cohesive manner so that the virtual planning for the optimal placement of dental implants can be clinically implemented [1–4]. The benefits for patients can be decreased operating time, flapless procedures [5, 6] with reduced postoperative pain and swelling, and immediate temporization [7–9]. As a result of this digital revolution, surgeons can develop improved diagnosis, more accurate implant placement, and better long-term results. In depth understanding of clinical CBCT is essential for the diagnosis and treatment planning of dental implant patients. The evolution of CT scanning from fan beam to spiral methods [10, 11] (Fig. 5.1a, b) has allowed the development of in-office cone beam CT (CBCT) scanners [12–15] (Fig. 5.2a–c) which are now a widely used dental imaging method. Stand up, lie down, sitting, and mobile CBCT units are available. CBCT is based on plain tomography which was developed in the 1930s by Vallebona [16]. Plain tomography allowed the sectioning of an anatomic structure from the surrounding organs as a plain radiographic series of images. At present, the Orthopantomograph provides panoramic images (Fig. 5.3) that are an example of continued use of plain tomography [17]. With the advent of computers, it became possible to further develop plain tomography into a more sophisticated form of 3D imaging. Hounsfield and Cormack independently developed the concept for CT scanning [18–21], for which they shared the Nobel Prize in 1979 [22, 23]. It was Hounsfield who actually created the first CT scanner that could image the brain. From this early unit, CT scanning of the whole body using the fan beam technique was later developed [24]. With newer computer and scintillator technological advances, spiral (helical) CT scanning machines were built [25, 26], and it is from helical scanners that CBCT is derived based on the work of Kalendar [27–29].

The basic mathematical method for CT scanning is the use of Radon's transform developed in 1917 [30] (Fig. 5.4), based on back projection geometry [31–34] (Fig. 5.5). The methods for calculating the algorithm are based on either the iterative reconstruction (IR) [35–37] or filtered back projection (FBP) [38, 39]. The FBP needs less time for computation [38, 39], while the IR results in fewer artifacts [35–37]. Computers provide the ability to mathematically analyze and create the reformatted images in various planes of axial, sagittal, and coronal projections (Figs. 5.6, 5.7, and 5.8), 2D panoramic (Fig. 5.9) and lateral cephalometric (Fig. 5.10) images as well as 3D (Fig. 5.11) and oblique sagittal reformatted images (Fig. 5.12) [40].

Cone beam CT allows patients to be scanned at a significant reduction in radiation exposure with powerful algorithms and lowered cancer risk compared to helical CT [41, 42]. With 72 million studies reported in the USA, CT contributes to the overall rise in radiation exposure to patients [43], when compared to plain radiography. The greatly increased exposure of populations to radiation in the developed countries from CT scans where large numbers of these imaging studies have been performed has led to considerable concern for increased cancer rates [44]. A direct correlation between the large increases in CT scans is related to the increased numbers of available medical CT scanners. Numerous reports have raised concern regarding increased cancer rates from increased CT imaging radiation [45]. However it is estimated that as a result of the high utilization of CT scanners, there are negligible increases in cancer as compared to those that result from background environmental radiation exposure. For example, it is estimated that 500 individuals will die from cancer as a result of radiation exposure from the approximately 600,000 abdominal and head

A.M. Greenberg (✉)
Division of Oral and Maxillofacial Surgery, Columbia University College of Dental Medicine, 18 East 48th Street Suite 1702, New York, NY 10017, USA
e-mail: nycimplant@aol.com

L.H. Sultan
Department of Surgery, Broward Health Medical Center, Fort Lauderdale, FL, USA

A.M. Greenberg (ed.), *Digital Technologies in Craniomaxillofacial Surgery*, https://doi.org/10.1007/978-1-4939-1532-3_5

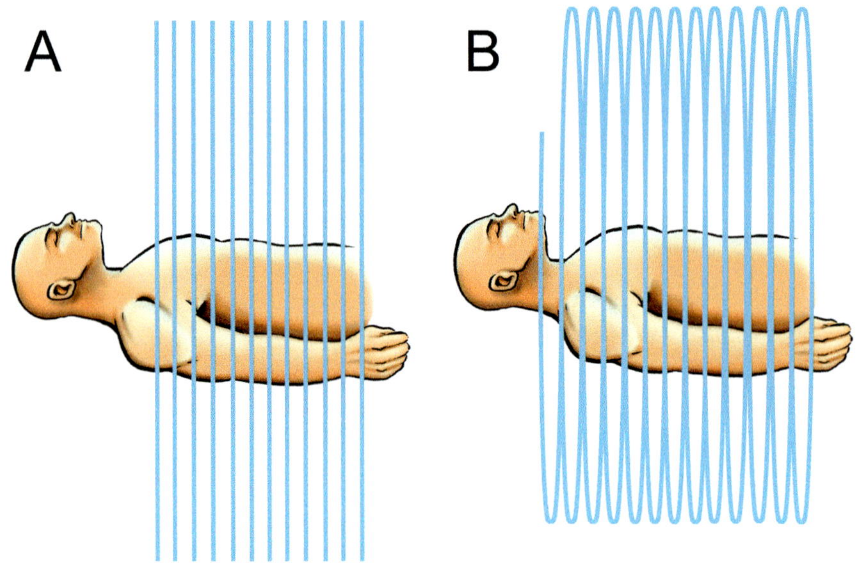

Fig. 5.1 (**a**) Fan beam CT and (**b**) helical (spiral) CT

CT examinations performed each year in children under 15 years of age in the USA [46].

A further understanding of the radiation exposure of patients from plain and CT radiography can be helpful in deciding when such studies are appropriate and to answer patient's concerns. Ludlow et al. [47] have reviewed that the radiation exposure from plain dental radiography effective doses as full-mouth exposures = 34.9–170.7 (μSv), bitewing = 5(μSv), and panoramic =14.2–24.3 (μSv) can be compared to the background annual radiation exposure from the environment = 3100 (μSv) [48]. Roberts et al. [49] have reported that CBCT radiation dosage is found to be full FOV (field of view) 206.2 (μSv), 13 cm FOV 133.9 (μSv), 6 cm FOV high-resolution maxilla 93.3 (μSv), 5 cm FOV high-resolution mandible 188.5 (μSv), 6 cm standard mandible 96.2 (μSv), and 6 cm standard maxilla 58.9 (μSv), The FOV radiation can vary between different CBCT machines from 51.7 to 193.4 (μSv). There appears to be considerable concern regarding the lack of uniformity and evidence-based understanding of various CBCT scanners' actual radiation doses [50]. Compared to a medical helical CT scan of the head = 2000 (μSv) [51], the average radiation dosage from CBCT is substantially lower at 5–10% (51.7–193.4 (μSv). Depending on the CBCT scanner and FOV, the radiation dosage equivalent to a multiple of panoramic radiographs ranges for a 12″ FOV scan from 2 to 4 (15–78 μSv) and a for a 9″ FOV scan 1–1 ½ (5–33 μSv) [47, 49]. A further reference is the greatly increased risk of cancer from radiation exposure from a full body scan, which has been compared to the rate in atomic bomb survivors [52].

The CBCT images have excellent bone window resolution but lack the soft tissue details of helical CT scans. These images have become essential to contemporary dental implant treatment because they allow the correct diagnosis, highly detailed representations of critical anatomic structures, precise measurements, and treatment planning in both 2D and 3D. CBCT through the use of Hounsfield units can also provide the determination as to whether the patient has suitable bone density. Hounsfield units [53] range from 0 to 1000 (bone =400+, water = 0, and air = 1000) [54].

The use of CBCT also provides imaging information regarding key anatomic structures such as the nasopalatine foramen [55] (Fig. 5.13a, b), mental foramina [56–58] (Fig. 5.14), mandibular canals [59, 60] (Fig. 5.15), and sinus cavity [61, 62] (Fig. 5.16a, b) positions. This allows the prevention of complications such as nerve injuries and injudicious sinus perforation. The presence of other dental or osseous pathology, whether impacted teeth [63–65] (Fig. 5.17a, b), cysts [66–68] (Fig. 5.18a–d), endodontic infections [69] (Fig. 5.19), periodontal disease [70] (Fig. 5.20a, b), dental caries [71] (Fig. 5.21), and malignant [72–74] (Fig. 5.22a, b) or benign tumors [75–87] (Fig. 5.23a–c), can also be visualized with CBCT.

The panoramic and reformatted oblique sagittal views are the most important for planning the placement of dental implants [88, 89]. The panoramic view allows a rapid survey of the patient's dental condition, general understanding of bone height, and the presence of pathology. Full field of view (FOV) machines provide panoramic views, while machines with more limited views do not. The reformatted oblique sagittal views allow detailed cross-sectional evaluation of the maxilla or mandible and provide information concerning the width and height of the bone [90]. These views can have the cuts adjusted to be narrower or wider. This allows the clinician the ability to measure the bone height and width to determine sizes of implants that can be placed, and whether localized bone graft augmentation is necessary. These views can also allow better evaluation of the posterior mandible with marking of the mandibular nerve, mental foramen, and incisive nerve branches (Fig. 5.24). It has been shown that there can be multiple branches of the mandibular nerve, vari-

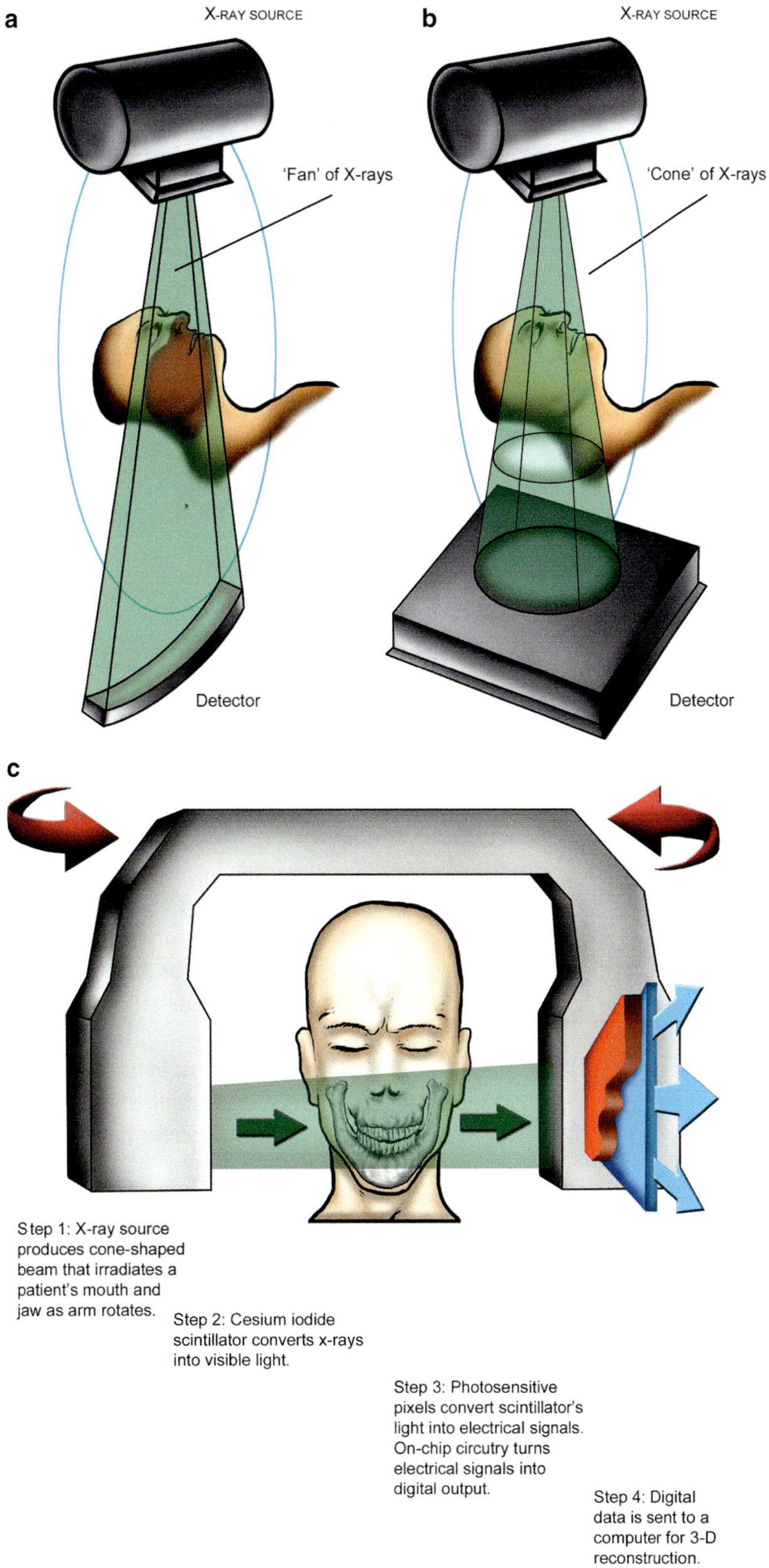

Fig. 5.2 (**a**) Fan beam CT scanner, (**b**) cone beam CT scanner, and (**c**) stand up/sitting flat plane scanner

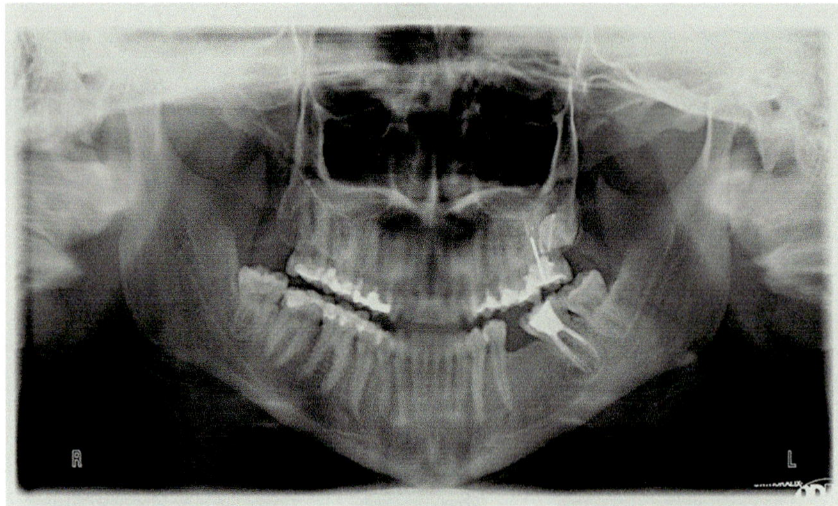

Fig. 5.3 Panoramic radiograph

$$Rf(L) = \int_L f(x)\,|dx|.$$

Fig. 5.4 Radon's transform formula

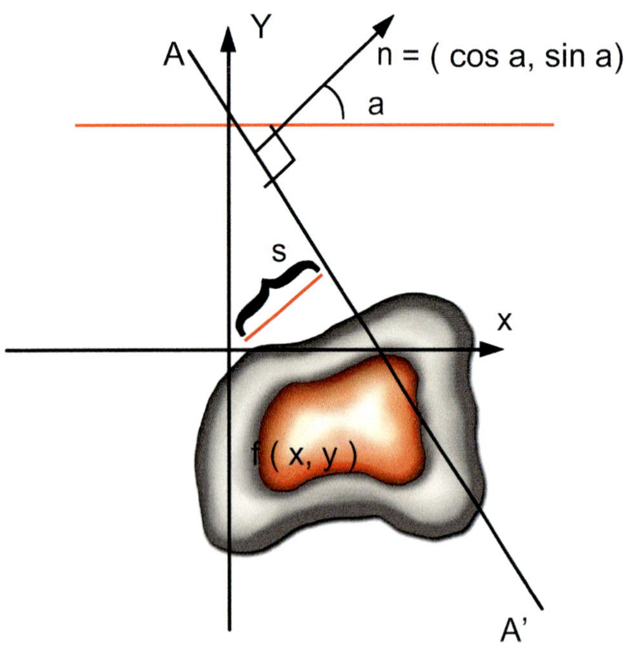

Fig. 5.5 Radon's transform back projection geometry

ation in the mental foramen position, and anterior loop of the mandibular nerve before exiting as the mental nerve [91]. Dual or bifid mandibular canals are noted in 15.6% of patients [92]. The mandibular incisive nerve is present in 93% of CBCT scans [93]. Accessory mental foramina can be found in 7% of patients CBCT images [94]. The reformatted oblique sagittal views can also be utilized in extraction cases for simultaneous implant placement whether preoperative or following removal of the tooth [95] (Fig. 5.25).

For dental implant planning, it is the oblique sagittal images (Fig. 5.26) that are the most important as they provide the cross-sectional images of the mandible or maxilla that provide both the height and width dimensions that are critical to planning dental implant position for trajectory and depth. These images can be matched to a 3D image of the bone and dental prosthesis in a virtual environment that permits a prosthetically driven placement of dental implants [96] (Fig. 5.27a, b). In this way, it is not just a matter of placing the dental implant where there is adequate bone, but also taking into consideration the ideal position of the dental implant for the fabrication of the individual crown or multiple unit prosthesis. This can also be useful in planning dental implant positions for screw versus cement retained restorations which have different trajectory positions relative to the prosthesis and dentition. Depth control allows the precise placement of dental implants for immediate restoration as in full-arch edentulous prosthesis such as "All on 4" types of cases [97] or for the avoidance of key anatomic structures such as the mandibular nerves, mental foramen, and maxillary sinuses [98]. Jenson et al. have reported on the "shelf technique" of bone reduction for immediate placement of dental implants and prosthesis [99, 100]. Modular templates with an outer framework containing a guideway can be utilized for bone reduction with a modular part containing the drill sleeves inserted for implant drill sequence and implant placement [101, 102].

These CBCT images can also be utilized in other software applications that can allow a STL output for fabrication of

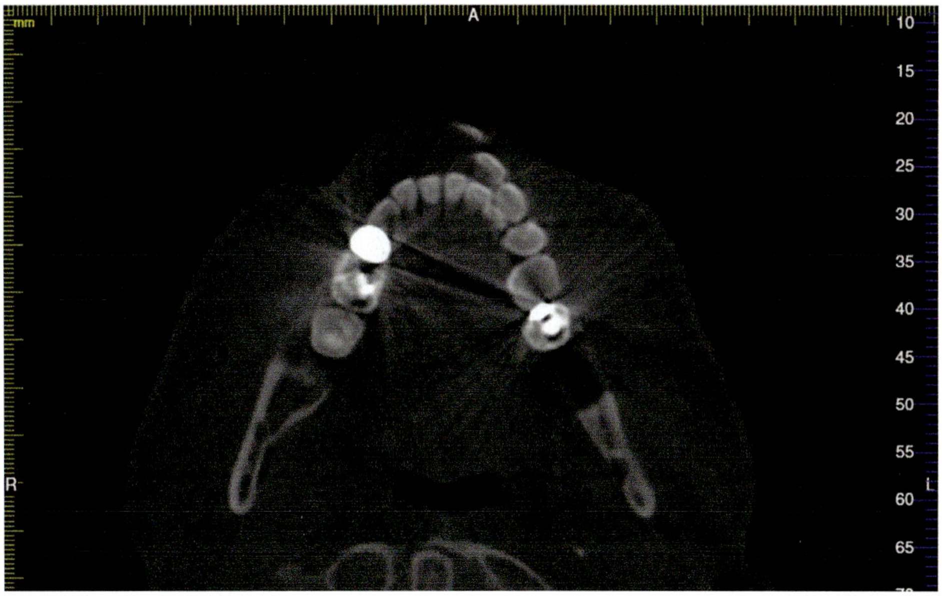

Fig. 5.6 CBCT axial view

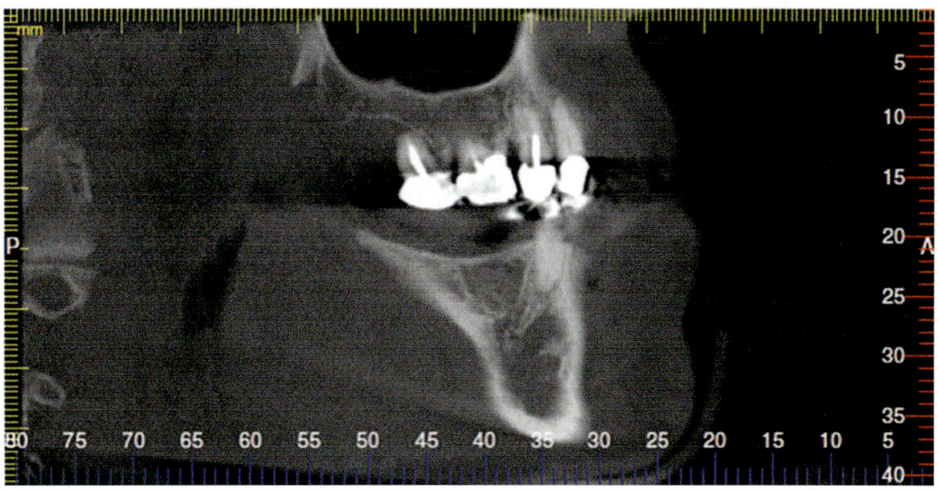

Fig. 5.7 CBCT sagittal view

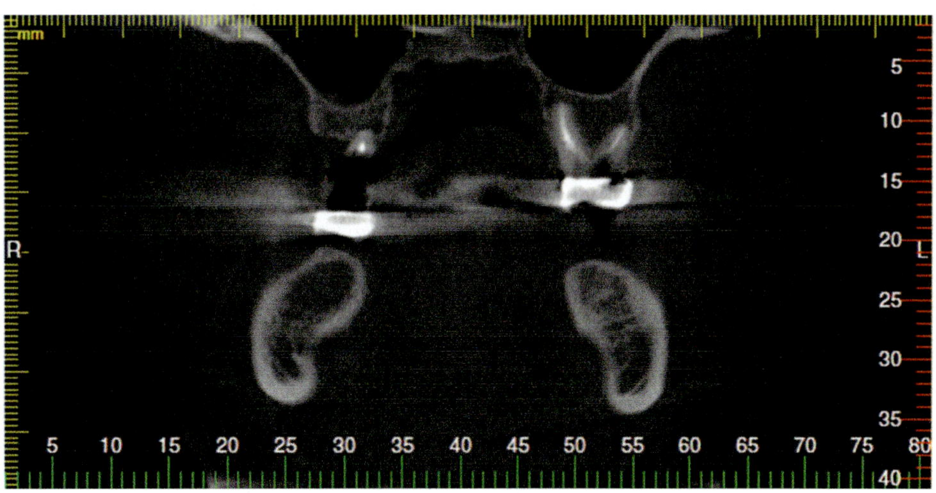

Fig. 5.8 CBCT coronal view

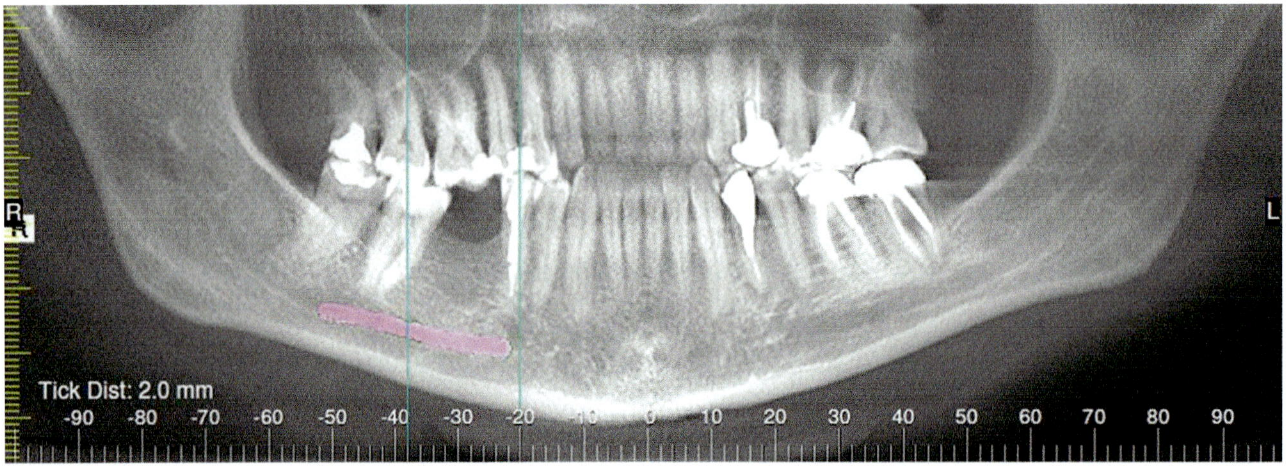

Fig. 5.9 CBCT panoramic view

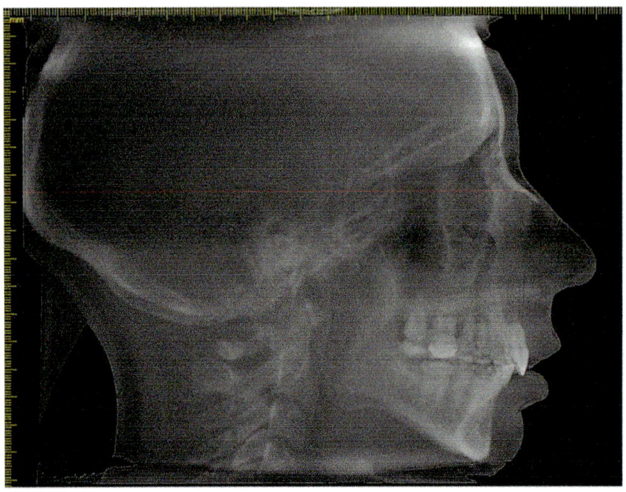

Fig. 5.10 CBCT lateral cephalometric view

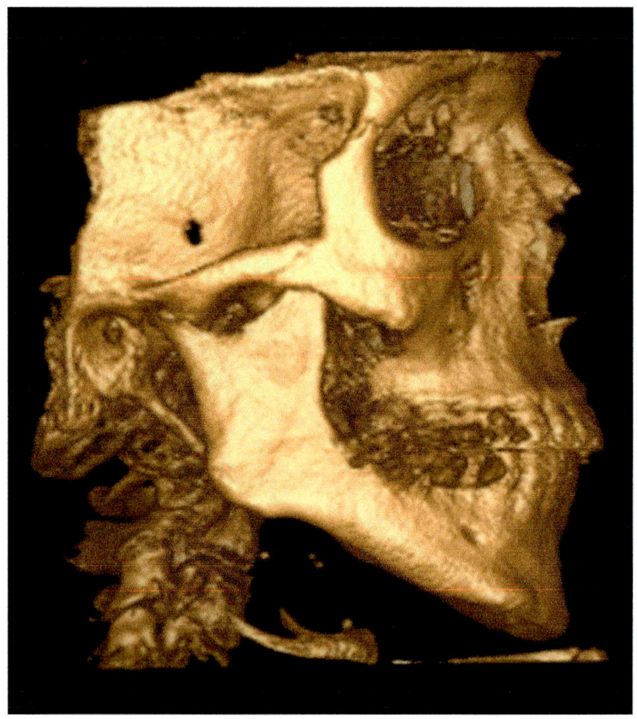

Fig. 5.11 CBCT 3D lateral view

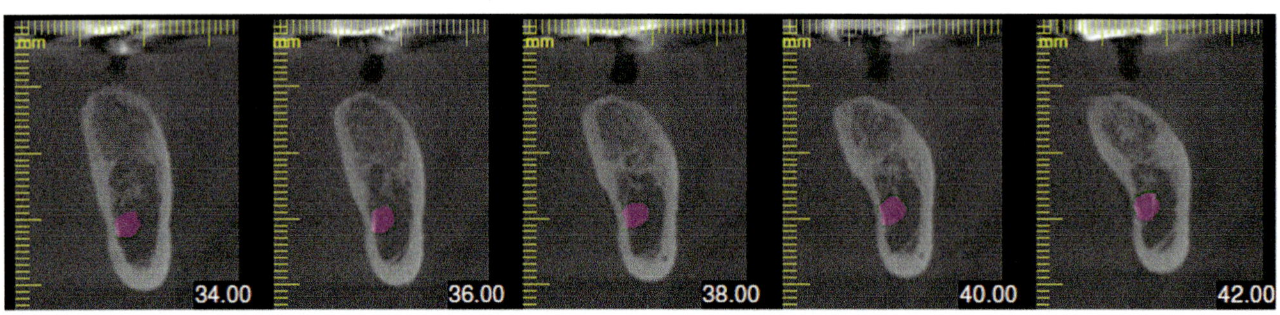

Fig. 5.12 CBCT reformatted oblique sagittal view of the mandible

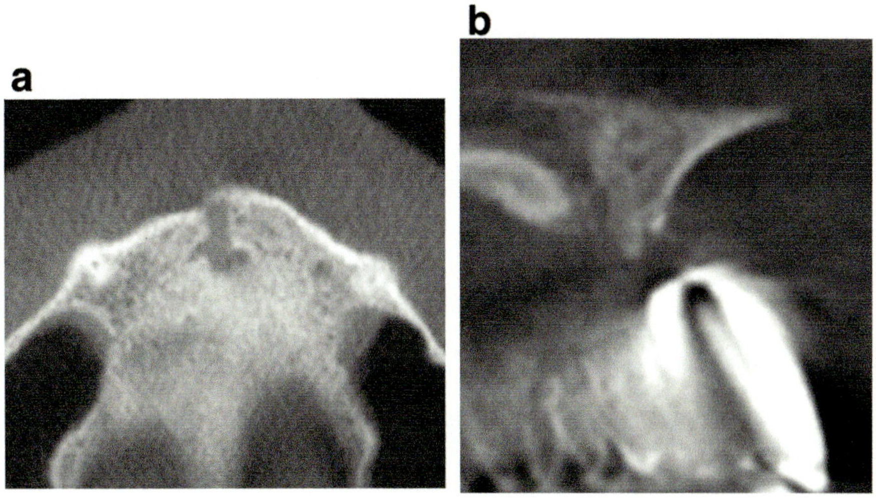

Fig. 5.13 CBCT (**a**) axial view incisive foramen and (**b**) sagittal view incisive foramen

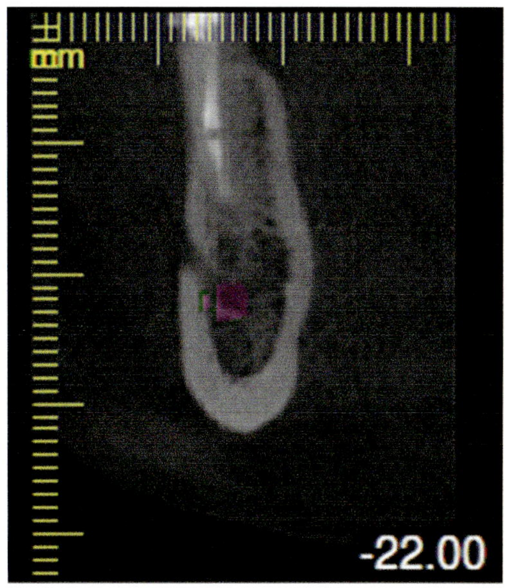

Fig. 5.14 CBCT sagittal view mental foramen

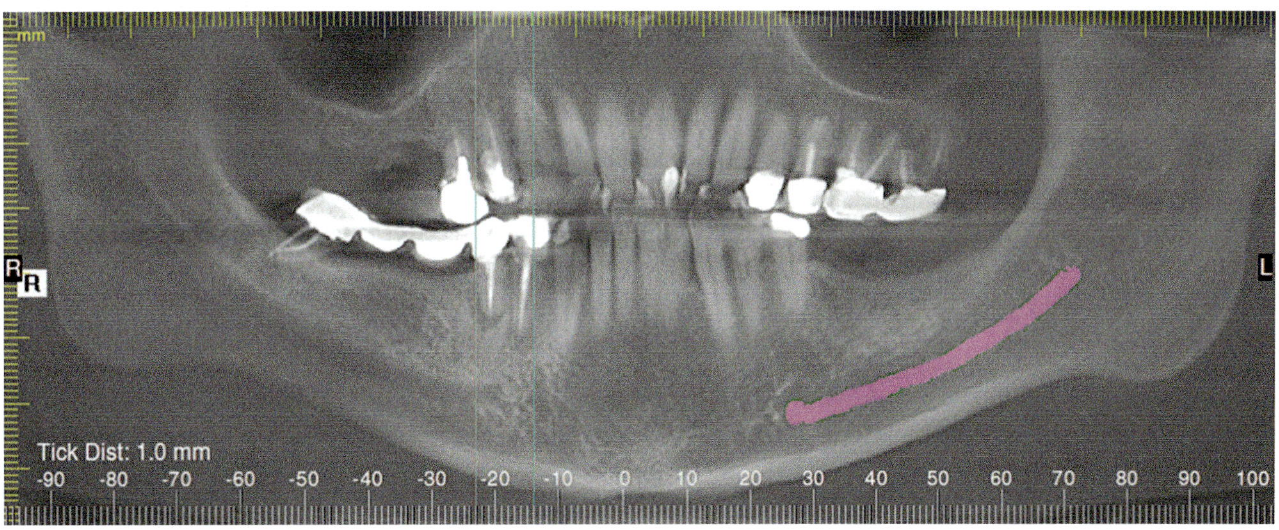

Fig. 5.15 CBCT panoramic view with marking of *left* mandibular canal

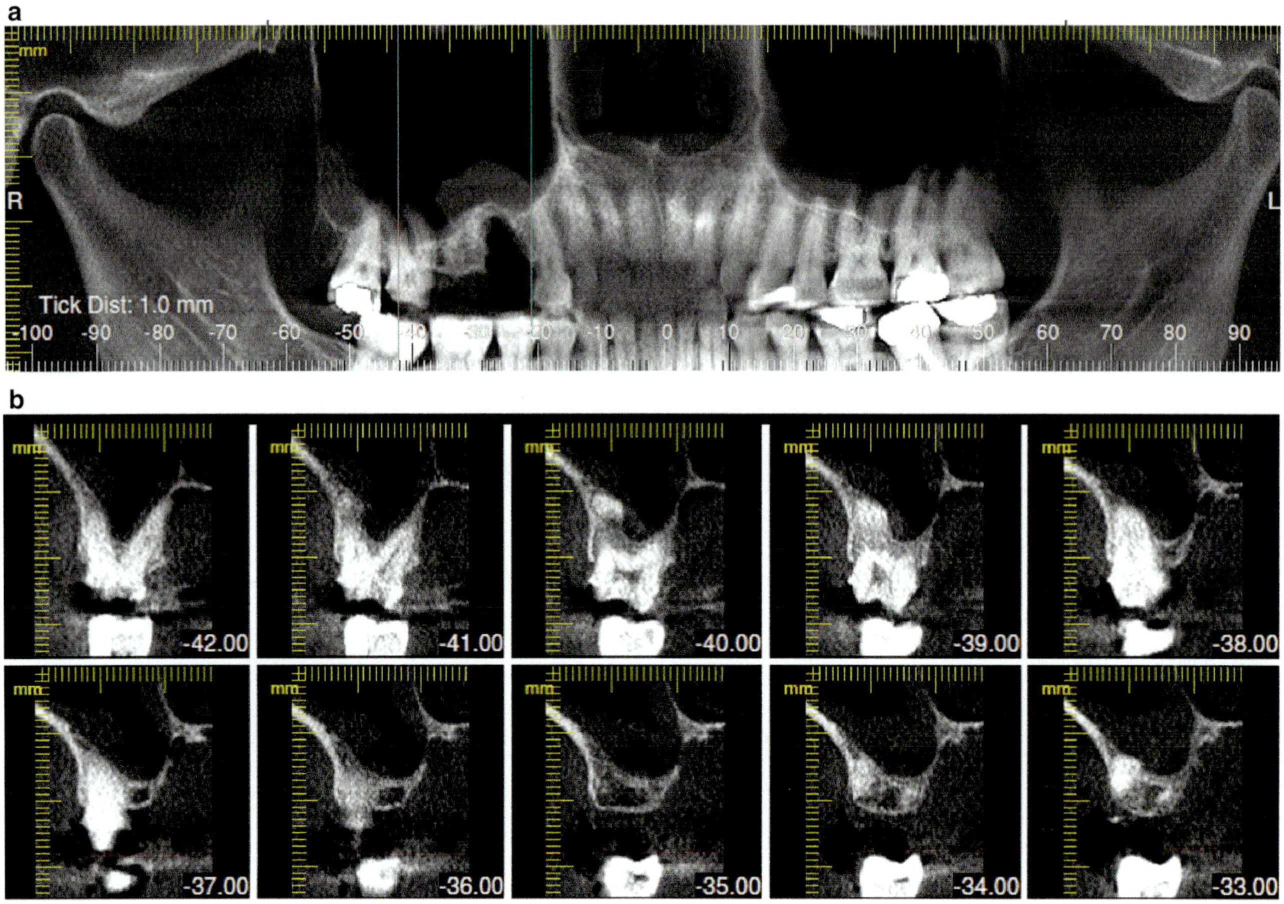

Fig. 5.16 (**a**) CBCT panoramic view of maxillary sinuses. (**b**) CBCT reformatted oblique sagittal view of the maxillary sinus. Note, right maxillary sinus floor mucosal thickening

custom patient-specific surgical drill guides by rapid printing or prototyping for clinical use (Fig. 5.28). The CT-based patient-specific surgical drill guide allows the surgeon to achieve the optimal implant positions through preoperative planning [103, 104]. The presurgical software planning includes the determination of adequate bone height and width, need for site development with bone grafting, whether as simple or complex alveolar ridge augmentation, sinus bone augmentation via indirect and direct techniques, sites for immediate extraction and implant placement, teeth with decay, and periodontal or endodontic infections [95].

The acquisition of the data can be from a variety of methods which can include single scan, dual scan, combined CT, and optical methods. Optical methods can include the intraoral scanning of the patient's dentition [105] (Fig. 5.29) or of a dental model. The data sets can be merged so as to manage the artifacts created from the scatter caused by radiation particles striking metallic dental restorations [106] (Fig. 5.30a, b). For the dual scan procedure, it is necessary to have a laboratory-fabricated radiographic template in which fiducial markers are placed (Fig. 5.31a, b). These markers can be made from gutta-percha or metal balls. These fiducial markers allow the merger of two data sets [99]. The first data set is of the patient with the radiographic template in the mouth correctly seated (Fig. 5.31c). The second data set is from imaging of the radiographic template by itself in a Styrofoam box (Fig. 5.32). The purpose of having two data sets is to produce an artifact free image of the radiographic template which can then be manipulated by the planning software to contain the implant trajectories, and a surgical drill guide is then rapid printed from the STL file. Artifacts are created from the gamma radiation striking the patient's dental metallic restorations which creates scatter effects in the 3D image that obscures the dental anatomy. Another method for the dual scanning process is to place the fiducial markers into the actual prosthesis which converts the removable partial or complete denture into a radiographic template. The two data sets are then uploaded to a fileshare at a vendor's website so that the data sets can be merged, converted, and then returned to the dentist for use in the planning software. In this way, a clean image of the patient's dentition free of artifacts allows prosthetic planning and rapid printing of an accurately fitting drill guide for tooth-borne cases.

Software planning allows for the conversion of the virtual image of the patient's bony anatomy and planned dental implant positions and depths through the fabrication of a sur-

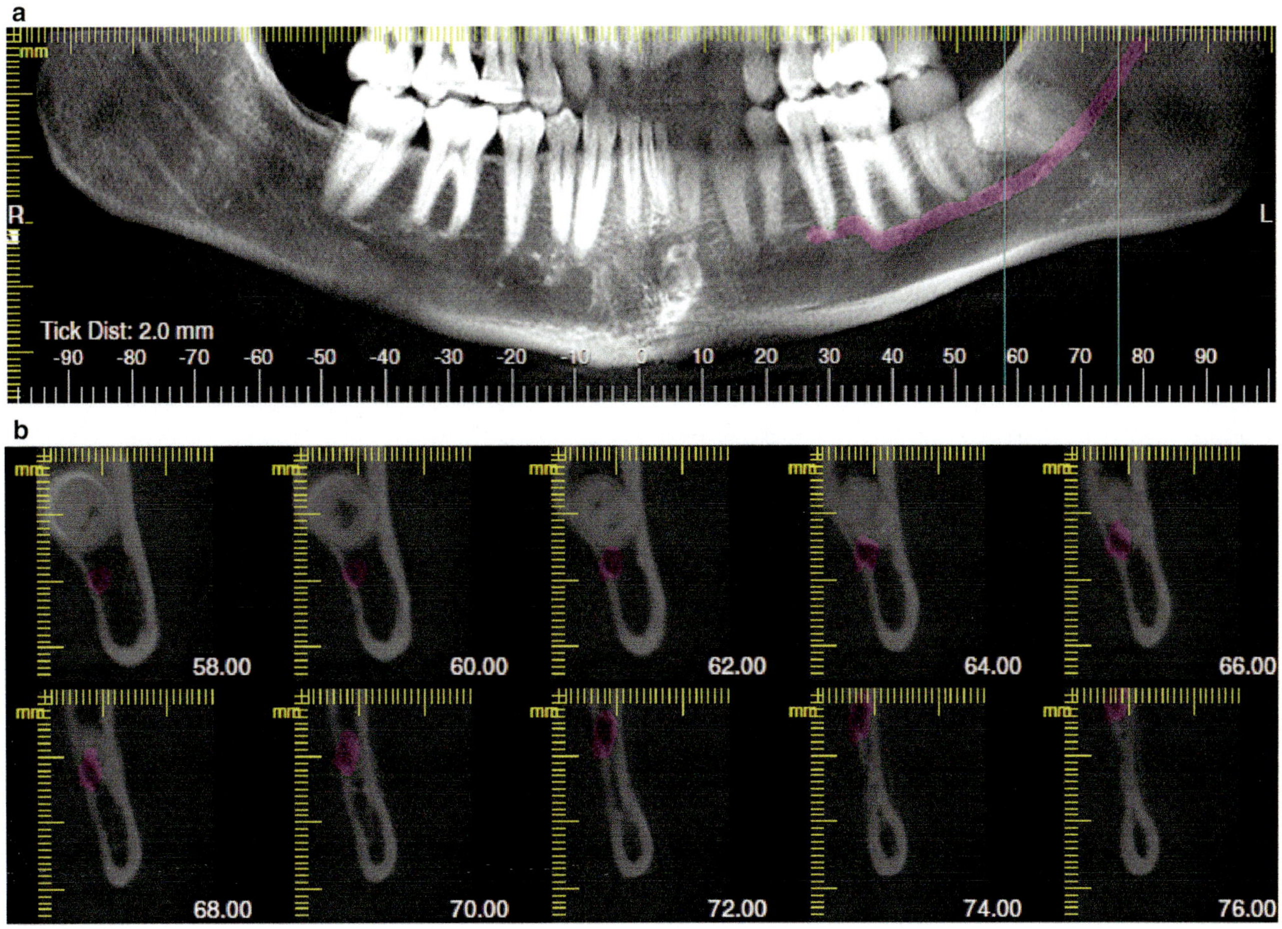

Fig. 5.17 (**a**) CBCT panoramic view of mandibular impacted *left* third molar with mandibular canal marking demonstrating intimate relationship with root apex. (**b**) CBCT reformatted oblique sagittal views of mandibular impacted *left* third molar with mandibular canal marking demonstrating intimate relationship with root apex

gical drill template produced by rapid manufacturing and rapid printing technologies [107] (Fig. 5.33). When it is converted from the virtual image by rapid printing, the actual surgical drill guide will have the precise information regarding the planned implant trajectories and surgical depth transferred to it. These guides can be bone-borne, tooth-borne, mucosal-borne, or a combination of seatings [108, 109]. Stabilization of surgical guides can be performed by nondominant hand or an assistant pressing the guide down (Fig. 5.40) or with surgical pins or screws (Fig. 5.34a–c). These screw or pin stabilizer channels can be planned in the software and produced in the surgical drill guide [107]. The drill guides have metal sleeves placed into the trajectories so that drill bits can be placed directly in them or through handles sized for different diameter drill bits. There are many manufacturers that provide their own CT-guided implant surgery drill kits (Fig. 5.35a–c). These kits provide all of the instrumentation necessary to perform CT-guided implant surgery with rapid printed drill guides. Once the drill guide has been fabricated, the first step is to place the metal drill sleeves into the surgical guide. These sleeves can have set diameters (Fig. 5.36a-e) which accommodate a specific drill bit width. In order to use different-sized drill bits, multiple surgical guides are printed, and each has a different diameter drill sleeve placed. The surgical guides are then changed during the drilling sequence. A master type of metal drill sleeve (Fig. 5.33 and 5.40) is to accommodate different drill handles which have specific drill bit diameters [109] (Fig. 5.37a–k), so that with a single drill guide, multiple drill bits can be used. If the software is also used to plan the exact implant depth, the top portion of the drill sleeve is placed at a height in a preset position in the drill guide so that when the drill bit is utilized, either a drill with a set stop is utilized or to a specific measurement mark in the drill bit (Fig. 5.38a–c). There are also implant mounts that can then allow the placement of the dental implant to a precise depth through the master sleeve (Fig. 5.39). In this manner, not only do they allow the drilling of the implant osteotomy to the precise trajectory and depth, but also allow the precise placement of the implant. This is accomplished with specially designed fixture

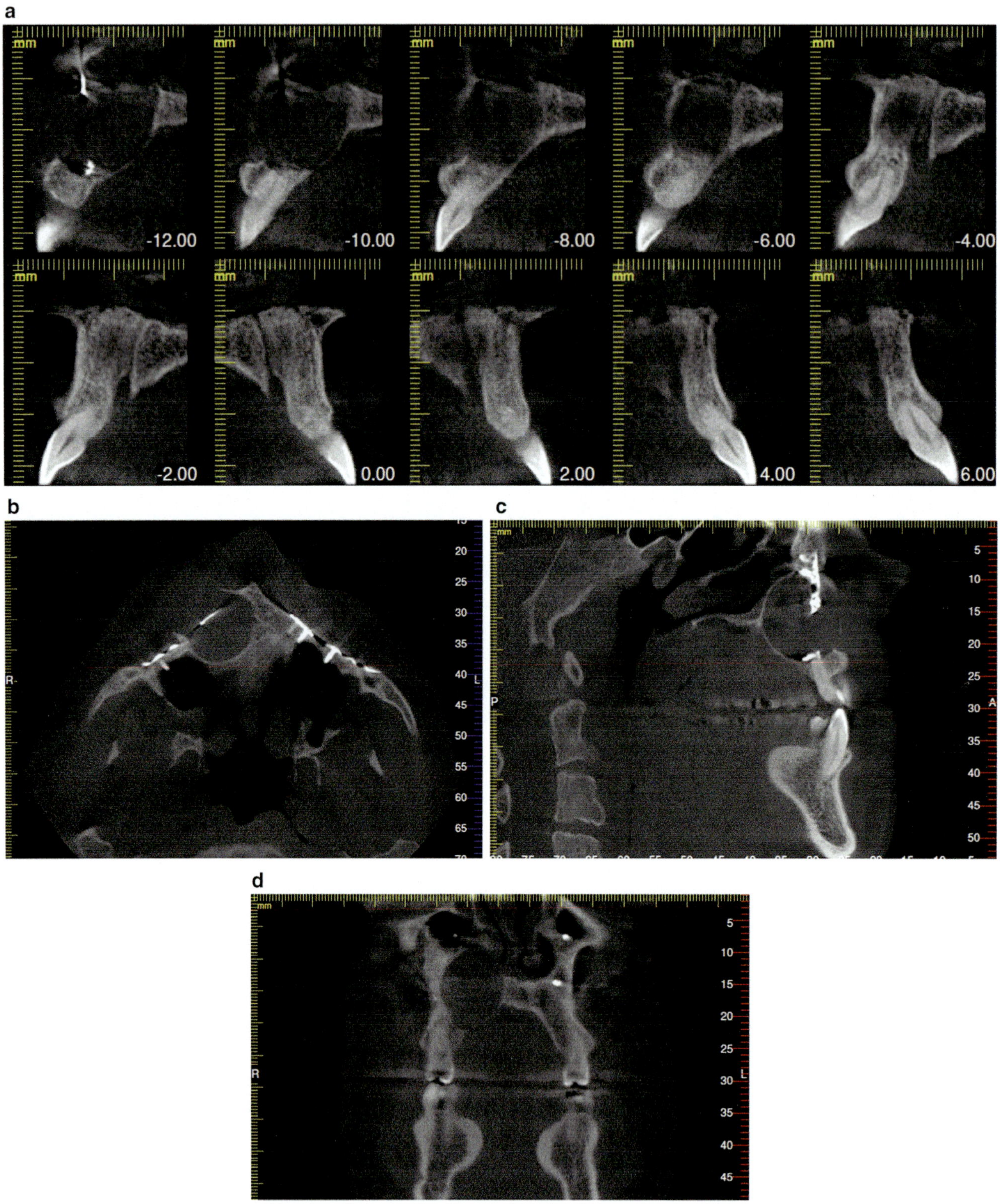

Fig. 5.18 (**a**) CBCT reformatted oblique sagittal view of *right* maxillary radicular cyst. (**b**) CBCT axial view of *right* maxillary radicular cyst. (**c**) CBCT sagittal view of *right* maxillary radicular cyst. (**d**) CBCT coronal view of *right* maxillary radicular cyst

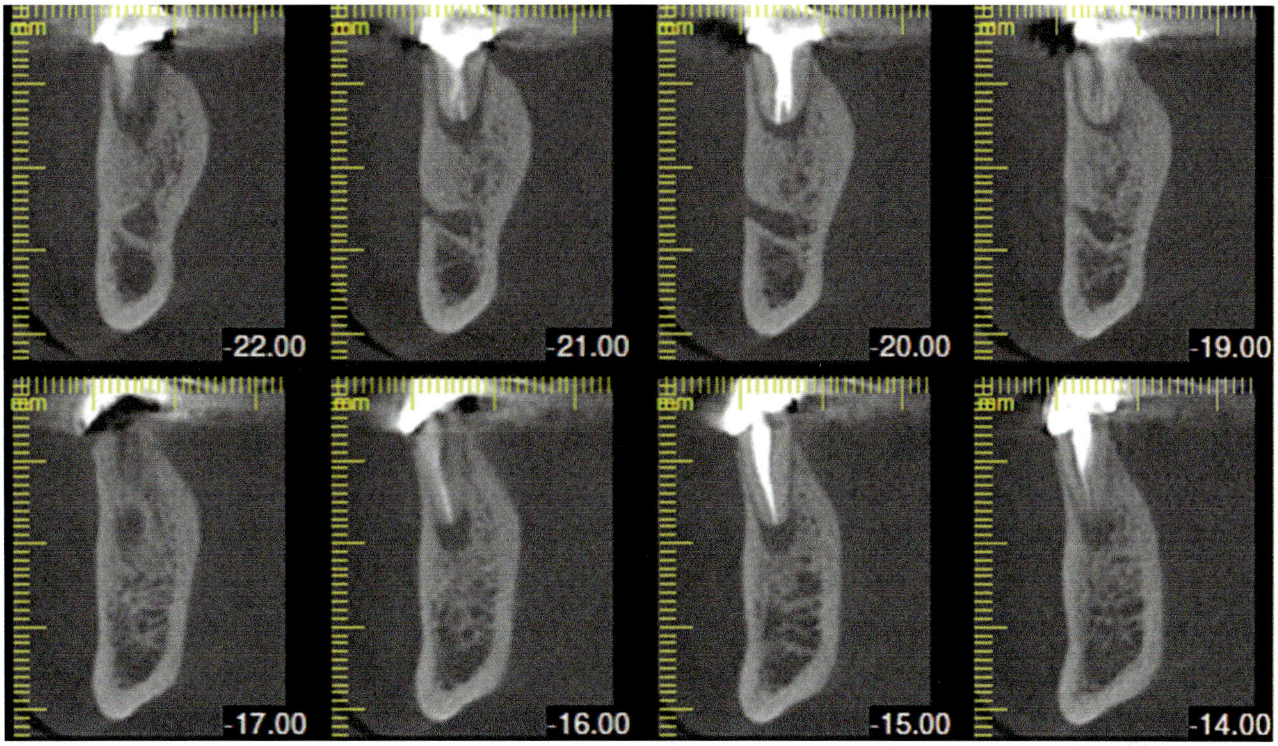

Fig. 5.19 CBCT reformatted oblique sagittal views of *right* mandibular first and second premolar endodontic infections with periapical radiolucencies

mounts that take into consideration the gingival height as well. In this manner, the dental implant(s) can be placed through the same drill sleeve of the surgical guide and can even provide stabilization of the guide as well.

When the surgical drill guide is received from the manufacturer, it is critical to check the fit of the appliance. This can be done by fitting the appliance onto a dental model. Sometimes the acrylic that surrounds the metal drill sleeves can be excessive and prevents the seating of the template on the dentition and needs to be judiciously trimmed away with an acrylic bur in a rotary instrument.

When the procedure begins, the first step after stabilizing the surgical drill guide (Fig. 5.40) is to use the mucosal punch to remove a core of gingiva if a flapless case is being performed (Fig. 5.41a–d); otherwise a flap is raised. Bone profilers (bone mill drill bits) can also be utilized if the crest of ridge has a knife edge (Fig. 5.42a–d). The drill sequence then begins and depths can be controlled. The drill handles are utilized to increase the diameters of the drill bits in the drilling technique (Fig.5.43). Once the osteotomies are completed, bone taps can be utilized if necessary for dense bone (Fig. 5.44a–d), after which countersinks can be utilized (Fig. 5.45a–d). After this step, the implants can then be inserted to correct depth via specialized implant mounts (Fig. 5.46a–c). If a two-stage procedure, cover screws or closure caps are placed; if single stage, either healing abutments or the prosthesis is then inserted.

Case Reports

Clinical examples of cases are presented so as to elaborate the technique of CT-guided dental implant placement.

C#17ase 1 (Figures 5.47–5.64)

A 22-year-old white male presented with left posterior mandibular swelling, which on CT scan revealed an expansile multiloculated lesion of the left posterior mandible associated with a third molar impacted tooth #17 and associated pericoronal radiolucency and compound odontoma (triple lesion). Biopsy demonstrated an ameloblastic fibroma. Because of the aggressive nature of the lesion and potential for malignant transformation, a left posterior segmental mandibulectomy with immediate iliac crest block bone graft was performed. After 1 year, the reconstruction plate was removed, and a tibial bone graft was performed to augment the width of the iliac crest graft. After 9 months, three dental implants were placed using CT guidance with a rapid printed surgical drill guide in the left posterior mandible and later restored as individual crowns (Restorative Dentistry by Dr. George Costaras, NY, NY).

Case 2 (Figures 5.65–5.91)

A 46-year-old male presented with anterior maxillary Class III occlusal ridge relationship with adequate maxillary bone height and width. Bilateral mandibular ramus corticocancellous block grafts with scraped bone and resorbable collagen membrane coverage placed on the buccal crestal surface to augment the region of teeth #7, 8, 9, and 10 to permit correct dental implant trajectories for a prosthetic restoration. Ten months following the bone graft was noted to have had adequate healing, virtual treatment planning was performed (ImplantMaster, iDent Imaging, Inc., New York, NY, USA), and following removal of bone fixation screws, four dental implants were placed at the sites of teeth #7, 8, 9, and 10 using CT guidance with a rapid printed surgical drill guide. The dental implants were later restored as a fixed bridge (Restorative Dentistry by Dr. Samuel Cohen, NY, NY, orthodontics by Dr. Bruce Greenberg, NY, NY).

a

b

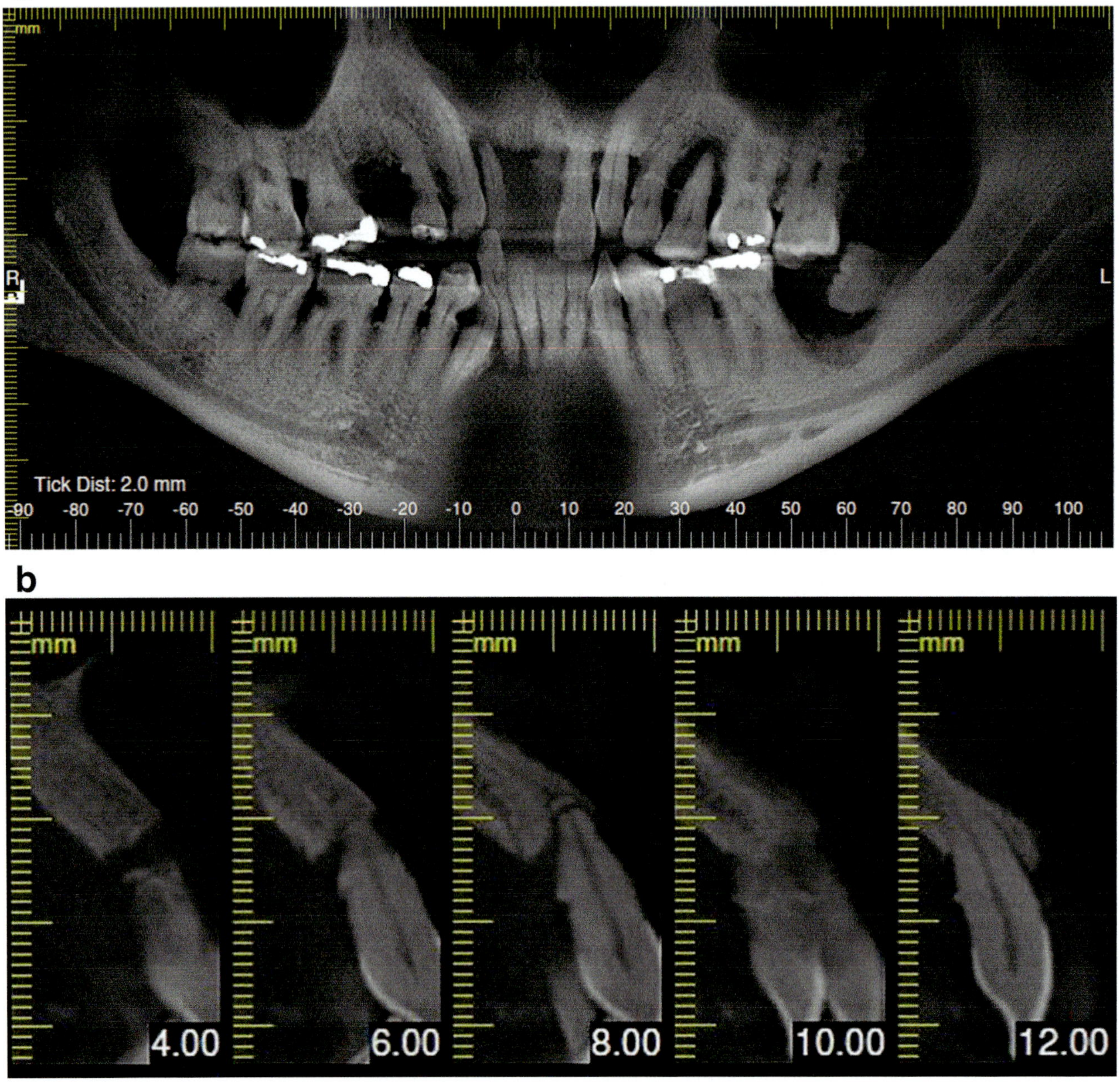

Fig. 5.20 (**a**) CBCT panoramic radiograph of generalized periodontal disease. (**b**) CBCT reformatted oblique sagittal views of anterior maxillary incisors with advanced periodontal disease and bone loss. (**c**) CBCT reformatted oblique sagittal views of anterior mandibular incisors with moderate periodontal disease and bone loss

c

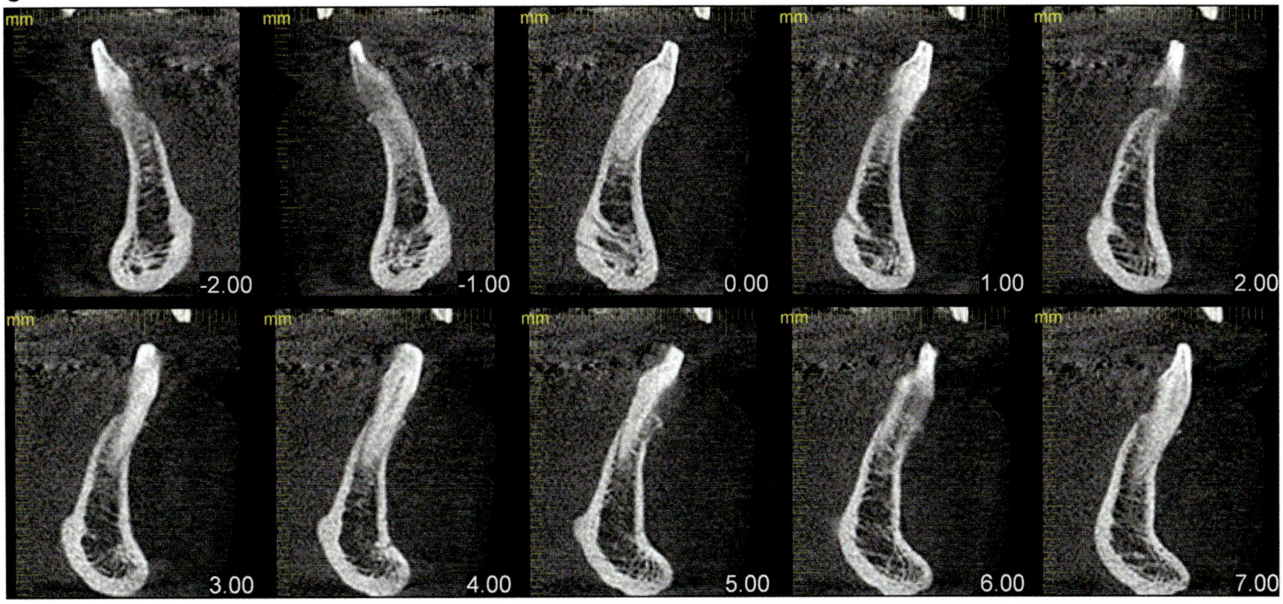

Fig. 5.20 (continued)

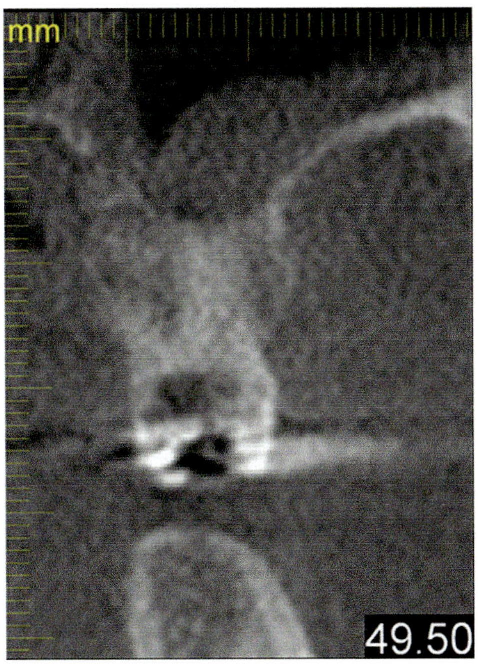

Fig. 5.21 CBCT reformatted oblique sagittal views of posterior maxillary molar with dental caries

Case 3 (Figures 5.92–5.113)

A 22-year-old male presented following orthodontic treatment with congenitally absent lateral incisors teeth #7 and 10 with adequate bone and interdental spacing for the placement of dental implants. After a CBCT was obtained with a radiographic template, virtual treatment planning was performed (ImplantMaster, iDent Imaging, Inc., New York, NY, USA), and two dental implants were placed at the sites of teeth #7 and 10 using CT guidance with a rapid printed surgical drill guide. The dental implants were later restored as individual crowns. (Restorative Dentistry by Dr. Joseph Haggar, NY, NY, orthodontics by Dr. Bruce Greenberg, NY, NY).

Case 4 (Figures 5.114–5.127)

A 58-year-old male presented with total edentulism for implant reconstruction with a chief complaint of loose fitting dentures. His medical history was significant for osteoporosis, hepatitis C, and porphyria. He desired an immediate load protocol over conventional bone grafting and implant placement. Clinical and imaging analysis revealed a severely atrophic maxilla and mandible. The maxilla demonstrated insufficient Zone I, II, and III bone for conventional implant placement. A computer-guided treatment plan was developed utilizing SIMPLANT Master software (Materialise, Dentsply, York, PA). A quad zygoma design with an additional anterior implant was developed to restore the severely atrophic maxilla. Nobel Biocare (Yorba Linda, CA) compatible SIMPLANT (Materialise, Dentsply, York, PA) surgical guides were designed with position and angulation control of the zygoma implants. Fixation screw holes were placed to stabilize the guides during drilling. Four zygomatic and single midline maxillary implants are in position according to the computer-guided plan. Closed tray impression coping was placed over angled multiunit abutments in preparation for polyvinylsiloxane impressions for provisional restorations. The patient also desired malar augmentation; bilateral malar Silastic implants were placed over resorbable barrier membranes prior to wound closure.

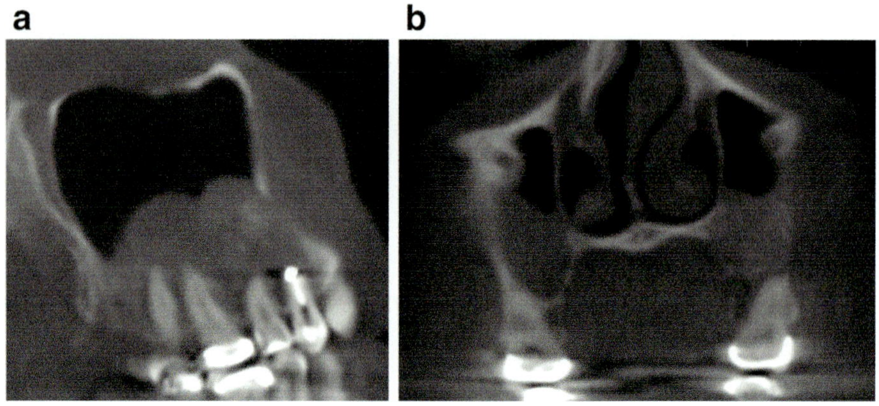

Fig. 5.22 (**a**) CBCT sagittal view of *left* maxillary osteosarcoma mixed radiolucent and radiopaque lesion involving the *left* maxillary sinus and root apices. (**b**) CBCT coronal view of *left* maxillary osteosarcoma mixed radiolucent and radiopaque lesion involving the *left* maxillary sinus

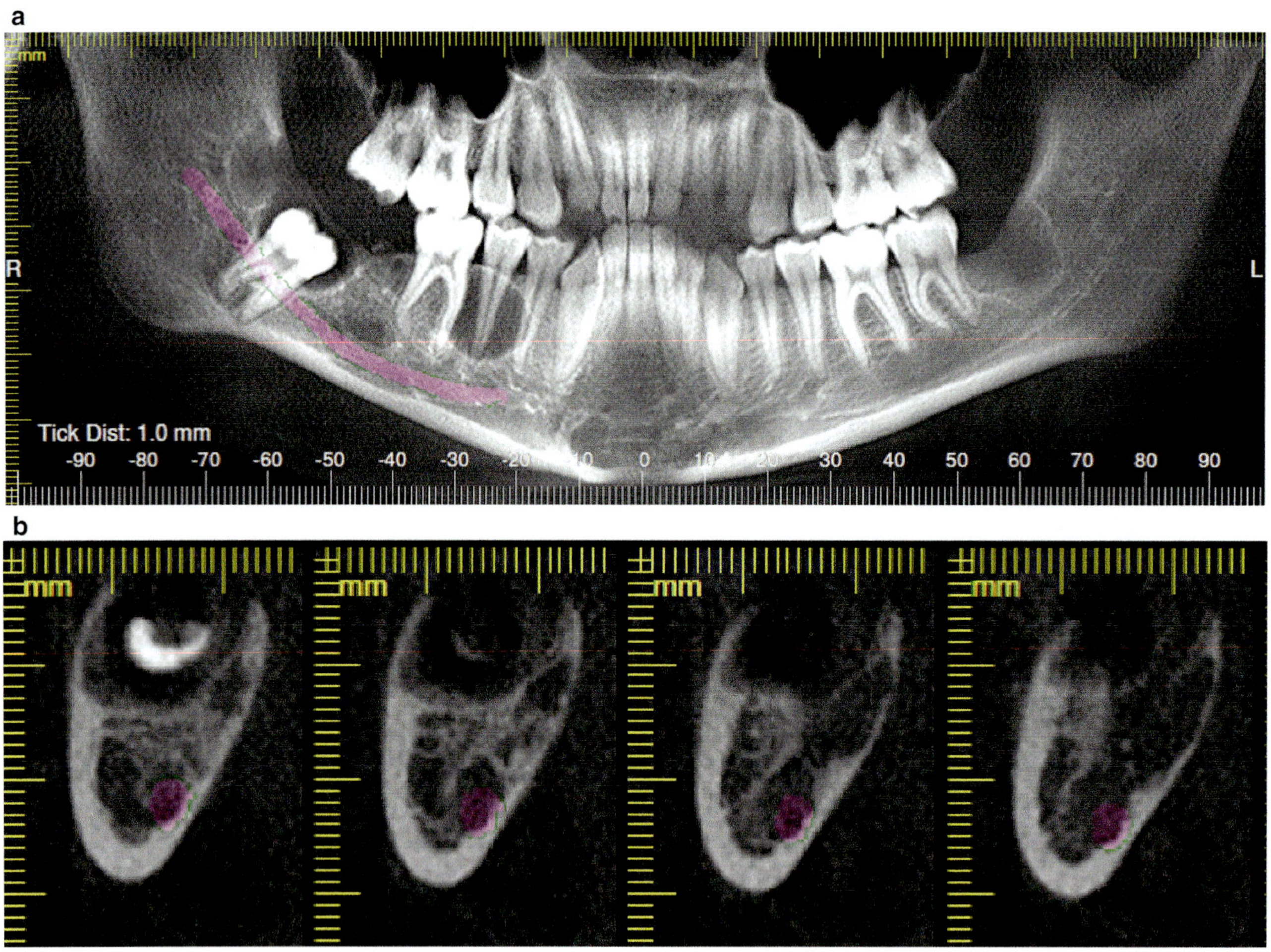

Fig. 5.23 (**a**) CBCT panoramic view of *right* mandibular impacted second molar with dentigerous cyst and ameloblastic fibro-odontoma in a 12-year-old female. (**b**) CBCT oblique sagittal view of *right* mandibular ameloblastic fibro-odontoma in a 12-year-old female with mixed radiopaque and radiolucent appearance. (**c**) Mandibular dentigerous cyst associated with impacted third molar

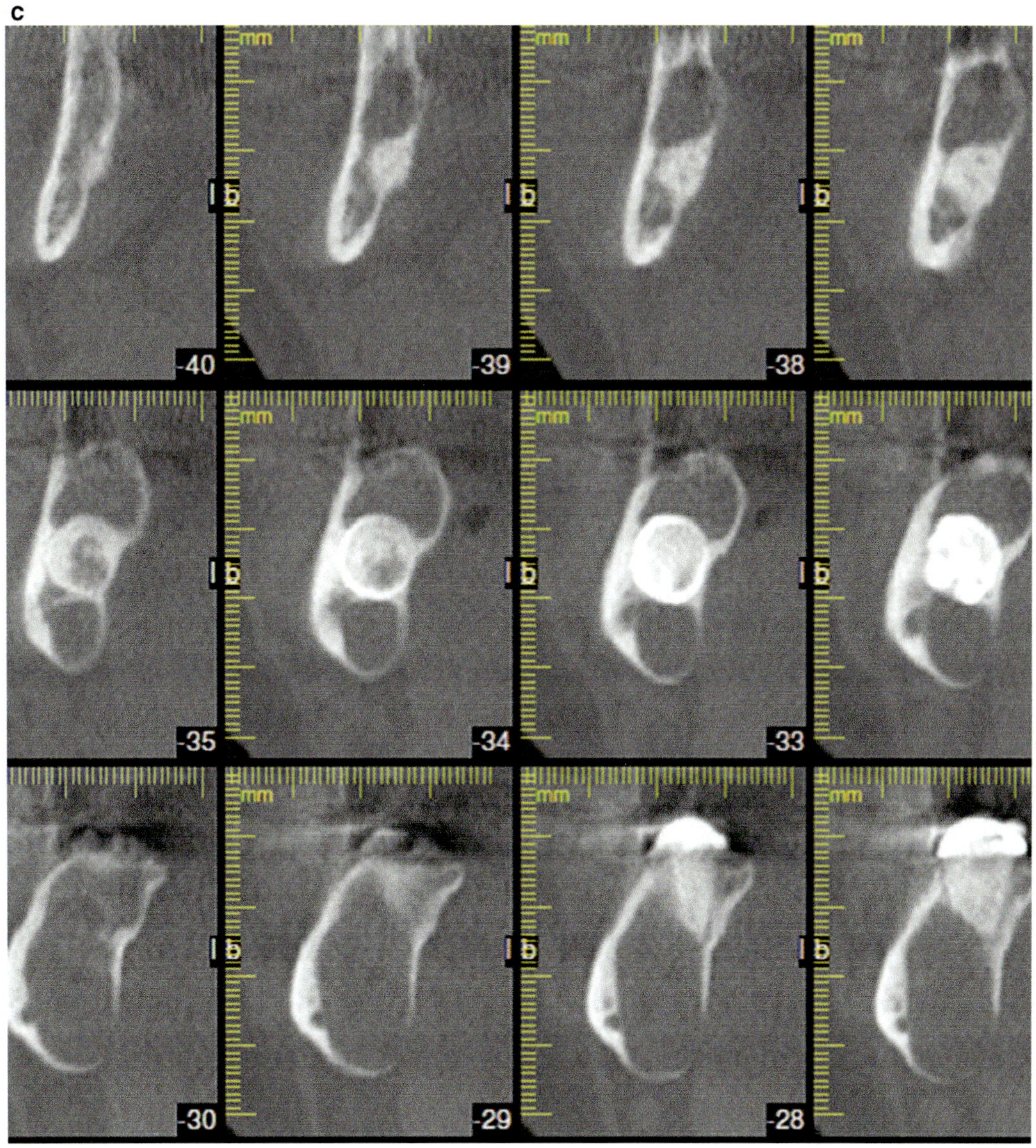

Fig. 5.23 (continued)

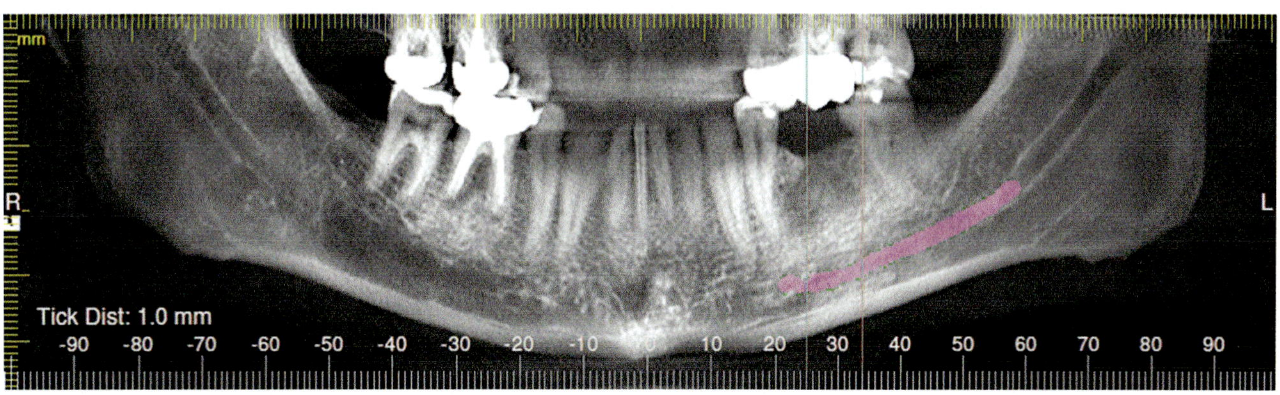

Fig. 5.24 CBCT panoramic radiograph of *left* mandibular missing first molar and marking of the *left* mandibular canal

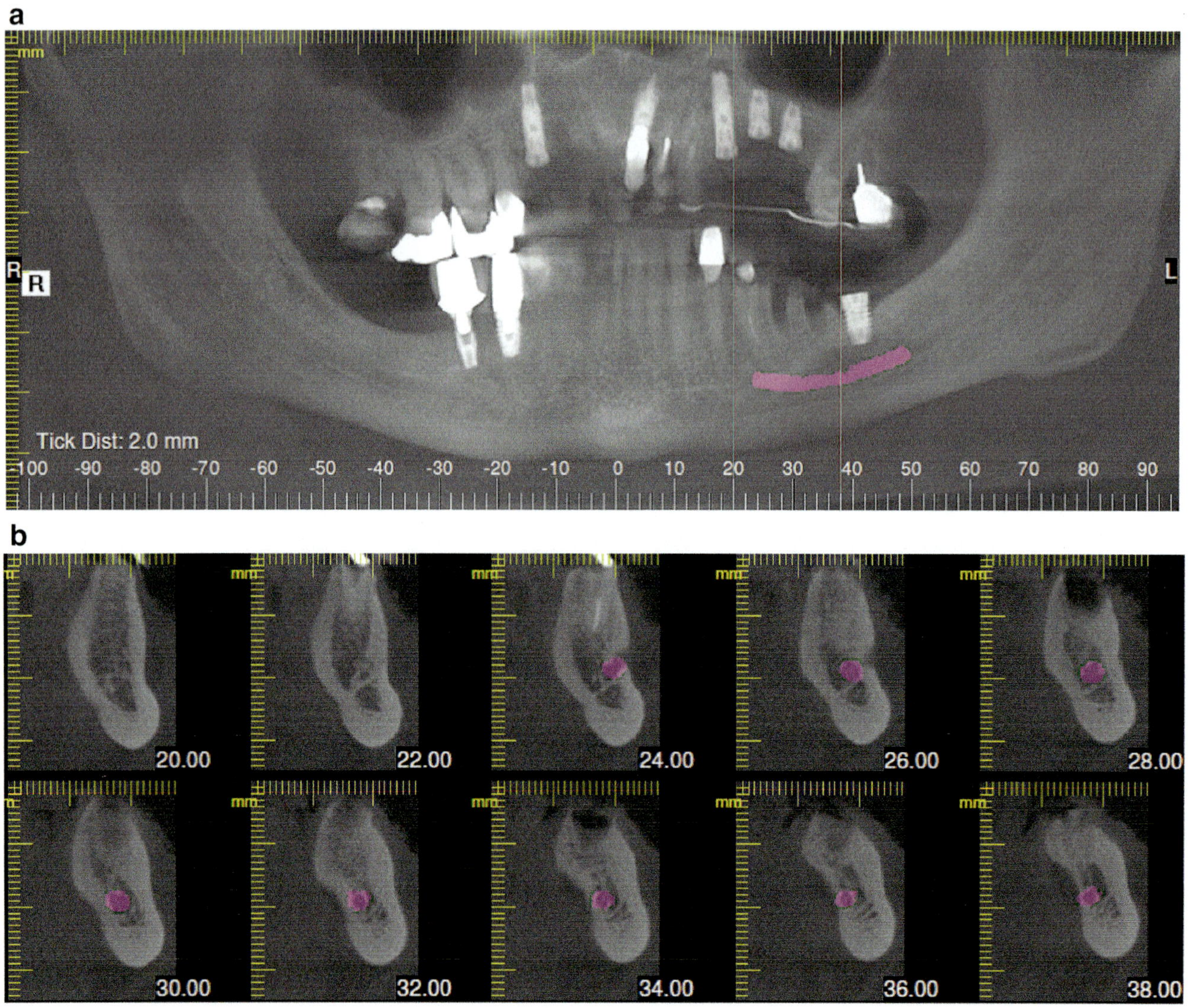

Fig. 5.25 (**a**) CBCT panoramic radiograph of *left* mandibular missing first molar tooth #19 immediately following extraction with marking of the *left* mandibular canal. (**b**) CBCT reformatted oblique sagittal views of *left* mandibular missing first molar immediately following extraction with marking of the *left* mandibular canal. Note previously placed dental implant tooth #18

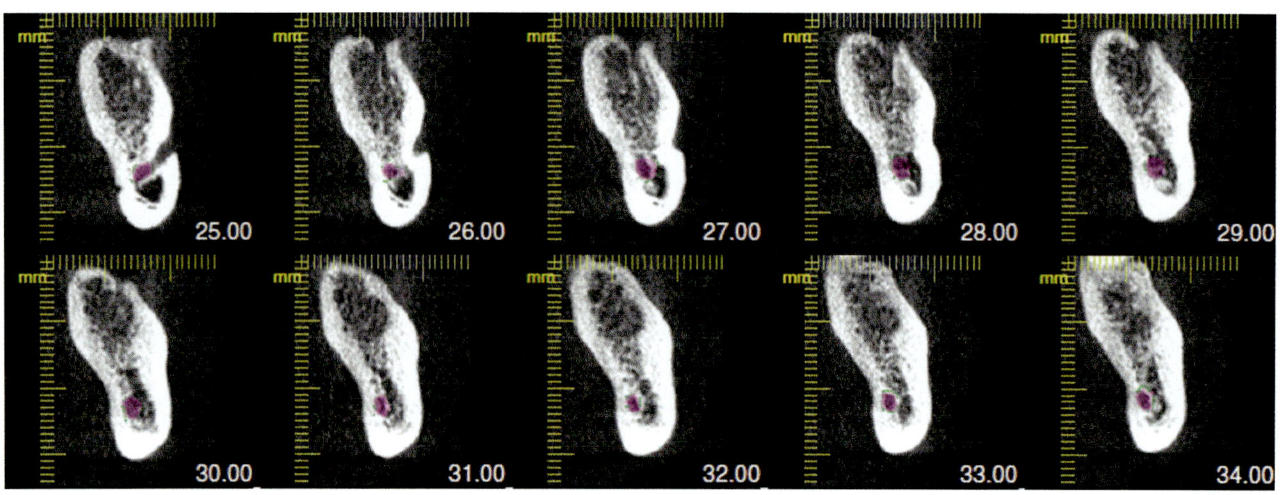

Fig. 5.26 CBCT reformatted oblique sagittal views of *left* mandibular missing first molar and marking of the *left* mandibular canal

a

b

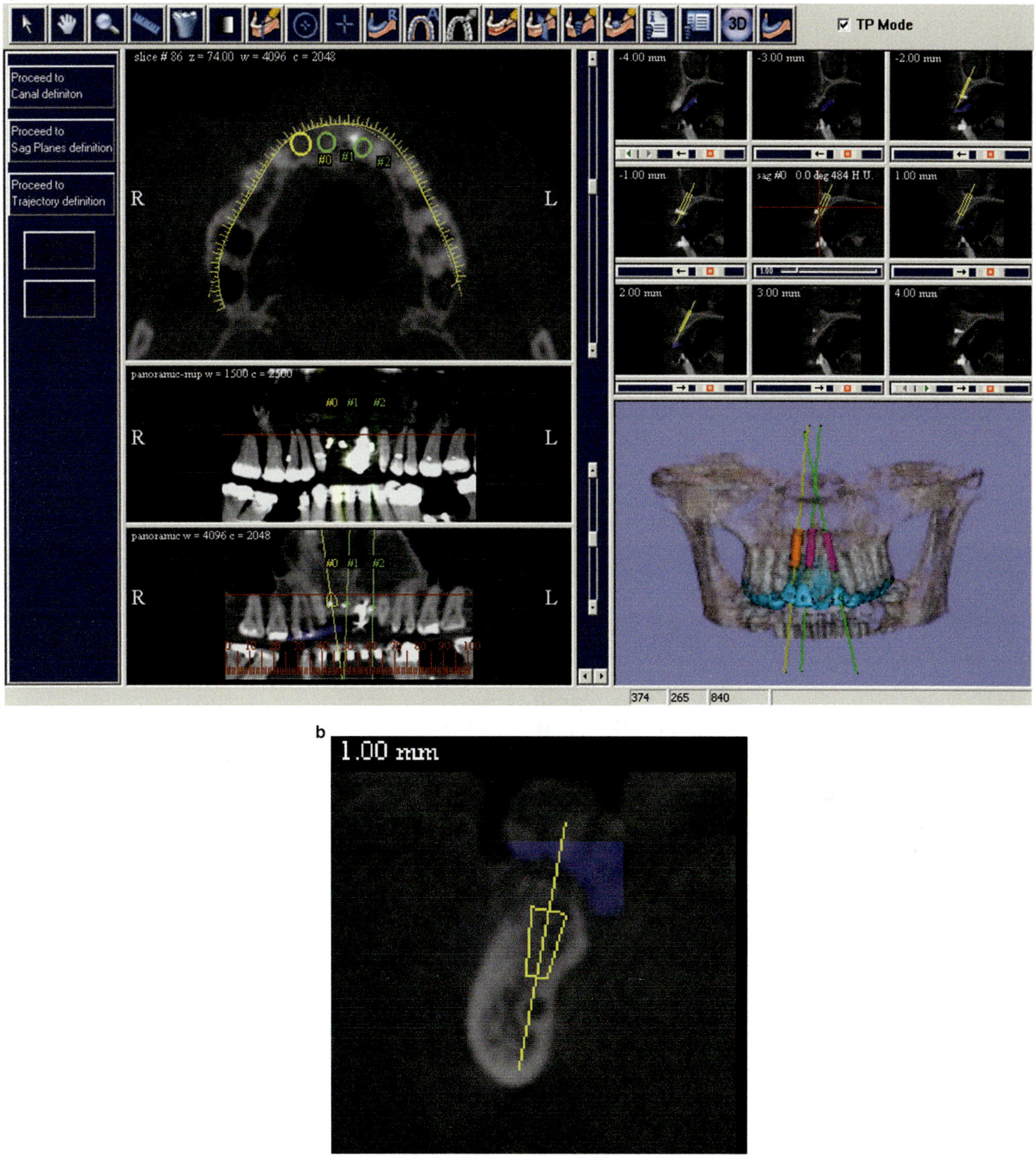

Fig. 5.27 (**a**) Virtual planning environment with superimposition of dental prosthesis contained within a radiographic surgical guide, maxilla, and planned dental implant trajectories (ImplantMaster, iDent Imaging, Inc., New York, NY, USA). (**b**) Virtual planning environment with superimposition of dental prosthesis contained within a radiographic surgical guide reformatted oblique sagittal view and planned dental implant trajectory (ImplantMaster, iDent Imaging, Inc., New York, NY, USA)

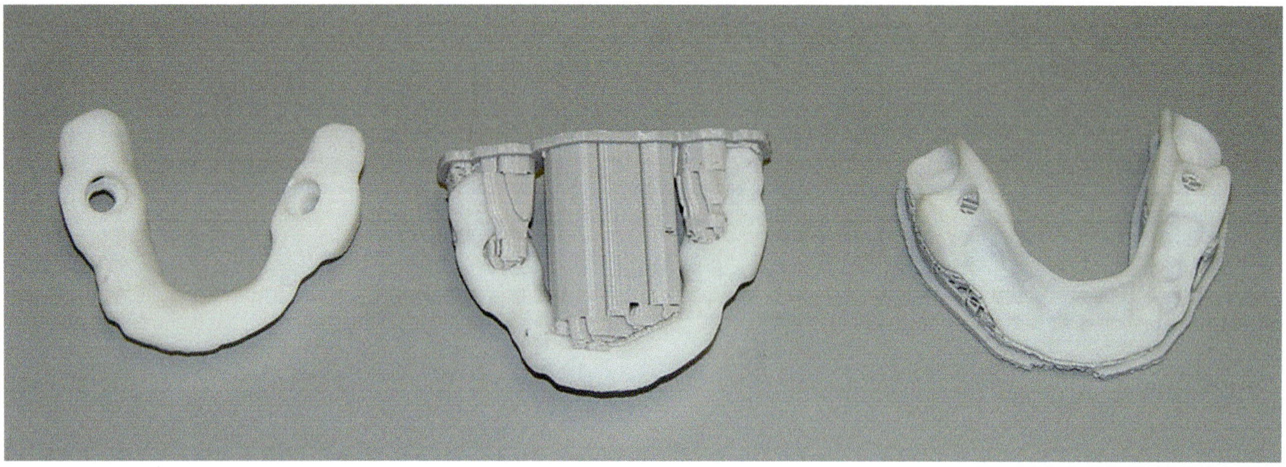

Fig. 5.28 Patient-specific rapid printed CT-guided surgical drill template with scaffolding from 3D printer still attached

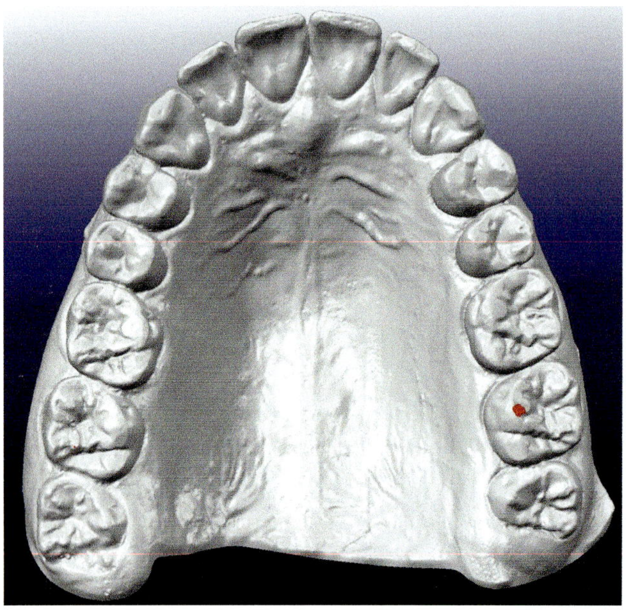

Fig. 5.29 Optical scan of dentition

A conventional All on 4 protocol was used in the mandible. A SIMPLANT bone-borne surgical guide offering depth control was fixated to the mandible. All implants were placed to a crestal level at 50 NCm of torque. Anterior conical and posterior angled multiunit abutments were placed in order to develop a favorable path of draw. Closed tray impression copings were then planed for impressions. The patient was fitted with metal reinforced provisional restorations the following day.

Case 5 (Figures 5.128–5.144)

A 35-year-old male presents with complaints of loose teeth and recurrent infections. Exam reveals generalized advanced periodontitis with a hopeless prognosis. CBCT confirmed the presence of adequate bone for the immediate removal of all remaining teeth and "All on 4" protocol which the patient elected. SIMPLANT Master software (Materialise, Dentsply, York, PA) was utilized to develop ideal implant placement utilizing the "All on 4" protocol. Segmentation was performed in order to exactly visualize alveolar topography for implant emergence in the cingulum region. SIMPLANT Nobel compatible surgical guides were designed and developed for implant placement with depth control in the maxilla and mandible. Full-arch extractions were performed and full-thickness flaps were developed, and the dental implants were placed using the surgical drill guides, after which the placement of the provisional implant-retained maxillary and mandibular prostheses was performed.

a b

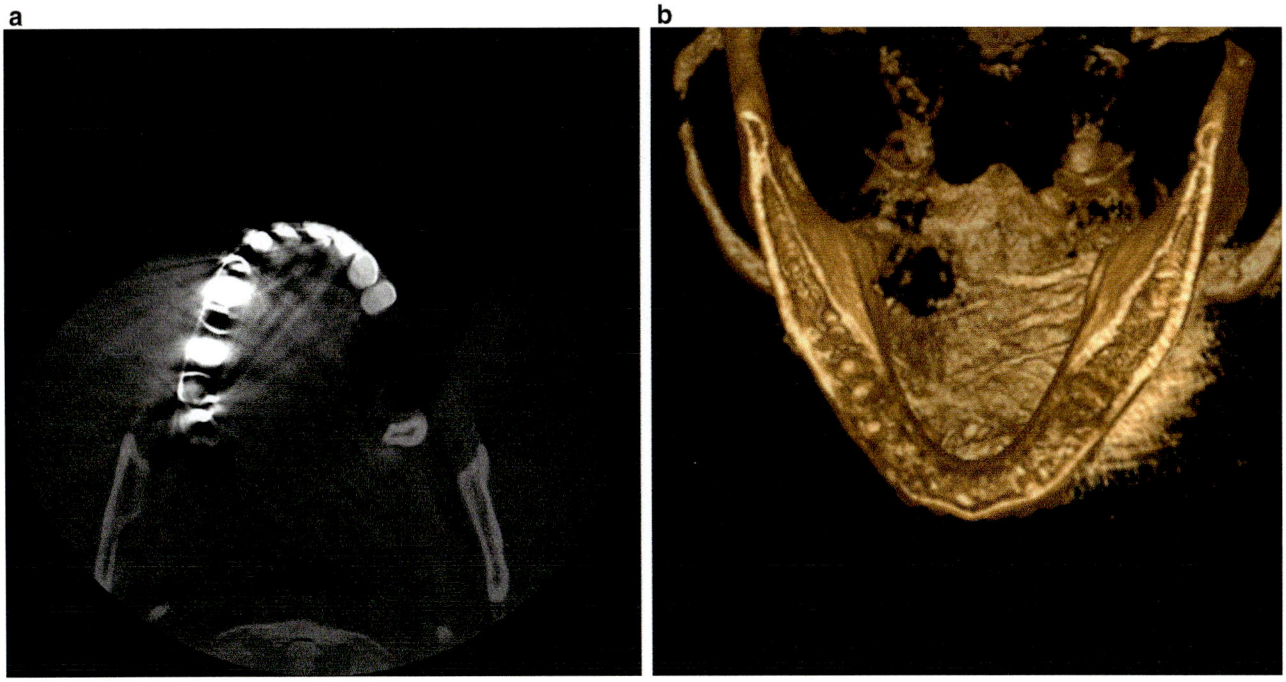

Fig. 5.30 (**a**) CBCT axial view of dental artifacts. (**b**) CBCT 3D view of dental artifacts

a b c

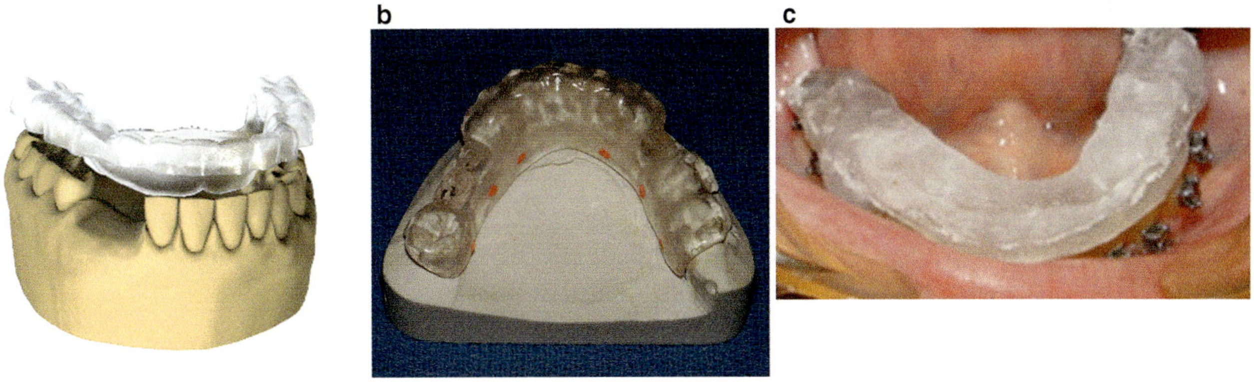

Fig. 5.31 (**a**, **b**) Laboratory-fabricated radiographic template **a** (Straumann USA, LLC, Andover, MA, USA. Used with permission). (**c**) Radiographic template seated in the mouth

Fig. 5.32 Radiographic template contained within Styrofoam box. Styrofoam does not appear in the CBCT image

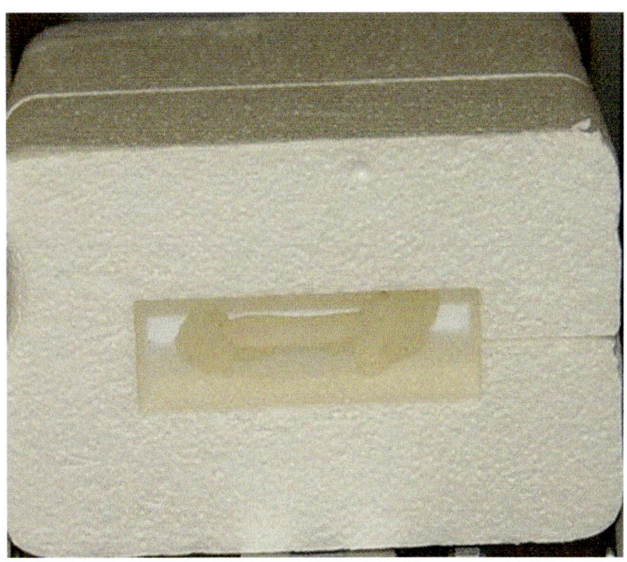

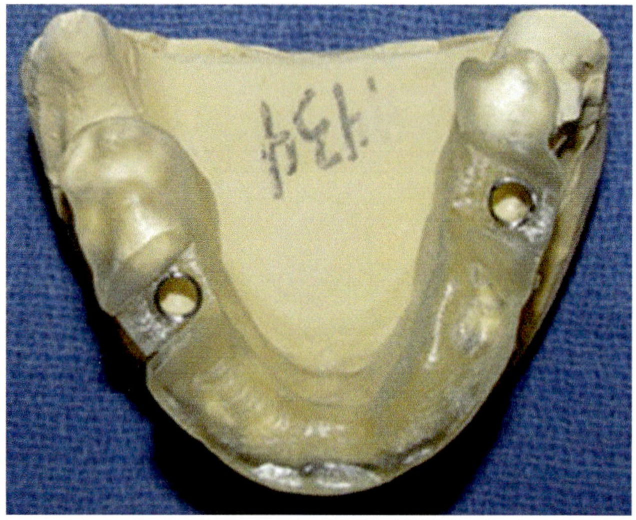

Fig. 5.33 Rapid printed surgical template with metal master drill sleeves

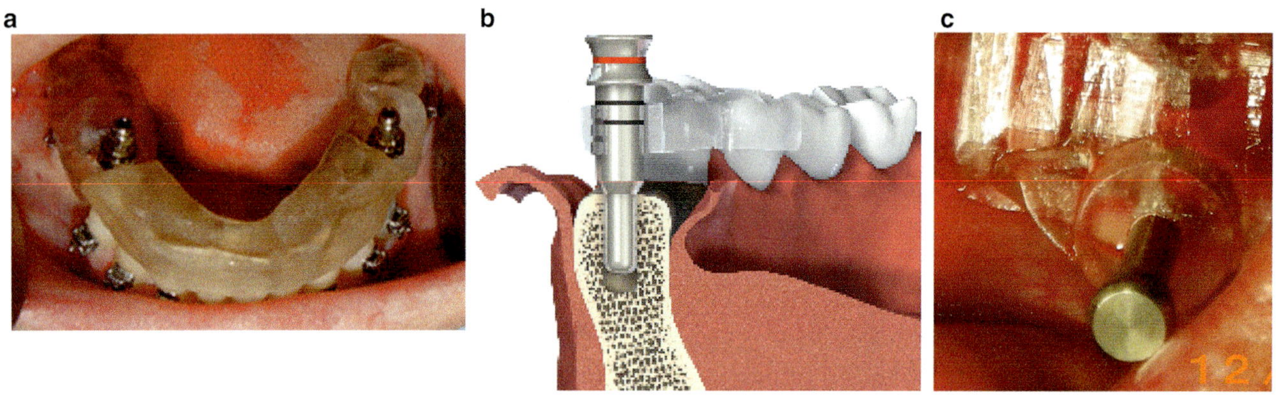

Fig. 5.34 (**a**) Fixation of surgical guide with placed dental implant fixture mounts using the Navigator system (Zimmer Biomet 3i, Palm Beach Gardens, FL, USA). (**b**) Fixation of surgical guide with stabilization pin (Straumann USA, LLC, Andover, MA, USA. Used with permission). (**c**) Fixation of surgical guide with stabilization pin (Nobel Biocare, Yorba Linda, CA, USA)

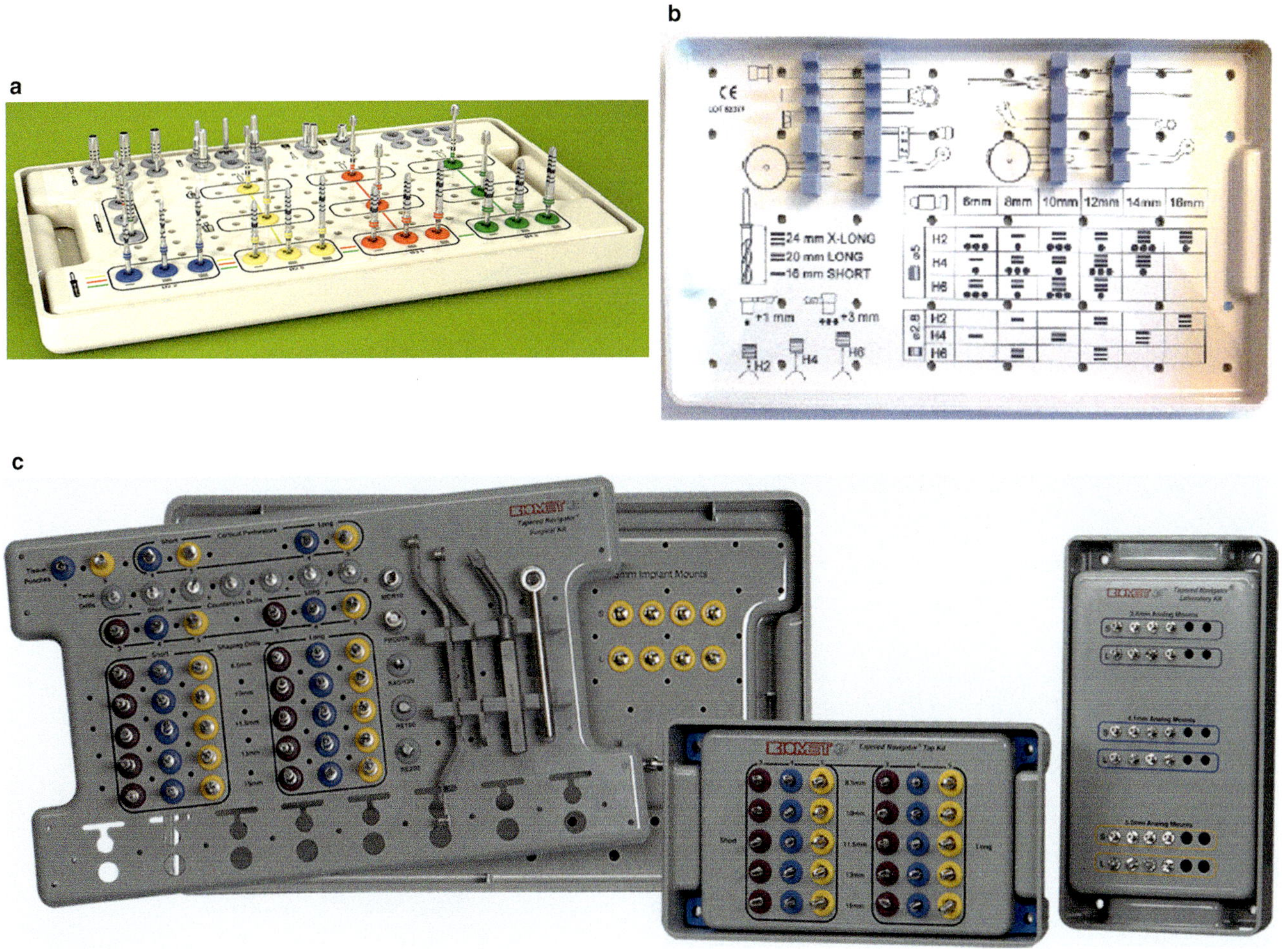

Fig. 5.35 Straumann graphic tray for CT-guided surgery: (**a**) upper tray; (**b**) lower tray (By permission Straumann USA, LLC, Andover, MA, USA); and (**c**) Zimmer Biomet 31 Navigator System (Zimmer Biomet 3i, Palm Beach Gardens, FL, USA)

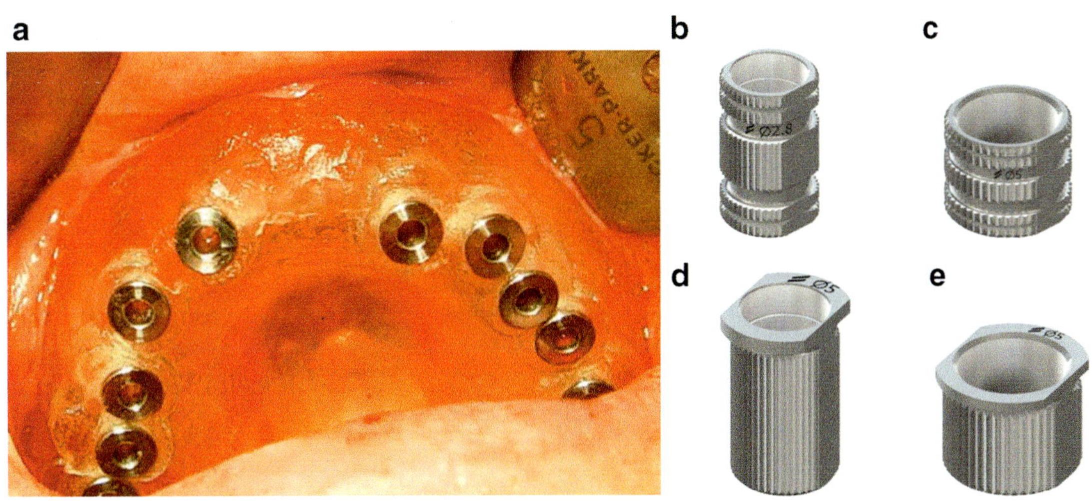

Fig. 5.36 (**a**) Surgical drill guide with 2.3 mm metal drill sleeves, and (Parts **b**–**e** (Straumann USA, LLC, Andover, MA, USA. Used with permission.) Drill guide narrow diameter drill sleeves. (**a**) 2.8 mm sleeve. (**b**) 5.0 mm sleeve. (**c**) Drill guide regular and wide diameter drill sleeves. (**d**) 2.8 mm T sleeve. (**e**) 5.0 mm T sleeve

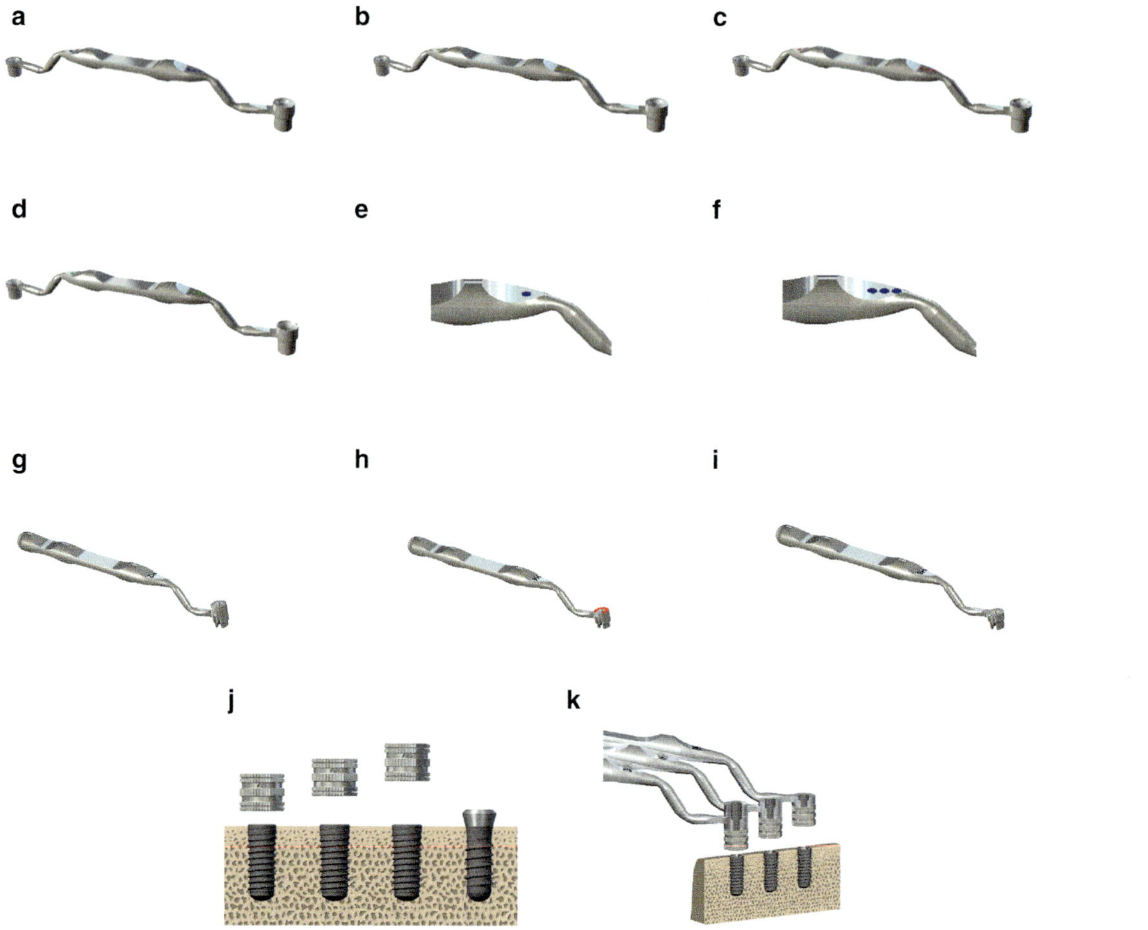

Fig. 5.37 (**a**) Drill handles dual ended. (Straumann USA, LLC, Andover, MA, USA. Used with permission.) (**a**) 2.2 mm. (**b**) 2.8 mm. (**c**) 3.2 mm. (**d**) 4.2 mm. (**b**) Markings at each drill handle end. (**e**) 1 dot = 1.0 mm. (**f**) 3 dots = 3.0 mm. (**c**) The C handles H2, H4, and H6 allow for heights of 2, 4, and 6 mm and allow the side placement of the drill bit into the sleeve which can accommodate limited jaw opening especially in the posterior maxilla or mandible. (**g**) C-handle H2. (**h**) C-handle H4. (**i**) C-handle H6. (**j**) Drill sleeves can be located at different tissue heights. (**k**) C handles accommodate different soft tissue heights

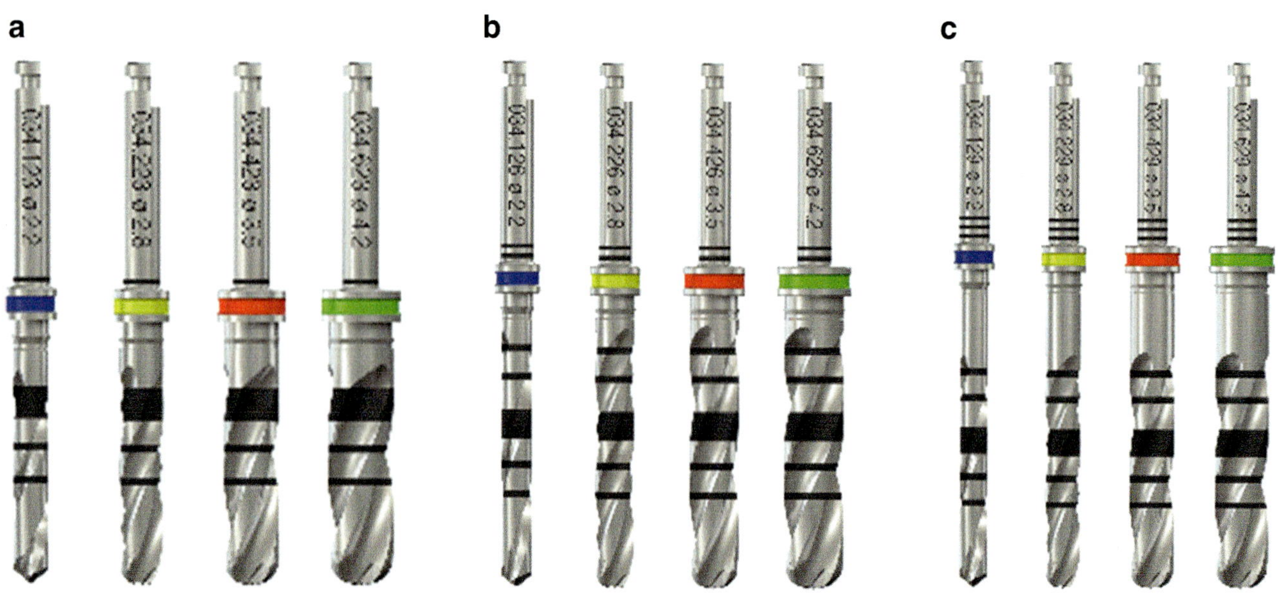

Fig. 5.38 Guided surgery pilot and twist drill bits. (Straumann USA, LLC, Andover, MA, USA. Used with permission.) (**a**) 32 mm. (**b**) 36 mm. (**c**) 40 mm

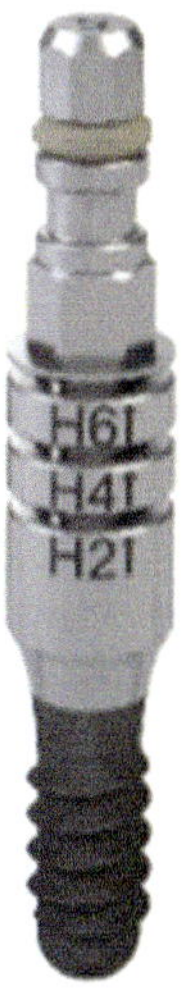

Fig. 5.39 The guided surgery implant transfer mount has notches with markings for gingiva height at H2 = 2.0 mm, H4 = 4.0 mm, and H6 = 6.0 mm. (Straumann USA, LLC, Andover, MA, USA. Used with permission.)

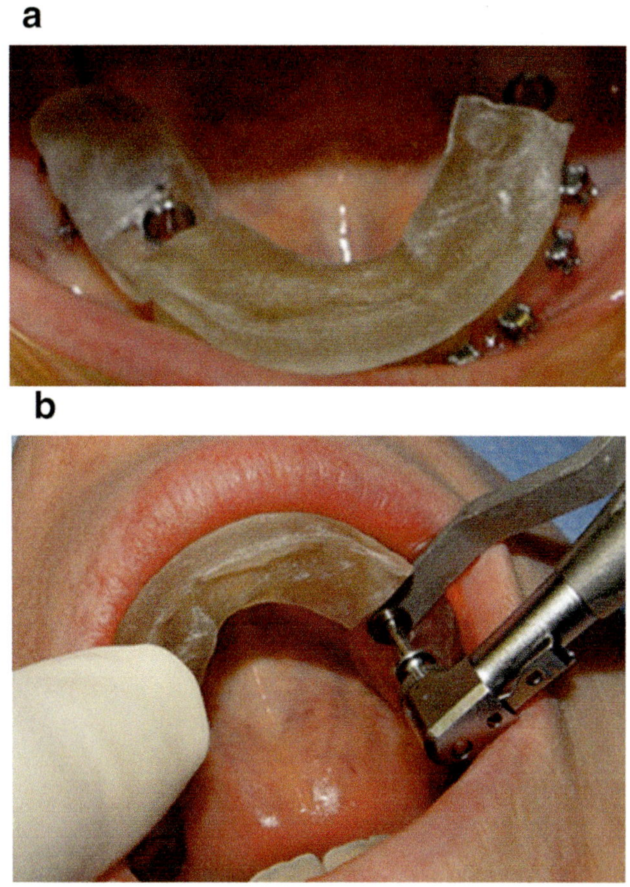

Fig. 5.40 (**a**) Mandibular surgical drill guide seated in place. (**b**) Mandibular surgical drill guide seated in place and stabilized with non-dominant hand while drilling through drill handle placed in master sleeve. (Zimmer Biomet 3i Navigator System, Palm Beach Gardens, Fl, USA)

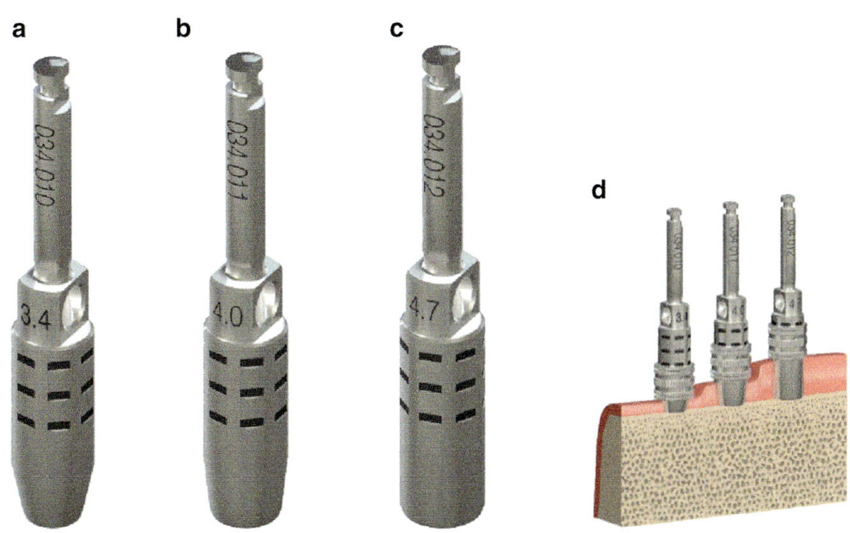

Fig. 5.41 Mucosa punches. (**a**) 3.4 mm diameter. (**b**) 4.0 mm diameter. (**c**) 4.7 mm diameter. (**d**) Mucosal punches with height markers at different soft tissue heights. (Straumann USA, LLC, Andover, MA, USA. Used with permission.)

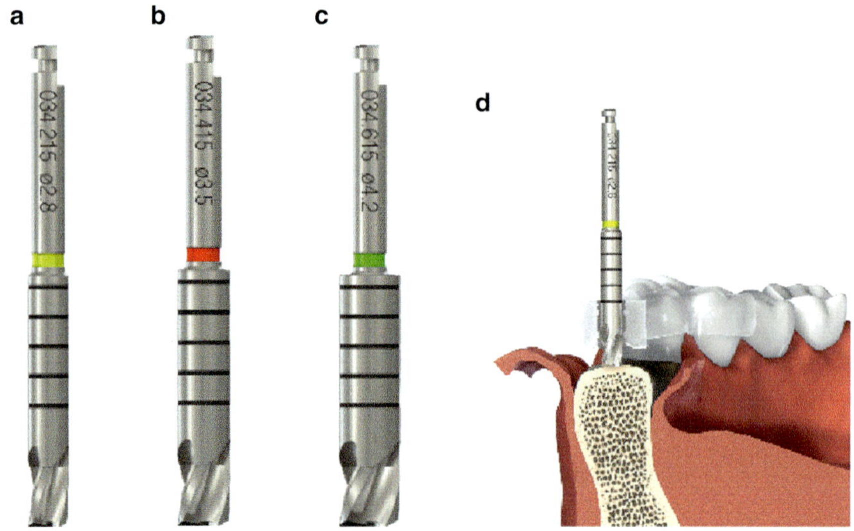

Fig. 5.42 Bone mill drill bits. (Straumann USA, LLC, Andover, MA, USA. Used with permission.) (**a**) 2.8 mm diameter. (**b**) 3.2 mm diameter. (**c**) 4.2 mm diameter. (**d**) Bone mill used in surgical guide

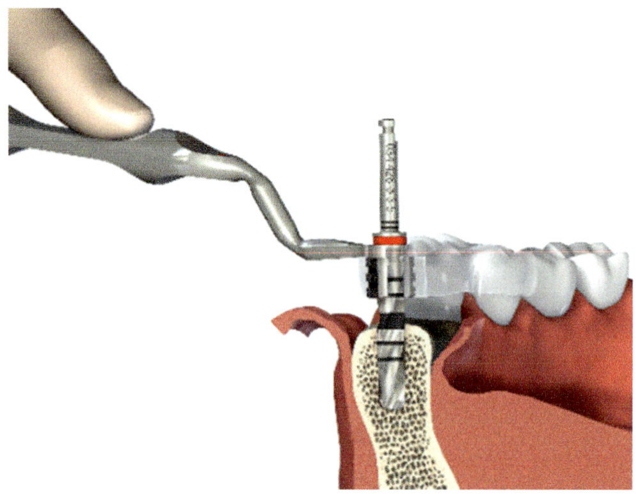

Fig. 5.43 Guided surgery twist drill through surgical drill template drill sleeve. (Straumann USA, LLC, Andover, MA, USA. Used with permission.)

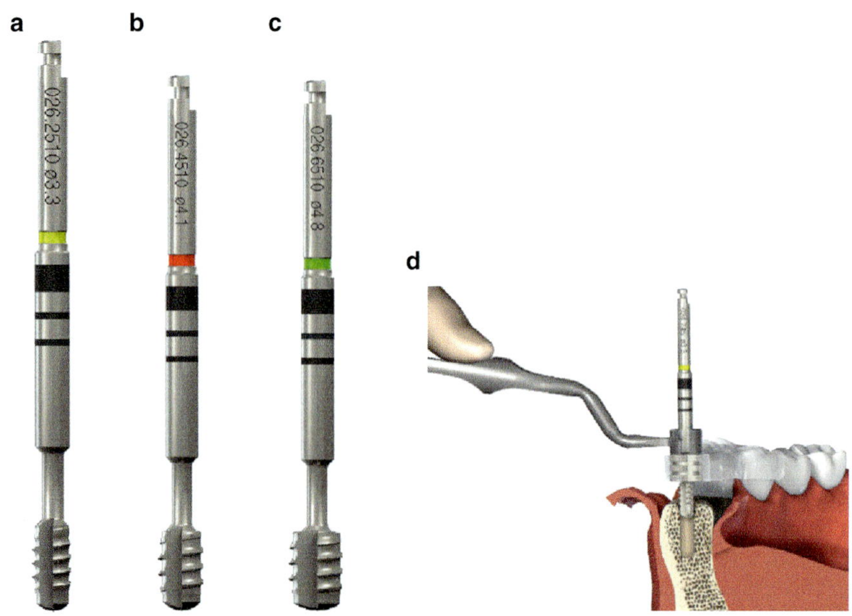

Fig. 5.44 Guided taps for standard and standard plus implants 42 mm lengths. (**a**) 3.3 mm. (**b**) 4.1 mm. (**c**) 4.8 mm. (**d**) Guided tap in use through surgical drill template. (Straumann USA, LLC, Andover, MA, USA. Used with permission.)

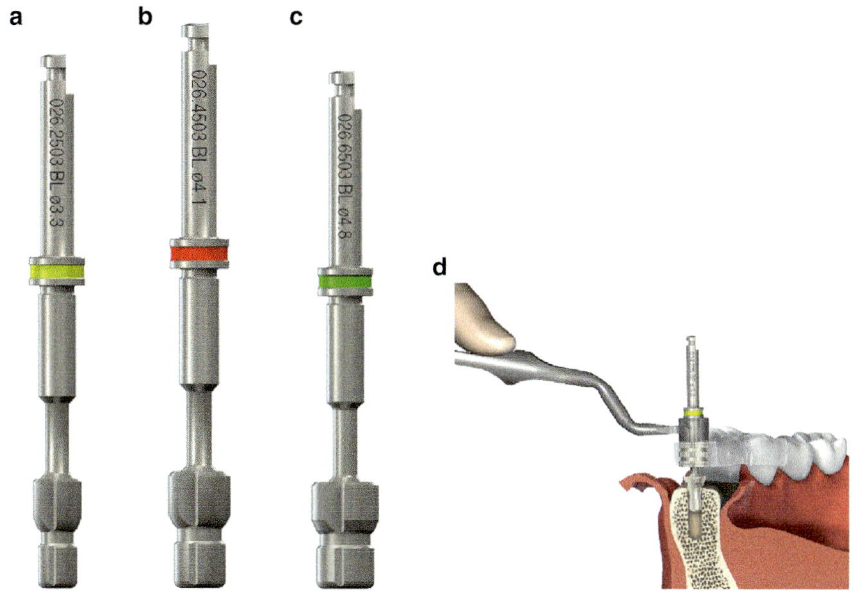

Fig. 5.45 Guided profile drills for bone level implants 37 mm lengths. (Straumann USA, LLC, Andover, MA, USA. Used with permission.) (**a**) 3.3 mm. (**b**) 4.1 mm. (**c**) 4.8 mm. (**d**) Guided profile drill in use through surgical drill template

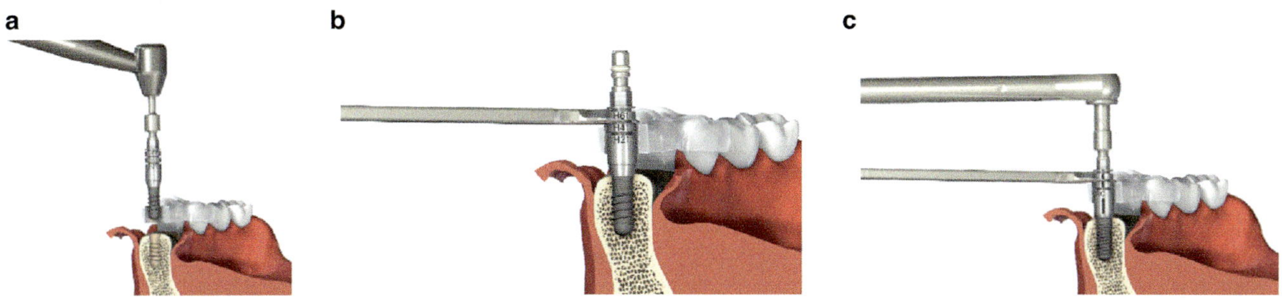

Fig. 5.46 Figure 5.46 Standard implant with a preattached guided surgery implant transfer mount. (Straumann USA, LLC, Andover, MA, USA. Used with permission.) (**a**) Rotary handpiece with adapter attached to standard implant with a preattached for placement guided surgery implant transfer mount though surgical drill template. (**b**) Stop key attached to notch of guided surgery implant transfer mount. (**c**) Ratchet tightening of the guided surgery implant with stop key attached to notch of transfer mount

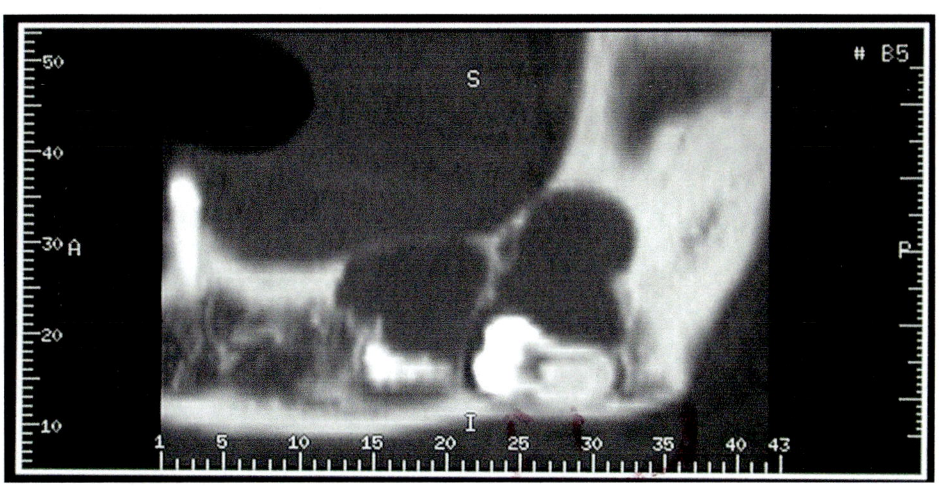

Fig. 5.47 CT scan panoramic view of *left* mandible large multiloculated radiolucent lesion with associated radiodensity and pericoronal radiolucency associated with impacted third molar tooth #17 (triple lesion)

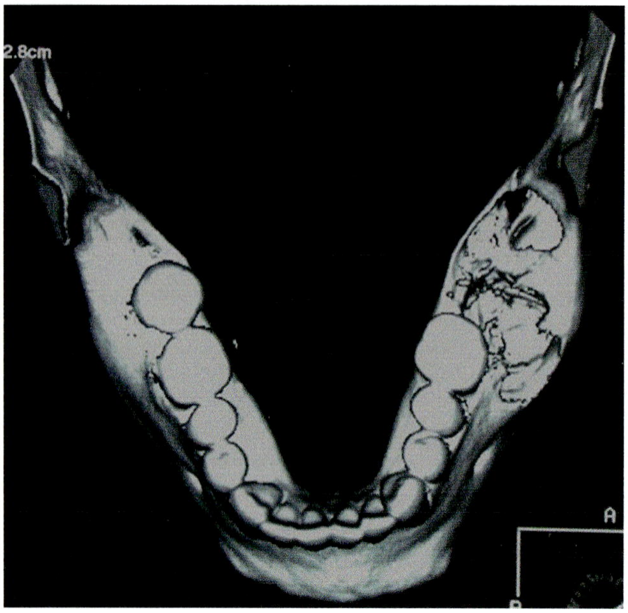

Fig. 5.48 Superior view of 3D CT scan of expansile lesion of the *left* posterior mandible (triple lesion)

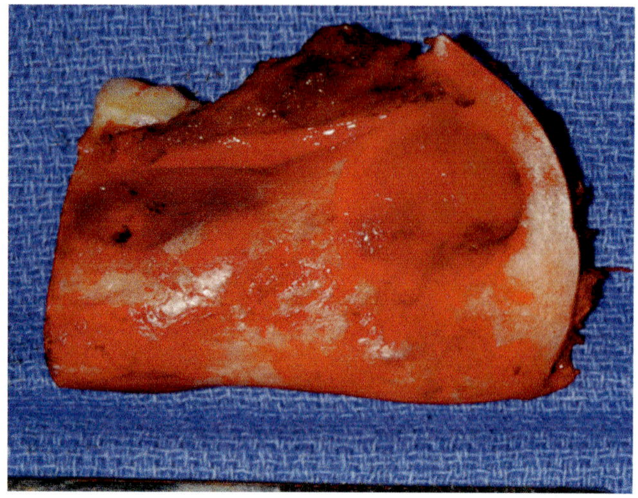

Fig. 5.50 Surgical specimen of *left* posterior partial mandibulectomy

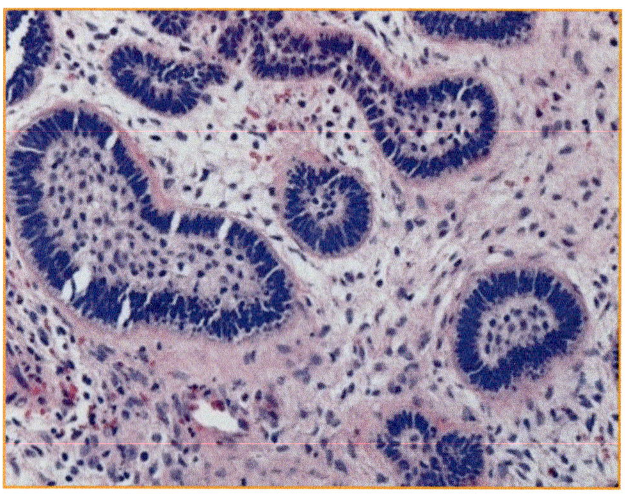

Fig. 5.49 H and E stained high power magnification of ameloblastic fibroma

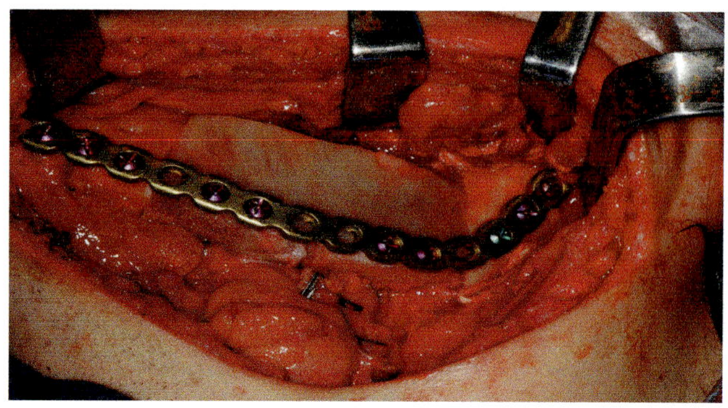

Fig. 5.51 Intraoperative view of *left* posterior mandible following partial mandibulectomy for ameloblastic fibroma and immediate free iliac crest block bone graft reconstruction with internal fixation (DuPuy Synthes Craniomaxillofacial, Paoli, PA, USA)

Fig. 5.52 Postoperative panoramic radiograph of *left* posterior mandible following partial mandibulectomy for ameloblastic fibroma and immediate free iliac crest block bone graft reconstruction with internal fixation (DuPuy Synthes Craniomaxillofacial, Paoli, PA, USA)

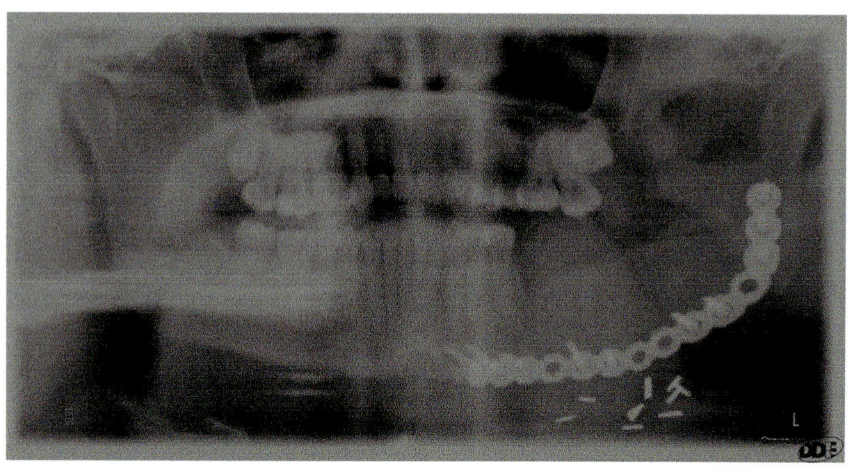

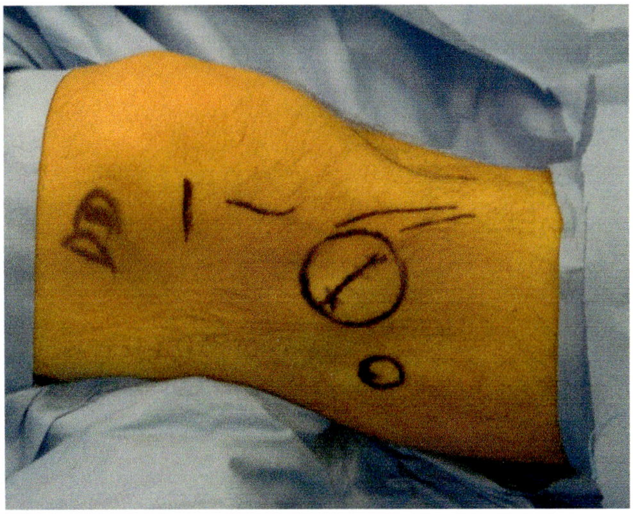

Fig. 5.53 Right knee marked for tibial bone graft harvest

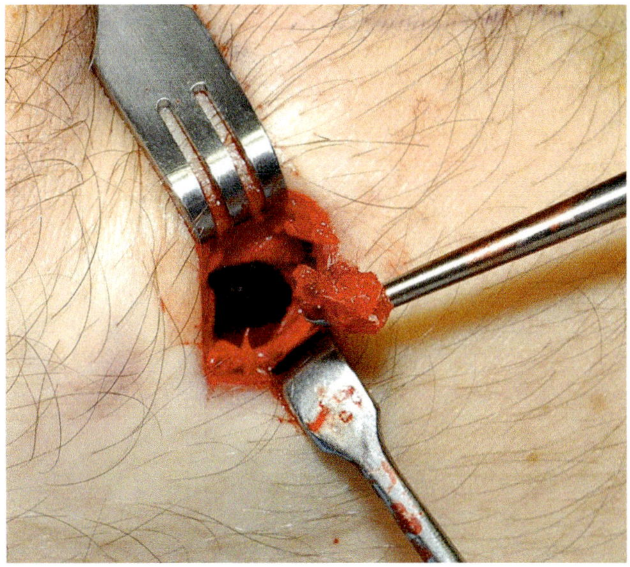

Fig. 5.54 Intraoperative tibial bone graft harvest

Fig. 5.55 Intraoperative view of *left* posterior mandible healed iliac crest reconstruction with bony union and tibial cancellous bone graft lateral augmentation and titanium mesh coverage (DuPuy Synthes Craniomaxillofacial, Paoli, PA)

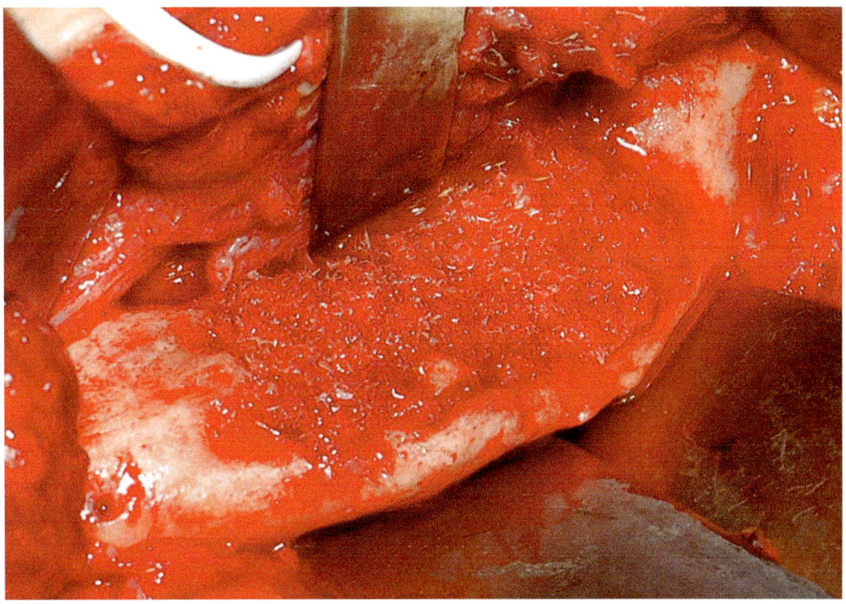

Fig. 5.56 Postoperative panoramic radiograph of *left* posterior mandible healed iliac crest reconstruction with bony union and tibial cancellous bone graft lateral augmentation and titanium mesh coverage (DuPuy Synthes Craniomaxillofacial, Paoli, PA)

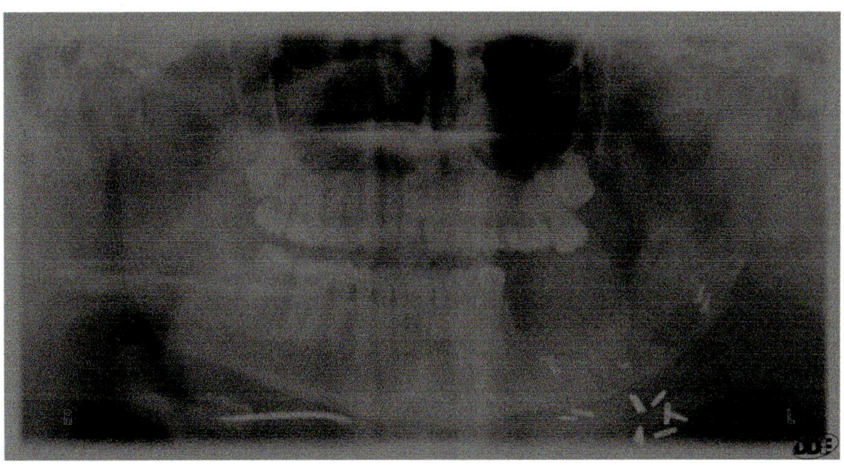

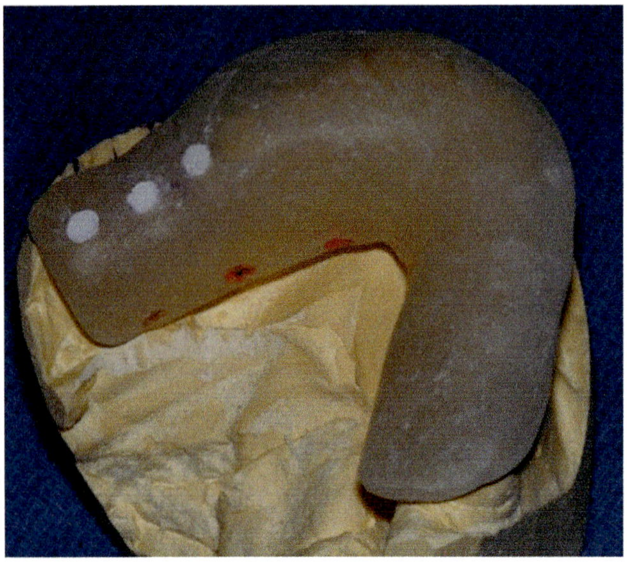

Fig. 5.57 Radiographic template for dual scan imaging

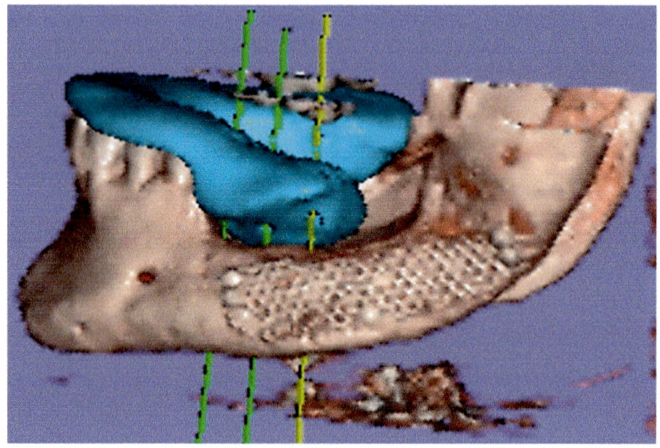

Fig. 5.59 Enlarged view of 3D representation of mandibular radiographic template with three dental implant trajectories (iDent Imaging, Inc., New York, NY, USA)

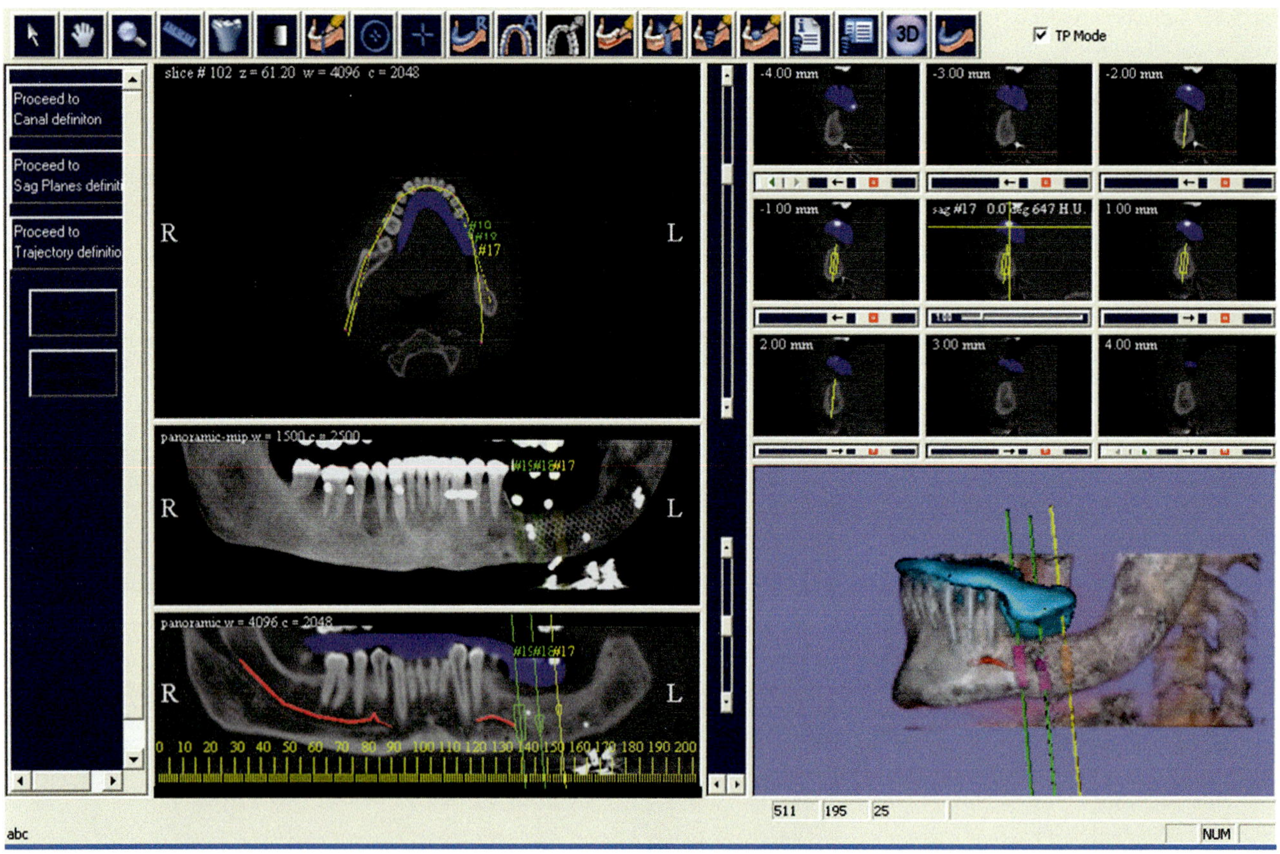

Fig. 5.58 Virtual planning with representation of radiographic template and trajectories for dental implants in the axial, oblique sagittal, and 3D images (iDent Imaging, Inc., New York, NY, USA)

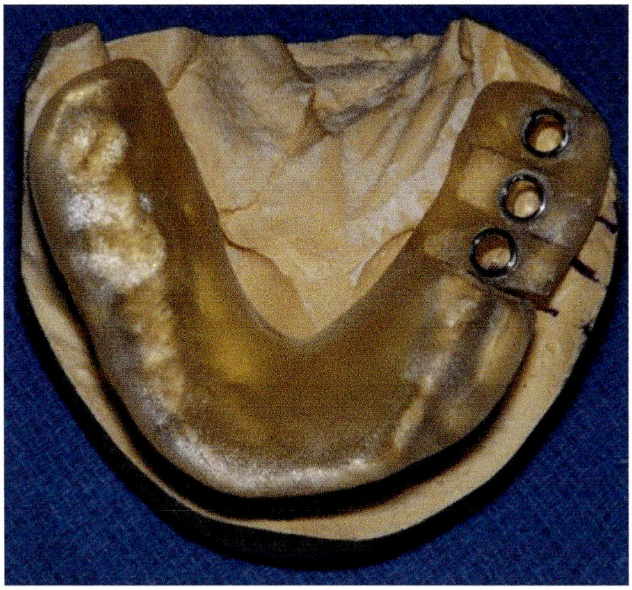

Fig. 5.60 Rapid printed mandibular CT surgical drill guide with master sleeves in place (iDent Imaging, Inc., New York, NY, USA)

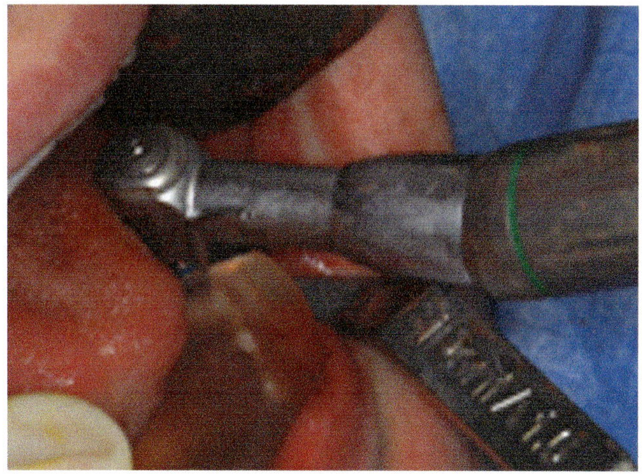

Fig. 5.62 Intraoperative view of drilling through master sleeve with drill handle within CT surgical drill guide

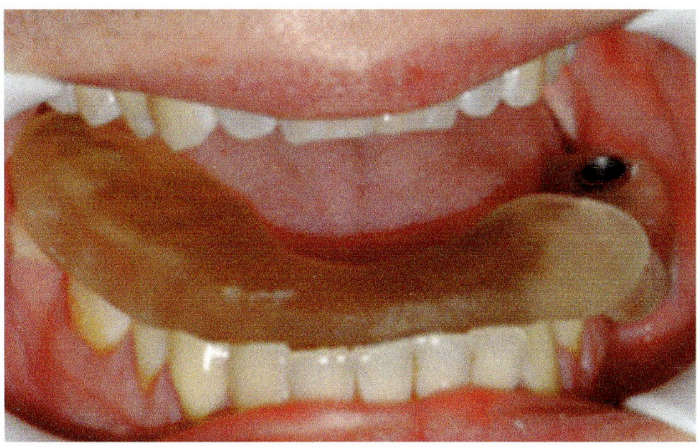

Fig. 5.61 Rapid printed CT surgical drill guide seated on mandibular dentition with satisfactory fit intraoral view

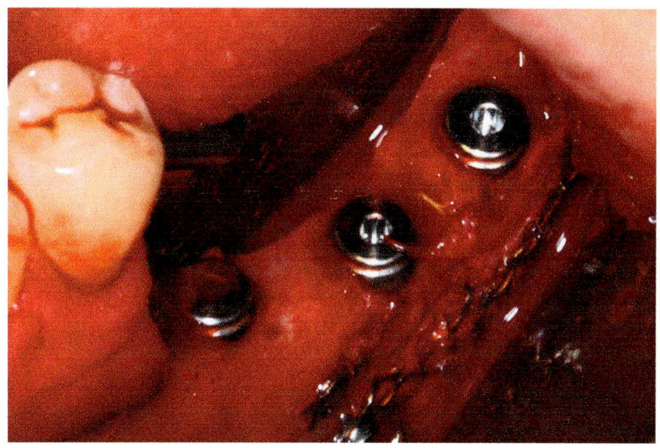

Fig. 5.63 Intraoperative view of three dental implants placed on the *left* posterior mandible (Keystone Dental, Burlington, MA, USA)

Fig. 5.64 Postoperative panoramic radiograph with implant-retained crowns. Note that the implant trajectories follow the virtual planning

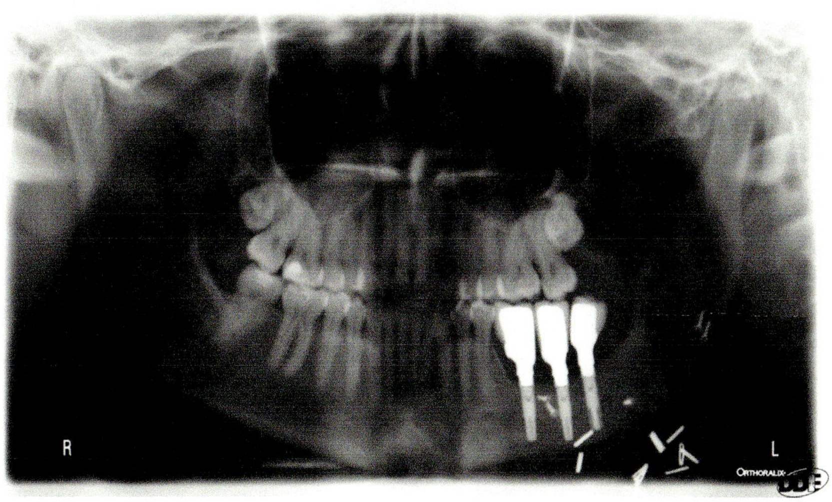

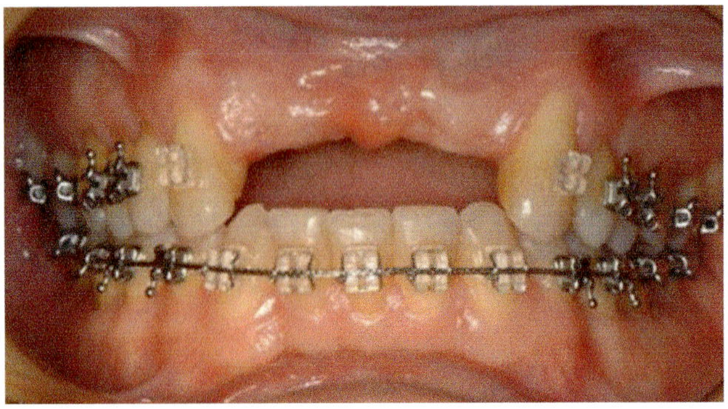

Fig. 5.65 Frontal view of partially edentulous occlusion missing teeth #7, 8, 9, and 10 with fixed orthodontic appliance

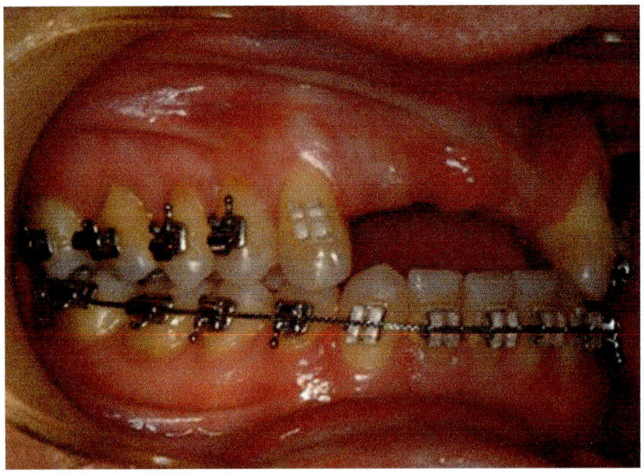

Fig. 5.66 Right frontal view of partially edentulous occlusion missing teeth #7, 8, 9, and 10 with fixed orthodontic appliance

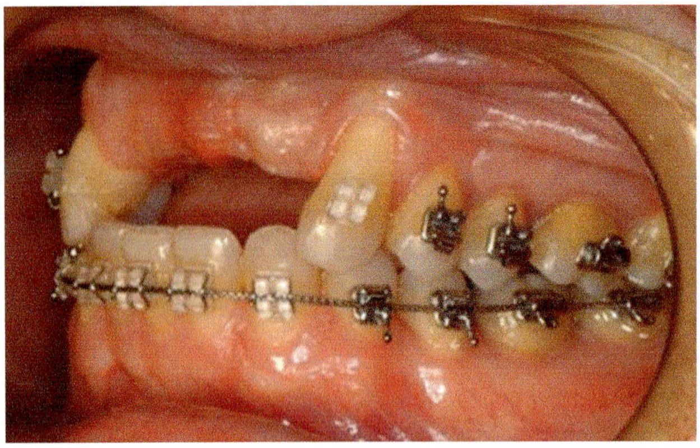

Fig. 5.67 Left frontal view of partially edentulous occlusion missing teeth #7, 8, 9, and 10 with fixed orthodontic appliance

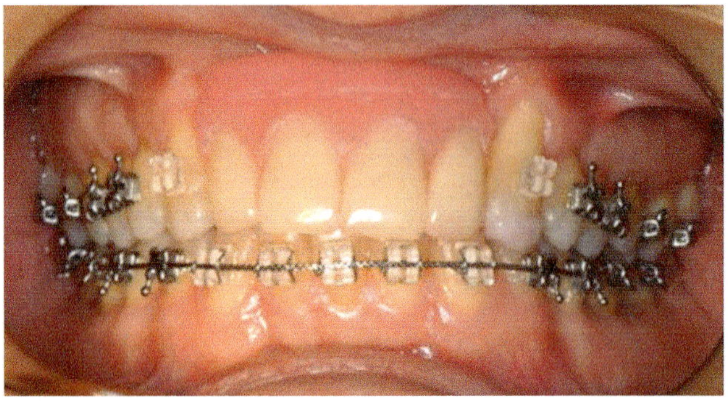

Fig. 5.68 Frontal view of ideal denture set up for partially edentulous occlusion missing teeth #7, 8, 9, and 10 with fixed orthodontic appliance

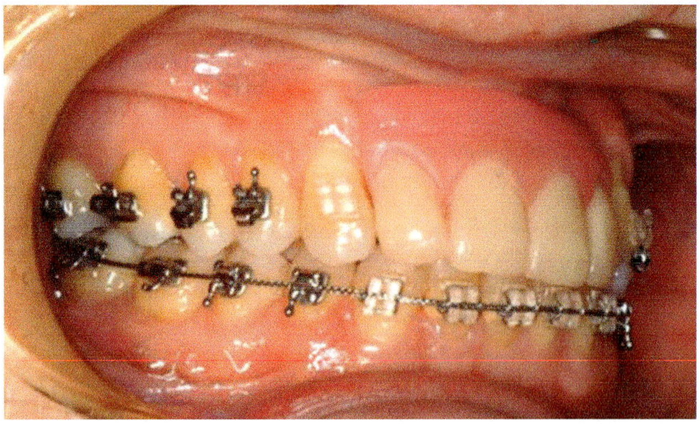

Fig. 5.69 Right frontal lateral view of ideal denture set up for partially edentulous occlusion missing teeth #7, 8, 9, and 10 with fixed orthodontic appliance

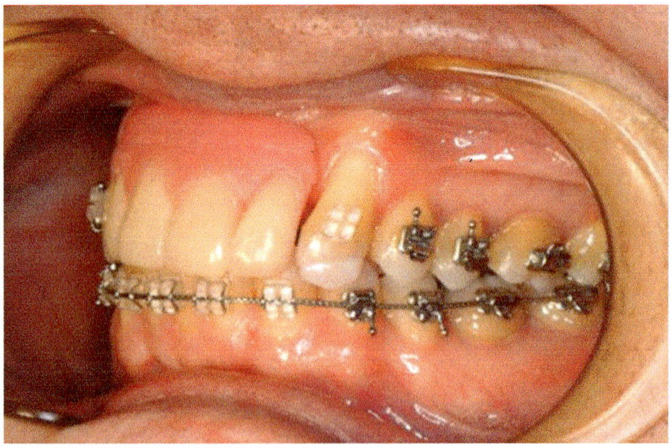

Fig. 5.70 Left frontal lateral view of ideal denture set up for partially edentulous occlusion missing teeth #7, 8, 9, and 10 with fixed orthodontic appliance

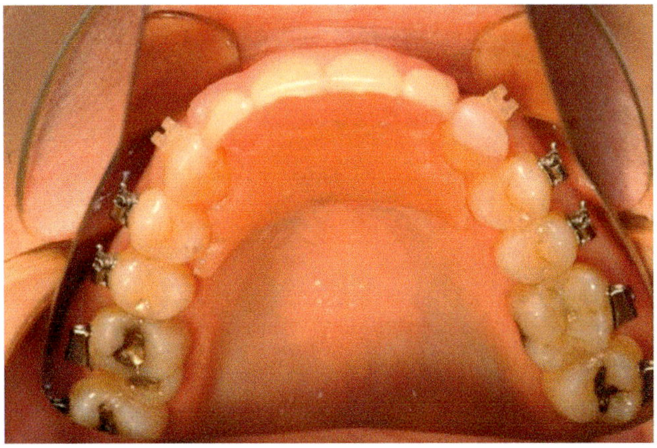

Fig. 5.71 Occlusal view of ideal denture set up for partially edentulous occlusion missing teeth #7, 8, 9, and 10 with fixed orthodontic appliance

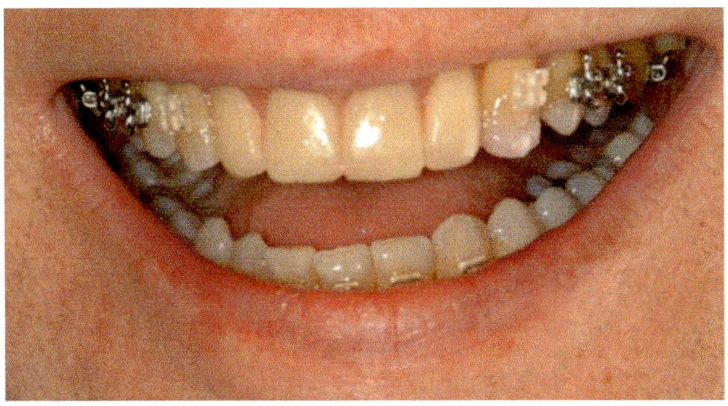

Fig. 5.72 Intraoral frontal lip draped view of ideal denture set up for partially edentulous occlusion missing teeth #7, 8, 9, and 10 with fixed orthodontic appliance

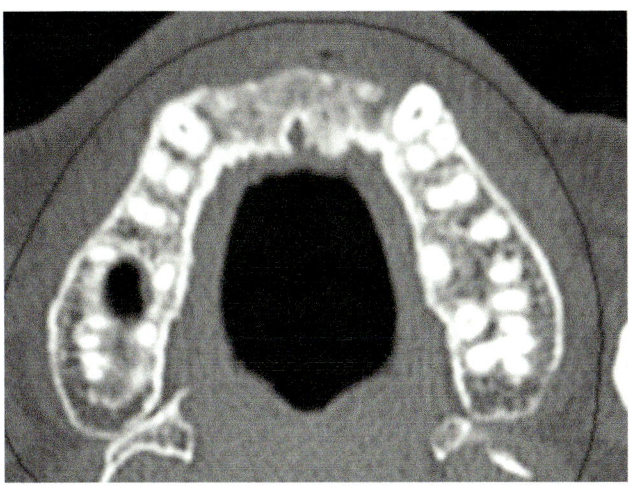

Fig. 5.73 Preoperative axial view of CT scan demonstrates adequate alveolar bone but in a Class III relationship

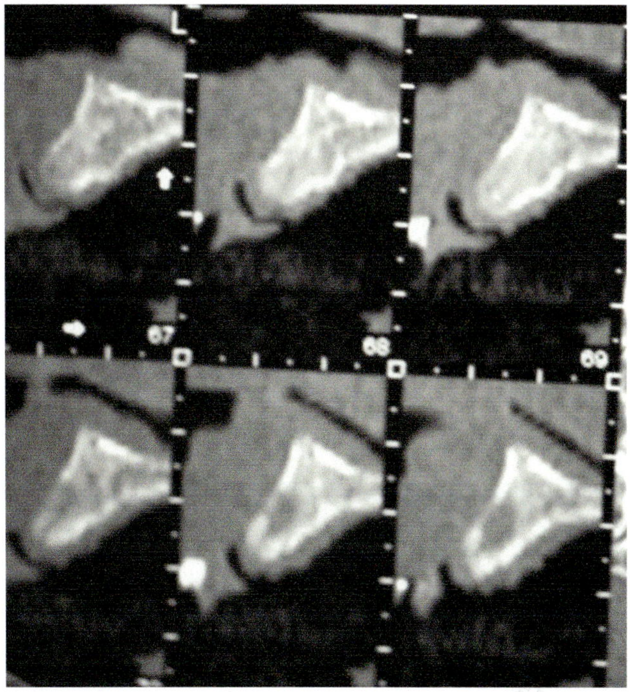

Fig. 5.74 Preoperative oblique sagittal view of anterior maxillary region

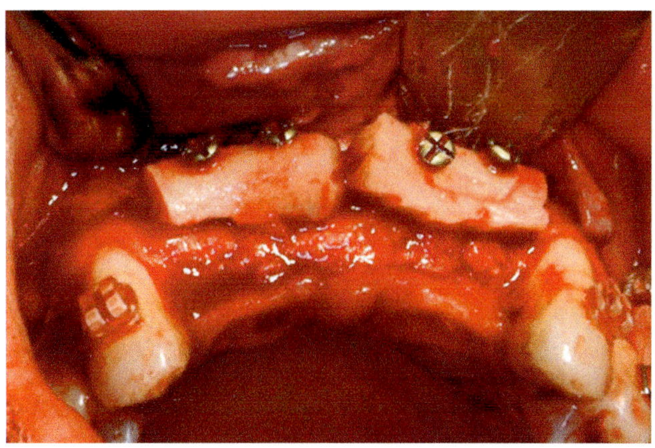

Fig. 5.75 Intraoperative view of bilateral mandibular ramus cortico-cancellous bone grafts to the anterior maxillary alveolar region teeth #7, 8, 9, and 10 with screw fixation (DuPuy Synthes Craniomaxillofacial, Paoli, PA, USA)

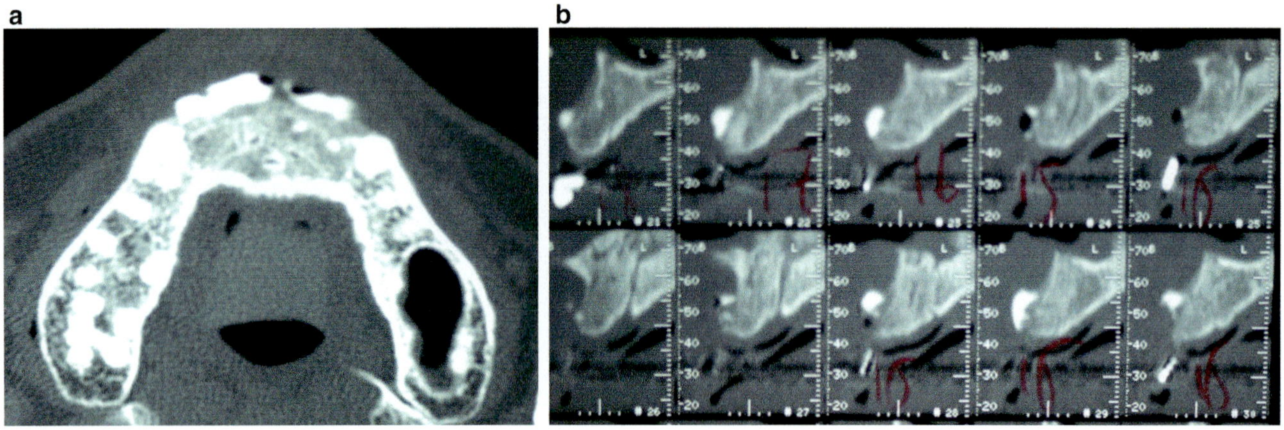

Fig. 5.76 Postoperative CT scan following bilateral mandibular ramus corticocancellous bone grafts to the anterior maxillary alveolar region teeth #7, 8, 9, and 10. (**a**) Axial view. (**b**) Oblique sagittal views

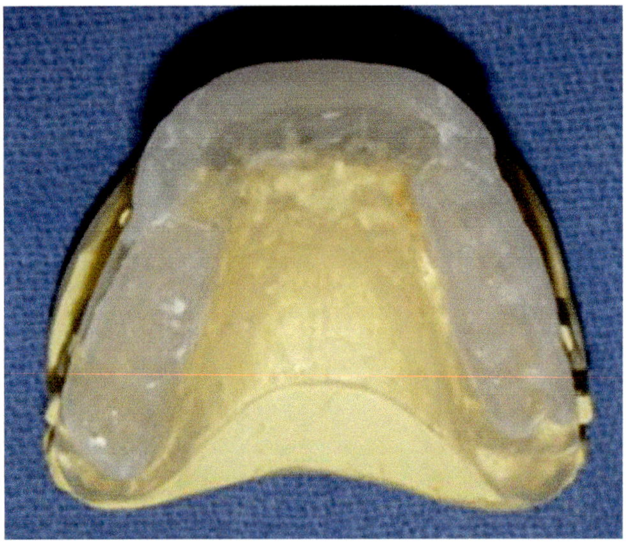

Fig. 5.77 Radiographic template

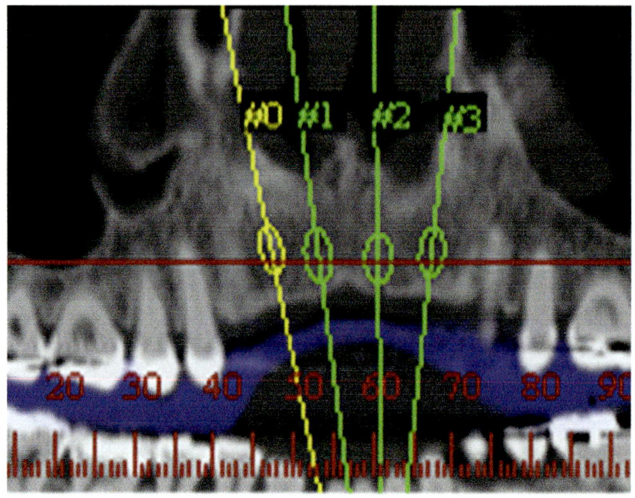

Fig. 5.79 Virtual planning environment with planned dental implant trajectories in panoramic view of the virtual planning environment (iDent Imaging, Inc., New York, NY, USA)

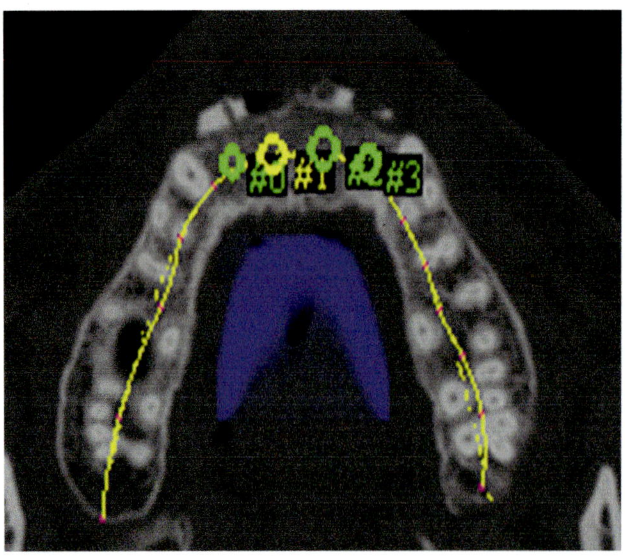

Fig. 5.78 Virtual planning environment axial view demonstrating ideal dental implant positions following anterior maxillary corticocancellous ramus bone grafting (iDent Imaging, Inc., New York, NY, USA)

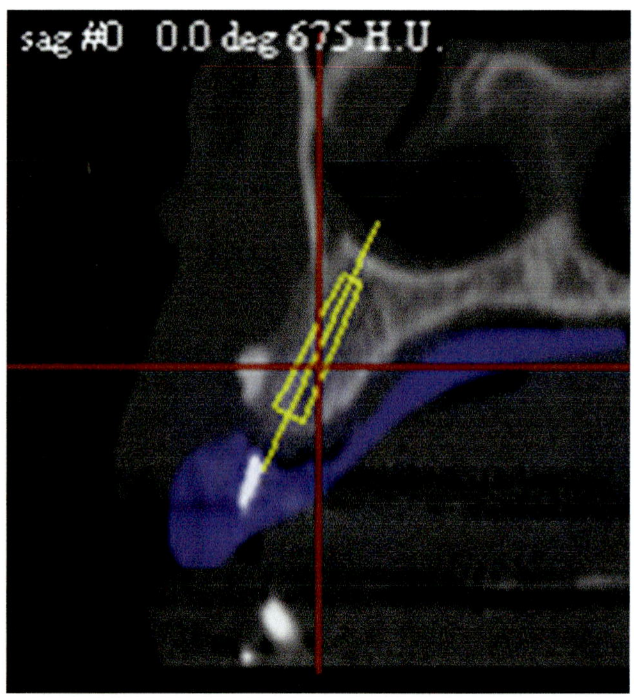

Fig. 5.80 Virtual planning environment oblique sagittal view of dental implant tooth #7 (iDent Imaging, Inc., New York, NY, USA)

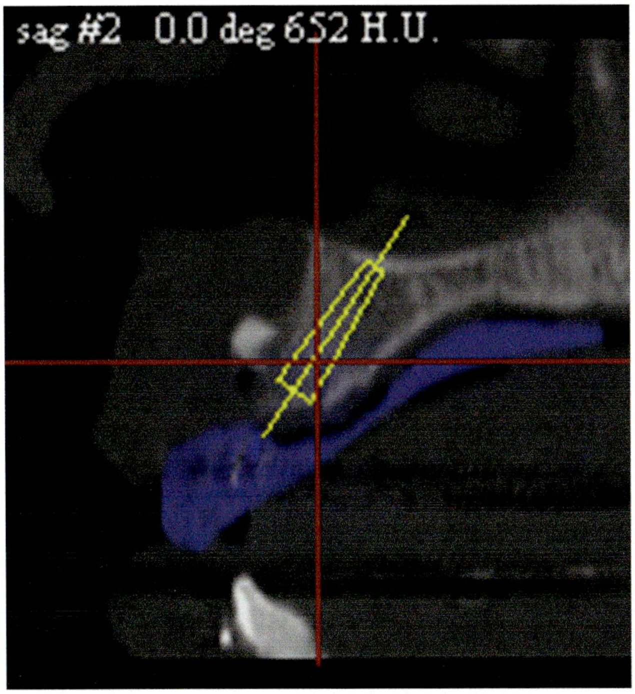

Fig. 5.81 Virtual planning environment oblique sagittal view of dental implant tooth #8 (iDent Imaging, Inc., New York, NY, USA)

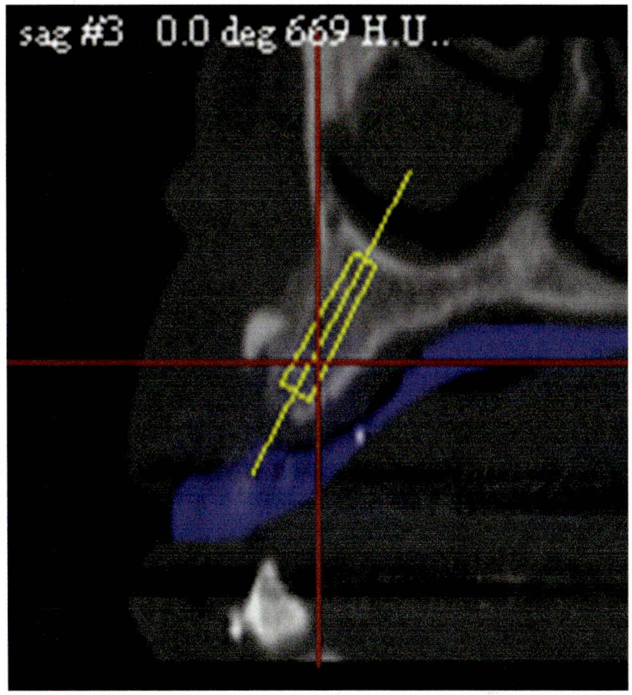

Fig. 5.83 Virtual planning environment oblique sagittal view of dental implant tooth #10 (iDent Imaging, Inc., New York, NY, USA)

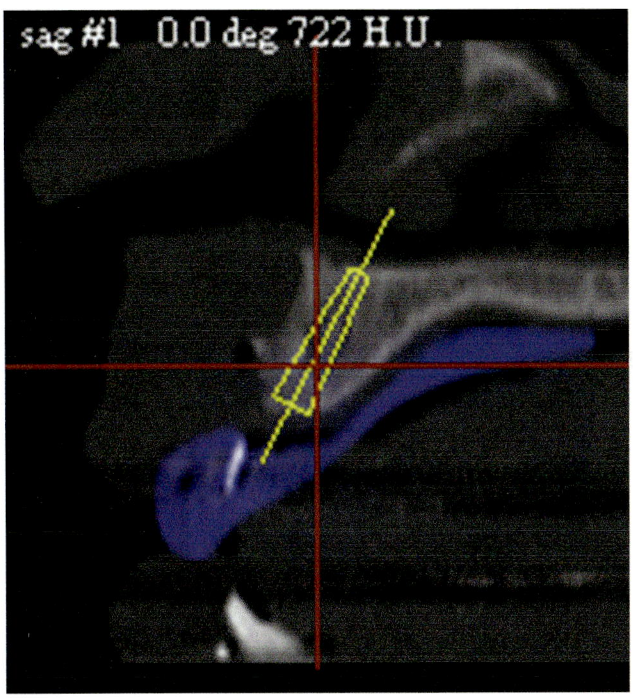

Fig. 5.82 Virtual planning environment oblique sagittal view of dental implant tooth #9 (iDent Imaging, Inc., New York, NY, USA)

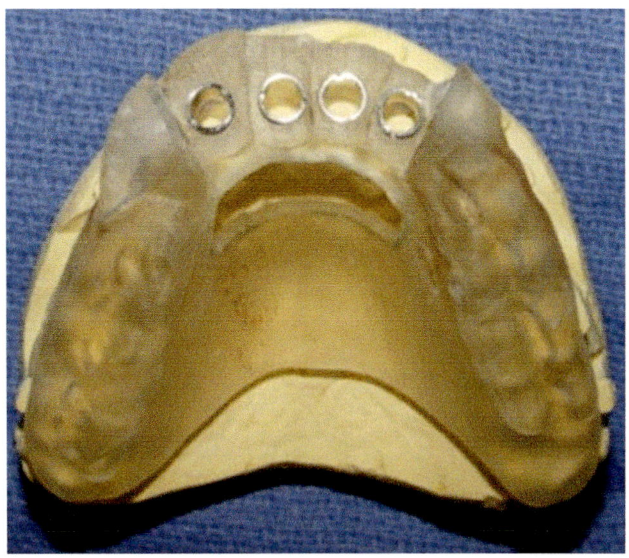

Fig. 5.84 Rapid printed CT surgical drill guide with palatal window for open flap for buccal bone reduction (iDent Imaging, Inc., New York, NY, USA)

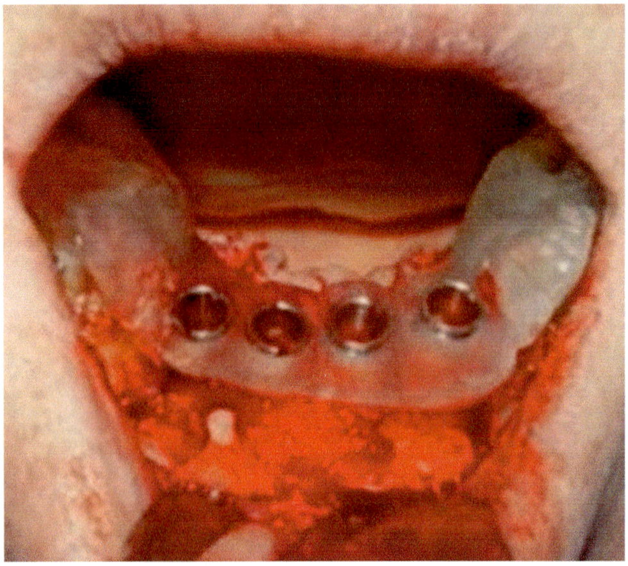

Fig. 5.85 Intraoperative view of rapid printed CT surgical drill guide with palatal window for open flap for buccal bone reduction seated on dentition and flap retracted through palatal window

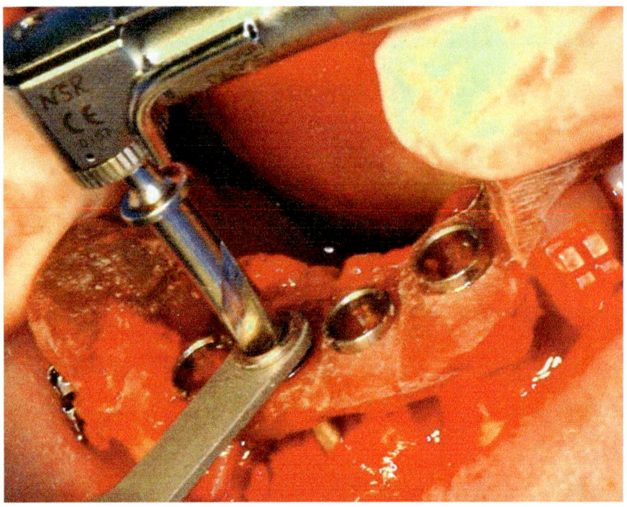

Fig. 5.86 Intraoperative of drilling through guide with drill handle

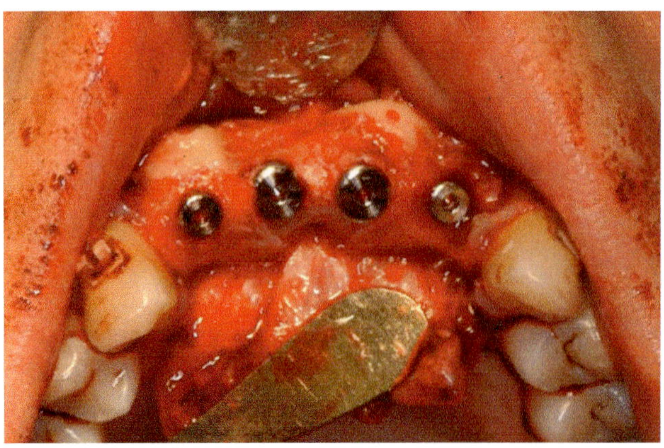

Fig. 5.87 Intraoperative view of dental implant placement with precise placement of implants in ideal positions teeth #7 (narrow diameter), #8 (regular diameter), #9 (regular diameter), and #10 (narrow diameter) (Zimmer Biomet 3i, Palm Beach Gardens, FL, USA)

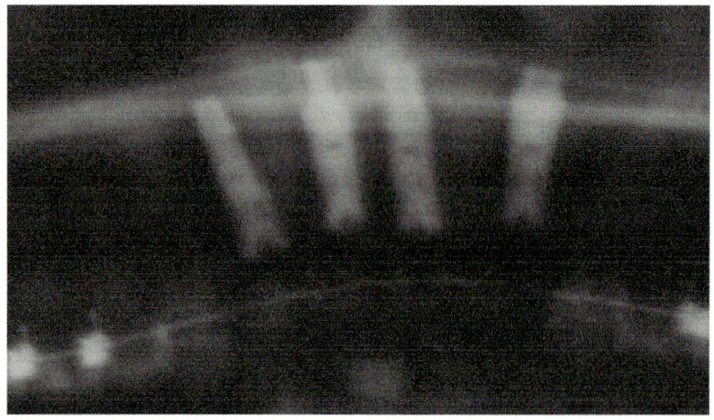

Fig. 5.88 Postoperative periapical radiograph demonstrates implant positions

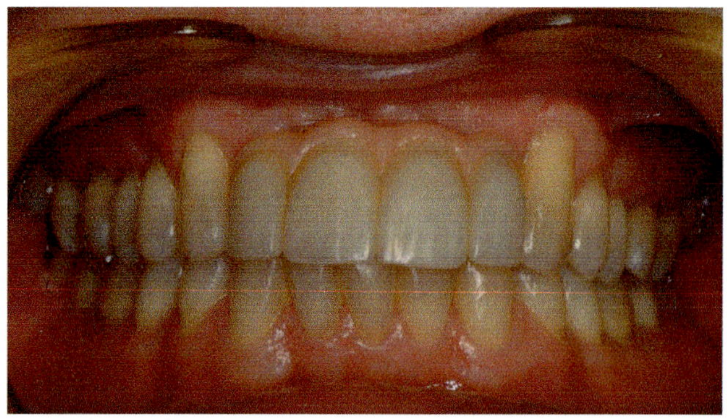

Fig. 5.89 Post treatment completion final prosthesis frontal view

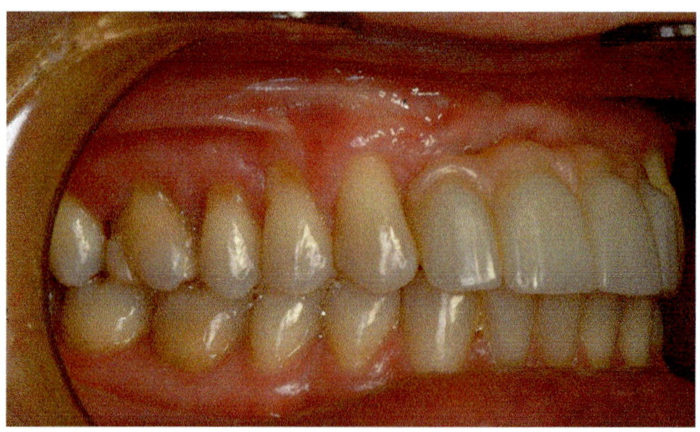

Fig. 5.90 Post treatment completion final prosthesis right lateral view

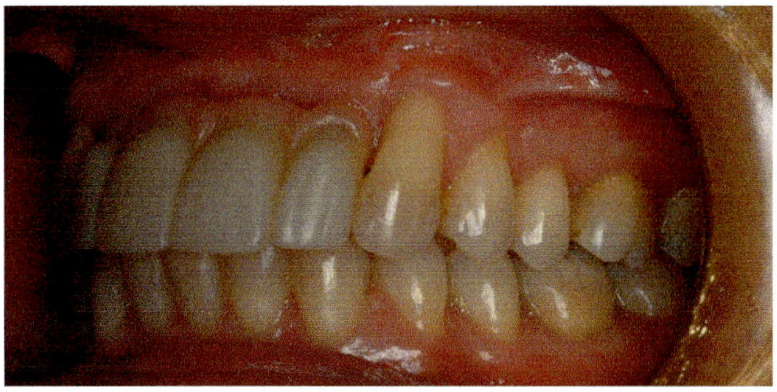

Fig. 5.91 Post treatment completion final prosthesis left lateral view

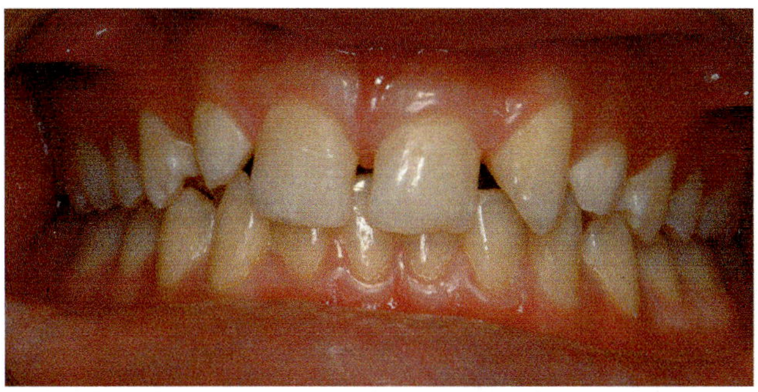

Fig. 5.92 Preoperative preorthodontic treatment frontal view

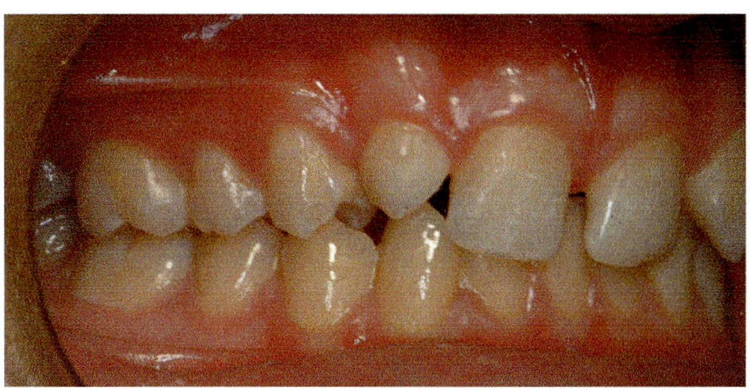

Fig. 5.93 Preoperative preorthodontic treatment frontal right view

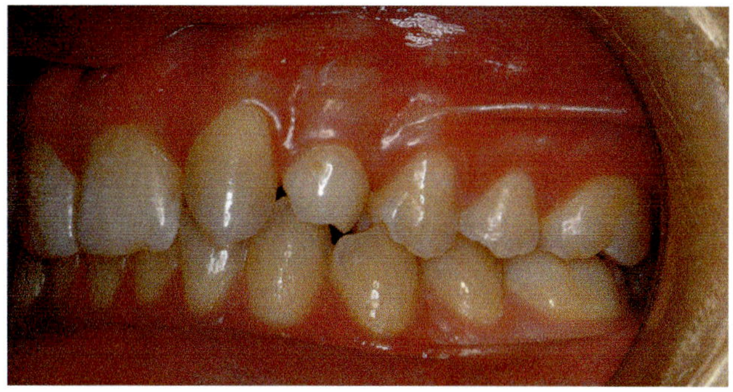

Fig. 5.94 Preoperative preorthodontic treatment frontal left view

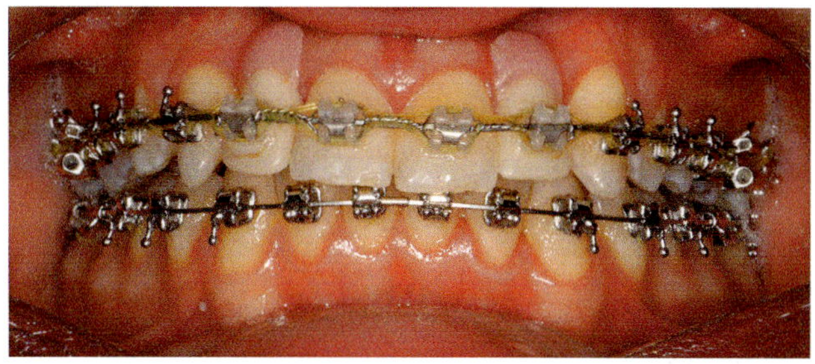

Fig. 5.95 Preoperative orthodontic treatment frontal view with space created for teeth #7 and 10 pontics

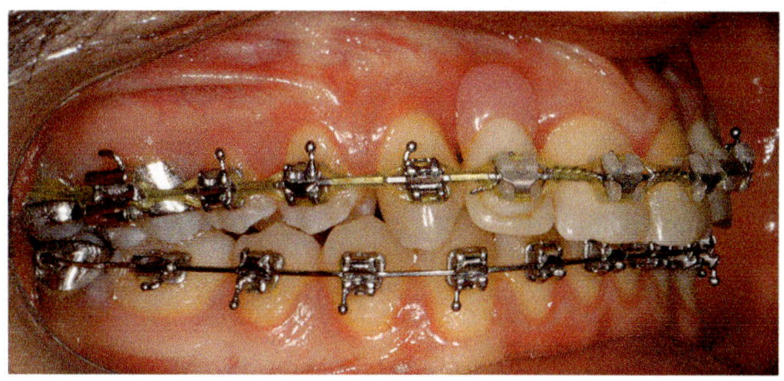

Fig. 5.96 Preoperative orthodontic treatment *right* lateral view with space created for tooth #7 pontic

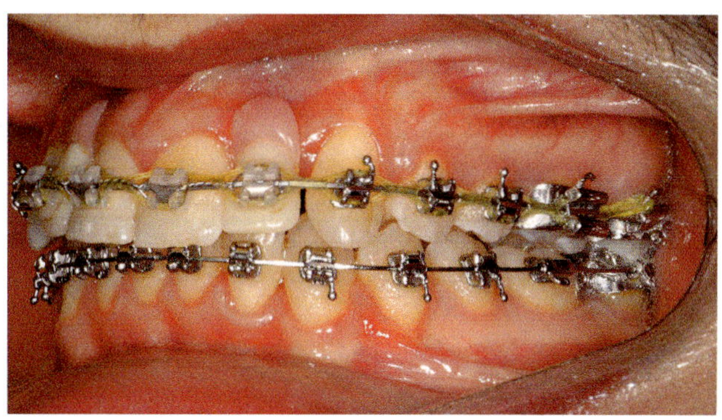

Fig. 5.97 Preoperative orthodontic treatment *left* lateral view with space created for tooth #10 pontic

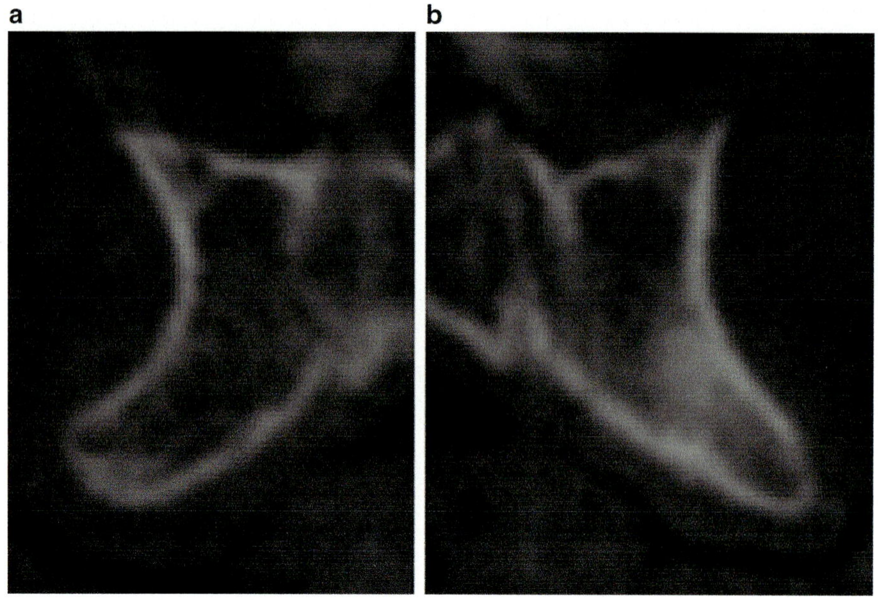

Fig. 5.98 (**a**) Preoperative CBCT oblique sagittal view tooth #7 adequate bone height and width. (**b**) Preoperative CBCT oblique sagittal view tooth #10 adequate bone height and width

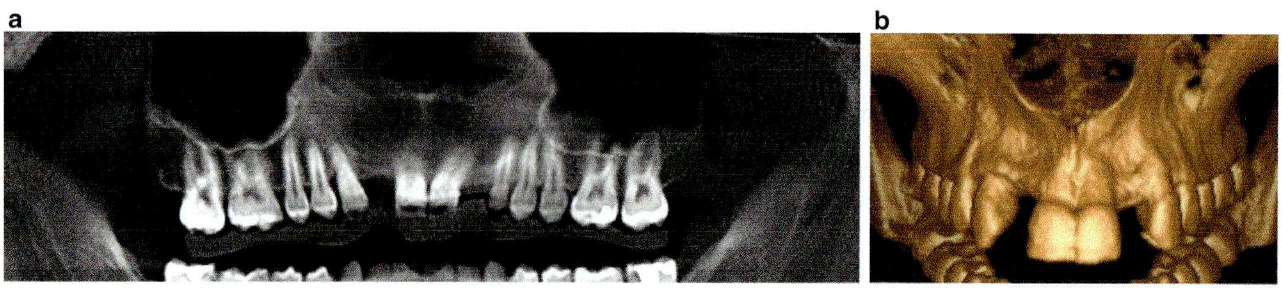

Fig. 5.99 (**a**) Preoperative panoramic radiograph. (**b**) 3D image of maxillary region facial view

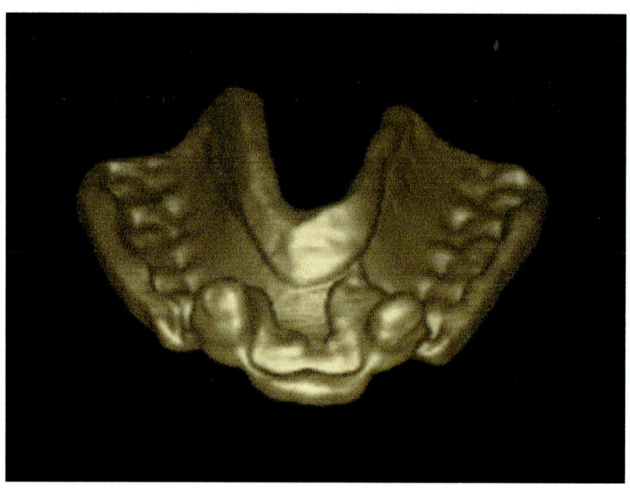

Fig. 5.100 Radiographic template

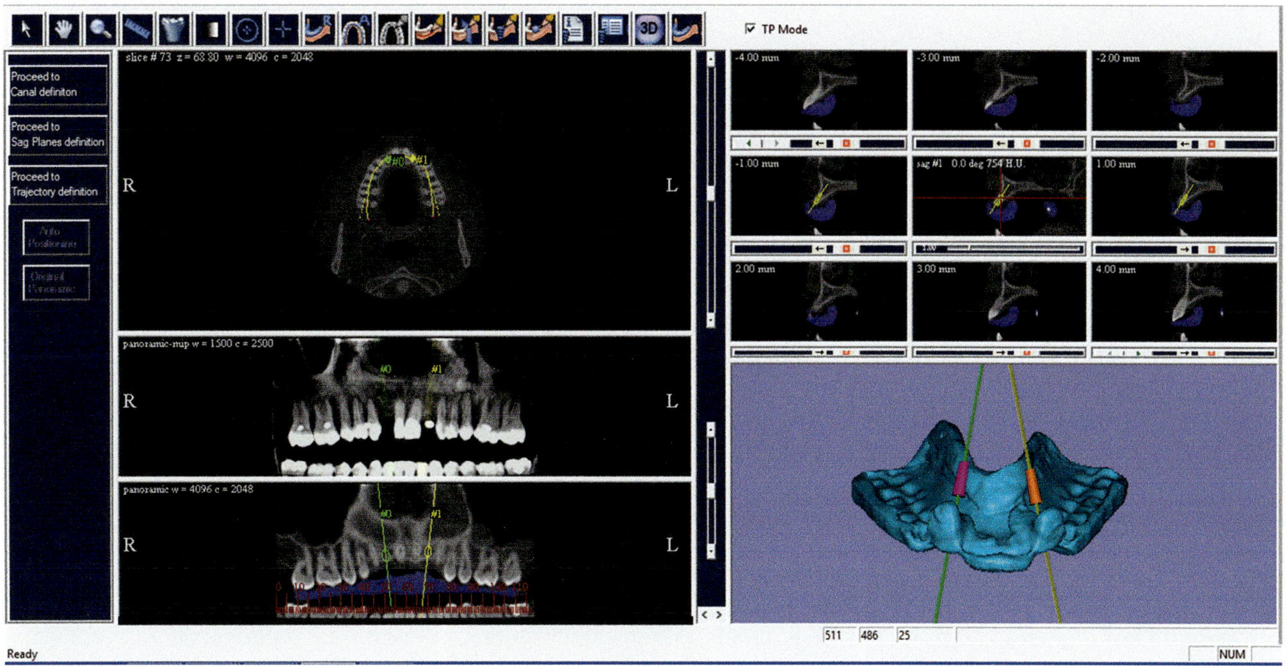

Fig. 5.101 Virtual planning environment 3D template with dental implant trajectories teeth #7 and 10 with panoramic and oblique sagittal views (iDent Imaging, Inc., New York, NY, USA)

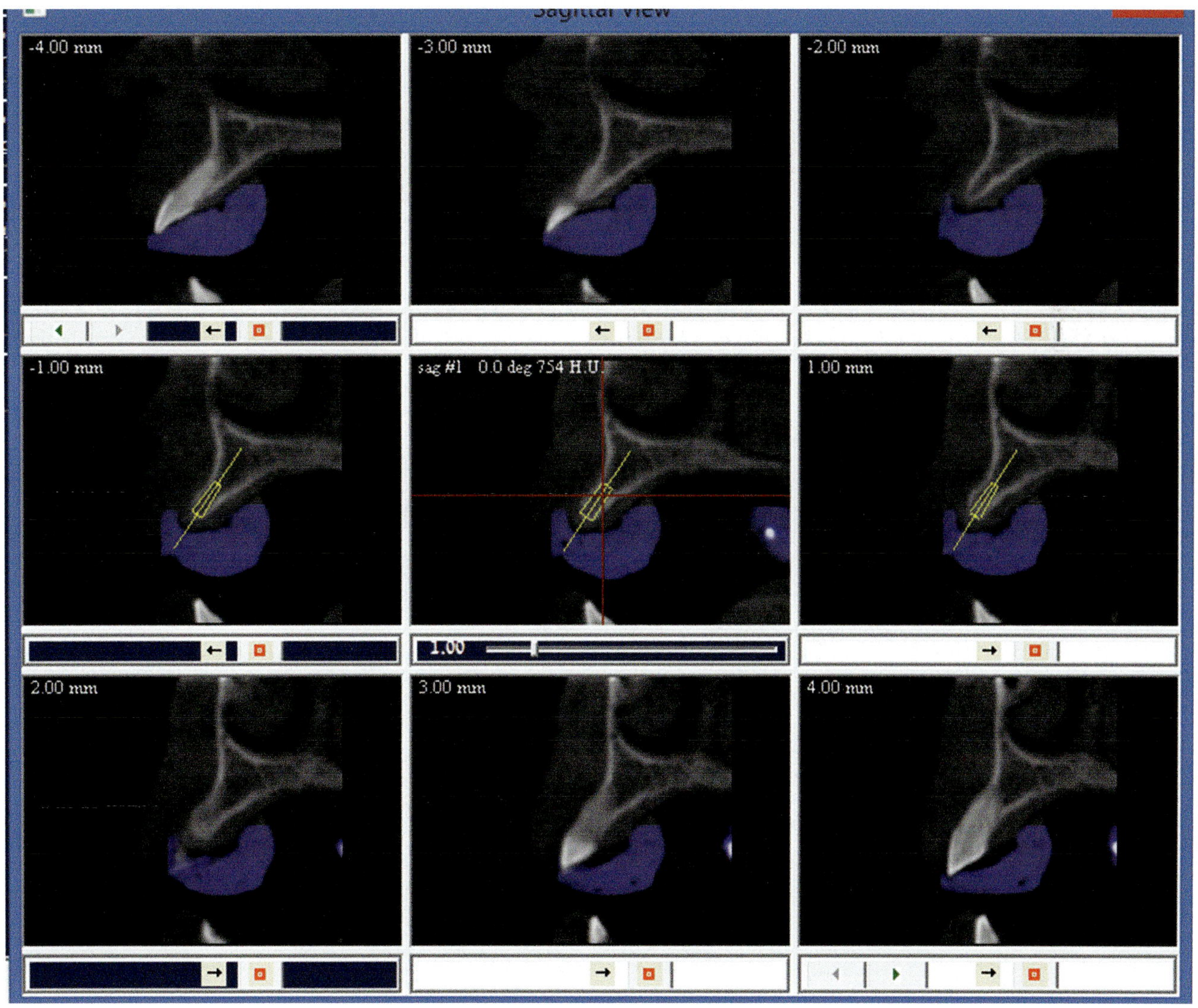

Fig. 5.102 Virtual planning environment radiographic template oblique sagittal views tooth #7 with dental implant trajectories (iDent Imaging, Inc., New York, NY, USA)

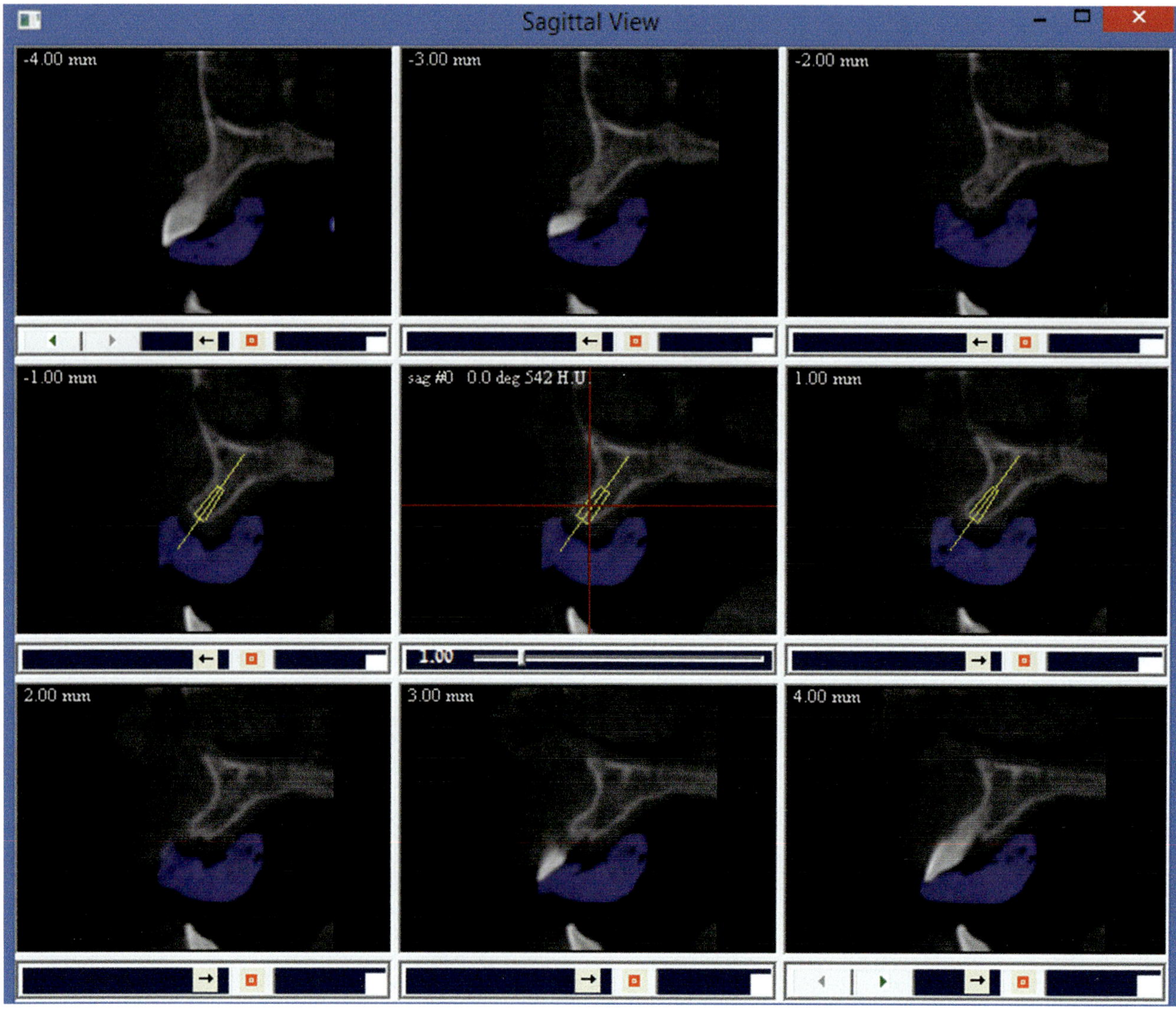

Fig. 5.103 Virtual planning environment radiographic template oblique sagittal views tooth #10 with dental implant trajectories (iDent Imaging, Inc., New York, NY, USA)

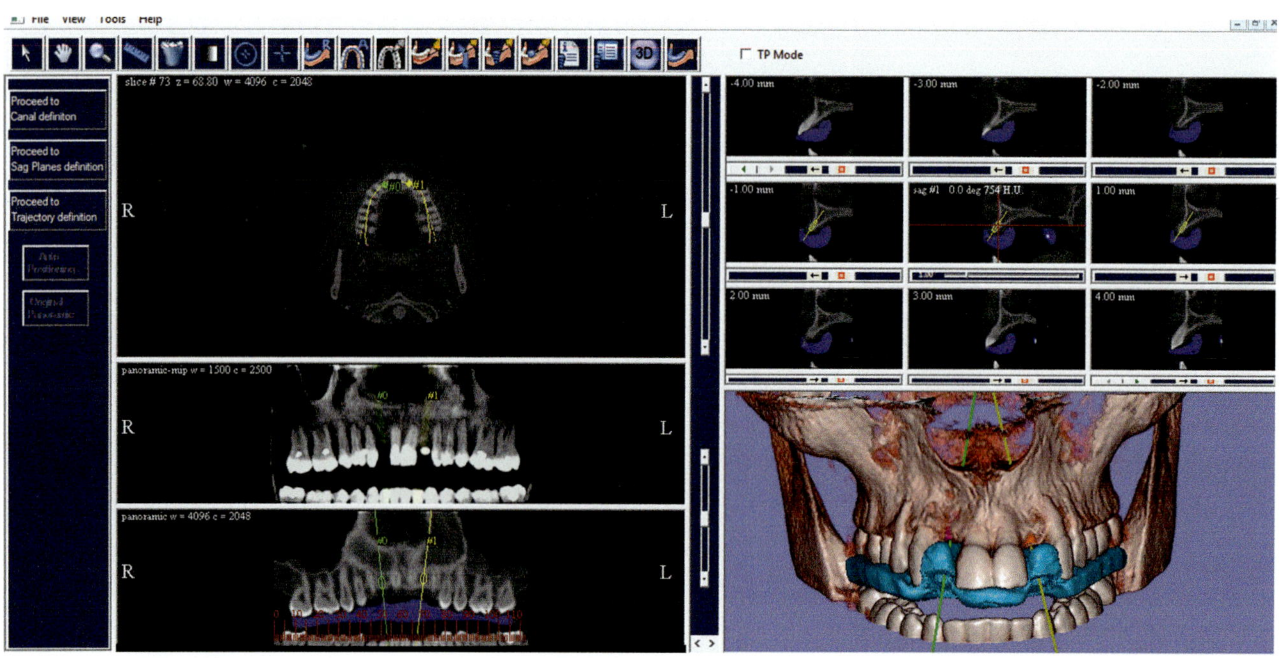

Fig. 5.104 Virtual planning environment with conversion of the radiographic template into the surgical template by digital subtraction of voxels with dental implant trajectories (iDent Imaging, Inc., New York, NY, USA)

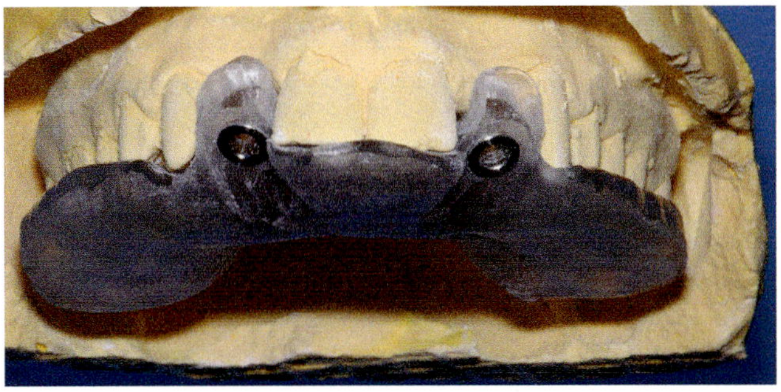

Fig. 5.105 Rapid printed surgical drill guide (iDent Imaging, Inc., New York, NY, USA)

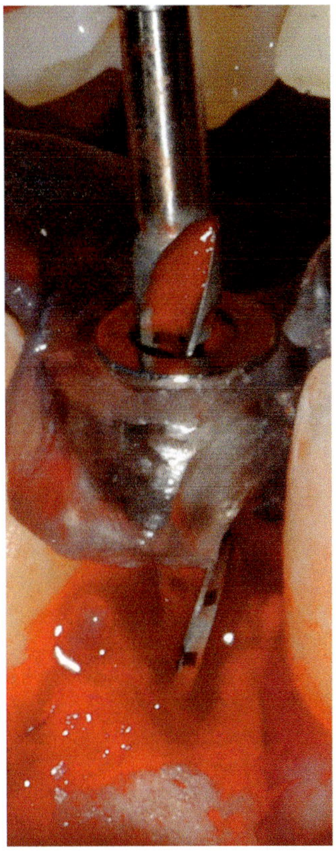

Fig. 5.106 Intraoperative view of drilling through master sleeve with handled drill guide within CT surgical drill guide

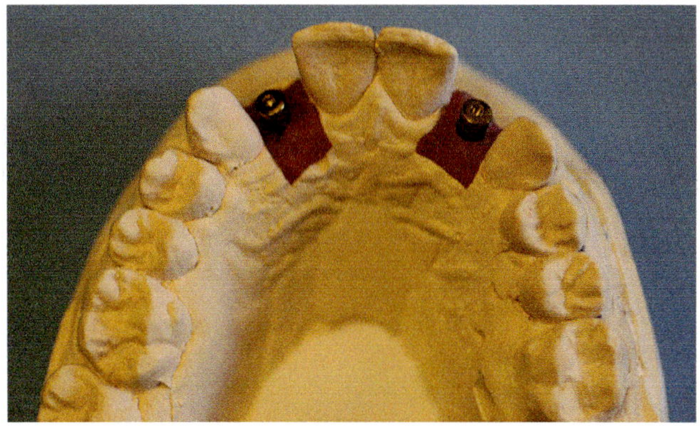

Fig. 5.108 Dental laboratory model demonstrating precise positions of dental implants #7 and 10 as per the surgical plan and surgical drill guide

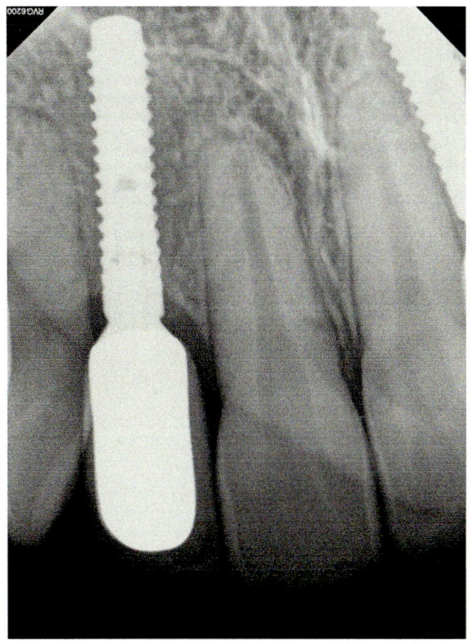

Fig. 5.109 Final postoperative PA radiograph of dental implant-retained crown maxillary *right* lateral incisor tooth #7

a b

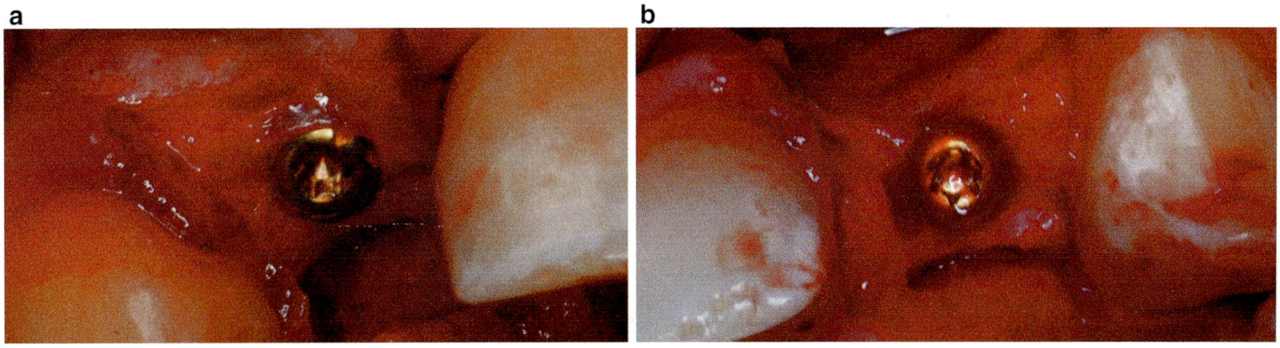

Fig. 5.107 (**a**) Intraoperative view of Straumann Bone Level Narrow Diameter dental implant (Straumann USA, LLC, Andover, MA, USA) placed maxillary *right* lateral incisor tooth #7. (**b**) Intraoperative view of Straumann Bone Level Narrow Diameter dental implant (Strauamnn USA, LLC, Andover, MA, USA) placed maxillary *left* lateral incisor tooth #10

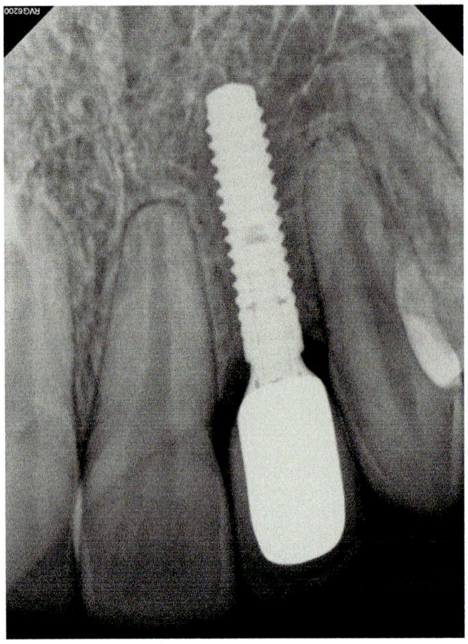

Fig. 5.110 Final postoperative PA radiograph of dental implant-retained crown maxillary *right* lateral incisor tooth #10

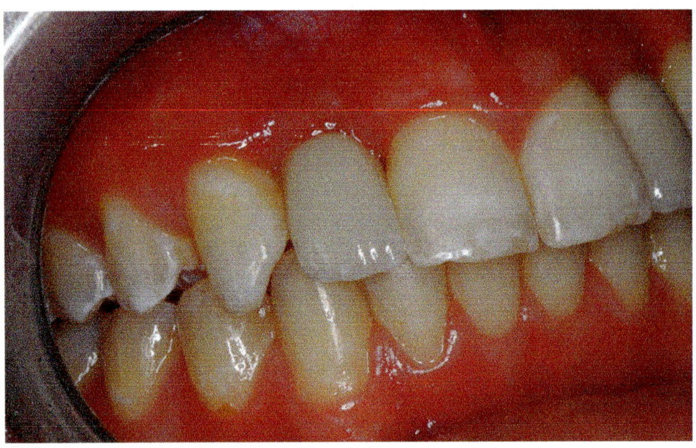

Fig. 5.111 Postoperative *right* facial view of dental implant-retained crown maxillary *right* lateral incisor tooth #7

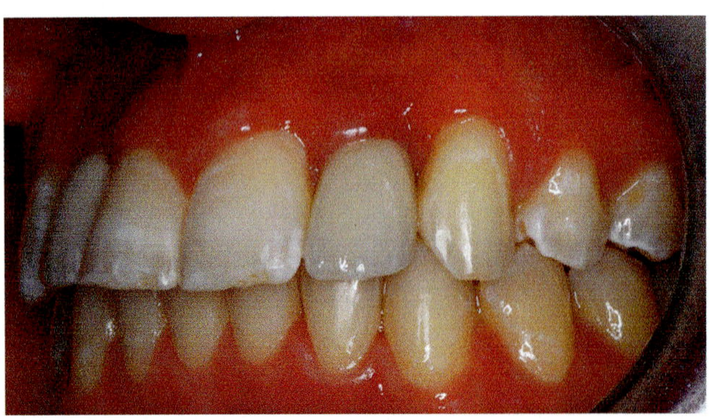

Fig. 5.112 Postoperative *left* facial view of dental implant-retained crown maxillary *left* lateral incisor tooth #10

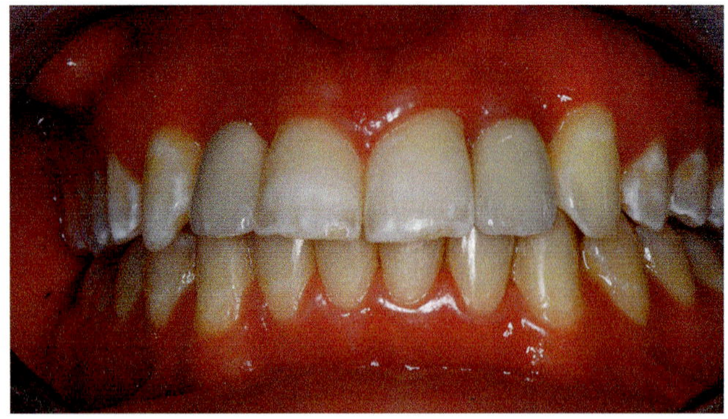

Fig. 5.113 Postoperative facial view of dental implant-retained crown maxillary *left* and *right* lateral incisors teeth #7 and 10

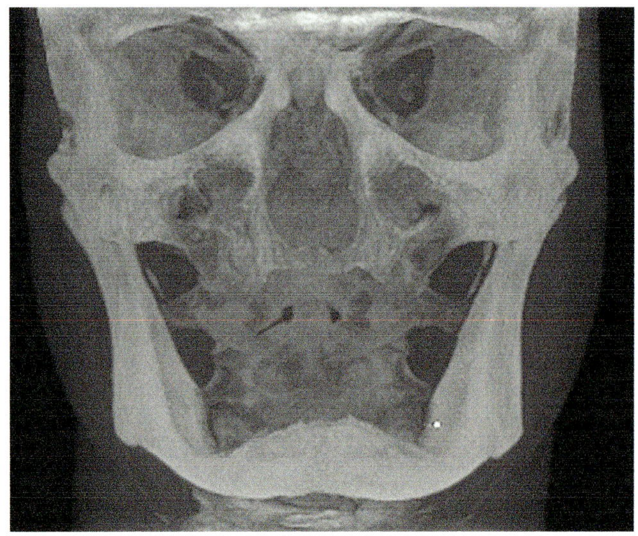

Fig. 5.114 Preoperative CBCT PA view of total edentulism with advanced alveolar atrophy

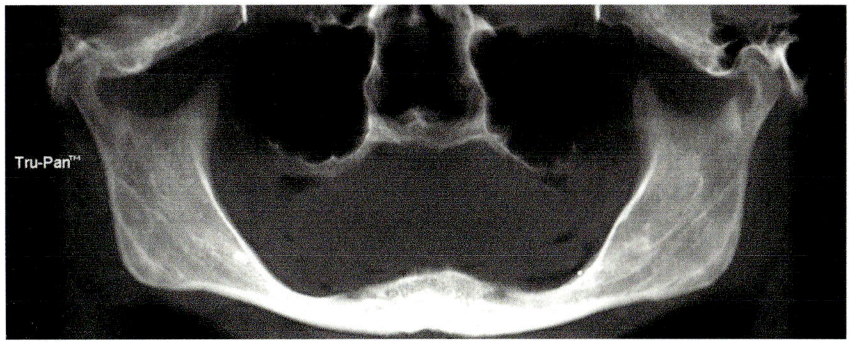

Fig. 5.115 Preoperative CBCT panoramic view of total edentulism with advanced alveolar atrophy

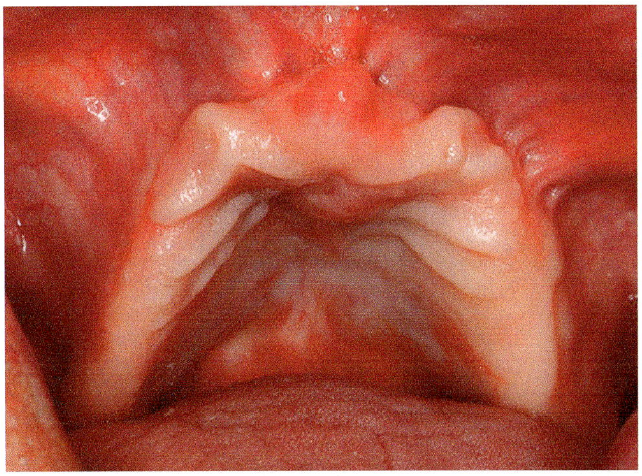

Fig. 5.116 Preoperative clinical frontal occlusal view of maxillary total edentulism

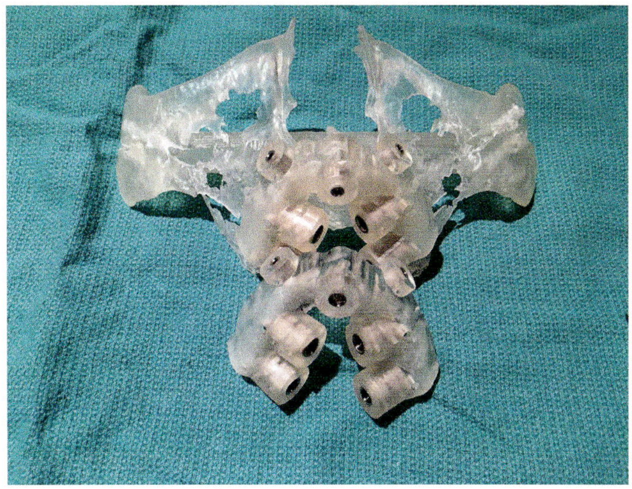

Fig. 5.118 Nobel Biocare compatible SIMPLANT (Materialise, Dentsply, York, PA, USA) sequential bone-borne surgical guides for four bilateral zygomatic implants with fixation screw holes which were placed to stabilize the guides during drilling and seating on 3D model

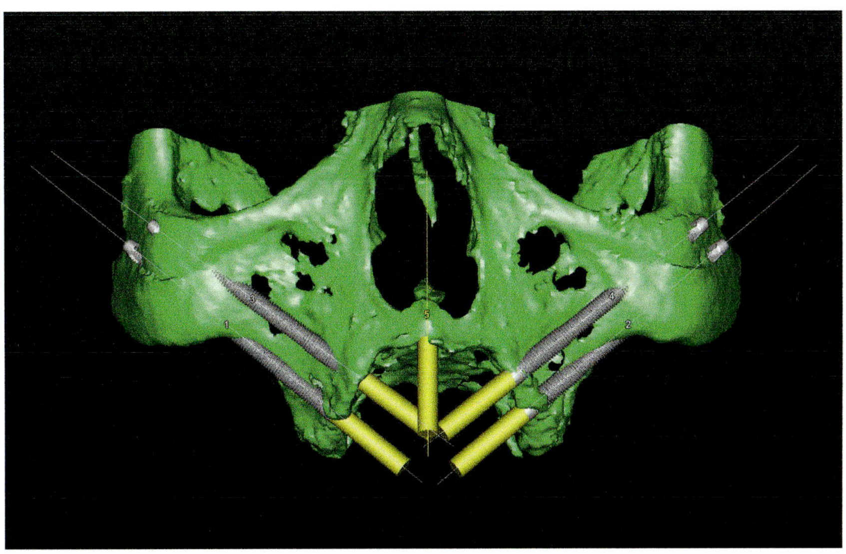

Fig. 5.117 Virtual treatment plan using SIMPLANT Master software (Materialise, Dentsply, York, PA, USA), with quad zygomatic implant design with an additional anterior midline implant to restore the severely atrophic maxilla

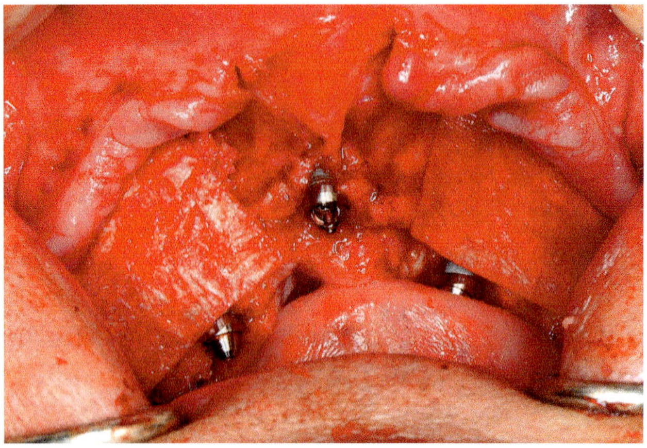

Fig. 5.119 Intraoperative view of four zygomatic and single midline maxillary implants which are in position with multiunit abutments in preparation for polyvinylsiloxane impressions for provisional restorations (Nobel Biocare, Yorba Linda, CA, USA)

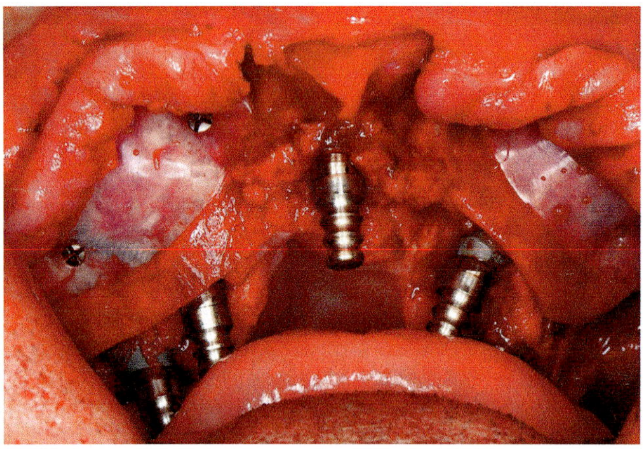

Fig. 5.120 Intraoperative view of four zygomatic and single midline maxillary implants which are in position according to the computer-guided plan. Closed tray impression coping was placed over angled multiunit abutments in preparation for polyvinylsiloxane impressions for provisional restorations. Bilateral malar augmentation with Silastic implants fixated with screws placed over resorbable barrier membranes prior to wound closure (Nobel Biocare, Yorba Linda, CA, USA)

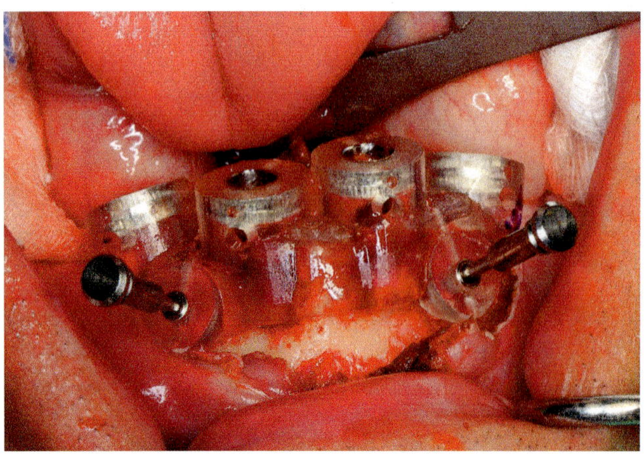

Fig. 5.121 Intraoperative view of mandibular bone-borne surgical guide with stabilization pins for "All on 4" implant placement (Materialise, Dentsply, York, PA, USA)

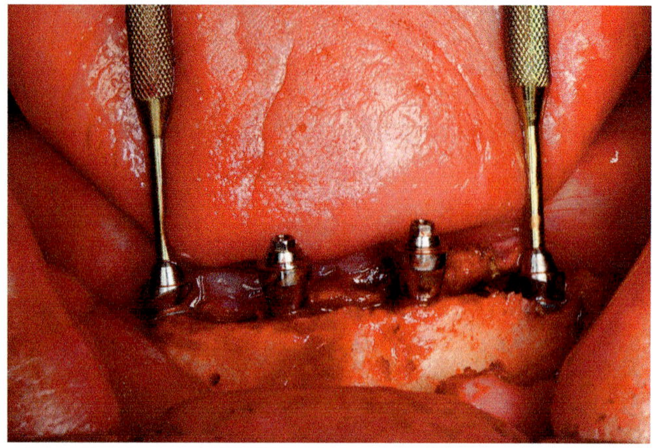

Fig. 5.122 Intraoperative view of four mandibular implants with placement of anterior conical and posterior angled multiunit abutments (Nobel Biocare, Yorba Linda, CA, USA)

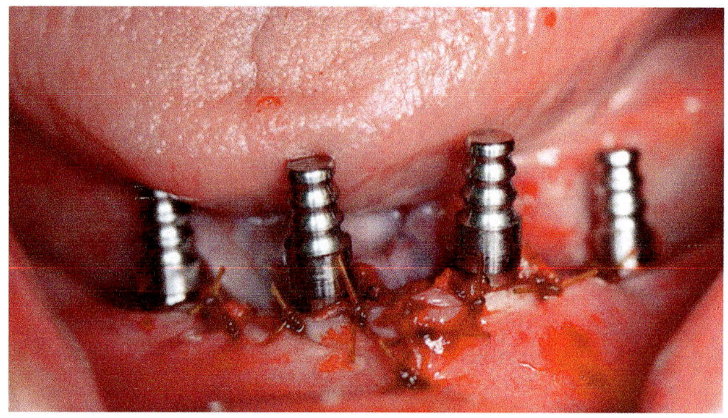

Fig. 5.123 Intraoperative view of four mandibular implants with placement of anterior conical and posterior angled multiunit abutments and placement of closed tray impression copings (Nobel Biocare, Yorba Linda, CA, USA)

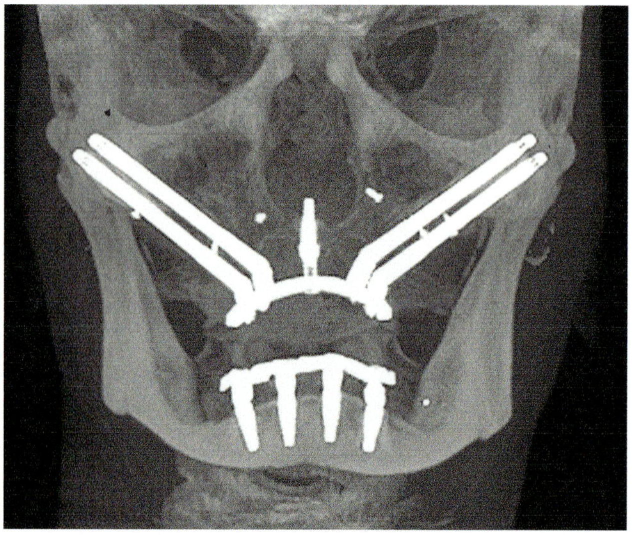

Fig. 5.124 Postoperative PA view of maxillary quad zygoma and single midline and mandibular conventional "All on 4" implant placement (Nobel Biocare, Yorba Linda, CA, USA)

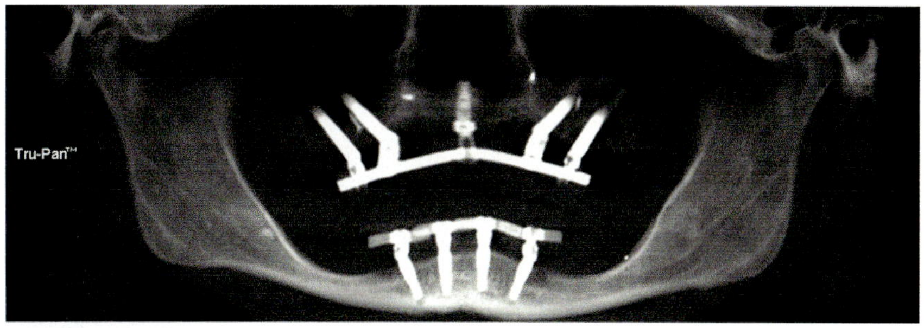

Fig. 5.125 Postoperative panoramic view of maxillary quad zygoma and single midline and mandibular conventional All on 4 implant placement

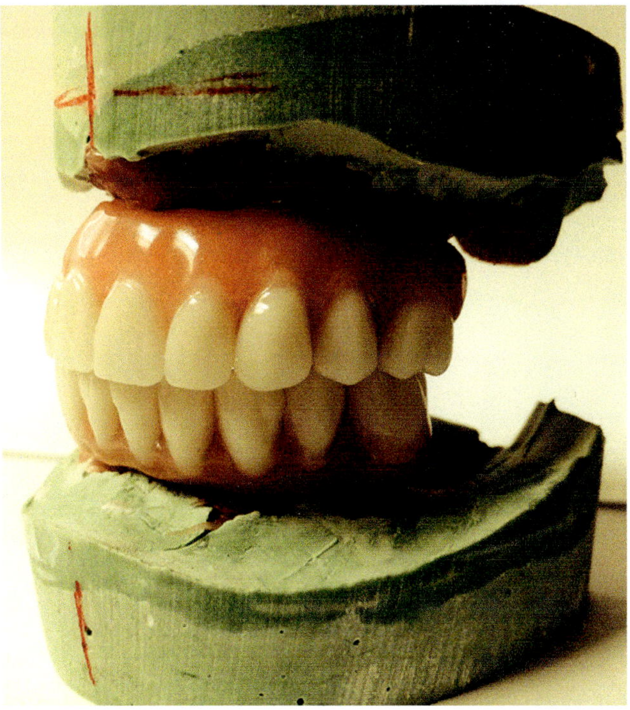

Fig. 5.126 Laboratory models of final maxillary quad zygoma and single midline and mandibular conventional All on 4 implant-retained prosthesis

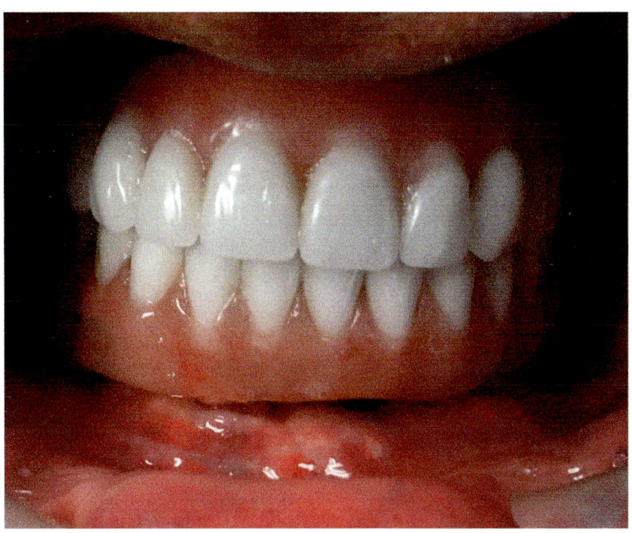

Fig. 5.127 Postoperative intraoral frontal view of final maxillary quad zygoma and single midline and mandibular conventional All on 4 implant-retained prosthesis which was placed on the first postoperative day

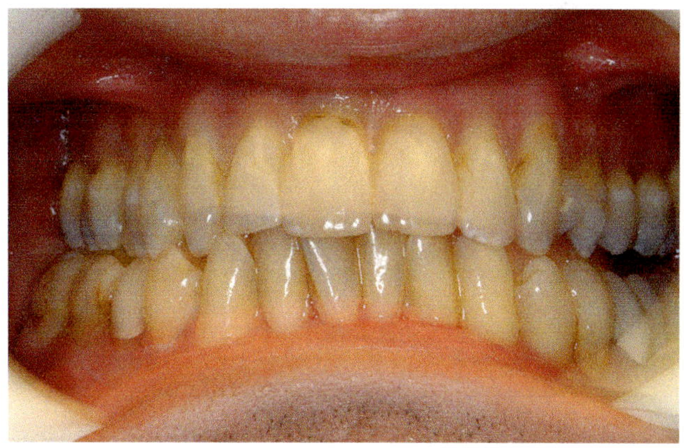

Fig. 5.128 Preoperative clinical frontal occlusal view of maxillary and mandibular failing dentition

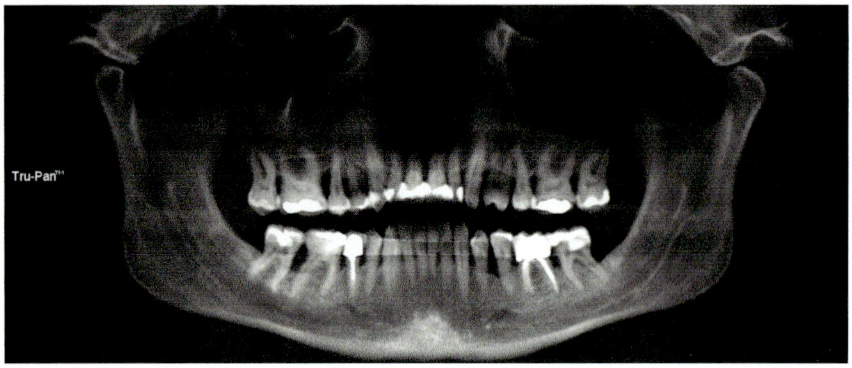

Fig. 5.129 Preoperative CBCT panoramic view of failed maxillary and mandibular dentition with generalized advanced periodontitis

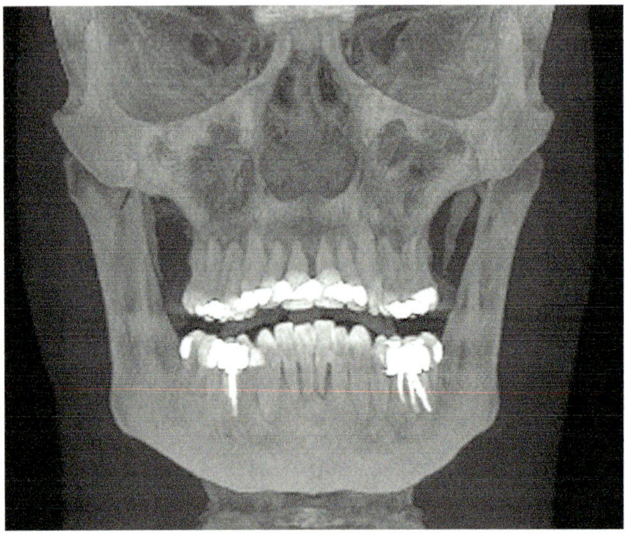

Fig. 5.130 Preoperative CBCT PA view of failed maxillary and mandibular dentition with generalized advanced periodontitis demonstrating adequate bone quality and quantity

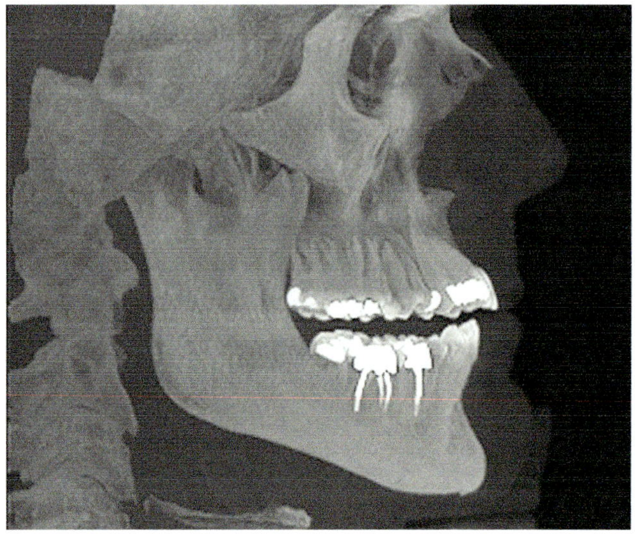

Fig. 5.131 Preoperative lateral cephalometric view of failed maxillary and mandibular dentition with generalized advanced periodontitis demonstrating adequate bone quality and quantity

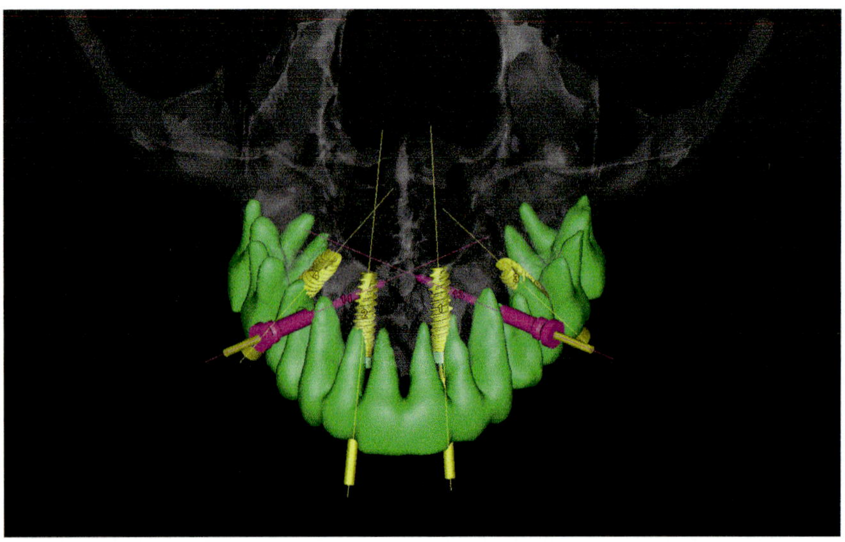

Fig. 5.132 Virtual treatment plan using SIMPLANT Master software (Materialise, Dentsply, York, PA, USA), demonstrating maxillary implant planning and two stabilization pin trajectories

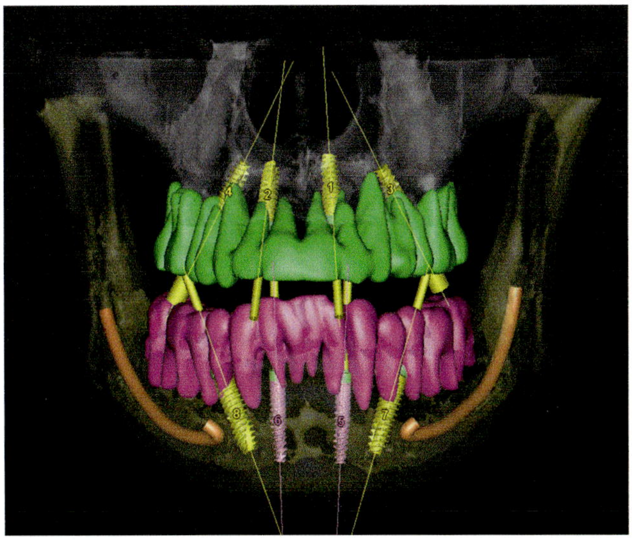

Fig. 5.133 Virtual treatment plan using SIMPLANT Master software (Materialise, Dentsply, York, PA, USA), frontal view demonstrating maxillary and mandibular "All on 4" implant planning and with prostheses and implant trajectories

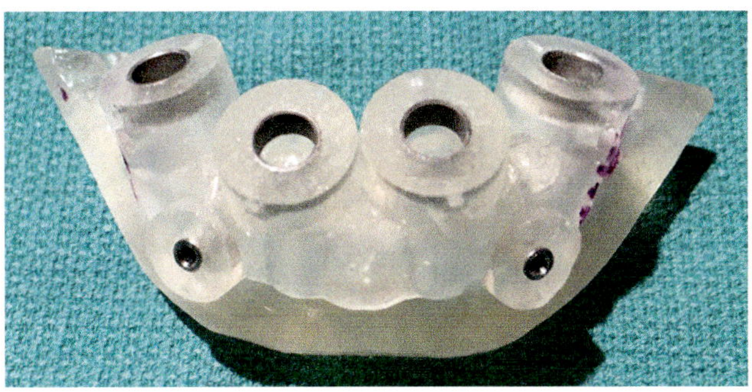

Fig. 5.134 Nobel Biocare (Yorba Linda, CA, USA) compatible SIMPLANT (Materialise, Dentsply, York, PA, USA) maxillary bone-borne surgical guide for four bilateral zygomatic implants with fixation screw holes which were placed to stabilize the guides during drilling

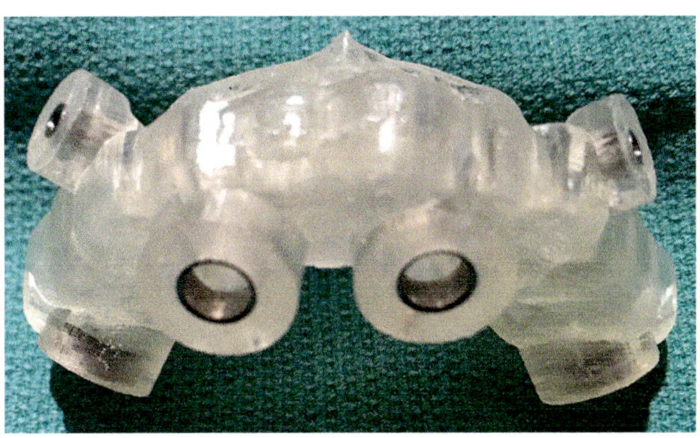

Fig. 5.135 Nobel Biocare (Yorba Linda, CA, USA) compatible SIMPLANT (Materialise, Dentsply, York, PA, USA) mandibular bone-borne surgical guide for four bilateral zygomatic implants with fixation screw holes which were placed to stabilize the guides during drilling

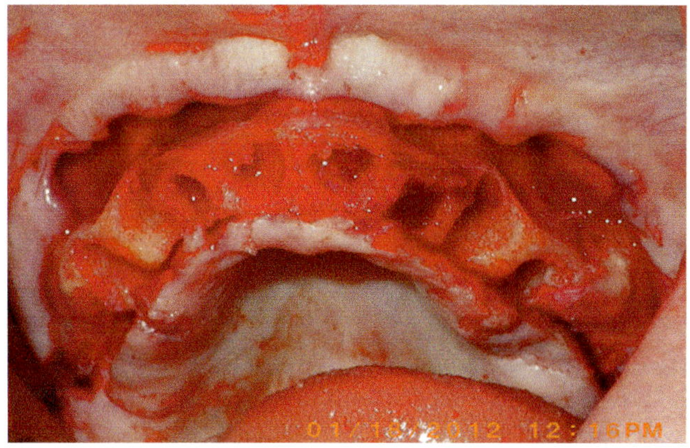

Fig. 5.136 Intraoperative view of maxillary alveolar ridge following removal of all remaining teeth and alveolectomy

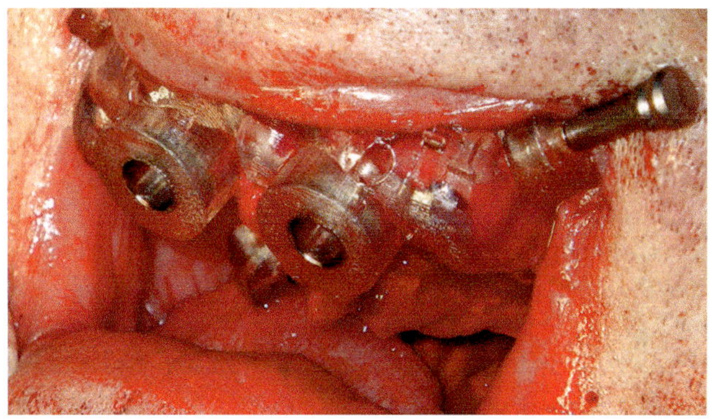

Fig. 5.137 Intraoperative view of maxillary bone-borne surgical guide with stabilization pins for "All on 4" implant placement (Materialise, Dentsply, York, PA, USA)

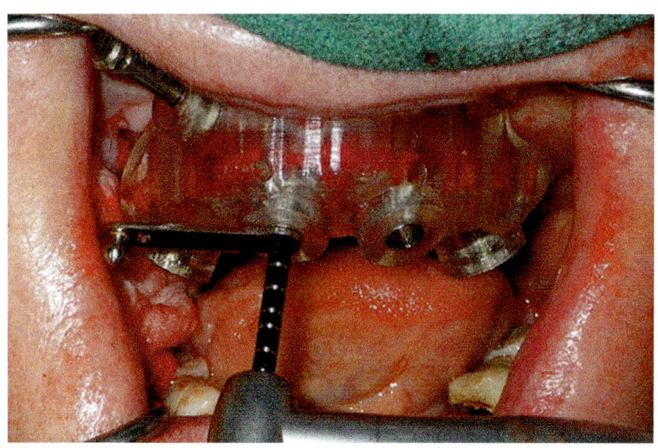

Fig. 5.138 Intraoperative view of maxillary bone-borne surgical guide with stabilization pins for "All on 4" implant placement drill sequence using drill handle (Materialise, Dentsply, York, PA, USA, Nobel Biocare, Yorba Linda, CA, USA)

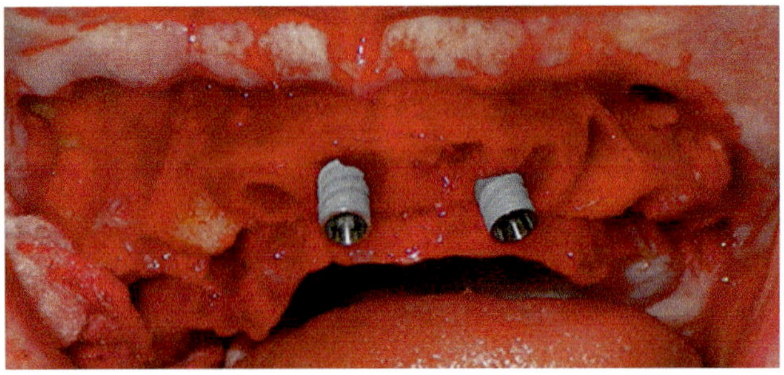

Fig. 5.139 Intraoperative view of initial placement of maxillary dental implants (Nobel Biocare, Yorba Linda, CA, USA)

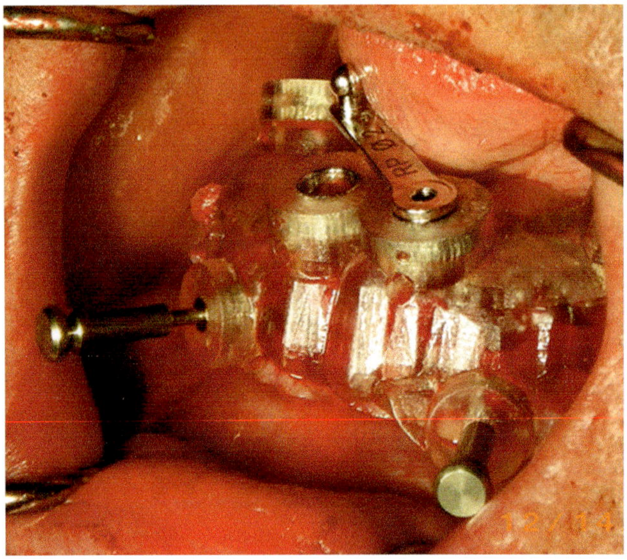

Fig. 5.140 Intraoperative view of mandibular bone-borne surgical guide with stabilization pins for "All on 4" implant placement (Nobel Biocare, Yorba Linda, CA, USA, Materialise, Dentsply, York, PA, USA)

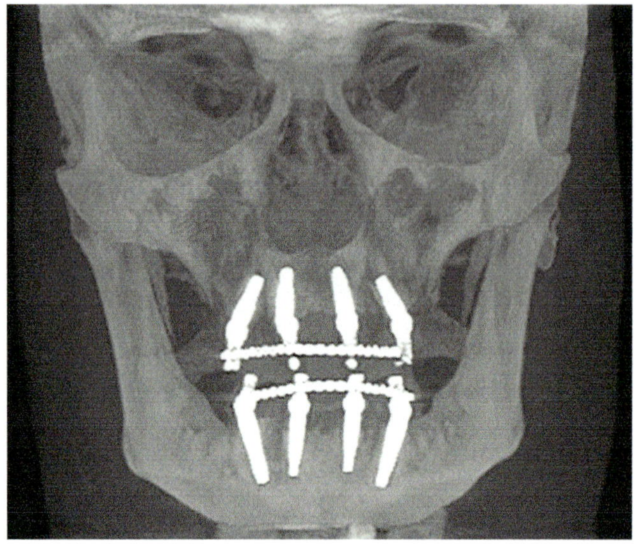

Fig. 5.142 Postoperative CBCT PA view of maxillary and mandibular "All on 4" implant placement with provisional restorations reinforced with metal bars

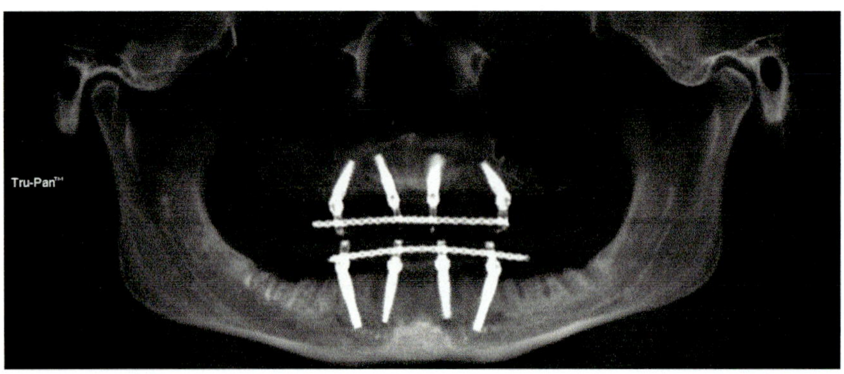

Fig. 5.141 Postoperative CBCT panoramic view of maxillary and mandibular "All on 4" implant placement with provisional restorations reinforced with metal bars

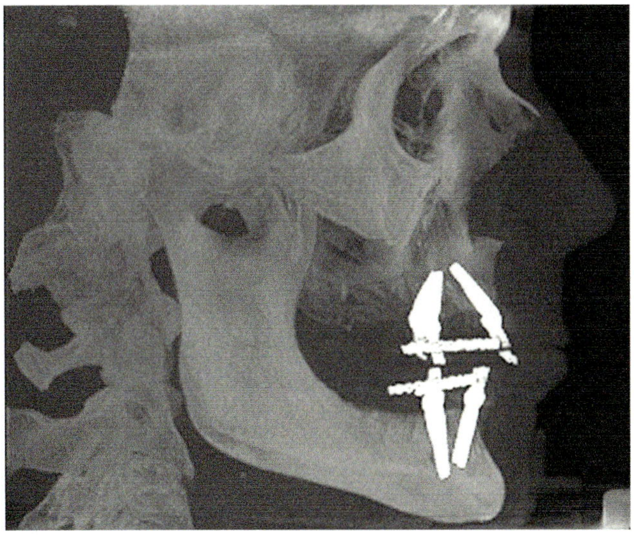

Fig. 5.143 Postoperative CBCT lateral cephalometric view of maxillary and mandibular "All on 4" implant placement with provisional restorations reinforced with metal bars (Nobel Biocare, Yorba Linda, CA, USA)

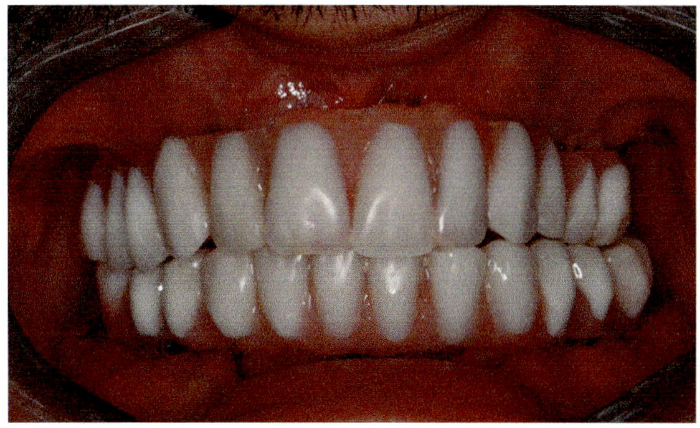

Fig. 5.144 Postoperative intraoral frontal view of final maxillary and mandibular "All on 4" implant placement with provisional restorations reinforced with metal bars

References

1. Klein M, Abrams M. Computer-guided surgery utilizing a computer-milled surgical template. Pract Proced Aesthet Dent. 2001 Mar;13(2):165–9.
2. Klein M, Cranin AN, Sirakian A. A computerized tomography (CT) scan appliance for optimal presurgical and preprosthetic planning of the implant patient. Pract Periodontics Aesthet Dent. 1993 Aug;5(6):33–9.
3. Tardieu PB, Vrielinck L, Escolano E, Henne M, Tardieu AL. Computer-assisted implant placement: scan template, simplant, surgiguide, and SAFE system. Int J Periodontics Restorative Dent. 2007 Apr;27(2):141–9.
4. Jacobs R, Adriansens A, Naert I, Quirynen M, Hermans R, van Steenberghe D. Predictability of reformatted computed tomography for pre-operative planning of endosseous implants. Dentomaxillofac Radiol. 1999;28(1):37–41. Clin Proc. 1996 Mar;71(3):288
5. van Steenberghe D, Glauser R, Blombäck U, Andersson M, Schutyser F, Pettersson A, Wendelhag I. A computed tomographic scan-derived customized surgical template and fixed prosthesis for flapless surgery and immediate loading of implants in fully edentulous maxillae: a prospective multicenter study. Clin Implant Dent Relat Res. 2005;7(Suppl 1):S111–20.
6. van Steenberghe D, Naert I, Andersson M, Brajnovic I, Van Cleynenbreugel J, Suetens P. A custom template and definitive prosthesis allowing immediate implant loading in the maxilla: a clinical report. Int J Oral Maxillofac Implants. 2002 Sep-Oct;17(5):663–70.
7. Tselios N, Parel SM, Jones JD. Immediate placement and immediate provisional abutment modeling in anterior single-tooth implant restorations using a CAD/CAM application: a clinical report. J Prosthet Dent. 2006 Mar;95(3):181–5.
8. Amorfini L, Storelli S, Romeo E. Rehabilitation of a dentate mandible requiring a full arch rehabilitation. Immediate loading of a fixed complete denture on implants placed with a bone supported surgical computer planned guide: case report. J Oral Implantol. 2011;37:106–13.
9. Turkyilmaz I, Suarez JC, Company AM. Immediate implant placement and provisional crown fabrication after a minimally invasive extraction of a peg-shaped maxillary lateral incisor: a clinical report. J Contemp Dent Pract. 2009 Sep 1;10(5):E073–80.
10. Rubin GD. Computed tomography: revolutionizing the practice of medicine for 40 years. Radiology. 2014 Nov;273(2 Suppl):S45–74.
11. Wesolowski JR, Lev MH. CT: history, technology, and clinical aspects. Semin Ultrasound CT MR. 2005 Dec;26(6):376–9.
12. Scarfe WC, Farman AG, Levin MD, Gane D. Essentials of maxillofacial cone beam computed tomography. Alpha Omegan. 2010 Jun;103(2):62–7.
13. Scarfe WC, Farman A, Sukovic P. Clinical applications of cone-beam computed tomography in dental practice. J Can Dent Assoc. 2006;72(1):75–80.
14. Ahmad M, Jenny J. Downie M application of cone beam computed tomography in oral and maxillofacial surgery. Aust Dent J. 2012 Mar;57(Suppl 1):82–94.
15. Chau AC, Fung K. Comparison of radiation dose for implant imaging using conventional spiral tomography, computed tomography, and cone-beam computed tomography. Oral Surg Oral Med Oral Pathol Oral Radiol Endod. 2009 Apr;107(4):559–65.
16. Oliva L. Alessandro Vallebona (1899–1987). Radiol Med. 1988 Jul-Aug;76(1–2):127–9.
17. Scarfe WC, Eraso FE, Farman AG. Characteristics of the Orthopantomograph OP 100. Dentomaxillofac Radiol. 1998 Jan;27(1):51–7.
18. Beckmann EC. Godfrey Newbold Hounsfield. Phys Today. 2005;58(3):84–5.
19. Oransky, Ivan (2004). "Sir Godfrey N. Hounsfield". Lancet 364 (9439): 1032.
20. Beckmann EC. CT scanning the early days. Br J Radiol. January 2006;79(937):5–8.
21. Shampo MA, Kyle RA. Allan Cormack – codeveloper of computed tomographic scanner. Mayo Clin Proc. 1996 Mar;71(3):288.
22. Raju TN. The Nobel chronicles. 1979: Allan MacLeod Cormack (b 1924); and Sir Godfrey Newbold Hounsfield (b 1919). Lancet. 1999;354(9190):1653.
23. Goodman LR. The Beatles, the Nobel prize, and CT scanning of the chest. Radiol Clin N Am. 2010 Jan;48(1):1–7.

24. Rogalla P, Kloeters C, Hein PA. CT technology overview: 64-slice and beyond. Radiol Clin N Am. 2009 Jan;47(1):1–11.
25. Sittig DF, Ash JS, Ledley RS. The story behind the development of the first whole-body computerized tomography scanner as told by Robert S Ledley. J Am Med Inform Assoc. 2006 Sep-Oct;13(5):465–9.
26. Alexander RE, Gunderman RB. EMI and the first CT scanner. J Am Coll Radiol. 2010 Oct;7(10):778–81.
27. Kalender WA, Seissler W, Klotz E, Vock P. Spiral volumetric CT with single-breathhold technique, continuous transport, and continuous scanner rotation. Radiology. 1990;176(1):181–3.
28. Kalender WA, Vock P, Polacin A, Soucek M. Spiral-CT: a new technique for volumetric scans. I. Basic principles and methodology. Rontgenpraxis. 1990 Sep;43(9):323–30.
29. Soucek M, Vock P, Daepp M, Kalender WA. Spiral-CT: a new technique for volumetric scans. II Potential clinical applications. Rontgenpraxis. 1990 Oct;43(10):365–75.
30. Hornich H. A tribute to Johann Radon. IEEE Trans Med Imaging. 1986;5(4):169.
31. Katsevich A. Analysis of an exact inversion algorithm for spiral cone-beam CT. Phys Med Biol. 2002 Aug 7;47(15):2583–97.
32. Schaller S, Flohr T, Steffen P. An efficient Fourier method for 3-D Radon inversion in exact cone-beam CT reconstruction. IEEE Trans Med Imaging. 1998 Apr;17(2):244–50.
33. Anastasio MA, Pan X, Clarkson E. Comments on the filtered backprojection algorithm, range conditions, and the pseudoinverse solution. IEEE Trans Med Imaging. 2001 Jun;20(6):539–42.
34. Morvidone M, Nguyen MK, Truong TT, Zaidi H. On the v-line Radon transform and its imaging applications. Int J Biomed Imaging. 2010;pii:208179. Epub 2010 Jul 13.
35. Zhang-O'Connor Y, Fessler JA. Fourier-based forward and back-projectors in iterative fan-beam tomographic image reconstruction. IEEE Trans Med Imaging. 2006 May;25(5):582–9.
36. Kordolaimi SD, et al. Introduction of an effective method for the optimization of CT protocols using iterative reconstruction algorithms: comparison with patient data. Am J Roentgenol. 2014;204(4):W434–9.
37. Brock RS, Docef A, Murphy MJ. Reconstruction of a cone-beam CT image via forward iterative projection matching. Med Phys. 2010 Dec;37(12):6212–20.
38. Pan X, Sidky EY, Vannier M. Why do commercial CT scanners still employ traditional, filtered back-projection for image reconstruction? Inverse Probl. 2009 Jan 1;25(12):1230009.
39. Kampp TD. The backprojection method applied to classical tomography. Med Phys. 1986 May-Jun;13(3):329–33.
40. Greenberg AM. Basics of cone-beam CT and CT guided dental implant surgery. Select Reading Oral Maxillofac Surg. 2011;19(5):1–48.
41. Pauwels R, Cockmartin L, Ivanauskaitė D, Urbonienė A, Gavala S, Donta C, Tsiklakis K, Jacobs R, Bosmans H, Bogaerts R, Horner K. SEDENTEXCT project Consortium. Estimating cancer risk from dental cone-beam CT exposures based on skin dosimetry. Phys Med Biol. 2014 Jul 21;59(14):3877–91.
42. Lee CY, Koval TM, Suzuki JB. Low dose radiation risks of CT and CBCT: reducing the fear and controversy. J Oral Implantol. 2015;41(5):e223–30.
43. Brenner DJ, Hall EJ. Computed tomography – an increasing source of radiation exposure. N Engl J Med. 2007 Nov 29;357(22):2277–84.
44. Berrington de González A, Mahesh M, Kim KP, et al. Projected cancer risks from computed tomographic scans performed in the United States in 2007. Arch Intern Med. December 2009;169(22):2071–7.
45. Shuryak I, Sachs RK, Brenner DJ. A new view of radiation induced cancer. Radiat Prot Dosim. 2011;143(2-4):358–64.
46. Brenner D, Elliston C, Hall E, Berdon W. Estimated risks of radiation-induced fatal cancer from pediatric CT. AJR Am J Roentgenol. 2001 Feb;176(2):289–96.
47. Ludlow JB, Davies-Ludlow LE, White SC. Patient risk related to common dental radiographic examination examinations: the impact of 2007 international commission on radiological protection recommendations regarding dose calculation. J Am Dent Assoc. 2008;139:1237–43.
48. National Council on Radiation Protection and Measurements. Ionizing radiation exposure of the population of the United States. Bethesda: National Council on Radiation Protection and Measurements; NCRP Report No. 160;2006.
49. Roberts JA, Drage NA, Davies J, Thomas JW. Effective dose from cone beam CT examinations in dentistry. Br J Radiol. 2009;82:35–40.
50. De Vos W, Casselman J, Swennen GR. Cone-beam computerized tomography (CBCT) imaging of the oral and maxillofacial region: a systematic review of the literature. Int J Oral Maxillofac Surg. 2009 Jun;38(6):609–25.
51. Mettler FA, Huda W, Yoshizumi TT, Mahesh M. Effective doses in radiology and diagnostic nuclear medicine: a catalog. Radiology. 2008;248(1):254–63.
52. Brenner DJ, Elliston CD. Estimated radiation risks potentially associated with full-body CT screening. Radiology. 2004 Sep;232(3):735–738. Epub 2004 Jul 23.
53. Brooks RA. A quantitative theory of the Hounsfield unit and its application to dual energy scanning. J Comput Assist Tomogr. 1977;1:487.
54. Greenberg AM. Cone beam computed tomography and diagnosis for dental implants. Oral Maxillofac Surg Clin North Am. 2015;27:185–202.
55. Mardinger O, Namani-Sadan N, Chaushu G, Schwartz-Arad D. Morphologic changes of the nasopalatine canal related to dental implantation: a radiologic study in different degrees of absorbed maxillae. J Periodontol. 2008 Sep;79(9):1659–62.
56. Soikkonen K, Wolf J, Ainamo A, Xie Q. Changes in the position of the mental foramen as a result of alveolar atrophy. J Oral Rehabil. 1995 Nov;22(11):831–3.
57. Bou Serhal C, Jacobs R, Flygare L, Quirynen M, van Steenberghe D. Perioperative validation of localisation of the mental foramen. Dentomaxillofac Radiol. 2002 Jan;31(1):39–43.
58. Carruth P, He J, Benson BW, Schneiderman ED. Analysis of the size and position of the mental foramen using the CS 9000 cone-beam computed tomographic unit. J Endod. 2015 Jul;41(7):1032–6.
59. Haas LF, Dutra K, Porporatti AL, Mezzomo LA, De Luca CG, Flores-Mir C, Corrêa M. Anatomical variations of mandibular canal detected by panoramic radiography and CT: a systematic review and meta-analysis. Dentomaxillofac Radiol. 2016;45(2):20150310.
60. Miles MS, Parks ET, Eckert GJ, Blanchard SB. Comparative evaluation of mandibular canal visibility on cross-sectional cone-beam CT images: a retrospective study. Dentomaxillofac Radiol. 2016;45(2):20150296.
61. Bornstein MM, Seiffert C, Maestre-Ferrín L, Fodich I, Jacobs R, Buser D, von Arx T. An analysis of frequency, morphology, and locations of maxillary sinus septa using cone beam computed tomography. Int J Oral Maxillofac Implants. 2016;31(2):280–7.
62. Neugebauer J, Ritter L, Mischkowski RA, Dreiseidler T, Scherer P, Ketterle M, Rothamel D, Zöller JE. Evaluation of maxillary sinus anatomy by cone-beam CT prior to sinus floor elevation. Int J Oral Maxillofac Implants. 2010 Mar-Apr;25(2):258–65.
63. Becker A, Chaushu S, Casap-Caspi N. Cone-beam computed tomography and the orthosurgical management of impacted teeth. J Am Dent Assoc. 2010 Oct;141(Suppl 3):14S–8S.
64. Ghaeminia H, Meijer GJ, Soehardi A, Borstlap WA, Mulder J, BergÃ SJ. Position of the impacted third molar in relation to the

mandibular canal. Diagnostic accuracy of cone beam computed tomography compared with panoramic radiography. Int J Oral Maxillofac Surg. 2009 Sep;38(9):964–71.
65. Katheria BC, Kau CH, Tate R, Chen JW, English J, Bouquot J. Effectiveness of impacted and supernumerary tooth diagnosis from traditional radiography versus cone beam computed tomography. Pediatr Dent. 2010 Jul-Aug;32(4):304–9.
66. Magnusson B, Borrman H. The paradental cyst a clinicopathologic study of 26 cases. Swed Dent J. 1995;19(1–2):1–7.
67. Weber AL. Imaging of cysts and odontogenic tumors of the jaw. Definition and classification. Radiol Clin N Am. 1993 Jan;31(1):101–20.
68. Baykul T, Saglam AA, Aydin U, Başak K. Incidence of cystic changes in radiographically normal impacted lower third molar follicles. Oral Surg Oral Med Oral Pathol Oral Radiol Endod. 2005 May;99(5):542–5.
69. Simon JH, Enciso R, Malfaz JM, Roges R, Bailey-Perry M, Patel A. Differential diagnosis of large periapical lesions using cone-beam computed tomography measurements and biopsy. J Endod. 2006 Sep;32(9):833–7.
70. Tyndall DA, Rathore S. Cone-beam CT diagnostic applications: caries, periodontal bone assessment, and endodontic applications. Dent Clin N Am. 2008;52(4):825–41.
71. Zhang ZL, Qu XM, Li G, Zhang ZY, Ma XC. The detection accuracies for proximal caries by cone-beam computerized tomography, film, and phosphor plates. Oral Surg Oral Med Oral Pathol Oral Radiol Endod. 2011 Jan;111(1):103–8.
72. Hariya Y, Yuasa K, Nakayama E, Kawazu T, Okamura K, Kanda S. Value of computed tomography findings in differentiating between intraosseous malignant tumors and osteomyelitis of the mandible affecting the masticator space. Oral Surg Oral Med Oral Pathol Oral Radiol Endod. 2003 Apr;95(4):503–9.
73. Hendrikx AW, Maal T, Dieleman F, Van Cann EM, Merkx MA. Cone beam CT in the assessment of mandibular invasion by oral squamous cell carcinoma: results of the preliminary study. Int J Oral Maxillofac Surg. 2010 May;39(5):436–9.
74. Closmann JJ, Schmidt BL. The use of cone beam computed tomography as an aid in evaluating and treatment planning for mandibular cancer. J Oral Maxillofac Surg. 2007 Apr;65(4):766–71.
75. Cassatly MG, Greenberg AM, Kopp WK. Bilateral giant cell granulomata of the mandible: report of case. J Am Dent Assoc. 1988 Nov;117(6):731–3.
76. Cohen MA, Hertzanu Y. Radiologic features, including those seen with computed tomography, of central giant cell granuloma of the jaws. Oral Surg Oral Med Oral Pathol. 1988 Feb;65(2):255–61.
77. DeTomasi D, Hann JR. Traumatic bone cyst: report of case. J Am Dent Assoc. 1985 Jul;111(1):56–7.
78. Marks R, Block M, Sanusi ID, et al. Unicystic ameloblastoma. Int J Oral Surg. 1983;12:186.
79. Singer SR, Mupparapu M, Philipone E. Cone-beam computed tomography findings in a case of plexiform ameloblastoma. Quintessence Int. 2009;40:627.
80. Araki M, Kameodka S, Matsumato N, et al. Usefulness of cone-beam computed tomography for odontogenic myxoma. Dentomaxillofac Radiol. 2007;36:423.
81. Madras J, Lapointe H. Keratocystic odontogenic tumor: reclassification of the odontogenic keratocyst from cyst to tumour. J Can Dent Assoc. 2008;74:165.
82. Kamel SG, Kau CH, Wong ME, Kennedy JW, English JD. The role of cone beam CT in the evaluation and management of a family with Gardner's syndrome. J Craniomaxillofac Surg. 2009 Dec;37(8):461–8.
83. Manganaro AM, Millett GV. Periapical cemental dysplasia. Gen Dent. 1996 Jul-Aug;44(4):336–9.
84. Ackermann GL, Altini M. The cementomas – a clinicopathological re-appraisal. J Dent Assoc S Afr. 1992 May;47(5):187–94.
85. Ribeiro AC, Carlos R, Díaz KP, Gouvêa AF, Vargas PA. Bilateral central ossifying fibroma affecting the mandible report of an uncommon case and critical review of the literature. Oral Surg Oral Med Oral Pathol Oral Radiol Endod. 2011 Feb;111(2):e21–6.
86. Cavalcanti MG, Ruprecht A, Vannier MW. Evaluation of an ossifying fibroma using three-dimensional computed tomography. Dentomaxillofac Radiol. 2001 Nov;30(6):342–345; J Oral Pathol Med. 2007 Aug;36(7):383–393.
87. Philipsen HP, Reichart PA, Siar CH, Ng KH, Lau SH, Zhang X, Dhanuthai K, Swasdison S, Jainkittivong A, Meer S, Jivan V, Altini M, Hazarey V, Ogawa I, Takata T, Taylor AA, Godoy H, Delgado WA, Carlos-Bregni R, Macias JF, Matsuzaka K, Sato D, Vargas PA, Adebayo ET. An updated clinical and epidemiological profile of the adenomatoid odontogenic tumour: a collaborative retrospective study. J Oral Pathol Med. 2007 Aug;36(7):383–93.
88. Alkhader M, Hudieb M. Comparison of mesiodistal space measurements of single-implant sites on panoramic and oblique images generated by cone-beam CT. Surg Radiol Anat. 2014 Apr;36(3):255–8.
89. Greenstein G, Carpentieri JR, Cavallaro J. Dental cone-beam scans: important anatomic views for the contemporary implant surgeon. Compend Contin Educ Dent. 2015 Nov-Dec;36(10):735–41.
90. Greenberg AM. Digital technologies for dental implant treatment planning and guided surgery. Oral Maxillofac Surg Clin North Am. 2015;27:319–40.
91. Uchida Y, Noguchi N, Goto M, Yamashita Y, Hanihara T, Takamori H, Sato I, Kawai T, Yosue T. Measurement of anterior loop length for the mandibular canal and diameter of the mandibular incisive canal to avoid nerve damage when installing endosseous implants in the interforaminal region: a second attempt introducing cone beam computed tomography. J Oral Maxillofac Surg. 2009 Apr;67(4):744–50.
92. Kuribayashi A, Watanabe H, Imaizumi A, Tantanapornkul W, Katakami K, Kurabayashi T. Bifid mandibular canals: cone beam computed tomography evaluation. Dentomaxillofac Radiol. 2010 May;39(4):235–9.
93. Jacobs R, Mraiwa N, van Steenberghe D, Gijbels F, Quirynen M. Appearance, location, course, and morphology of the mandibular incisive canal: an assessment on spiral CT scan. Dentomaxillofac Radiol. 2002 Sep;31(5):322–7.
94. Naitoh M, Hiraiwa Y, Aimiya H, Gotoh K, Ariji E. Accessory mental foramen assessment using cone-beam computed tomography. Oral Surg Oral Med Oral Pathol Oral Radiol Endod. 2009 Feb;107(2):289–94.
95. De Santis D, Canton LC, Cucchi A, Zanotti G, Pistoia E, Nocini PF. Computer-assisted surgery in the lower jaw: double surgical guide for immediately loaded implants in postextractive sites-technical notes and a case report. J Oral Implantol. 2010;36(1):61–8.
96. Rosenfeld AL, Mandelaris GA, Tardieu PB. Prosthetically directed implant placement using computer software to ensure precise placement and predictable prosthetic outcomes. Part 1: diagnostics, imaging, and collaborative accountability. Int J Periodontics Restorative Dent. 2006 Jun;26(3):215–21.
97. Maló P, Rangert B, Nobre M. All-on-4 immediate-function concept with Brånemark system implants for completely edentulous maxillae: a 1-year retrospective clinical study. Clin Implant Dent Relat Res. 2005;7(Suppl 1):S88–94.
98. Tolstunov L, Thai D, Arellano L. Implant-guided volumetric analysis of edentulous maxillary bone with cone-beam computerized tomography scan. Maxillary sinus pneumatization classification. J Oral Implantol. 2012 Aug;38(4):377–90.
99. Jensen OT, Adams MW, Cottam JR, Parel SM, Phillips WR 3rd. The all on 4 shelf: mandible. J Oral Maxillofac Surg. 2011 Jan;69(1):175–81.

100. Jensen OT, Adams MW, Cottam JR, Parel SM, Phillips WR 3rd. The all-on-4 shelf: maxilla. J Oral Maxillofac Surg. 2010 Oct;68(10):2520–7.
101. US 9,050,665.
102. US 8,750,590.
103. Valente F, Schiroli G, Sbrenna A. Accuracy of computer-aided oral implant surgery: a clinical and radiographic study. Int J Oral Maxillofac Implants. 2009 Mar-Apr;24(2):234–42.
104. Pomares C. A retrospective study of edentulous patients rehabilitated according to the 'all-on-four' or the 'all-on-six' immediate function concept using flapless computer-guided implant surgery. Eur J Oral Implantol. 2010 Summer;3(2):155–63.
105. Flügge TV, Nelson K, Schmelzeisen R, Metzger MC. Three-dimensional plotting and printing of an implant drilling guide: simplifying guided implant surgery. J Oral Maxillofac Surg. 2013 Aug;71(8):1340–6.
106. Nardi C, Borri C, Regini F, Calistri L, Castellani A, Lorini C, Colagrande S. Metal and motion artifacts by cone beam computed tomography (CBCT) in dental and maxillofacial study. Radiol Med. 2015 Jul;120(7):618–26.
107. Van de Wiele G, Teughels W, Vercruyssen M, Coucke W, Temmerman A, Quirynen M. The accuracy of guided surgery via mucosa-supported stereolithographic surgical templates in the hands of surgeons with little experience. Clin Oral Implants Res. 2015 Dec;26(12):1489–94.
108. Turbush SK. Turkyilmaz I accuracy of three different types of stereolithographic surgical guide in implant placement: an in vitro study. J Prosthet Dent. 2012 Sep;108(3):181–8.
109. Greenberg AM, Nelson K. Basic dental implantology. In: Greenberg AM, Schmelzeisen R, editors. Craniomaxillofacial Reconstructive and Corrective Bone Surgery. 2nd ed. New York: Springer Verlag; 2018, In press.

Virtual Surgical Planning for Orthognathic Surgery

6

Vincent Carrao, Mohammad Tofigh, and Alex M. Greenberg

Introduction

Orthognathic surgery is a fascinating and powerful treatment modality to provide correction for patients with dentofacial deformities. These complex surgical procedures require accurate diagnosis, appropriate treatment planning, and precise surgical execution.

The first mandibular osteotomies were first performed in the mid-1800s by Simon P. Hullihan [1] who operated the first subapical osteotomy. There was an evolution to the vertical ramus osteotomies in the 1930s by Lane and others and the bilateral sagittal split osteotomies performed in the 1950s and 1960s by Trauner, Obwegeser, and DalPont [1]. The maxillary LeFort classification dates to the early 1900s with progressive advances in surgical technique by Bell and others over time leading to the LeFort I down fracture in the 1970s [1].

Orthognathic surgery has developed over time into a routine procedure, allowing it to be performed on a regular basis, and has become a safe and effective surgical procedure for skeletal facial deformities.

Traditionally, the diagnostic methods for orthognathic surgery have included detailed pre-orthodontic and preoperative clinical examination, plain radiographic analysis, and dental casts. The diagnostic workup is performed with articulator-mounted dental models, standard facial photography, panoramic dental radiograph, and traced posterior-anterior (PA) and lateral cephalometric radiographs followed by analysis techniques using various established norms. The surgical plan is then determined based on the analyzed data and the use of "model surgery." Model surgery includes the cutting, repositioning, and fixation of stone models mounted on a semi-adjustable articulator. Surgical splints are then hand fabricated in this process and used intraoperatively to guide the positioning of the maxilla and/or mandible. When combined with well-executed surgical technique, traditional orthognathic planning has proven to be safe, and a reasonably accurate method for the correction of dentofacial deformities.

Virtual Surgical Planning

The use of traditional model surgery for orthognathic surgery has harbored many inaccuracies related to surgical planning. These inaccuracies stem from the attempt to transfer from dental models the exact spatial relationship of the three-dimensional maxillomandibular complex to the semi-adjustable articulator. Diagnosing and accurately transferring the exact anterior-posterior and transverse positions of the maxilla, occlusal plane angle, and any existing cant of maxilla (the yaw, pitch, and roll) are not only cumbersome but also somewhat inaccurate [2]. The inaccuracy is inherent as part of human error, device error, and unavoidable volumetric expansion of materials such as plaster, wax, and glue. The standard articulator is designed to represent the average "normal" cranio-maxillofacial relationship and bilateral temporomandibular joint functional anatomy. This is problematic for patients with dentofacial deformities who often present with anatomical relationships that may significantly deviate from the norms. Furthermore, two-dimensional radiography can fail to adequately reveal complex anatomic variations and asymmetries of the facial skeleton. Identification of landmarks on cephalometric radiographs, especially for overlapping structures in an asymmetric patient can be inconsistent. Two-dimensional imaging provides insufficient information about condylar abnormalities, bone thickness in areas of interest, and exact spatial position

V. Carrao (✉)
Division of Oral and Maxillofacial Surgery, The Mount Sinai Hospital, Icahn School of Medicine at Mount Sinai, 1 Gustave Levy Place, New York, NY, USA
e-mail: vincent.carrao@mountsinai.org

M. Tofigh
Private Practive, Oral and Maxillofacial Surgery, New York, NY, USA

A.M. Greenberg
Division of Oral and Maxillofacial Surgery, Columbia University College of Dental Medicine, 18 East 48th Street Suite 1702, New York, NY 10017, USA
e-mail: nycimplant@aol.com

A.M. Greenberg (ed.), *Digital Technologies in Craniomaxillofacial Surgery*, https://doi.org/10.1007/978-1-4939-1532-3_6

of important structures. In addition, image distortion and magnification errors may be sources of error [3]. Precision of the surgical outcome in orthognathic surgery requires a detailed appreciation of patient's true anatomy and accurate planning. Limitations of 2D imaging, facebow transfer, and cast model surgery can lead to imprecise and inadequate diagnostic data gathering, inaccurate treatment planning, and suboptimal results, (especially in complex cases), even in the hands of the most experienced surgeons [4, 5]. Lastly, the large number of hours spent by the practitioner on the preoperative workup can be a discouraging factor.

Virtual surgical planning (VSP) for orthognathic surgery is a form of computer-assisted surgery that has developed from the various fields such as neurosurgery, orthopedic surgery, sinus surgery, dental implantology, and prosthodontics [6–8]. VSP has been made possible by the general advances in imaging technology, especially with the advent of 3D CT scanning in the 1970s and the subsequent improvements upon the resolution and accuracy of the software algorithms to generate 3D representations of soft and hard tissues. Computer-assisted surgery may involve preoperative planning in the form of manufactured stereolithographic models or by virtual surgical planning. In addition, computer-assisted surgery can include intraoperative navigation for complex reconstructive and corrective cranio-maxillofacial surgery [9, 10].

Virtual surgical planning (VSP) plays a role in both diagnostic as well as planning phases of orthognathic surgery. It uses digital imaging technology in the form of 3D computed tomography (CT) or cone beam computed tomography (CBCT) and 3D laser surface scanning of dental cast models (or directly from the patient's dentition) merged to capture the patients' exact anatomy. When combined with the traditional clinical examination and cephalometric analysis, one can arrive at a comprehensive diagnostic picture of the patient. The various maxillary and mandibular osteotomy techniques are performed to virtually simulate the surgical movements which upon completion computer-aided design/computer-aided manufacturing (CAD/CAM) technology is then utilized to design and fabricate surgical cutting and positioning guides.

The Virtual Surgical Planning (VSP) Process

A thorough discussion is held with the patient, assessing in detail pertinent subjective goals, chief complaints and expectations, history of dental and orthodontic treatment, as well as medical, surgical, and family history. A complete review of systems is performed with particular emphasis on sleep, speech, breathing, mastication, swallowing, orofacial pain, and oral habits. In our center, the clinical examination begins with complete dentofacial data gathering including TMJ examination, nasal and oral airway, dental, occlusal, and facial measurements and relationships, and soft tissue assessment. High-quality clinical photographs are obtained in natural head position in repose and with full animation in lateral, frontal, and 3/4 views, as well as intraoral views. A photograph is taken with a wooden tongue depressor placed against the maxillary canines and held by the patient to capture any obvious cant of the maxilla. Full-face CBCT of the patient in standing position is obtained. We prefer the CBCT imaging with the patient in an upright position to avoid the effect of gravity on the soft tissues, as well as for its reduced radiation dose compared to standard CT. Although panoramic and lateral cephalometric 2D radiographs can be generated from the CBCT, we obtain standard panoramic and plain lateral and posterior-anterior cephalometric views. The cephalometric radiographs are easily calibrated, traced, and analyzed by digital tracing and analysis software, which serves as a baseline or reference for comparison to postoperative imaging. A minimum of two sets of maxillary and mandibular alginate impressions are taken and poured with orthodontic stone or die stone. A bite registration and facebow registration are no longer obtained, as they are unnecessary.

The occlusion of trimmed dental cast-models is evaluated to assess the need for segmentation of the maxilla and/or occlusal adjustment. Segmentation of the maxilla can correct limited (<7 mm) transverse maxillary deficiencies or unleveled arches in comparison to the mandibular arch. When indicated, one maxillary cast can be segmented in two or more pieces and set in the desired position using rigid sticky wax or glue. The standard desired position of the maxillary cast is Class I occlusion in maximum intercuspation, unless otherwise indicated. The second maxillary cast is only needed to serve as reference for any occlusal adjustments or in case of unforeseen damage to the first cast during segmentation.

Once the desired occlusion is achieved with the dental casts, they are mounted on a Galetti articulator (Fig. 6.1) in the desired occlusal relationship. A thin layer of Vaseline is applied on all the teeth, and a bite registration is obtained using polyvinyl siloxane (PVS) bite registration material. The bite registration record is removed after setting, and the occlusion is checked again to ensure it is the desired final occlusion. The casts are unmounted from the articulator and placed into occlusion with the bite registration record secured in between, along with the uncut maxillary cast and they are shipped to the company for optical scanning and data merge with the CT data. An online meeting is then scheduled for the actual virtual surgical planning (VSP). Time can be saved by informing the technician of what type of maxillary and mandibular osteotomies are to be performed, thus allowing for virtual preparation prior to the planning session. The CT data is uploaded to the company website with Digital Imaging and Communications in Medicine (DICOM) format (Table 6.1).

Prior to the online meeting, the DICOM data is reconstructed in 3D, providing accurate skeletal and soft tissue rendering. The dental casts are scanned with surface to surface registration superimposed on the 3D reconstruction to provide high-resolution dental anatomy. The reason for scanning and registration of the dental casts is due to limitations

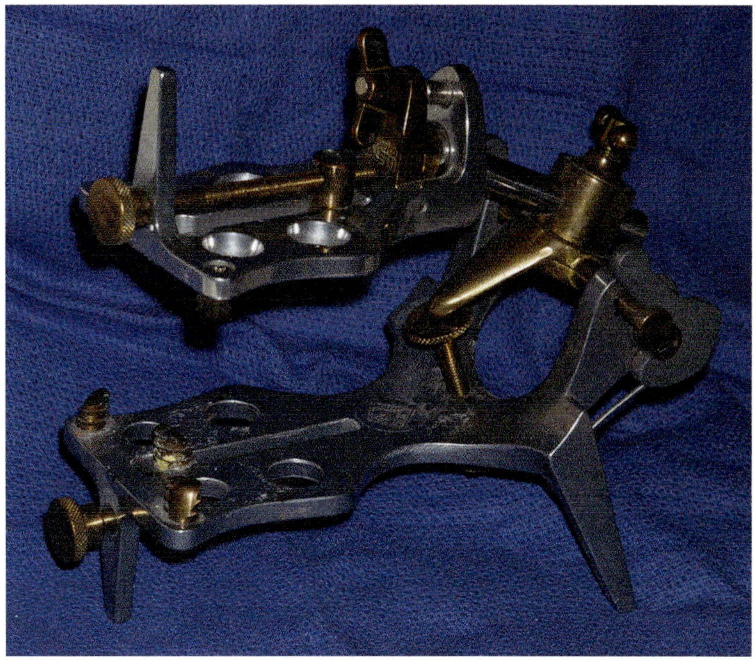

Fig. 6.1 Galetti articulator

Table 6.1 Examples of companies with VSP and CAD/CAM services

Companies performing VSP
Materialise, Plymouth, MI, USA
3D Systems Healthcare, Rockhill, SC, USA
ProtoMed, Santa Clara, CA, USA

of today's CT technology to accurately capture the complex dental anatomy which is obscured by streak artifacts created by metallic brackets, wires, and dental restorations.

During the online planning meeting, desired osteotomies and skeletal movements are virtually created. Our preferred approach is maxilla-first surgery, where by the maxilla is moved to the desired position based on the previously gathered clinical data (patient expectations, clinical measurements, facial and cephalometric analysis). Attention is paid to dental and facial midlines, presence of cants, and need for differential impactions (the roll, yaw, and pitch). The maxilla can be pivoted against any desired point of rotation with immediate visualization of the amount of interosseous gaps, overlaps, and degree of movement to the tenth of millimeters or angular degrees.

Although surgical guides can be fabricated for segmentation of the maxilla, we usually do not find them necessary. However, in cases of TMJ implant reconstruction, inverted-L mandibular osteotomies and interosseous bone grafting, or genioplasty for correction of an asymmetric chin, we find that cutting and positioning guides can be very helpful. The intermediate and final splints are generated with the use of CAD/CAM technology. They can be separate or as in the sandwich technique. If large skeletal movements are planned (such as in maxillomandibular advancement for the treatment of severe obstructive sleep apnea), a thick intermediate splint can be helpful as it facilitates the intraoperative intermaxillary fixation. The stability of a multi-piece maxilla can be improved by designing lingual lips that fit against the lingual surface of maxillary posterior teeth. A palatal strap with desired amount of clearance from palatal mucosa may be added for further strength.

Preparing for Orthognathic Surgery

Orthognathic surgery has many facets that need to be looked at carefully and performed correctly to achieve a good outcome. Each one of these facets must be addressed individually and then brought together as a whole to produce the desired result. So there are multiple steps that we review as surgeons when we approach a patient that presents for orthognathic surgery. What should our thought process be and how we then translate that information to the patient's understanding and surgical success. It should include the following:

- Patient presentation
- Patient workup
- Diagnosis
- Communication with the orthodontic team
- Surgical planning
- Surgery
- Postoperative care
- Final records

Patient Presentation

When patients present for a surgical consultation, they may or may not have a good idea what a proposed surgery may involve or entail. It is our responsibility as surgeons to inform the patient of the diagnosis in detail and in language the patient can understand. Once we feel confident that the patient understands the diagnosis, we must then offer all possible treatment options available. Some solutions may not include a surgical procedure to correct the patients presenting diagnosis; however, more often than not, when a patient presents with a maxillary/mandibular skeletal deformity, the proposed solution will be somewhere in the surgical realm. The surgeon's consultation then will have to include the preoperative course, the operative procedure, risks and benefits, complications, long-term prognosis, and postoperative care. The importance of informing the patient and achieving realistic expectations requires good communiction which cannot be overemphasized.

The consultation must stress; that orthognathic surgery is a team effort; thus, working closely with the orthodontist is of utmost importance, whether it be surgery first or orthodontics first. The conversation should continue in an open dialog format leading the discussion in a logical manner informing the patient of the initial workup including facial measurements, intraoral exam, photos, X-rays, maxillary/mandibular arch impressions, and a bite registration. An analysis is then performed with the information that is gathered to render a diagnosis, which will then move toward the development of a surgical plan. The surgical plan is devised and executed leading to the postoperative phase of treatment with finalization of orthodontics and long-term stability. We should stress to the patient that part of our armamentarium is the utilization of virtual surgical planning, which includes 3D renderings of the patient's anatomy and the proposed bony movements. These images can also be instrumental in patient education and understanding the actual surgical procedure prior to having the operative procedure performed. The patient should be informed that 3D predicted images are highly accurate but may not be an exact representation of the final outcome.

Patient Workup

The workup should be done in a meticulous systematic fashion. If it is done in a haphazard way, it is possible to make crucial mistakes that can lead to an altered diagnosis or errors related to the surgical procedure. Thus, obtaining accurate records is essential to the success of orthognathic surgery. The records obtained will be used as a representation of the patient as we move forward in the process of developing a diagnosis and ultimately the surgical plan. A cephalometric analysis of the X-rays is performed, and the models are articulated with the bite registration obtained. The photographs are another key element essential to the process. Intraoral photographs help us ensure that our mounted models are articulated correctly, and they give us information regarding the patients smile line, and the resting lip line which helps in the diagnosis of anterior vertical discrepancy. It provides a reference for the evaluation of the patient's facial midline and dental midlines, as well as a reference for any facial asymmetries. The actual facial and intraoral measurements obtained during the physical exam are utilized to ensure that all of the aforementioned data is correct. We can now incorporate the many different data sources we have obtained and integrate them into a final diagnosis.

Diagnosis

We must always remember that the diagnosis of a facial skeletal deformity is ultimately a clinical decision. One cannot utilize cephalograms or CT scans to provide a diagnosis without correlating the actual physical findings.

When developing the diagnosis, we must think of all the skeletal discrepancies in three dimensions, the vertical, horizontal, and anterior posterior planes. This is the only way to obtain the correct diagnosis and develop a good surgical plan, thus allowing us to address all aspects of the skeletal deformity requiring correction.

It is also important to note that prior to utilizing our VSP software, we need to have the correct preliminary diagnosis and have formulated a surgical plan. In other words we should already know the basic maxillary/mandibular surgical technique to be performed and the movements planned for the surgical correction that we formulated from our diagnosis. The surgical plan is then inputted into the 3D virtual planning environment software to show what the result of our surgery will produce in three dimensions: the exact bony movements and their measurements.

VSP has become an essential tool as an adjunct to our cognitive ability to develop a diagnosis and derive a surgical plan that will produce the best result. There may also be considerations for facial implants, and bone grafting as it relates to contour deformities of dentofacial deformities and craniofacial disorders.

Communication with the Orthodontic Team

The team approach in orthognathic surgery is paramount to obtaining the best possible outcome for the patient. Open communication with the orthodontic team regarding the following key points will allow the patient, the surgeon, and orthodontist to have a clear view of the surgical process and plan:

- Initial diagnosis
- Removal of third molars and other teeth agreed upon by the orthodontist and the surgeon
- Beginning of orthodontic treatment
- Developing a surgical/orthodontic plan
- Time required for orthodontic movement prior to surgery
- Placement of final rectangular wire and surgical hooks
- Final models

- CBCT within 6 months
- Virtual surgical planning (VSP)
- Surgery
- Postoperative care
- Postoperative orthodontics and long term retention

When the practitioners maintain sufficient dialog and a high level of communication, the patient's overall treatment will lead to a satisfactory outcome and a satisfied patient.

Virtual Surgical Planning

Once we have finalized the diagnosis and surgical plan, it is possible to proceed with the VSP and observe the bony movements in three dimensions. The VSP is usually performed 2–3 weeks before surgery after the final rectangular wire has been placed by the orthodontist. Stone models are obtained and placed in corrected occlusion with wax or polyether bite. If necessary models are sectioned and segments fixated with sticky wax or glue and then sent directly to the company to optically scan and merge into the VSP software. A sterolithographic model (if desired) can be obtained from the CBCT DICOM data which is uploaded by fileshare to the company. Once the company has both the dental models and CBCT DICOM data, an online meeting time can be scheduled to perform the virtual surgery and prepare to make surgical guides and splints.

As the movements are done virtually in a three-dimensional environment, one can readily see the relationship of the bony segments as they are moved into the planned position with measurements and provides an accurate view of the jaw position and possible bone interferences. For maxillary osteotomies, this allows simulation of advancement, impaction, differential movement, segmentation, cant correction, interferences, the amount of bone to removed, and overlap of segments. The mandibular osteotomies have the same advantage post movement; whether an intraoral vertical ramus osteotomy (IVRO), bilateral mandibular ramus sagittal split osteotomies (BSSO), or anterior horizontal mandibular osteotomy (AHMO). One can determine areas of premature contact, areas of adequate contact, and areas without contact. This information is invaluable to the surgeon regarding the surgical plan. If the preplanned movements are not appropriate for good bone approximation and healing, it would be an indication to modify the surgical approach or alter the plan to obtain a stable result.

When evaluating the final position of the upper and lower jaw in three dimensions, it becomes clear whether to make rotational movements and/or yaw changes that will improve the final outcome. Prior to VSP there was little to no control over these types of movements. With the help of VSP, we can make these additional movements, thus helping us in the operating room and to improve our outcomes.

For single jaw surgery, whether in the mandible or the maxilla, only a final splint needs to be fabricated, while for two jaw surgery, an intermediate and final splint is needed. Genioplasty positional splints also can be fabricated. Specifications for the splints can include the depth of indentation of the dentition, the width of the buccal flange, and optional wiring holes. VSP can also provide soft tissue changes in 2D and 3D images.

Surgery

When entering the operating room as surgeons, we like to have an accurate plan that can be executed swiftly with precision, with the confidence that we can achieve our surgical goals with patient safety and the best possible outcomes. With the use of VSP, we are able to have great confidence in our plan and decisions. All surgery still depends on knowledge of surgical anatomy and impeccable decision making while in the operating room. Thus, we always need to rely on our education, and surgical judgement and experience to be successful. Knowing where to make incisions and accurate osteotomies determines good surgical and functional results. As time progresses and technology becomes more integrated into medicine and surgery, we may continue to grow in confidence and rely on more accurate surgical adjuncts. Greater core knowledge of the patient's 3D skeletal anatomy reduces complications during surgical procedures. VSP thus saves considerable time during the surgical planning when compared to traditional model surgery, which has shown to be highly accurate, and surgery more efficient with the decision making planned well in advance. This reduces planning and operating time, which is better for surgeons and patients, and can be a cost savings for the delivery setting whether in the hospital, ambulatory surgery center, or private office.

Postoperative Care

The first 6 weeks post orthognathic surgery is an important time for patient care and a successful outcome of the surgery. The patient should be evaluated weekly for occlusal stability and/or stability of maxillary/mandibular fixation if jaws are wired shut. Monitoring nutritional status, wound care, and maxillary pedicle perfusion are essential aspects of postoperative care. The use of guiding elastics can be an important modality during the healing phase.

Postoperative radiographs on the first day may include panoramic, lateral cephalometric, PA cephalometric, or a 3D cone beam to evaluate:

- Soft tissue profile changes
- Position of the bony segments
- Condylar position in the fossa

- Hardware placement
- Possible injury to the roots of teeth
- Oral pharyngeal airway changes
- Compare movements to preoperative VSP
- Proper splint position and fit

If maxillomandibular fixation is utilized or splint removal is required, follow-up radiographs can also be performed 4–6 weeks postoperatively to evaluate the stability of the movements.

Orthodontic evaluation can begin as early as 1 week postoperatively depending on the team's preferences. However, postsurgical orthodontic forces are usually not applied for 6–7 weeks. Frequency of surgical follow-up during the 3–6 months, postoperative orthodontic treatment is also team dependent. Upon de-bonding, patients are given retainers; removable or fixed for long term orthodontic retention.

Final Records

Approximately 1 year following orthognathic surgery, the patient will return for final records which should include CBCT, panoramic radiograph, lateral cephalometric radiograph, models, and photos. These are utilized to compare the movements to the preoperative plan, the immediate postoperative results and to evaluate stability of the result, for healing of the segments and relapse. The final record taking session also completes the patient record from the initial consultation to the probable discharge of the patient from surgical care. The session will usually include:

- Physical exam
  - Facial appearance
    - Anterior posterior view
    - Lateral view
    - Three-fourths view
  - Mandibular mobility and jaw opening
  - TMJ
    - Clicking, popping, or crepitation
    - Muscles of mastication tenderness
    - TMJ tenderness
    - Headaches
  - Cranial nerve
    - V2
    - V3
  - Occlusion
  - Dental injuries (endodontic and periodontic)
- Photos
  - Facial views
  - Intra oral
- Radiographs
  - Plain films
    - Lateral ceph
    - PA ceph
    - Panoramic
    - Periapical
  - 3D cone beam

Pros and Cons of Virtual Surgical Planning

Pros

- Accuracy
  - Bone movements
  - Measurements of movements
  - Osteotomy design
- 3D view of the bony segments
  - Overlap
  - Bony gaps
  - Interferences
  - Asymmetries
  - Midlines
    - Rotation
    - Bodily shifts
  - Maxillary impaction
    - Rotation Point
      - ANS
      - Incisal edge
    - Bodily/differential movements
- Fabrication
  - Intermediate occlusal splints
  - Final occlusal splints
  - Cutting guides
  - Positional jigs
  - Simulated graft wedges
    - Size
    - Shape
- Time
  - Decreased
    - Less model surgery
    - No splint fabrication
    - Decreased radiographic analysis and prediction tracing
    - Improved presurgical understanding of patients bony anatomy
    - OR time

Cons

- Cost
  - Increased
    - CT scan
    - Shipping

    - Models
    - Bite
    - CT CD
    - Splints
    - Guides
    - Plans
- Teaching
    - Less model surgery
    - No splint fabrication
    - Improved 3D visualization
    - Research tool
- Back up
    - No ability to fabricate a backup splint unless stone or 3D printed models are available.

3D Virtual Surgical Planning

Maxillary and Mandibular Movements

VSP is performed in a virtual 3D environment utilizing the patient's CT scan data merged with optical scan data of the dental occlusion. To begin the process of VSP a 3D image of the preoperative facial skeleton is observed (Fig. 6.2). This image can be rotated and viewed from all sides. Based on a prediction tracing of a lateral cephalometric radiograph, desired positions for single or double jaw osteotomy segments can be planned. Commonly the maxilla is operated first at the Lefort I level and repositioned based on the intact mandible (Figs. 1.6a–n and 6.3). For double jaw osteotomies. once the position of the maxilla is established, whether as a single piece or in a segmental osteotomy, the mandible undergoes virtual vertical or sagittal split osteotomies and is set in position in the correct dental occlusion (Fig. 6.4). If genioplasty is to be performed, an anterior horizontal mandibular osteotomy is virtually performed and the inferior segment positioned (Fig. 6.5). The software provides precise measurements of the osteotomy cuts and movements (Figs. 6.6a, b and 6.7). Lateral cephalometric reference angle measurements can be incorporated into the planning (Fig. 6.8). For a double jaw case, the intermediate splint is virtually created as an STL file for CAD/CAM fabrication, usually via 3D printing (Fig. 6.9). STL files for CAD/CAM fabrication of the final splint is then virtually created for single or double jaw osteotomies (Fig. 6.10). Wire holes for the final splint can be digitally created. Cutting guides for all osteotomies can be also be created. As examples, a Genioplasty cutting guide (Fig. 6.11), and a positioning guide for Genioplasty (Fig. 6.12) are seen.

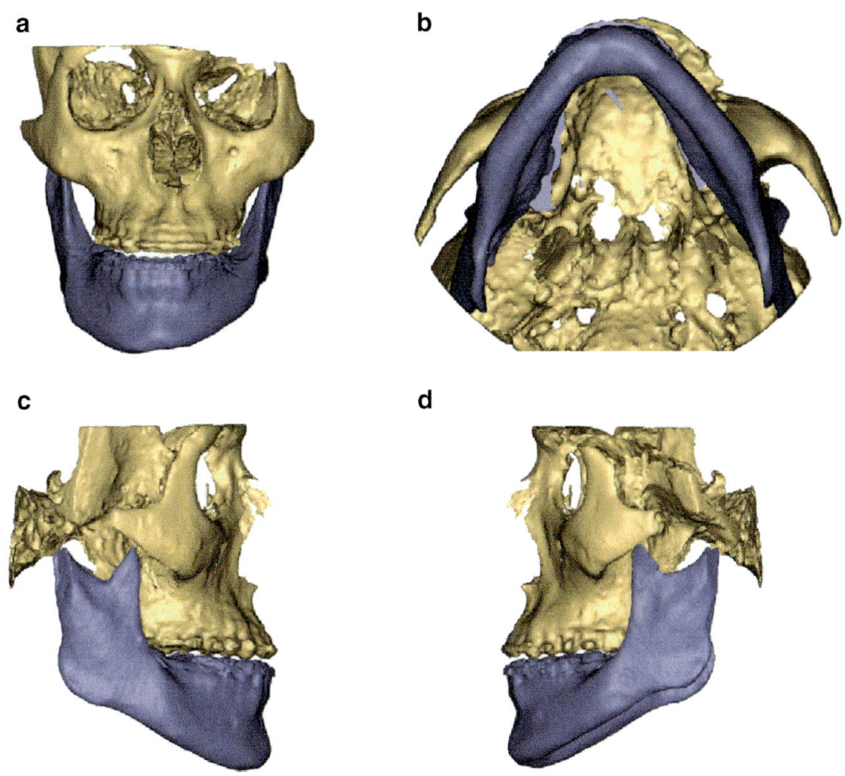

Fig. 6.2 VSP preoperative anatomy: Class III skeletal malocclusion with mandibular prognathism and deviation to the right frontal view. (**a**) Frontal view 3D (**b**) Inferior view 3D (**c**) Right lateral 3D (**d**) Left lateral 3D (Proplan, DuPuy Synthes Craniomaxillofacial, Paoli, PA, USA)

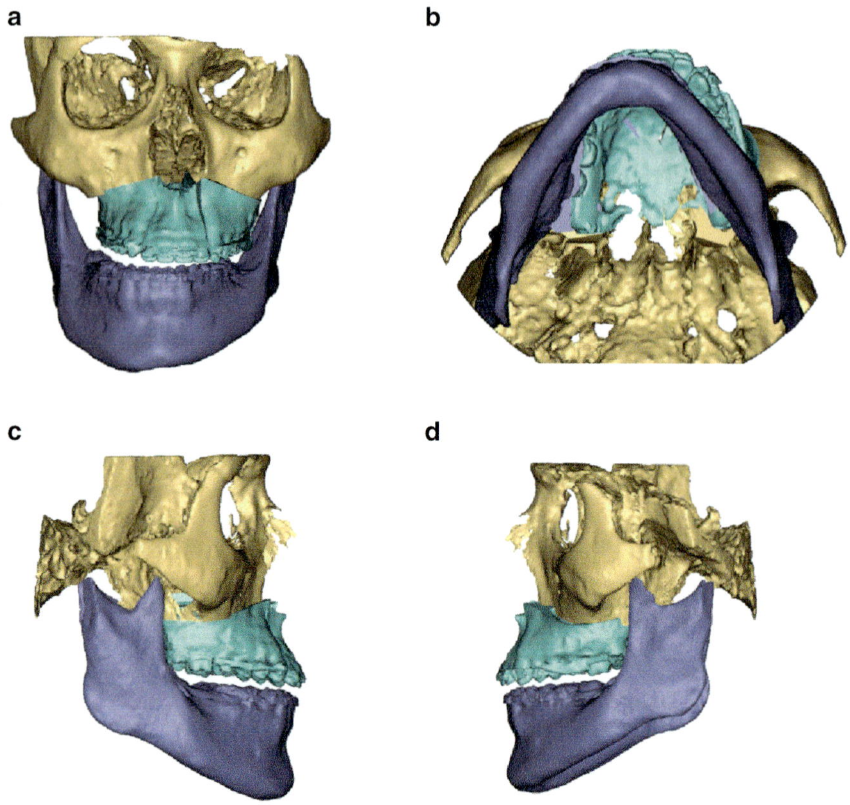

Fig. 6.3 VSP planned LeFort I maxillary movement for Class III skeletal malocclusion with mandibular prognathism and deviation to the right. For a single jaw osteotomy of the maxilla, from this set final position of the maxilla a final splint can be fabricated. For a double jaw, planning would continue with the mandibular osteotomies. (**a**) Frontal view 3D (**b**) Inferior view 3D (**c**) Right lateral 3D (**d**) Left lateral 3D. (Proplan, DuPuy Synthes Craniomaxillofacial, Paoli, PA, USA)

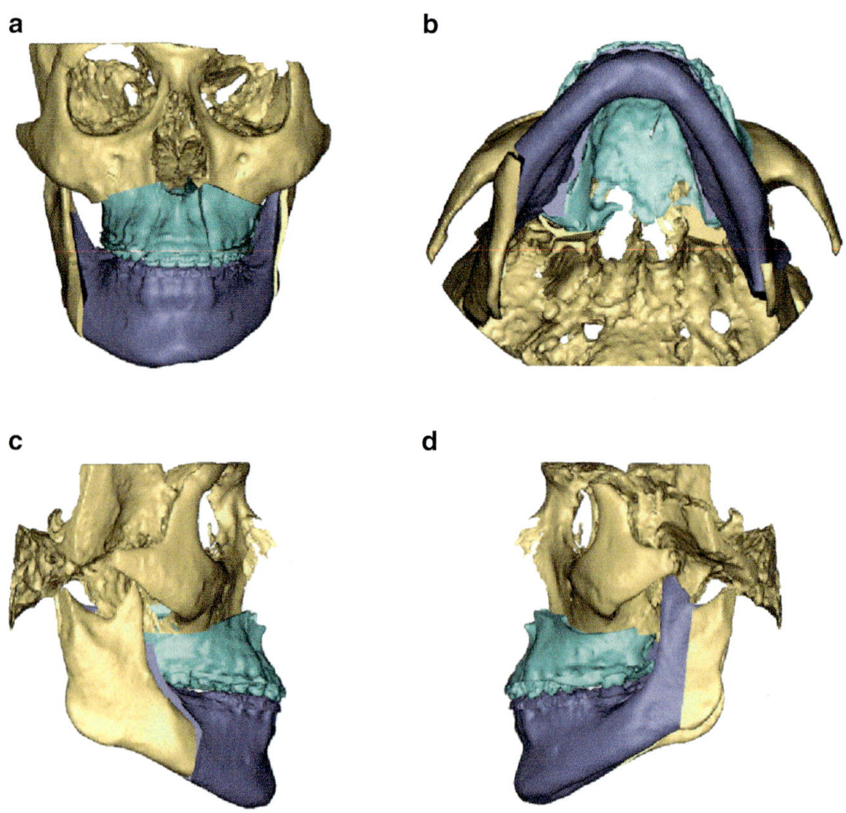

Fig. 6.4 VSP planned mandibular movement with a right sagittal split ramus and left vertical ramus osteotomies as it relates to the new LeFort I maxillary position for Class III skeletal malocclusion with mandibular prognathism and deviation to the right. (**a**) Frontal view 3D (**b**) inferior view 3D (**c**) right lateral 3D (**d**) left lateral 3D. (Proplan, DuPuy Synthes Craniomaxillofacial, Paoli, PA, USA)

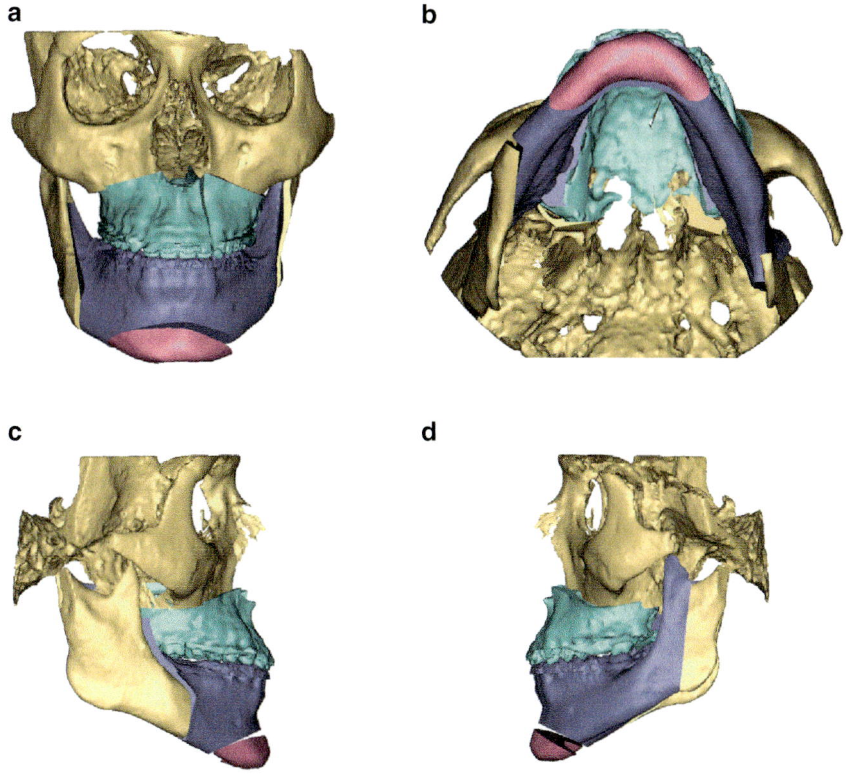

Fig. 6.5 VSP planned genioplasty as it relates to the LeFort I and mandibular movement with a right sagittal split ramus and left vertical ramus osteotomies for Class III skeletal malocclusion with mandibular prognathism and deviation to the right. (**a**) Frontal view 3D (**b**) inferior view 3D (**c**) right lateral 3D (**d**) left lateral 3D. (Proplan, DuPuy Synthes Craniomaxillofacial, Paoli, PA, USA)

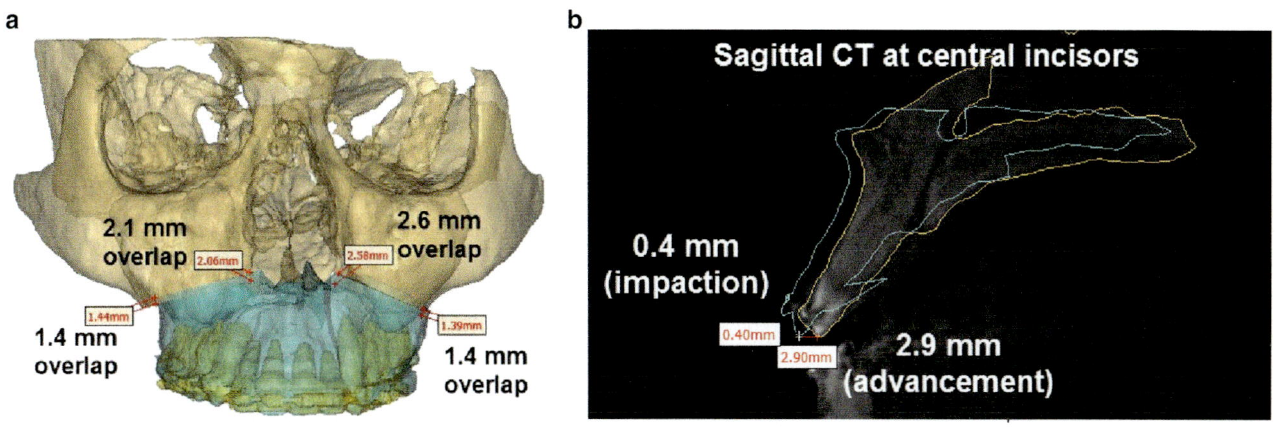

Fig. 6.6 VSP planned LeFort I maxillary movement with overlap measurements. (**a**) Frontal 3D view (**b**) sagittal 2D view. (Proplan, DuPuy Synthes Craniomaxillofacial, Paoli, PA, USA)

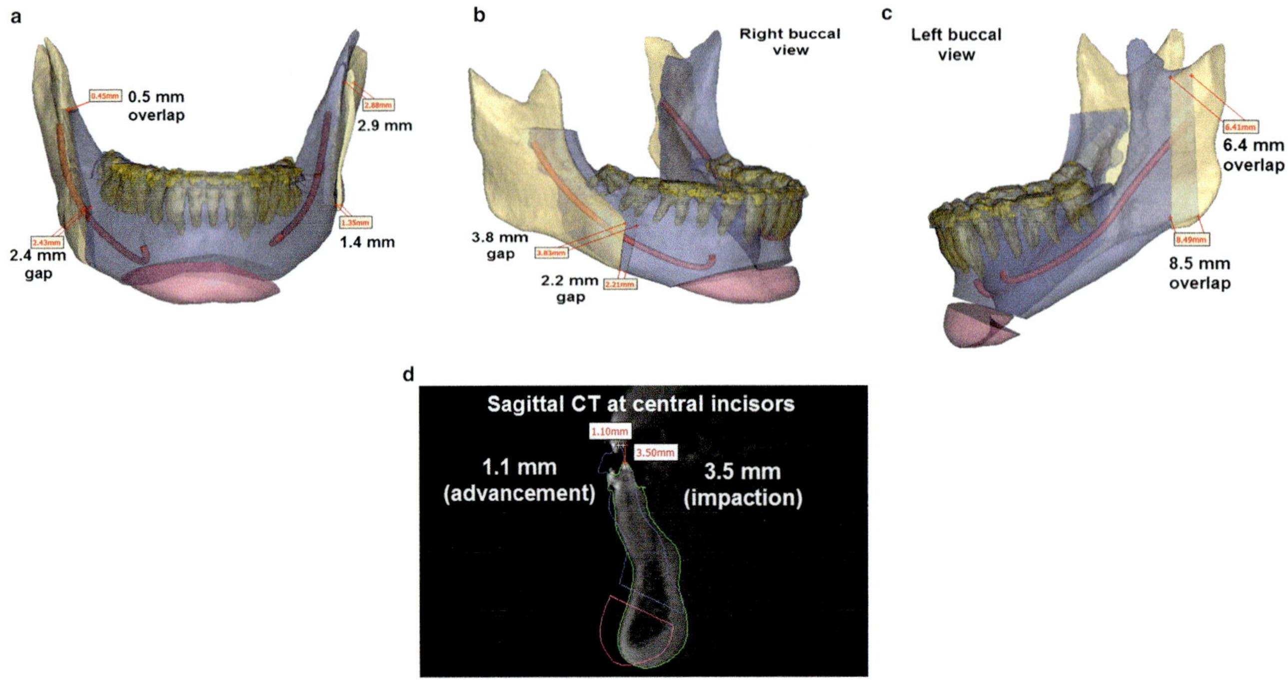

Fig. 6.7 VSP planned mandibular movement measurements with mandibular canal marking with a right sagittal split ramus, left vertical ramus, and genioplasty osteotomies as it relates to the new maxillary position for Class III skeletal malocclusion with mandibular prognathism and deviation to the right frontal view. (**a**) frontal view 3D (**b**) right lateral view 3D (**c**) left lateral 3D view (**d**) sagittal 2D view. (Proplan, DuPuy Synthes Craniomaxillofacial, Paoli, PA, USA)

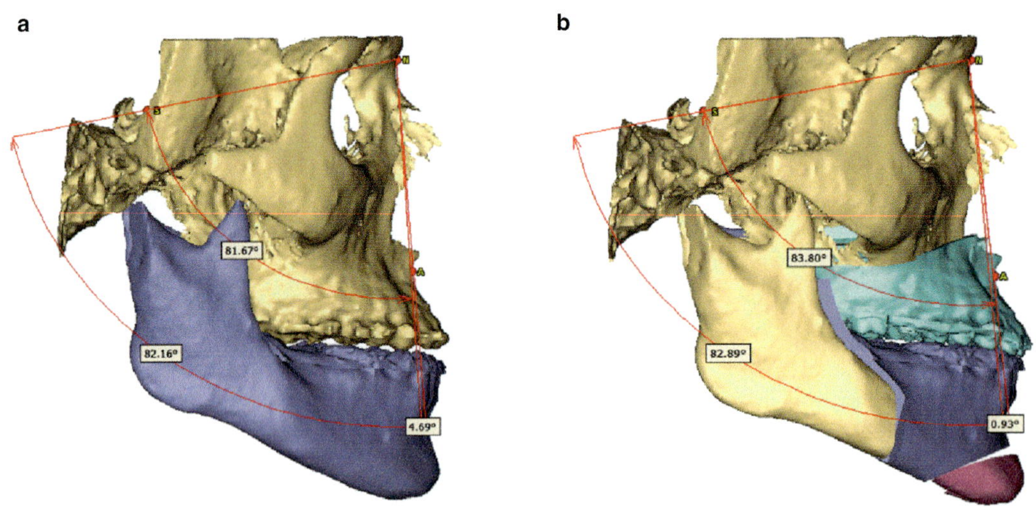

Fig. 6.8 VSP lateral cephalometric reference angle measurements preoperative and planned movements for a LeFort I, right sagittal split ramus, left vertical ramus, and genioplasty osteotomies as it relates to the new maxillary position for Class III skeletal malocclusion with mandibular prognathism and deviation to the right frontal view. (**a**) Right lateral preoperative view 3D (**b**) right lateral planned 3D view. (Proplan, DuPuy Synthes Craniomaxillofacial, Paoli, PA, USA)

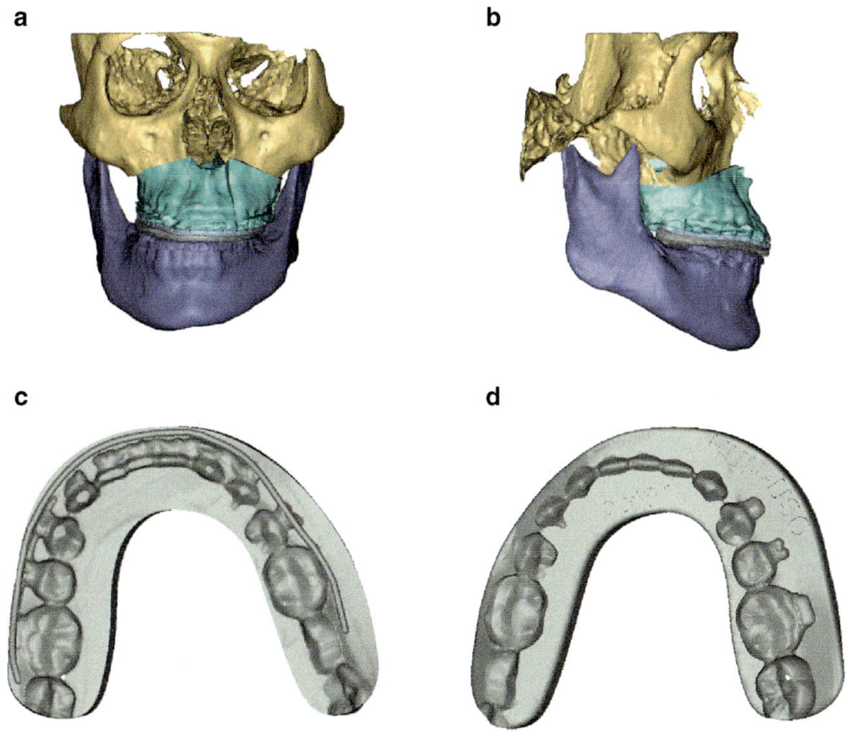

Fig. 6.9 VSP virtual intermediate splint fabrication for planned mandibular movement measurements with a right sagittal split ramus, left vertical ramus, and genioplasty osteotomies as it relates to the new maxillary position for Class III skeletal malocclusion with mandibular prognathism and deviation to the right frontal view. (**a**) Frontal view 3D (**b**) left lateral view 3D (**c**) intermediate splint superior view (**d**) intermediate splint inferior view. (Proplan, DuPuy Synthes Craniomaxillofacial, Paoli, PA, USA)

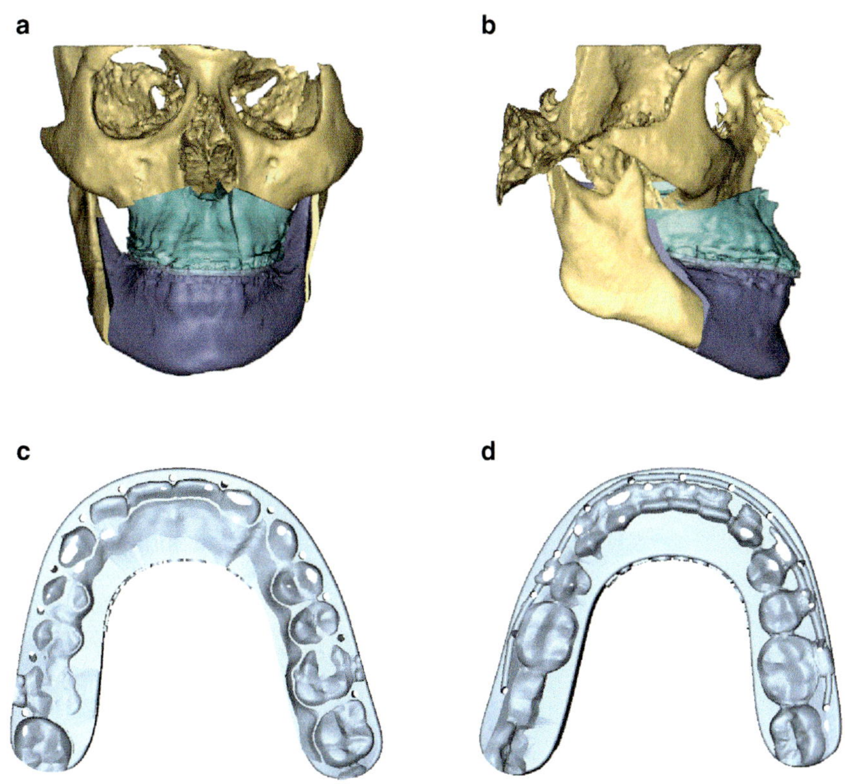

Fig. 6.10 VSP virtual final splint fabrication for planned mandibular movement measurements with a right sagittal split ramus, left vertical ramus, and genioplasty osteotomies as it relates to the new maxillary position for Class III skeletal malocclusion with mandibular prognathism and deviation to the right frontal view. (**a**) Frontal view 3D (**b**) left lateral view 3D (**c**) final splint superior view (**d**) final splint inferior view. (Proplan, DuPuy Synthes Craniomaxillofacial, Paoli, PA, USA)

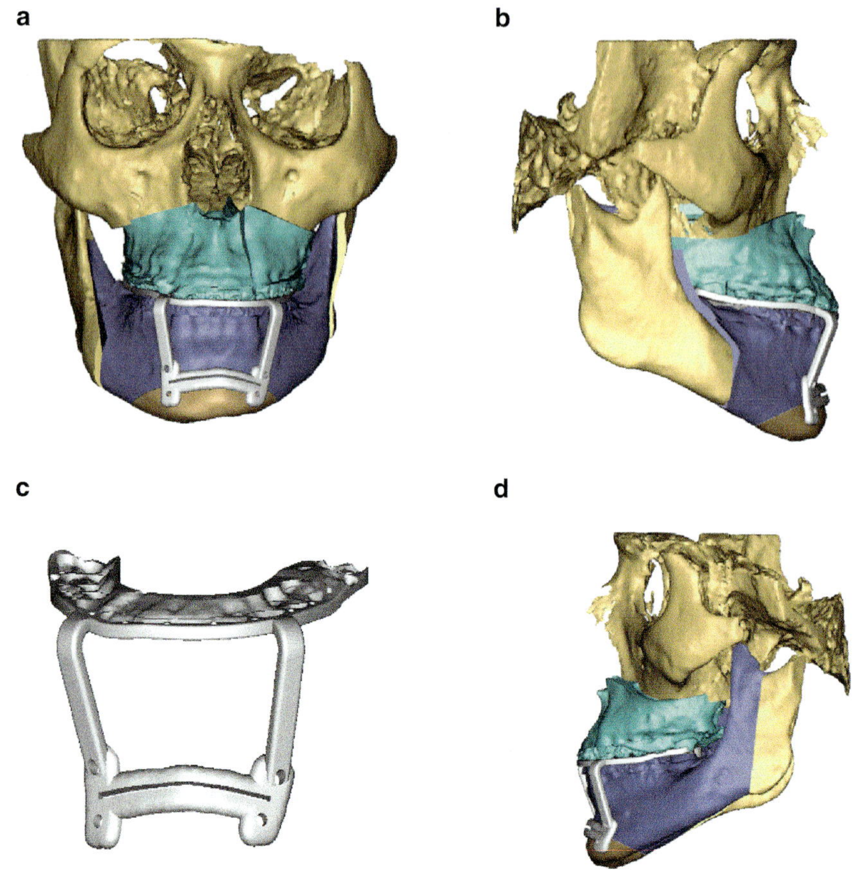

Fig. 6.11 VSP cutting guide for genioplasty as it relates to the LeFort I and mandibular movement with a right sagittal split ramus and left vertical ramus osteotomies for Class III skeletal malocclusion with mandibular prognathism and deviation to the right. (**a**) Frontal view 3D (**b**) right lateral view 3D (**c**) cutting guide 3D frontal view (**d**) left lateral 3D view. (Proplan, DuPuy Synthes Craniomaxillofacial, Paoli, PA, USA)

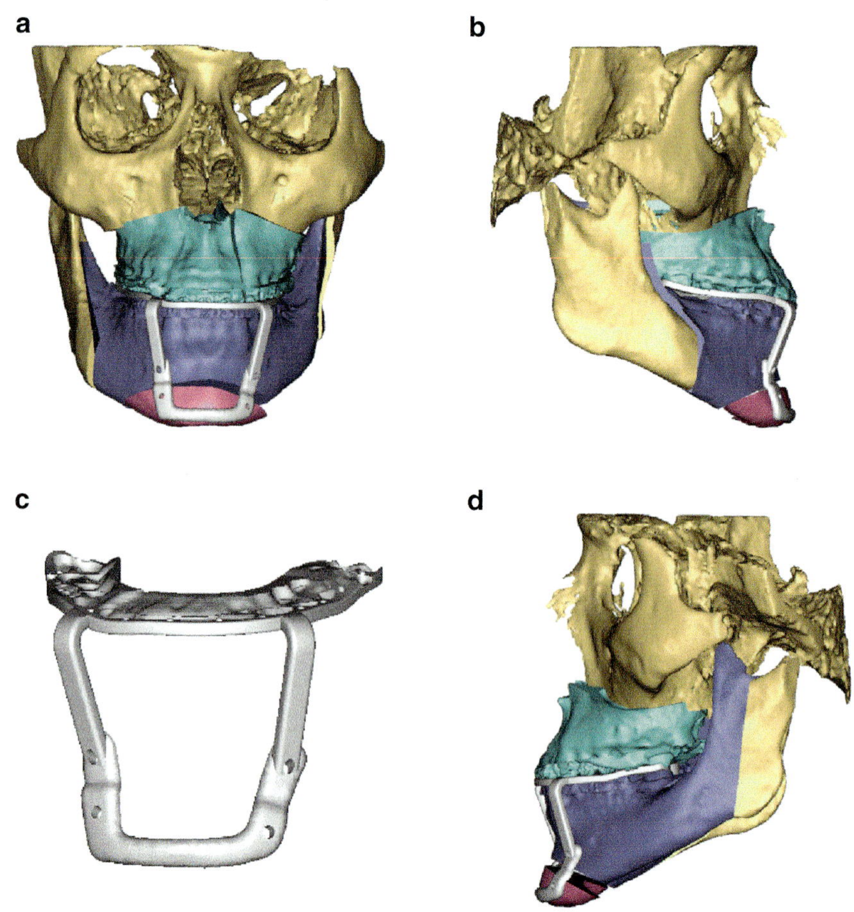

Fig. 6.12 VSP positioning guide for genioplasty as it relates to the LeFort I and mandibular movement with a right sagittal split ramus and left vertical ramus osteotomies for Class III skeletal malocclusion with mandibular prognathism and deviation to the right. Drill holes in guide allow fixation of the inferior genioplasty segment for rigid fixation. (**a**) Frontal view 3D (**b**) right lateral view 3D (**c**) positioning guide frontal 3D view (**d**) left lateral 3D view. (Proplan, DuPuy Synthes Craniomaxillofacial, Paoli, PA, USA)

Surgical Cases Planned with Digital Technology

Case 1 Figures 6.13–6.71

Twenty-eight year-old female presented with Class III skeletal malocclusion with mandibular prognathism and deviation to the right and bilateral midfacial and malar hypoplasia, following presurgical orthodontics.

Surgical plan was for LeFort I osteotomy, bilateral mandibular vertical ramus osteotomies, genioplasty, and bilateral malar implants. VSP (Proplan, DePuy Synthes Craniomaxillofacial, Paoli, PA, USA) was utilized to plan and fabricate custom intermediate and final splints. Bilateral Medpor zygomatic implant (Stryker, Kalamazoo, MI, USA) with DePuy Synthes screw fixation (DePuy Synthes Craniomaxillofacial, Paoli, PA, USA) was performed. Satisfactory postsurgical facial esthetic and occlusal result are demonstrated. (Surgery: Alex M. Greenberg, DDS, New York, NY, Orthodontics: Dr. Ronald Schwalb, New York, NY, USA).

Case 2 Figures 6.72–6.122

A 20 year-old female with possible diagnosis of Churg–Strauss syndrome presented with severe bilateral mandibular condylar resorption and mandibular retrognathia and retrogenia with Class II skeletal malocclusion. The plan was for LeFort I osteotomy, bilateral mandibular total joint prostheses, and genioplasty. An integrated planning process with VSP (Medical Modelling, Golden, CO, USA) to plan the surgery and fabricate custom intermediate and final splints, and the custom fabrication of the bilateral total TMJ prostheses (TMJ Concepts, Ventura, CA, USA) was utilized. Surgery was performed with a satisfactory facial esthetic, and occlusal result was achieved. A postoperative high level of occlusal stability is seen at 4 weeks and 1 year. (Surgery: Alex M Greenberg, DDS, Michael Perrino, DDS, MD, Assistant Professor, Oral and Maxillofacial Surgery, Columbia University College of Dental Medicine, Maher Jandali Rifai, DMD, MD, Chief Resident, Oral and Maxillofacial Surgery, Columbia University College of Dental Medicine, New York, NY, USA, Orthodontics: Dr. Shirley Lew, Private Practice, Brooklyn, NY, USA).

Patient-Specific Surgical Guides and Bone Plates

Patient-specific surgical guides for osteotomies and custom prebent bone plates can now be virtually planned and 3D printed from Titanium Grade 2 using laser melting process (Figs. 6.123, 6.124, 6.125, and 6.126).

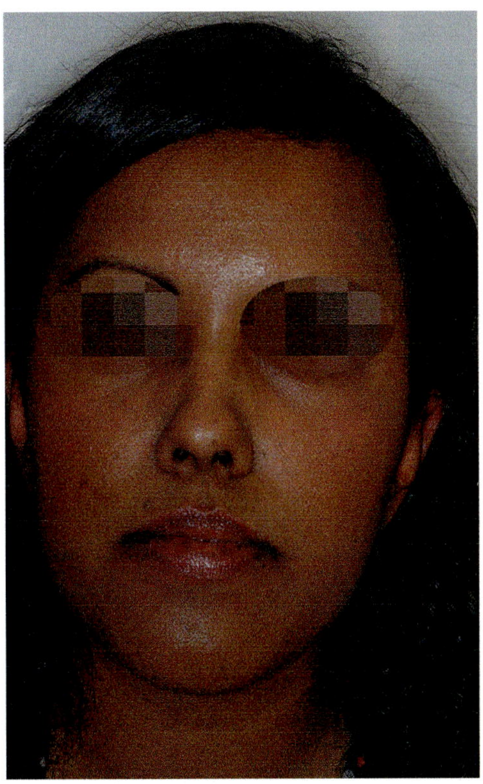

Fig. 6.13 Preoperative Class III malocclusion with mandibular hyperplasia facial view

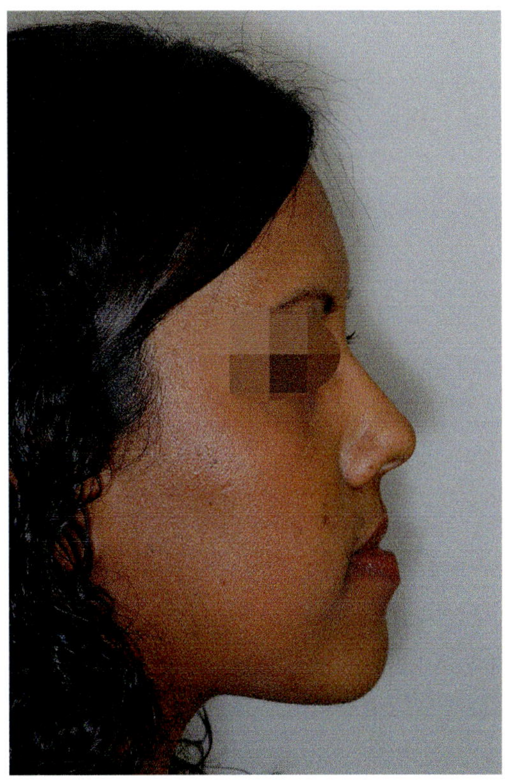

Fig. 6.14 Preoperative Class III malocclusion with mandibular hyperplasia right lateral facial view

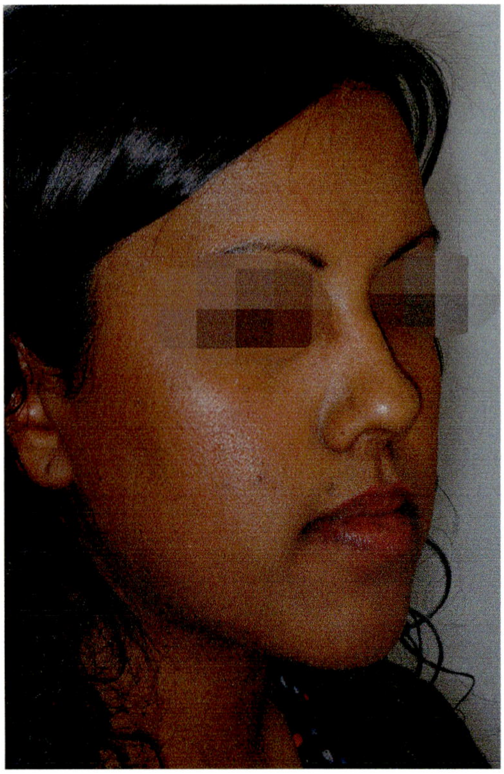

Fig. 6.15 3 Preoperative Class III malocclusion with mandibular hyperplasia right 3/4 facial view

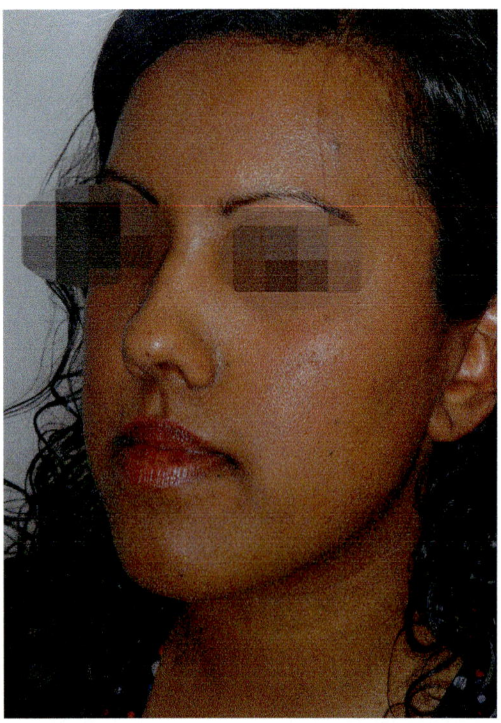

Fig. 6.16 Preoperative Class III malocclusion with mandibular hyperplasia left 3/4 facial view

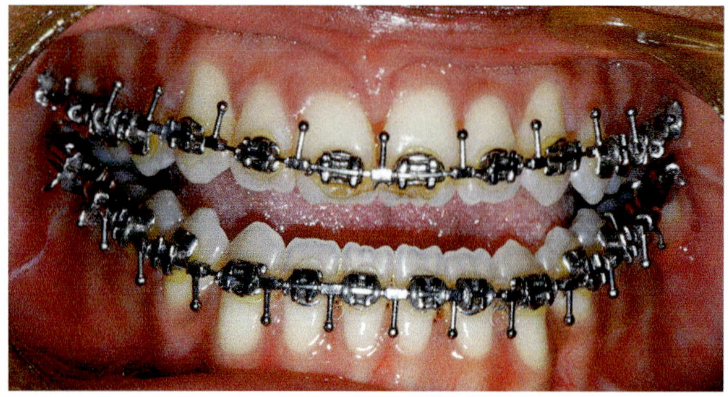

Fig. 6.17 Preoperative Class III malocclusion with surgical orthodontic appliance frontal occlusal view

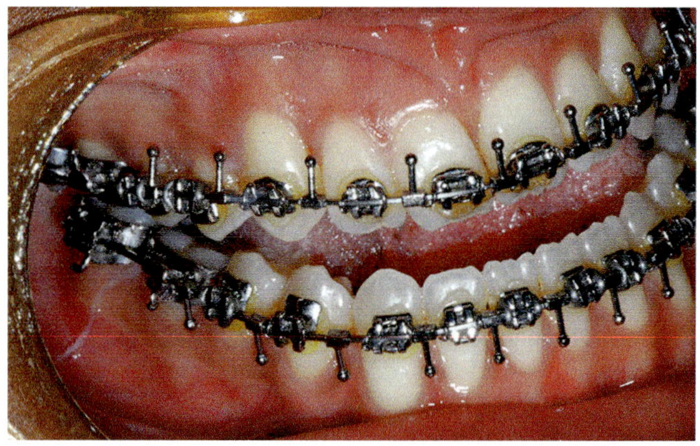

Fig. 6.18 Preoperative Class III malocclusion with surgical orthodontic appliance right lateral occlusal view

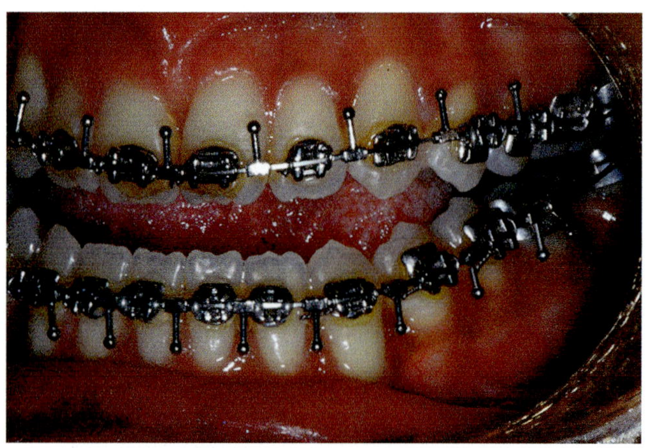

Fig. 6.19 Preoperative Class III malocclusion with surgical orthodontic appliance left lateral occlusal view

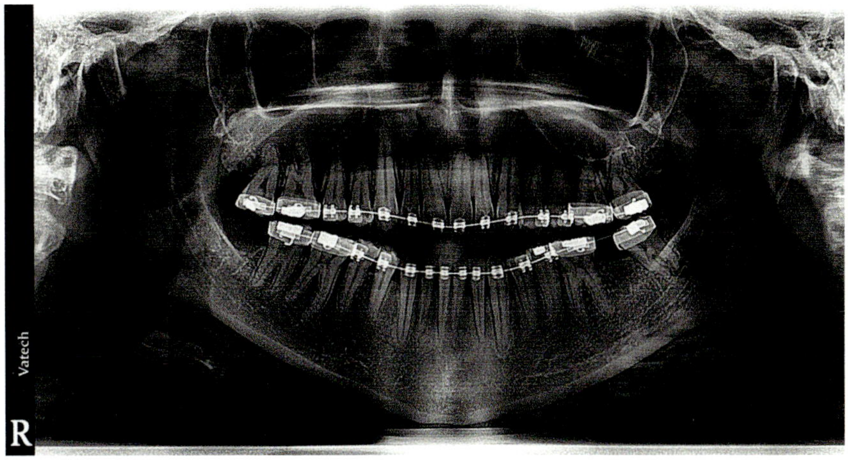

Fig. 6.20 Preoperative panoramic radiograph

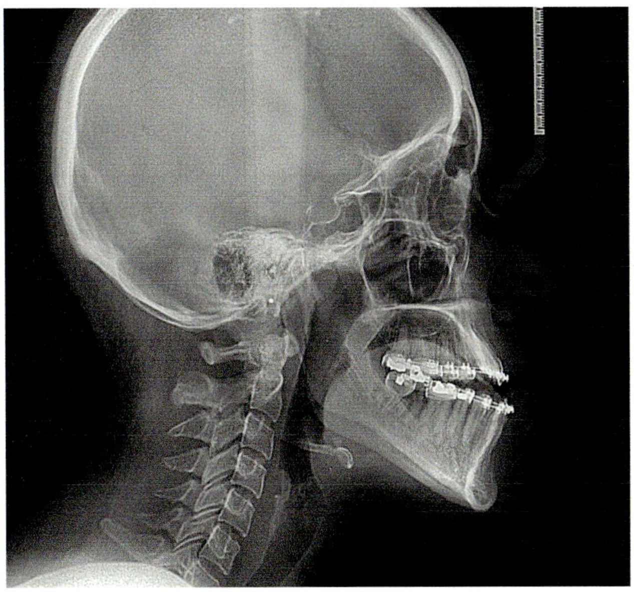

Fig. 6.21 Preoperative lateral cephalometric radiograph

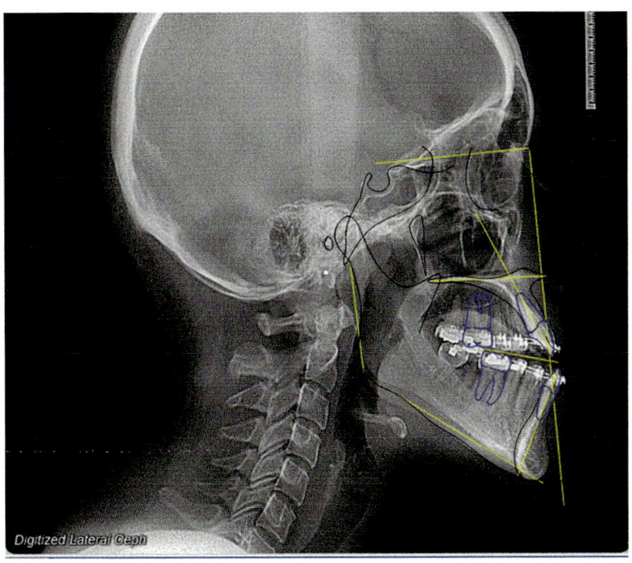

Fig. 6.22 Preoperative lateral cephalometric radiograph tracing for COGS analysis

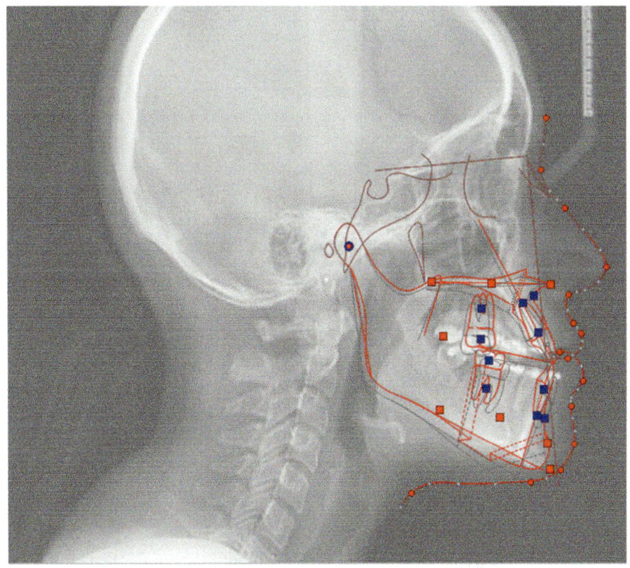

Fig. 6.23 Lateral cephalometric radiograph prediction tracing for LeFort I osteotomy, bilateral mandibular vertical ramus osteotomies, genioplasty, and bilateral malar implants

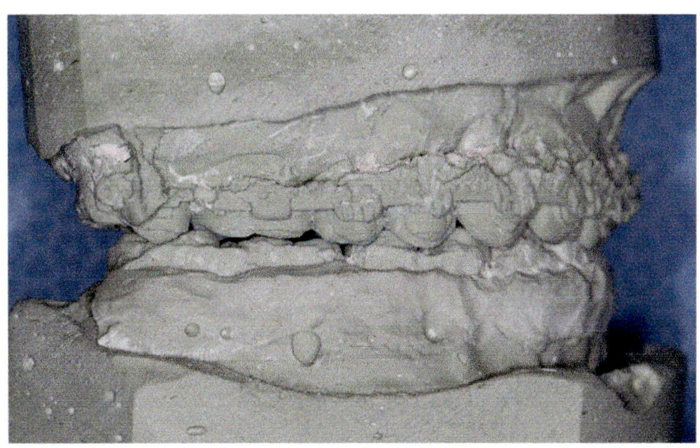

Fig. 6.24 Dental casts with planned Class I occlusion

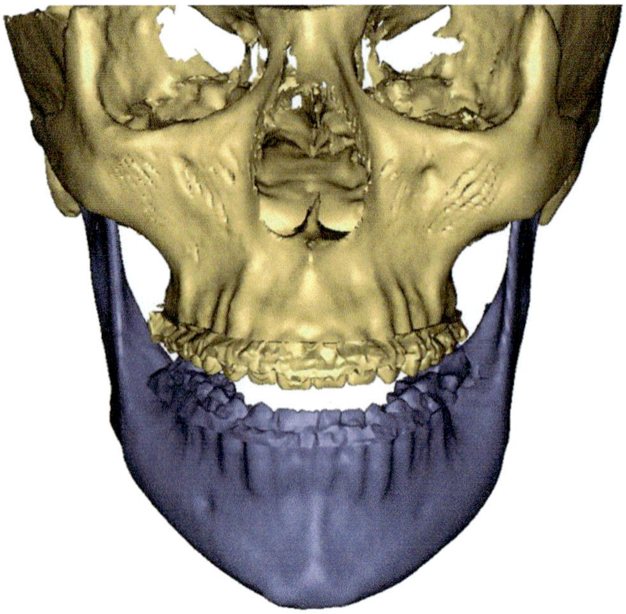

Fig. 6.25 VSP preoperative 3D frontal view. (Proplan, DuPuy Synthes Craniomaxillofacial, Paoli, PA, USA)

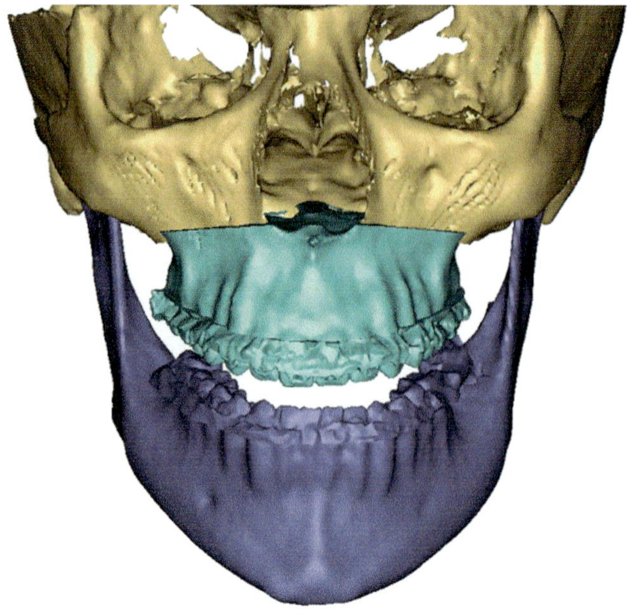

Fig. 6.27 VSP 3D simulated LeFort I maxillary impaction movement frontal view. (Proplan, DuPuy Synthes Craniomaxillofacial, Paoli, PA, USA)

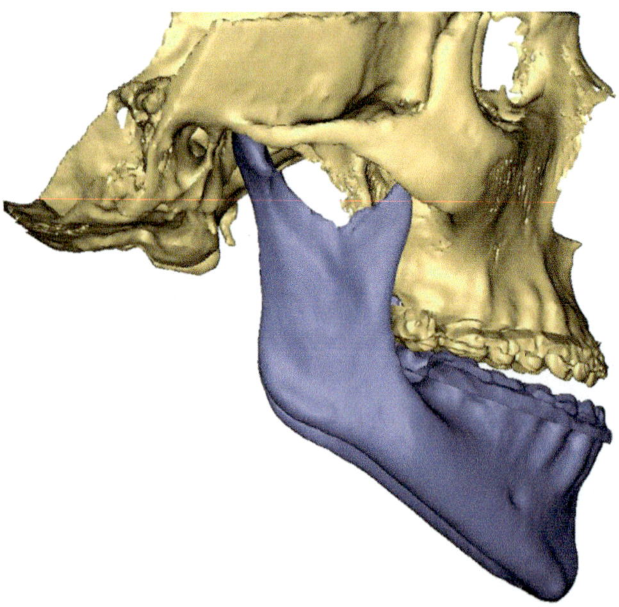

Fig. 6.26 VSP preoperative right lateral 3D view. (Proplan, DuPuy Synthes Craniomaxillofacial, Paoli, PA, USA)

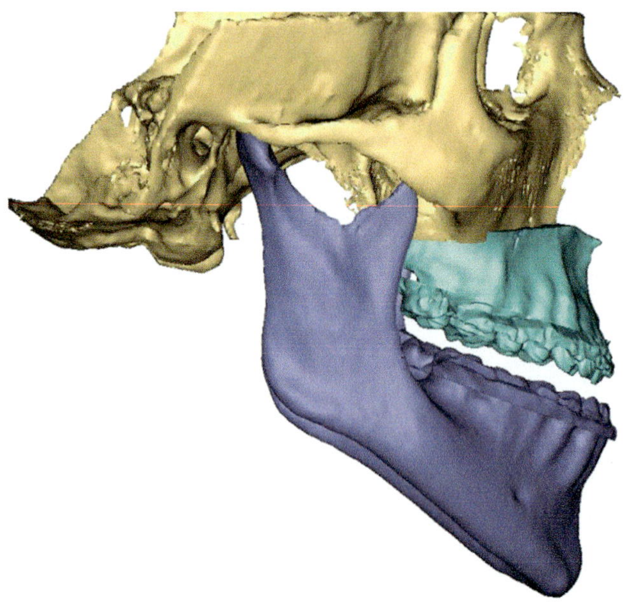

Fig. 6.28 VSP 3D simulated LeFort I maxillary impaction movement right lateral view. (Proplan, DuPuy Synthes Craniomaxillofacial, Paoli, PA, USA)

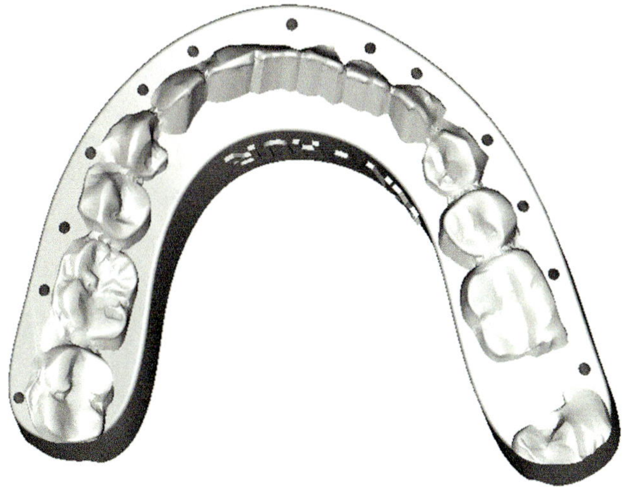

Fig. 6.29 VSP 3D simulated intermediate occlusal splint inferior mandibular view. (Proplan, DuPuy Synthes Craniomaxillofacial, Paoli, PA, USA)

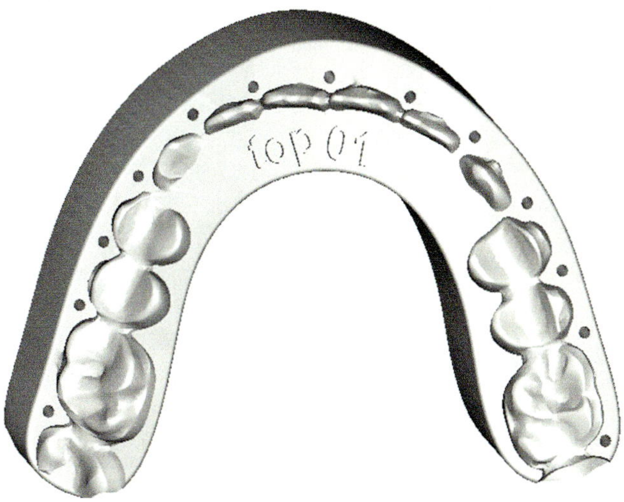

Fig. 6.30 VSP 3D simulated intermediate occlusal splint superior maxillary view. (Proplan, DuPuy Synthes Craniomaxillofacial, Paoli, PA, USA)

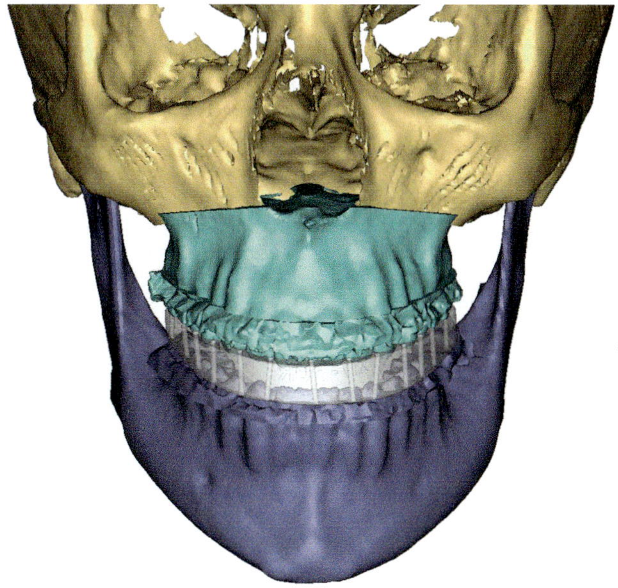

Fig. 6.31 VSP 3D simulated LeFort I maxillary movement with intermediate occlusal splint frontal view. (Proplan, DuPuy Synthes Craniomaxillofacial, Paoli, PA, USA)

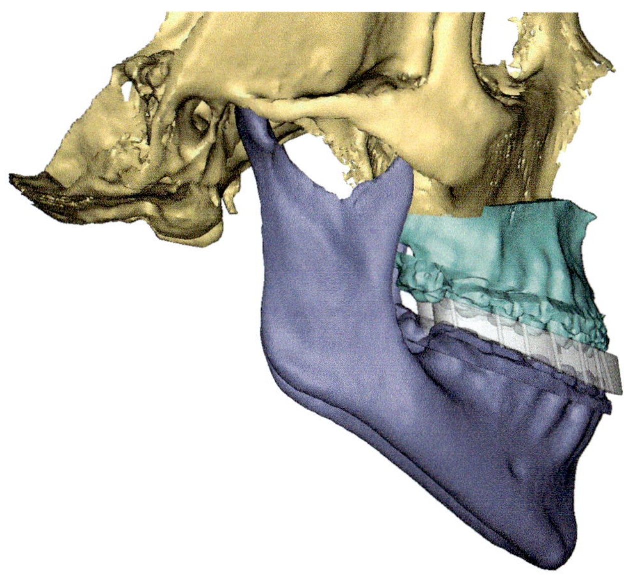

Fig. 6.32 VSP 3D simulated LeFort I maxillary movement with intermediate occlusal splint right lateral view. (Proplan, DuPuy Synthes Craniomaxillofacial, Paoli, PA, USA)

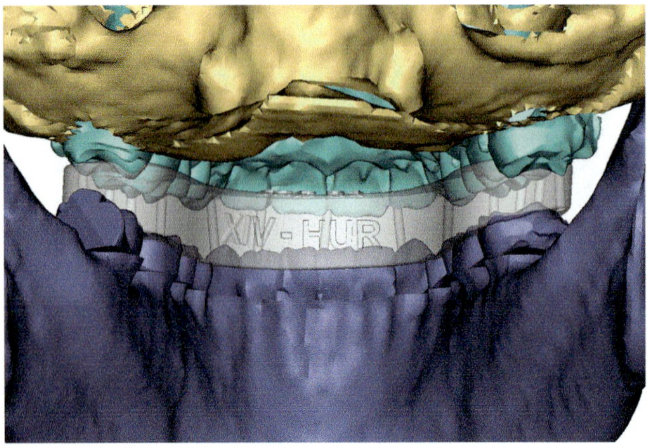

Fig. 6.33 VSP 3D simulated LeFort I maxillary movement with intermediate occlusal splint lingual view. (Proplan, DuPuy Synthes Craniomaxillofacial, Paoli, PA, USA)

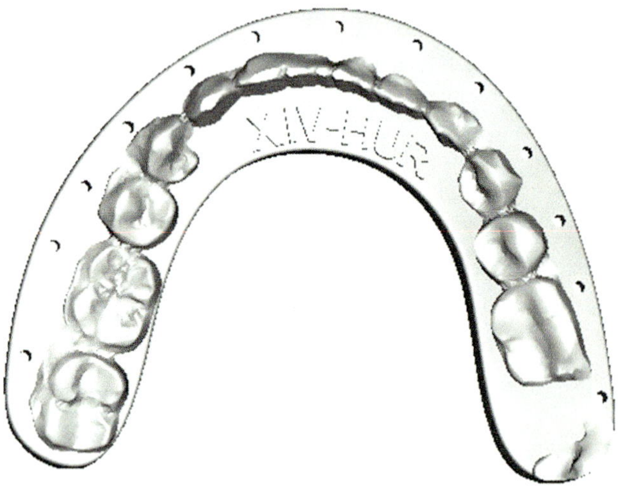

Fig. 6.34 VSP 3D simulated final occlusal splint inferior mandibular view. (Proplan, DuPuy Synthes Craniomaxillofacial, Paoli, PA, USA)

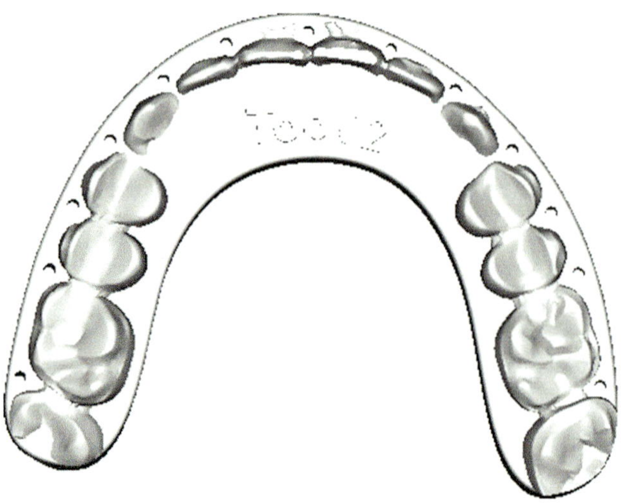

Fig. 6.35 VSP 3D simulated final occlusal splint superior maxillary view. (Proplan, DuPuy Synthes Craniomaxillofacial, Paoli, PA, USA)

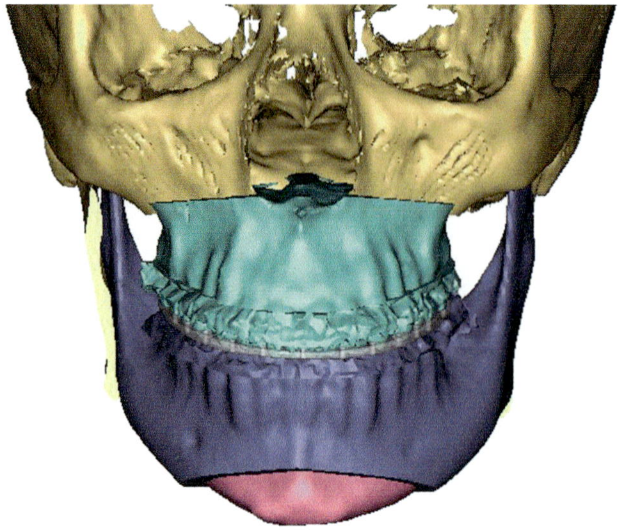

Fig. 6.36 VSP 3D simulated LeFort I osteotomy, bilateral mandibular vertical ramus osteotomies, and reduction genioplasty movements with final occlusal splint frontal view. (Proplan, DuPuy Synthes Craniomaxillofacial, Paoli, PA, USA)

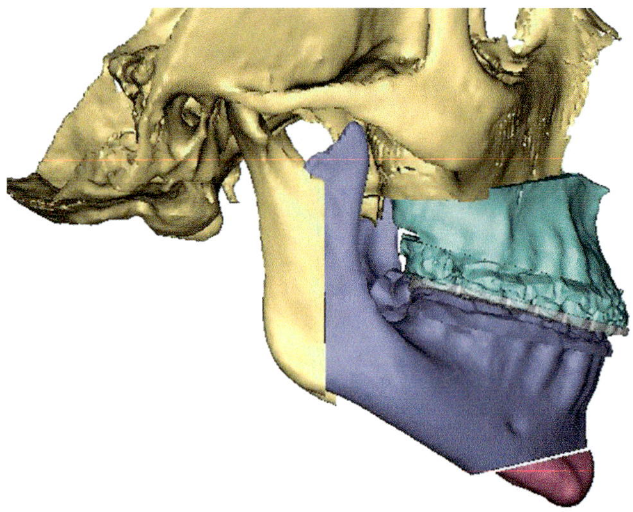

Fig. 6.37 VSP 3D simulated LeFort I osteotomy, bilateral mandibular vertical ramus osteotomies, and reduction genioplasty movements with final occlusal splint right lateral view (Proplan, DuPuy Synthes Craniomaxillofacial, Paoli, PA, USA)

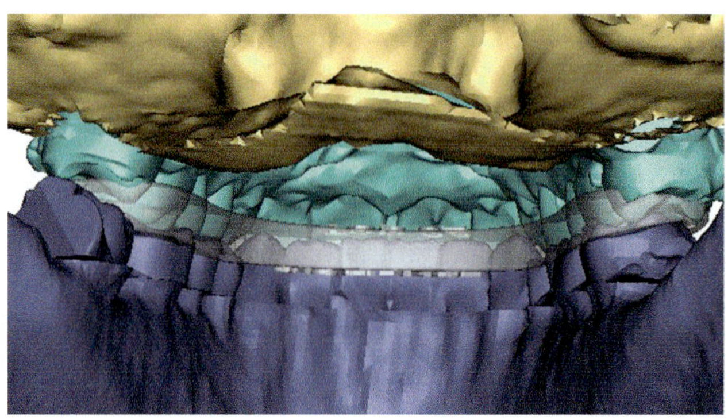

Fig. 6.38 VSP 3D simulated LeFort I osteotomy, bilateral mandibular vertical ramus osteotomies, and genioplasty movements with final occlusal splint lingual view (Proplan, DuPuy Synthes Craniomaxillofacial, Paoli, PA, USA)

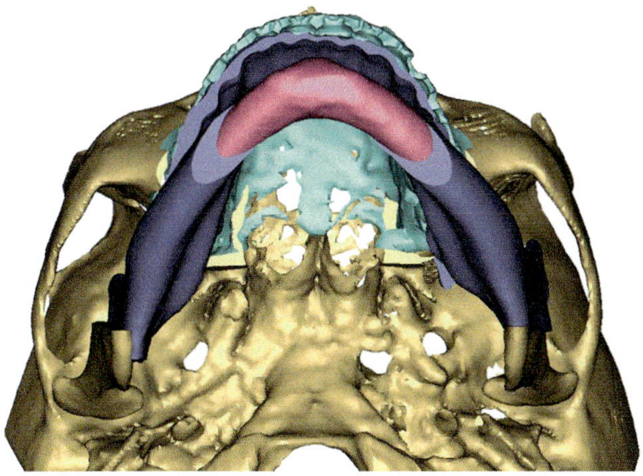

Fig. 6.39 VSP 3D simulated LeFort I osteotomy, bilateral mandibular vertical ramus osteotomies, and genioplasty movements with final occlusal splint inferior submental view (Proplan, DuPuy Synthes Craniomaxillofacial, Paoli, PA, USA)

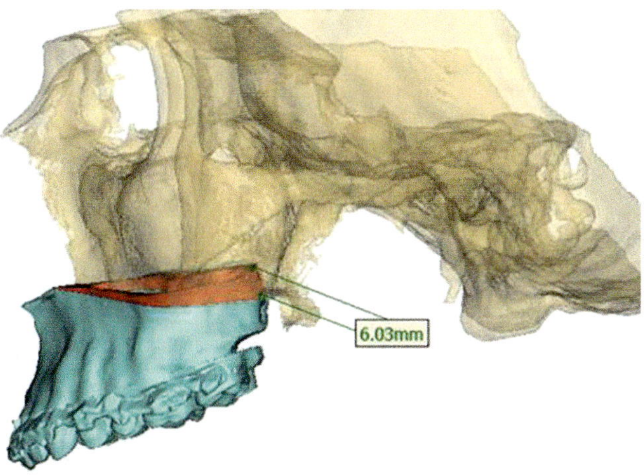

Fig. 6.40 VSP 3D simulated LeFort I osteotomy wedge excision left lateral view (Proplan, DuPuy Synthes Craniomaxillofacial, Paoli, PA, USA)

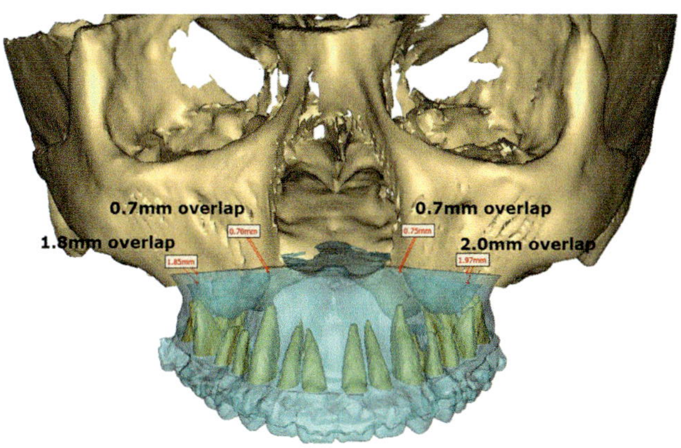

Fig. 6.41 VSP 3D simulated LeFort I osteotomy wedge excision with tooth roots and maxillary movement in frontal view (Proplan, DuPuy Synthes Craniomaxillofacial, Paoli, PA, USA)

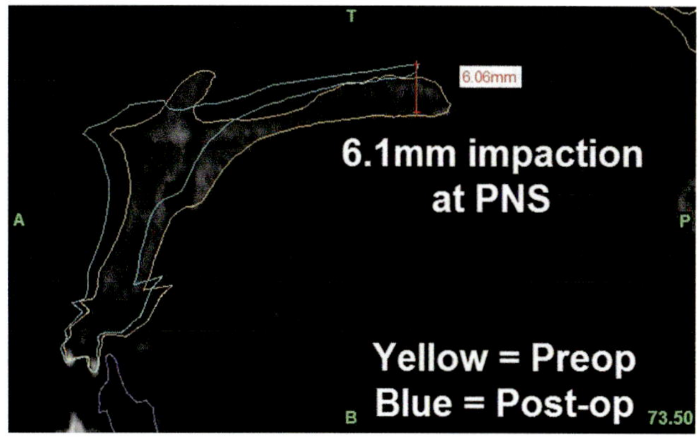

Fig. 6.42 VSP 3D simulated LeFort I osteotomy wedge excision with maxillary movement and measurements in sagittal view (Proplan, DuPuy Synthes Craniomaxillofacial, Paoli, PA, USA)

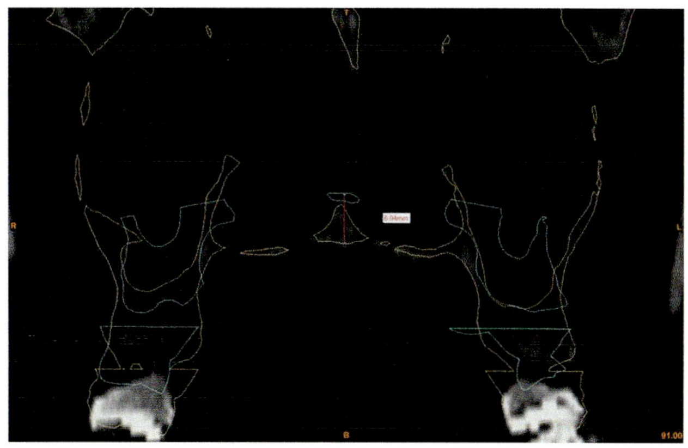

Fig. 6.43 VSP 3D simulated LeFort I osteotomy wedge excision with maxillary movement and measurements in coronal view (Proplan, DuPuy Synthes Craniomaxillofacial, Paoli, PA, USA)

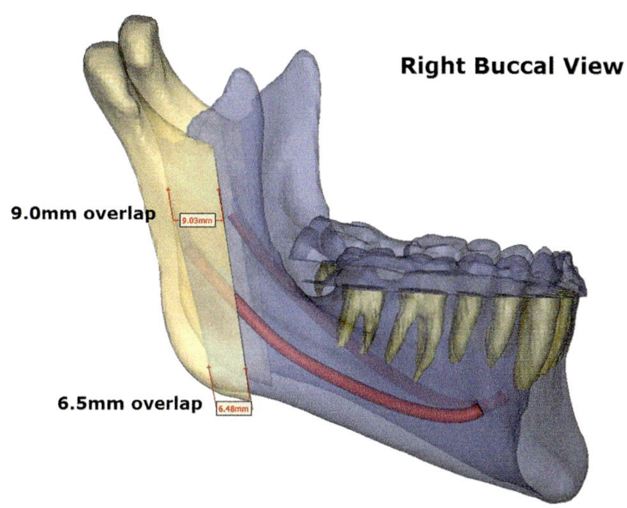

Fig. 6.44 VSP 3D simulated mandibular vertical ramus osteotomies movement with overlap of segments right lateral view (Proplan, DuPuy Synthes Craniomaxillofacial, Paoli, PA, USA)

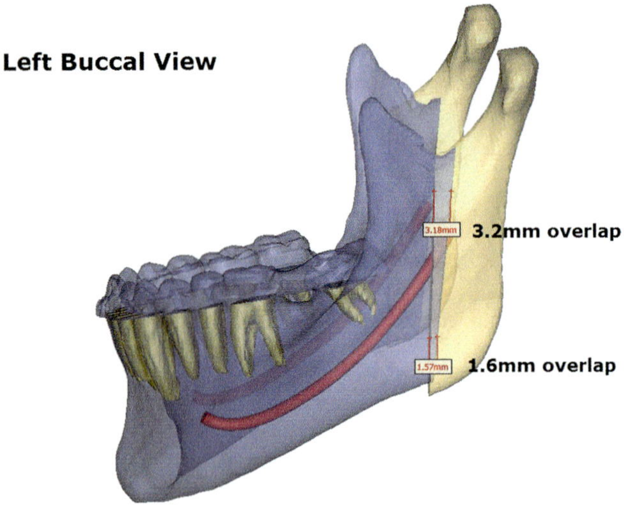

Fig. 6.45 VSP 3D simulated mandibular vertical ramus osteotomies movement with overlap of segments left lateral view (Proplan, DuPuy Synthes Craniomaxillofacial, Paoli, PA, USA)

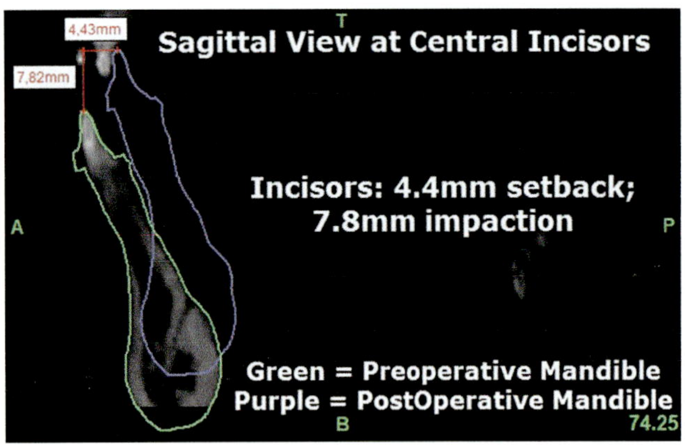

Fig. 6.46 VSP 3D simulated mandibular vertical ramus osteotomies movement with measurement of setback sagittal 2D view (Proplan, DuPuy Synthes Craniomaxillofacial, Paoli, PA, USA)

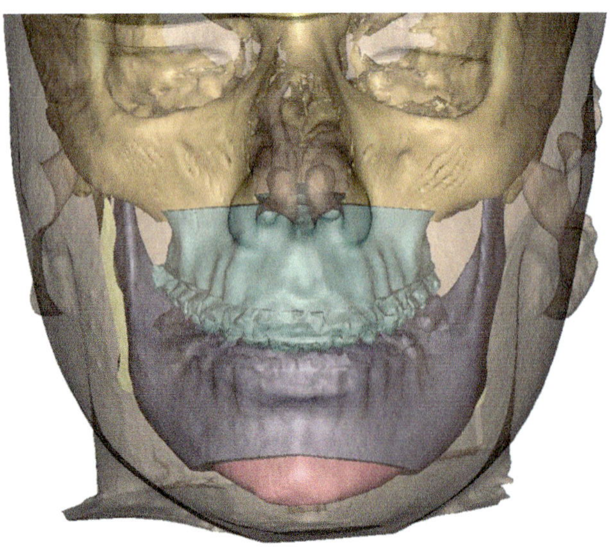

Fig. 6.47 VSP 3D simulated LeFort I osteotomy, bilateral mandibular vertical ramus osteotomies, and genioplasty movements soft tissue superimposed over bone window frontal view (Proplan, DuPuy Synthes Craniomaxillofacial, Paoli, PA, USA)

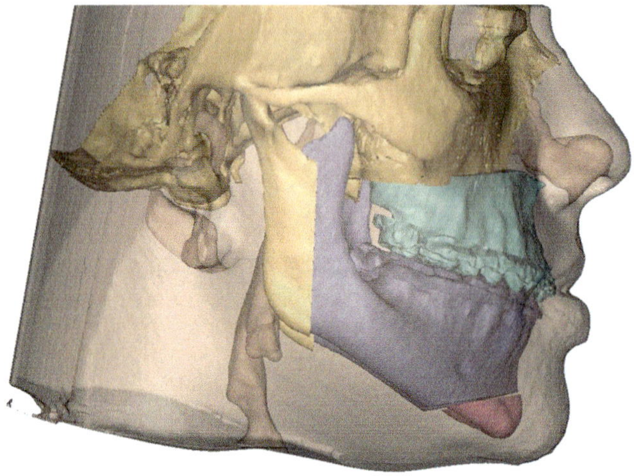

Fig. 6.48 VSP 3D simulated LeFort I osteotomy, bilateral mandibular vertical ramus osteotomies, and genioplasty movements soft tissue superimposed over bone window right lateral view (Proplan, DuPuy Synthes Craniomaxillofacial, Paoli, PA, USA)

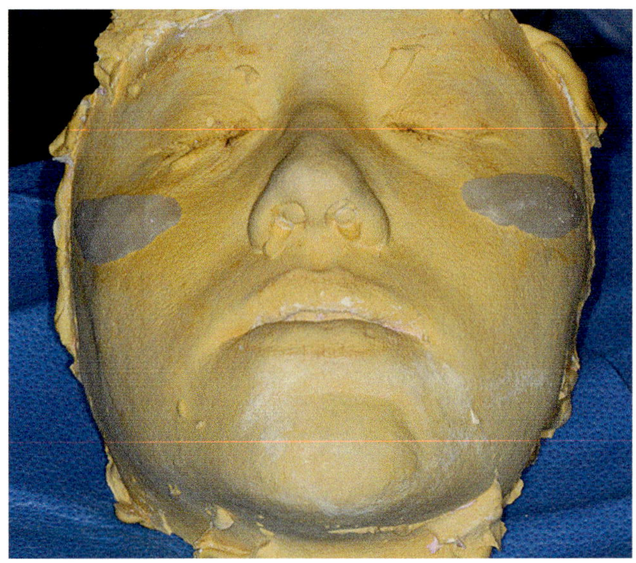

Fig. 6.49 Facial moulage with simulated wax zygomatic implant augmentation

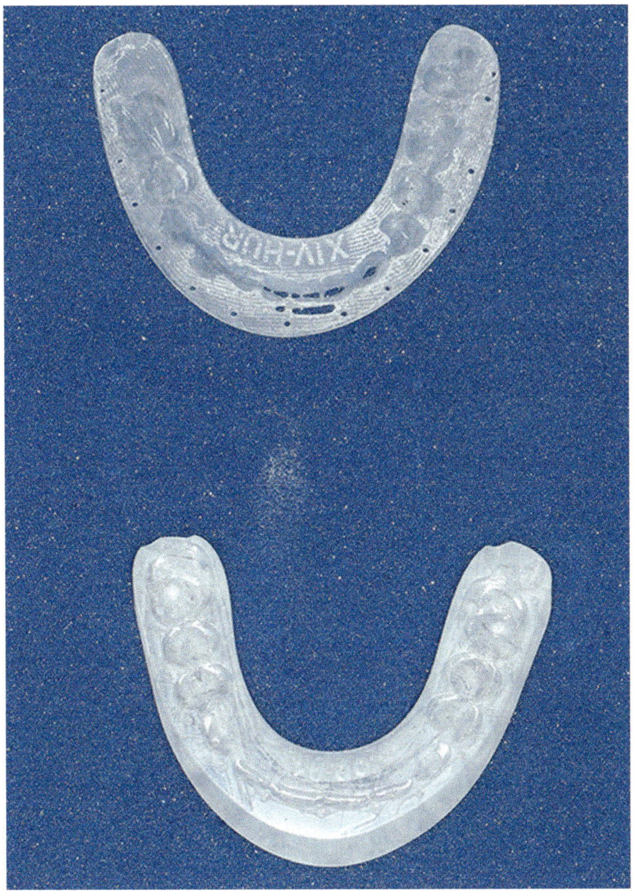

Fig. 6.50 Rapid printed final occlusal splint (*upper*) and intermediate splint (*lower*) (Proplan, DuPuy Synthes Craniomaxillofacial, Paoli, PA, USA)

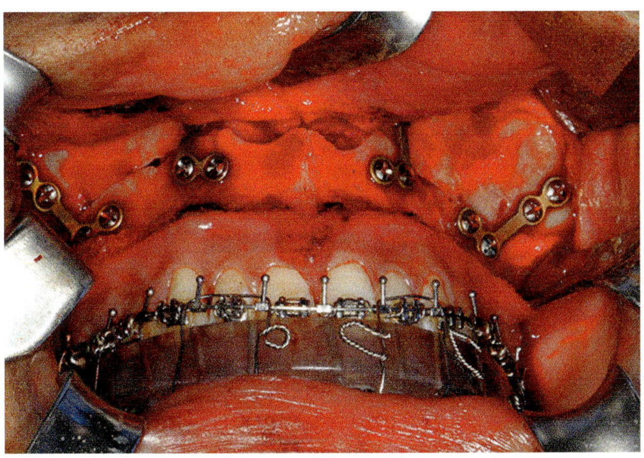

Fig. 6.51 Intraoperative view of intermediate splint with maxillomandibular fixation and completion of LeFort I osteotomy and internal fixation with four miniplate fixation bilateral zygomatic and nasomaxillary buttresses (DePuy Synthes Craniomaxillofacial, Paoli, PA, USA)

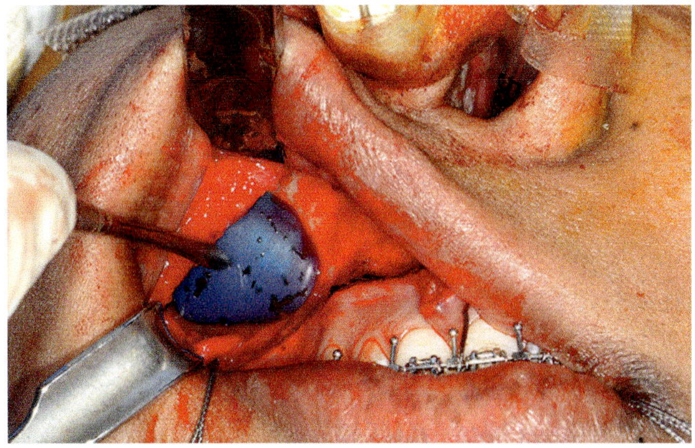

Fig. 6.52 Intraoperative view of right Medpor zygomatic implant sizer (Stryker, Kalamazoo, MI, USA)

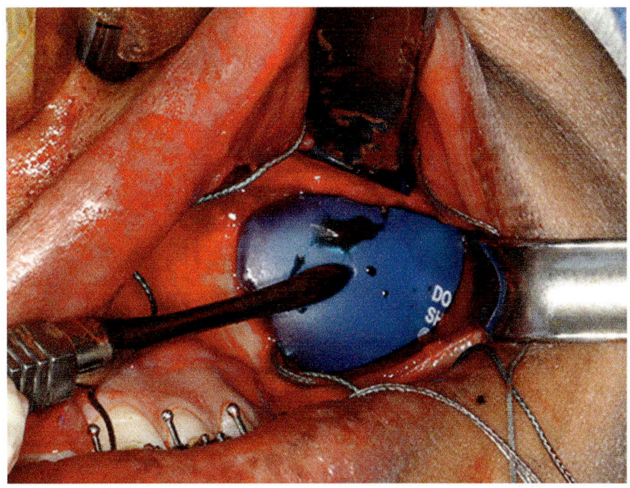

Fig. 6.53 Intraoperative view of left Medpor zygomatic implant sizer (Stryker, Kalamazoo, MI, USA)

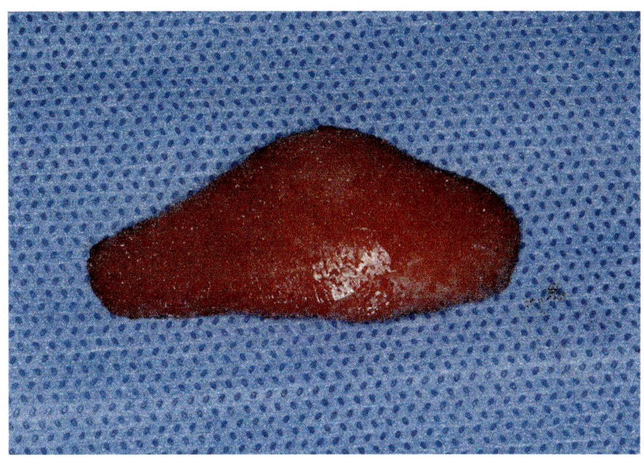

Fig. 6.54 Intraoperative view of right hand carved Medpor zygomatic implant (Stryker, Kalamazoo, MI, USA)

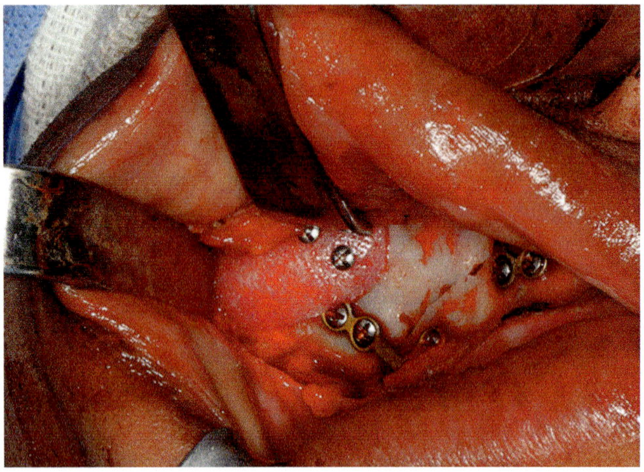

Fig. 6.55 Intraoperative view of right Medpor zygomatic implant (Stryker, Kalamazoo, MI, USA.) with screw fixation (DePuy Synthes Craniomaxillofacial, Paoli, PA, USA)

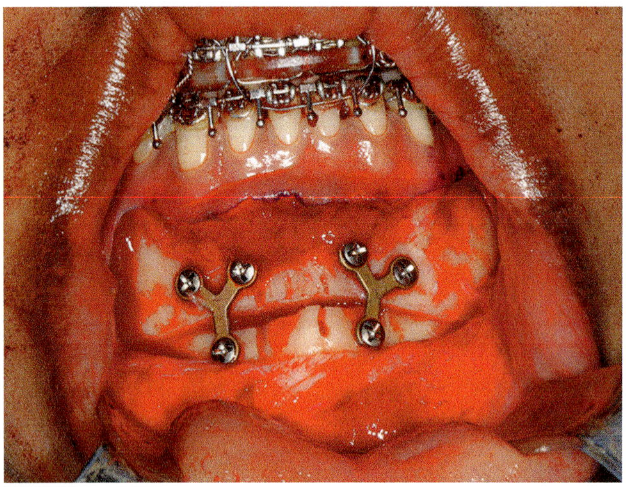

Fig. 6.56 Intraoperative view of genioplasty with two miniplate fixation (DePuy Synthes Craniomaxillofacial, Paoli, PA, USA)

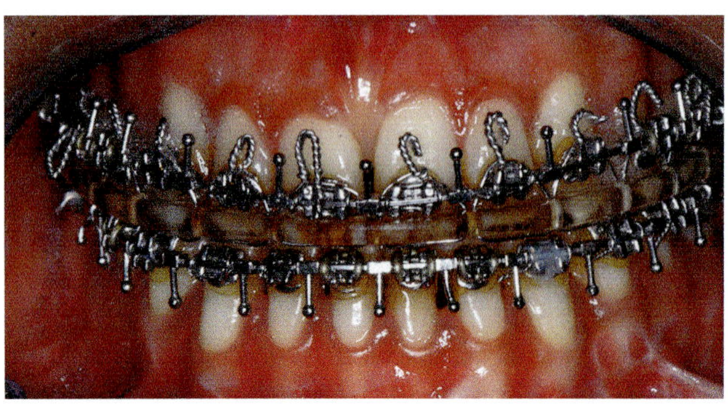

Fig. 6.57 Final occlusal splint frontal view

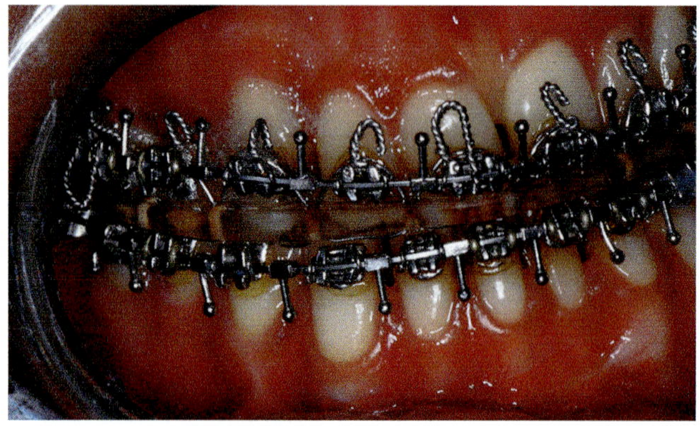

Fig. 6.58 Final occlusal splint right lateral view

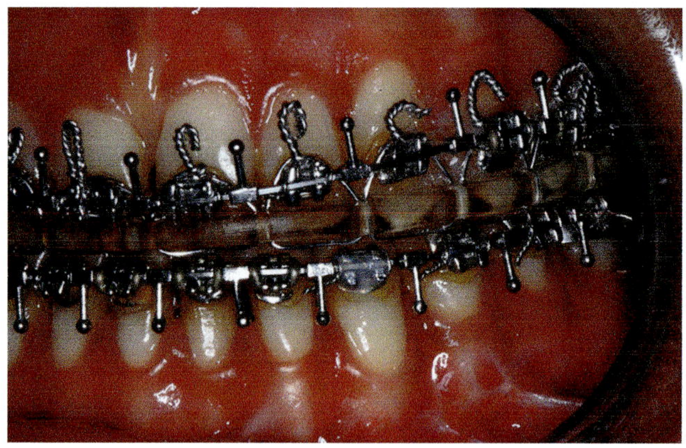

Fig. 6.59 Final occlusal splint left lateral view

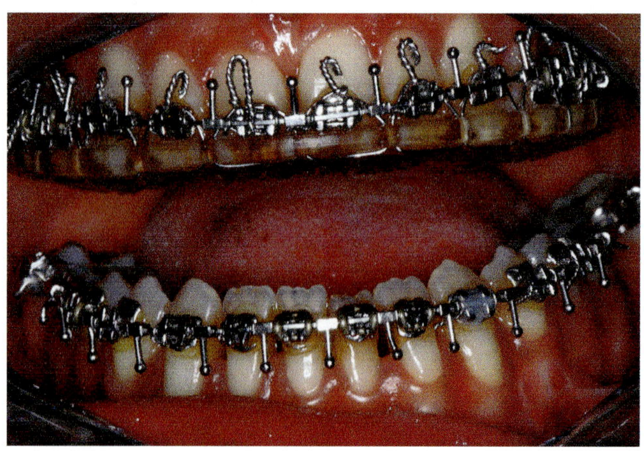

Fig. 6.60 Final occlusal splint post release of maxillomandibular fixation demonstrating satisfactory alignment on opening frontal view

Fig. 6.61 Postoperative 1 day lateral cephalometric radiograph LeFort I maxillary osteotomy, bilateral mandibular vertical ramus osteotomies, and genioplasty with final occlusal splint in maxillomandibular fixation

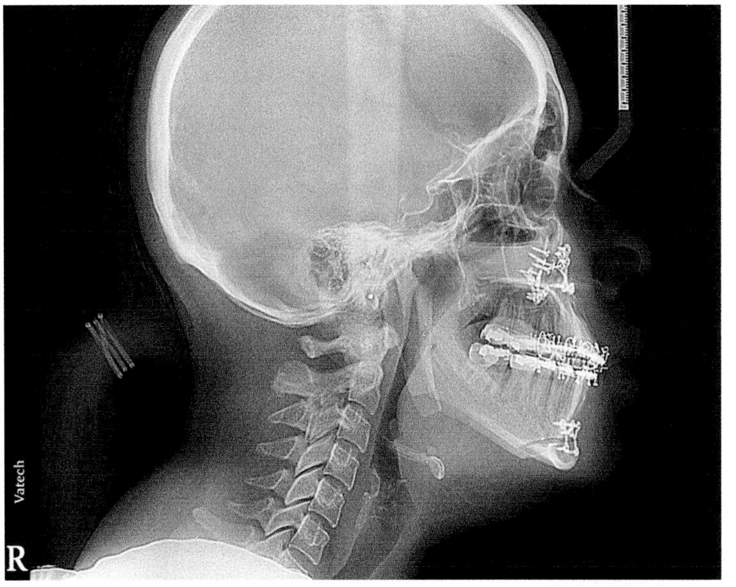

Fig. 6.62 Postoperative 1 day PA cephalometric radiograph LeFort I maxillary osteotomy, bilateral mandibular vertical ramus osteotomies, and genioplasty with final occlusal splint in maxillomandibular fixation

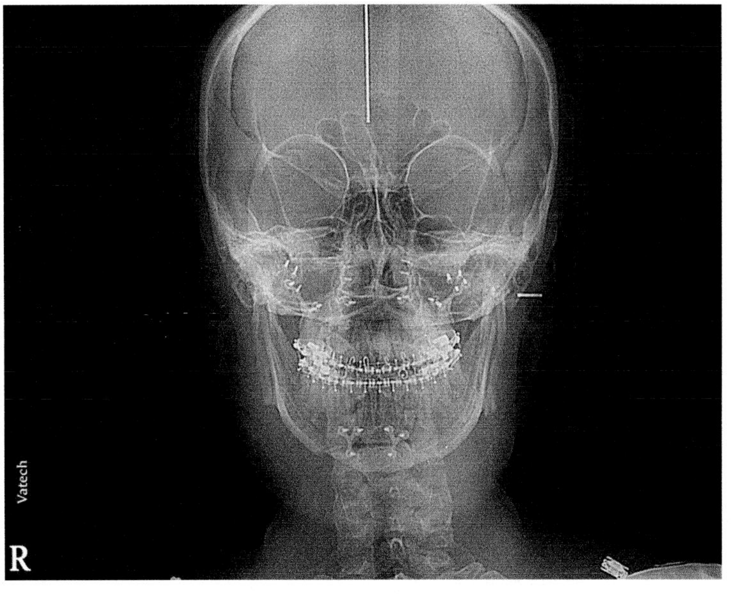

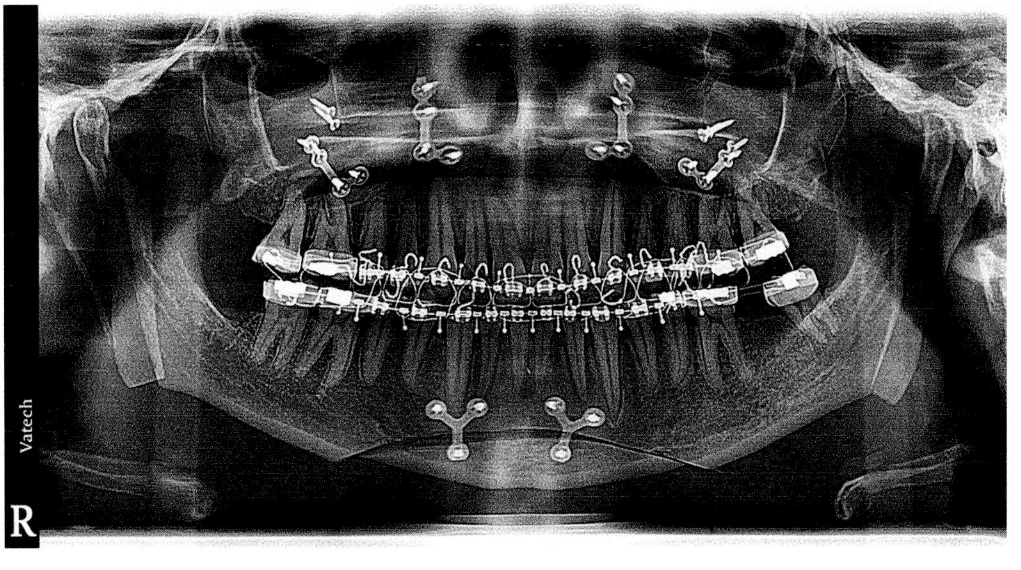

Fig. 6.63 Postoperative 1 day panoramic radiograph LeFort I maxillary osteotomy, bilateral mandibular vertical ramus osteotomies, and genioplasty with final occlusal splint in maxillomandibular fixation

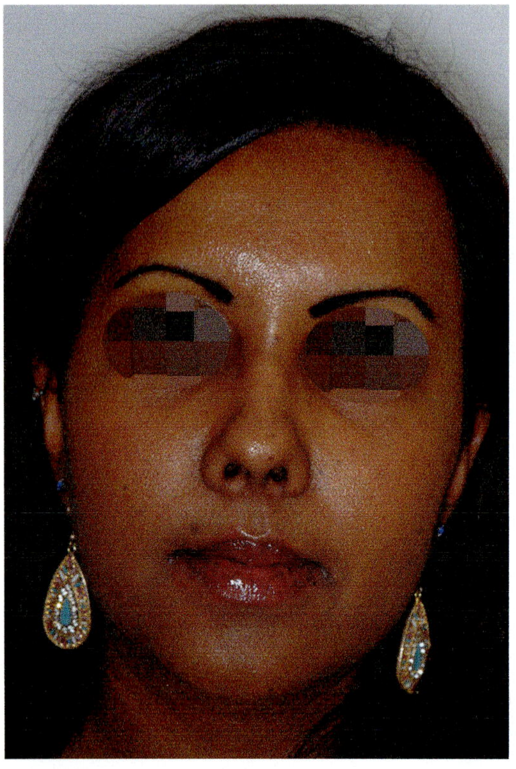

Fig. 6.64 Postoperative frontal facial view

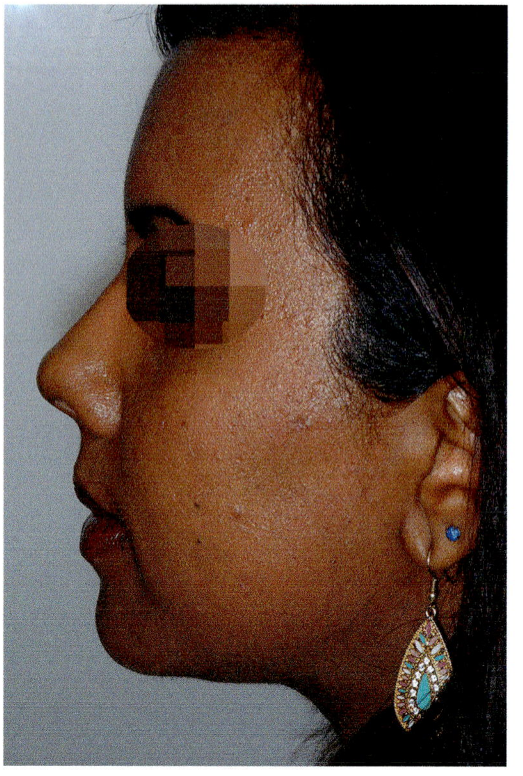

Fig. 6.66 Postoperative left lateral facial view

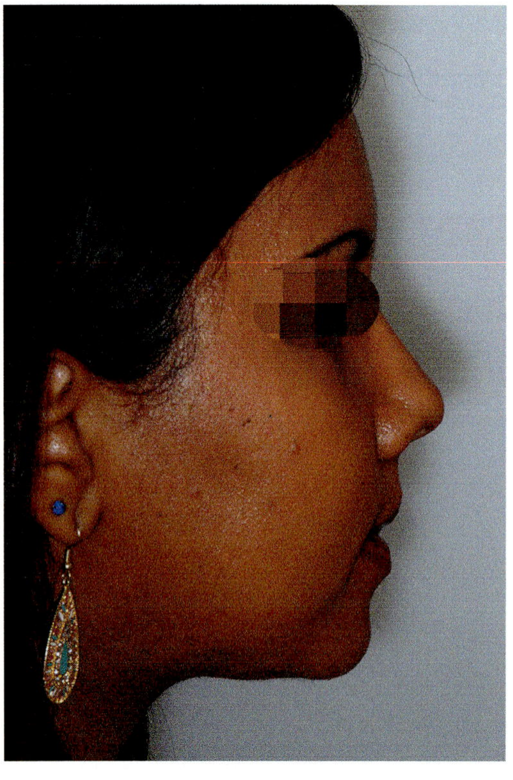

Fig. 6.65 Postoperative right lateral facial view

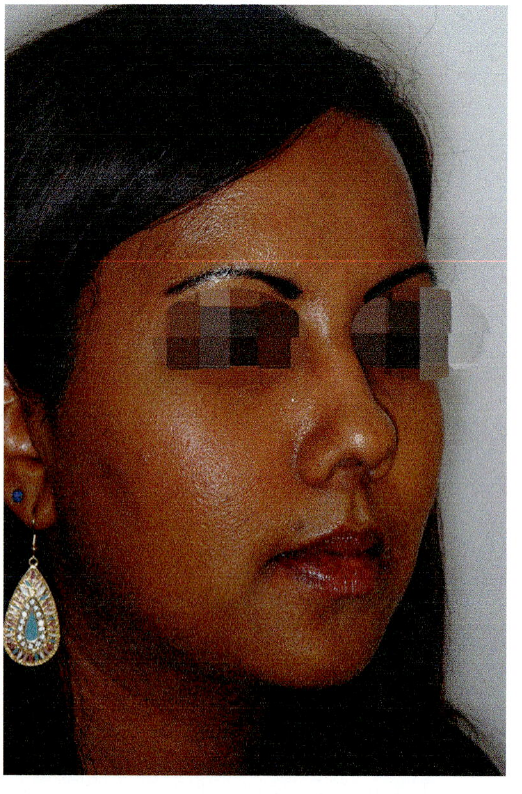

Fig. 6.67 Postoperative right 3/4 facial view

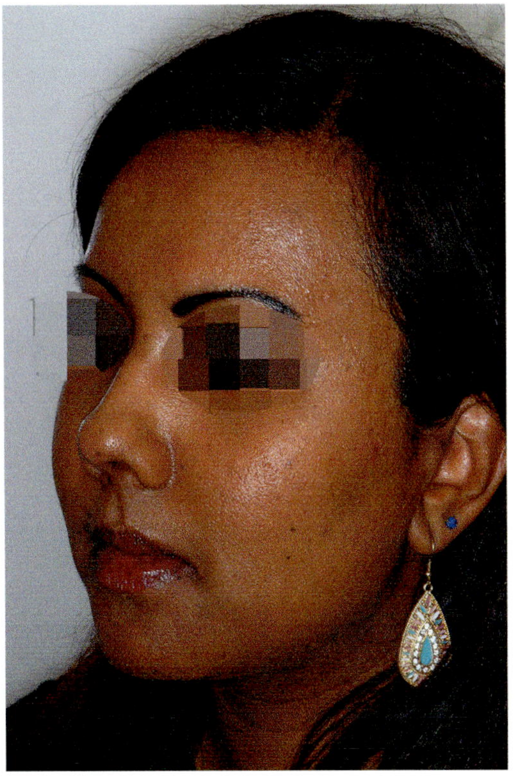

Fig. 6.68 Postoperative left 3/4 facial view

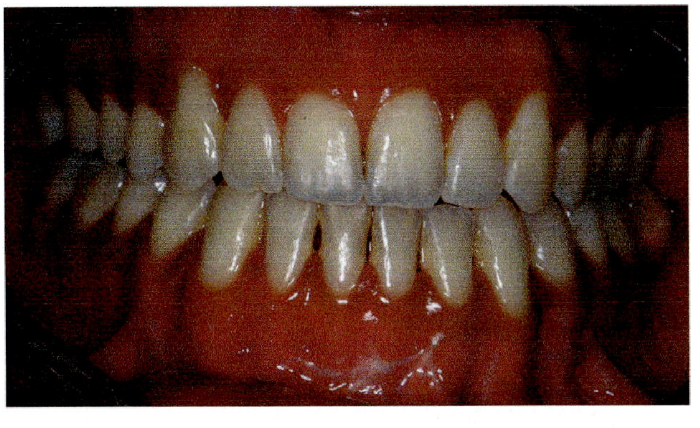

Fig. 6.69 Postoperative final occlusion frontal view

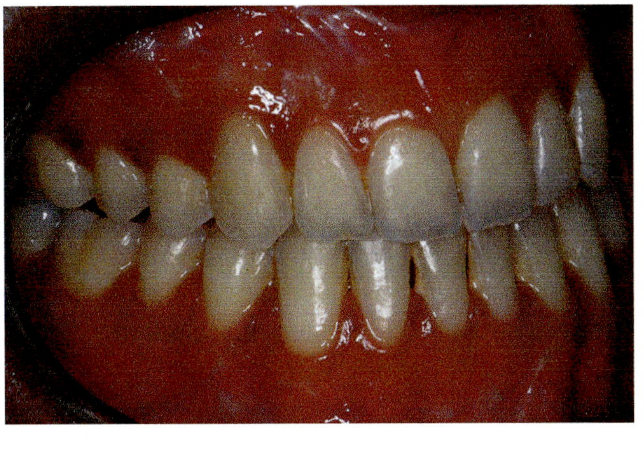

Fig. 6.70 Postoperative final occlusion right lateral view

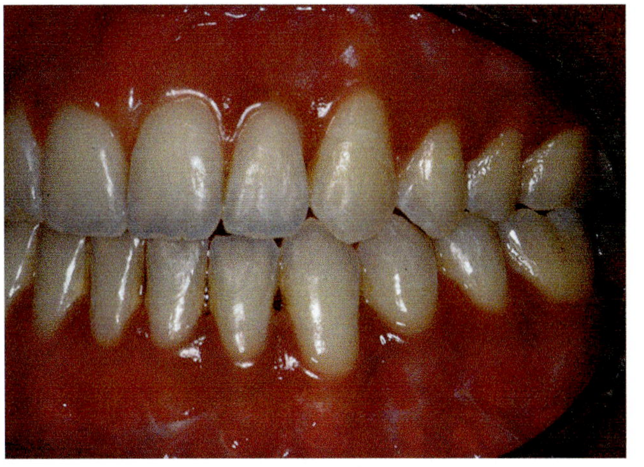

Fig. 6.71 Postoperative final occlusion left lateral view

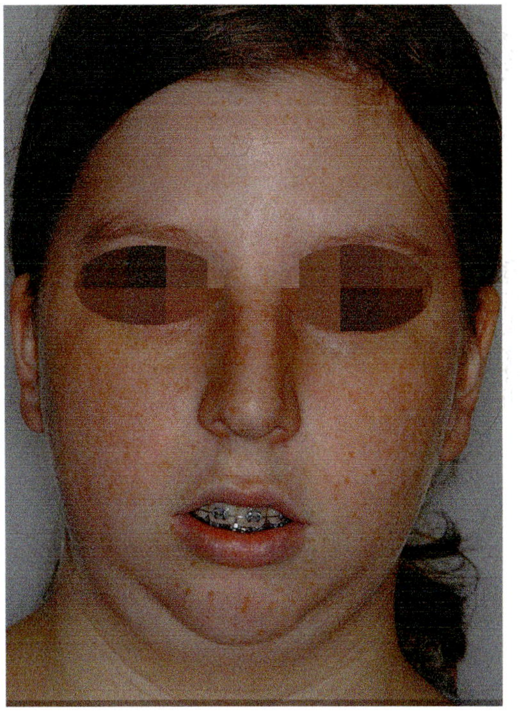

Fig. 6.72 Preoperative Class II malocclusion with mandibular hypoplasia facial view

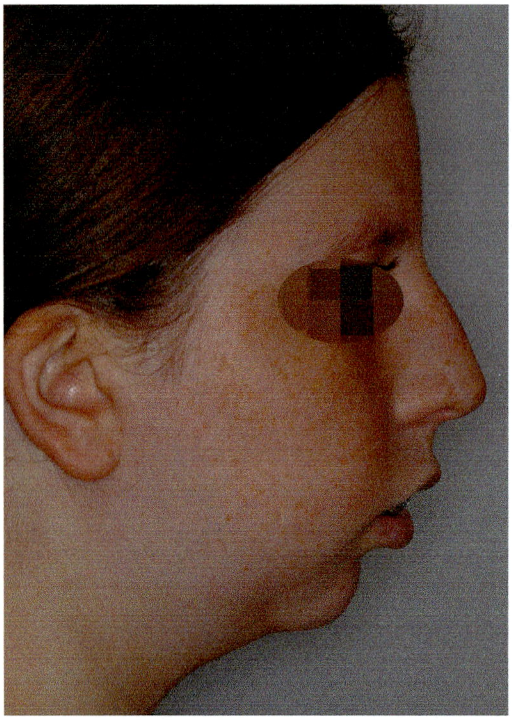

Fig. 6.73 Preoperative Class II malocclusion with mandibular hypoplasia right lateral facial view

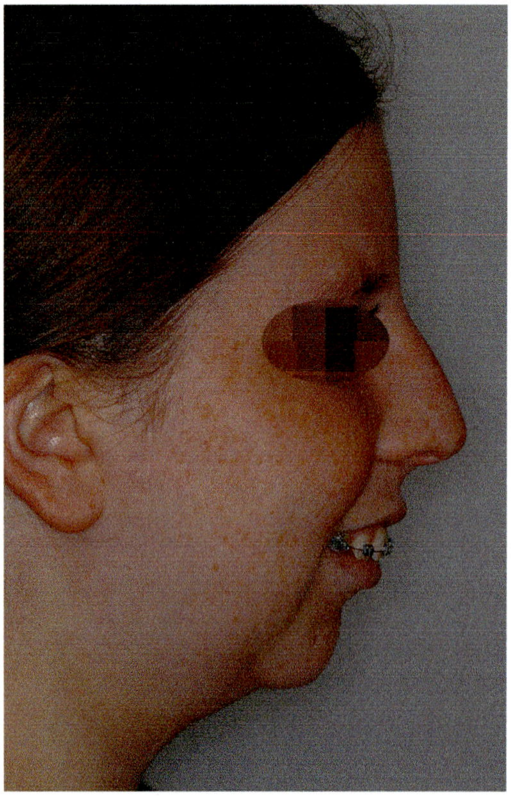

Fig. 6.74 Preoperative Class II malocclusion with mandibular hypoplasia right lateral facial view with smile

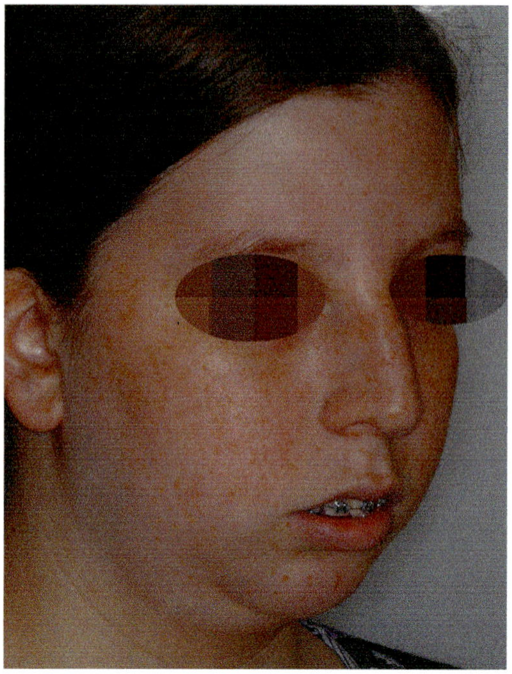

Fig. 6.75 Preoperative Class II malocclusion with mandibular hypoplasia right 3/4 facial view

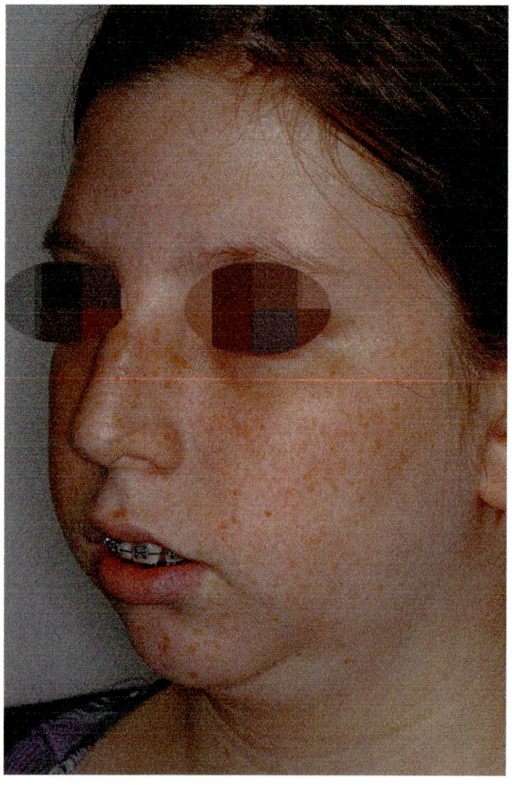

Fig. 6.76 Preoperative Class II malocclusion with mandibular hypoplasia left 3/4 facial view

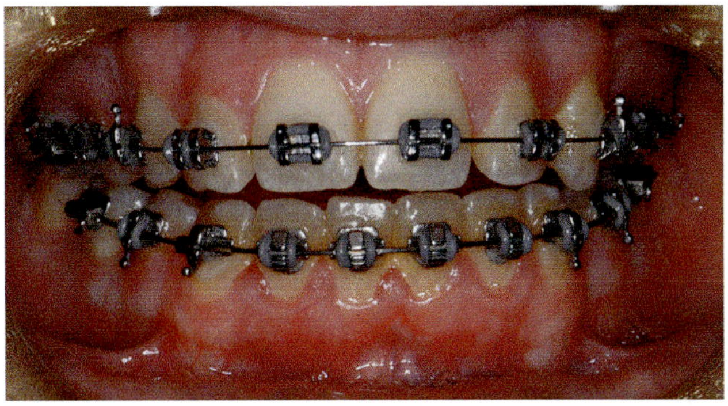

Fig. 6.77 Preoperative Class II malocclusion frontal occlusal view

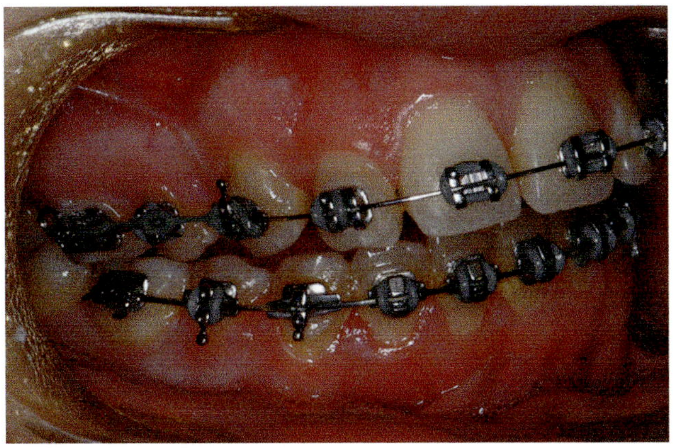

Fig. 6.78 Preoperative Class II malocclusion right lateral occlusal view

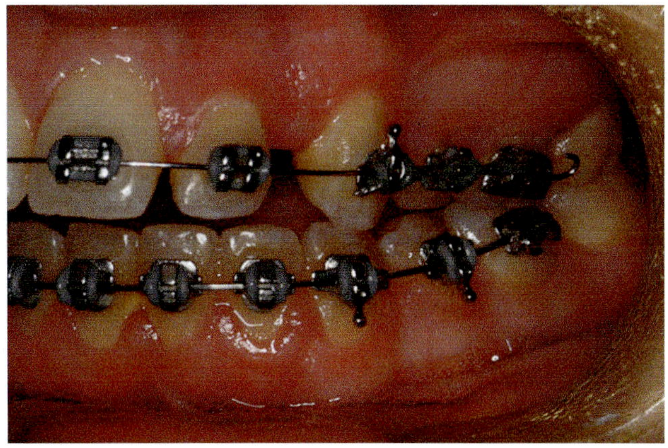

Fig. 6.79 Preoperative Class II malocclusion left lateral occlusal view

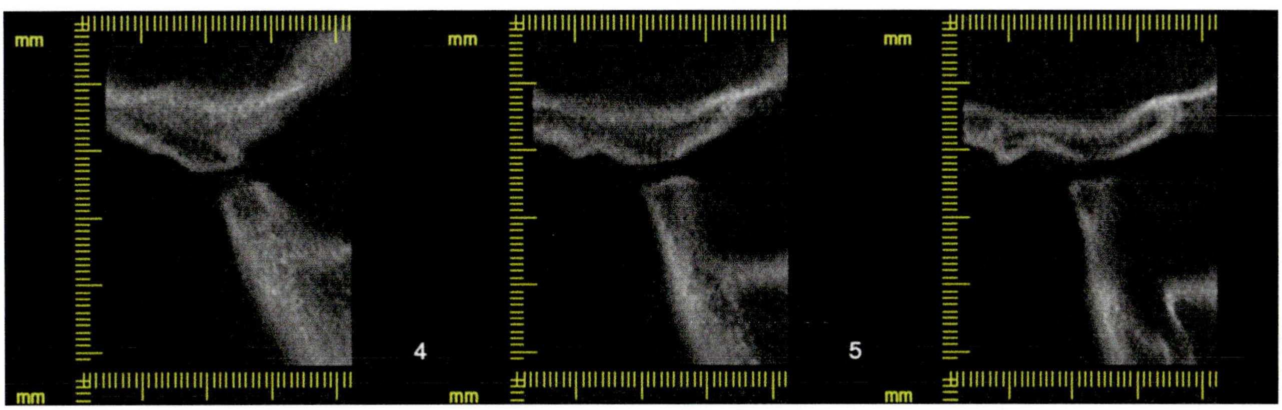

Fig. 6.80 Preoperative right CBCT TMJ views with advanced condylar resorption

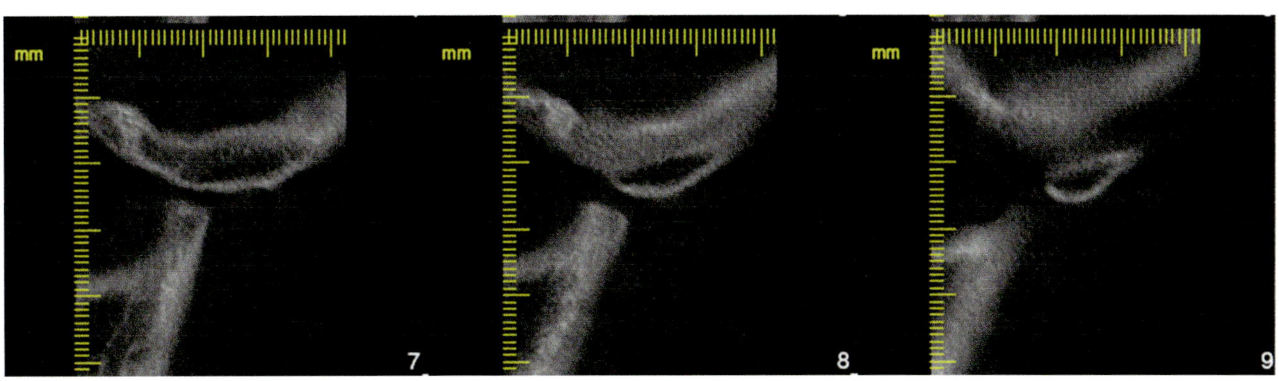

Fig. 6.81 Preoperative left CBCT TMJ views with advanced condylar resorption

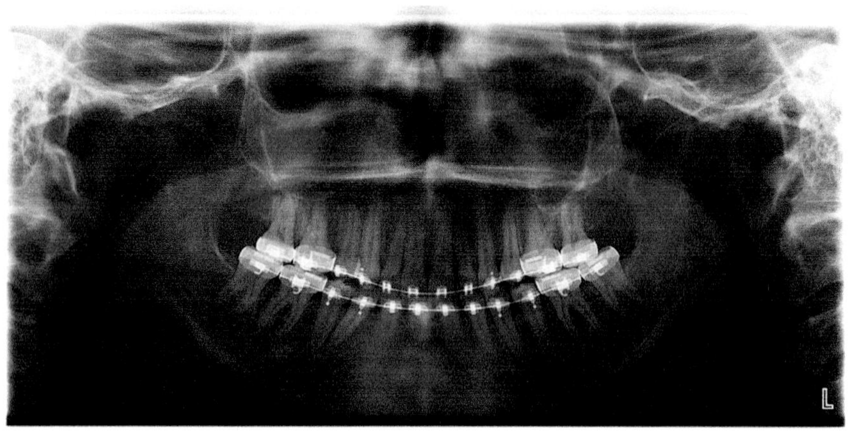

Fig. 6.82 Preoperative panoramic radiograph

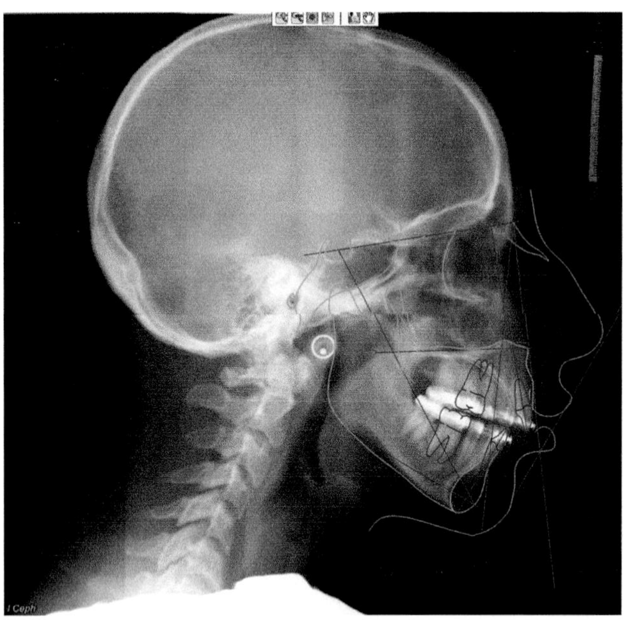

Fig. 6.83 Preoperative lateral cephalometric radiograph tracing for COGS analysis

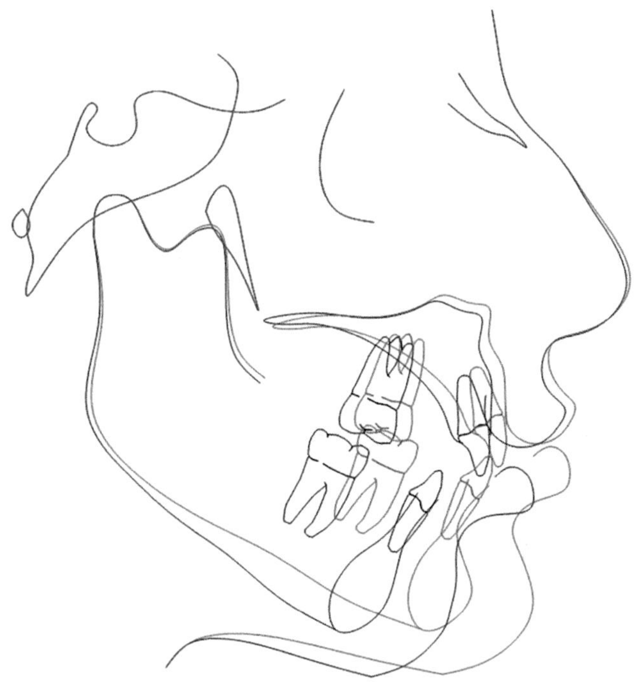

Fig. 6.84 Lateral cephalometric radiograph prediction tracing for LeFort I osteotomy, bilateral mandibular total joint replacements with advancement genioplasty

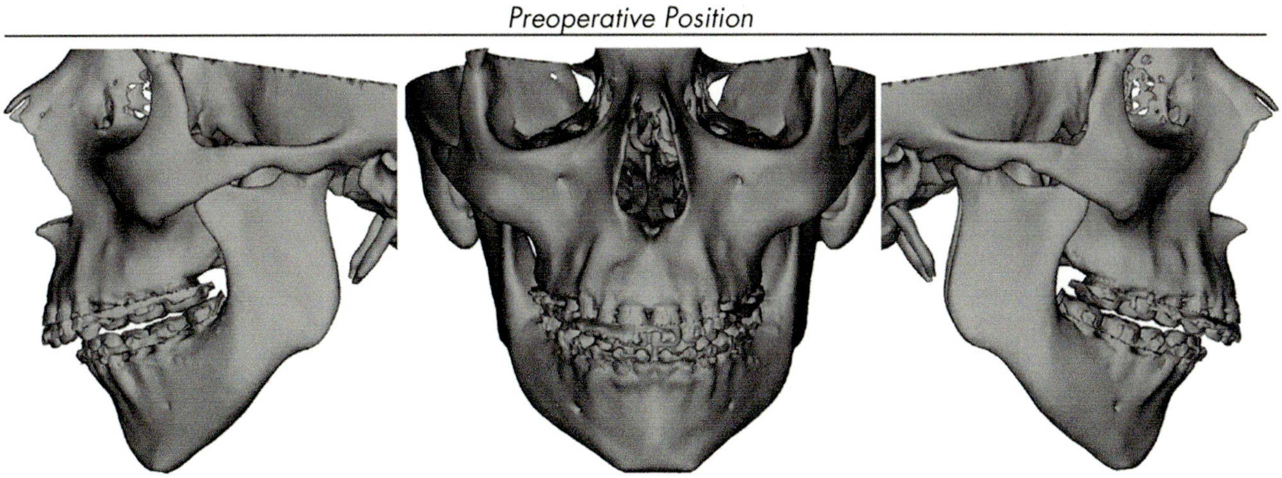

Fig. 6.85 VSP 3D preoperative right lateral, frontal, and left lateral skull views. (3D Systems Healthcare, Rock Hill, SC, USA)

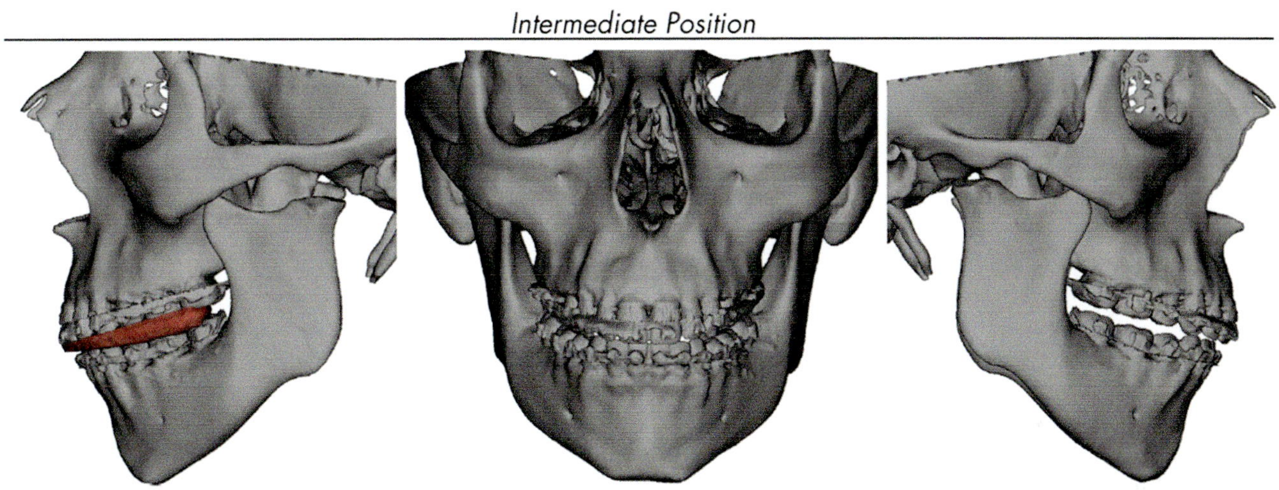

Fig. 6.86 VSP 3D operative plan with intermediate splint for setting of the mandibular total joint prosthesis right lateral, frontal, and left lateral skull views. (3D Systems Healthcare, Rock Hill, SC, USA)

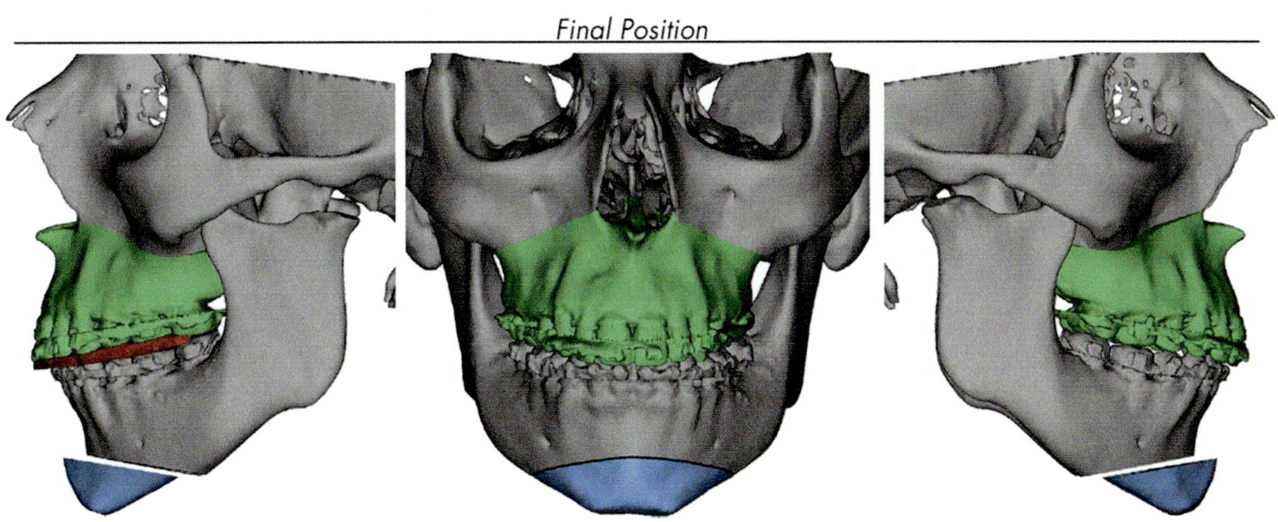

Fig. 6.87 VSP 3D operative plan with final splint and position of LeFort I osteotomy, mandible, and genioplasty with final splint for setting of the mandibular total joint prosthesis right lateral, frontal, and left lateral skull views. (3D Systems Healthcare, Rock Hill, SC, USA)

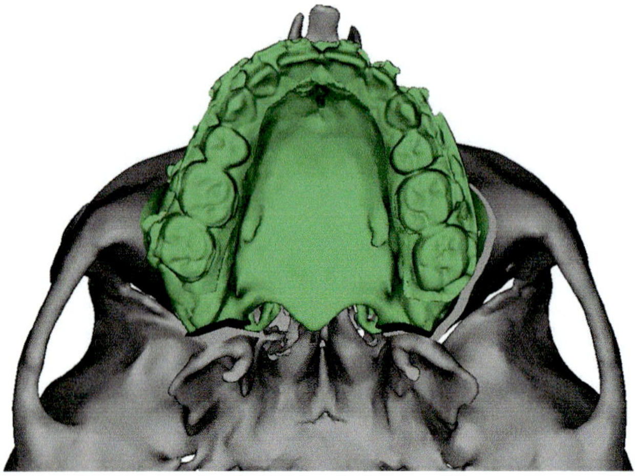

Fig. 6.88 VSP 3D LeFort I osteotomy final position inferior view. (3D Systems Healthcare, Rock Hill, SC, USA)

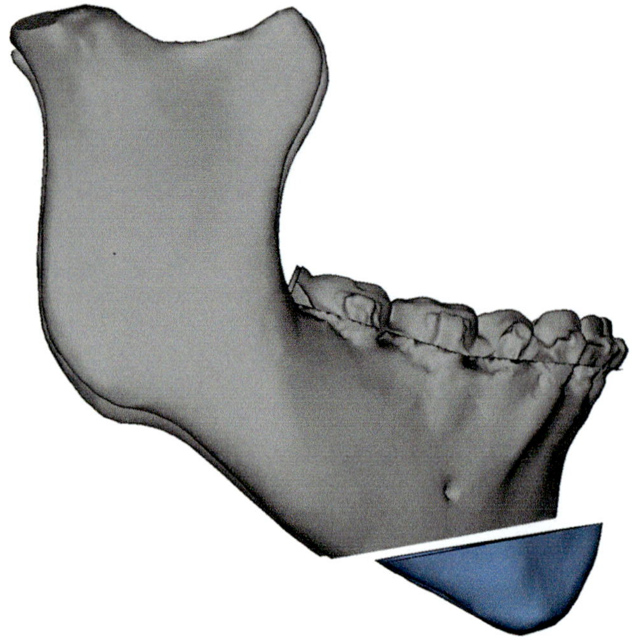

Fig. 6.90 VSP 3D genioplasty final position right lateral view. (3D Systems Healthcare, Rock Hill, SC, USA)

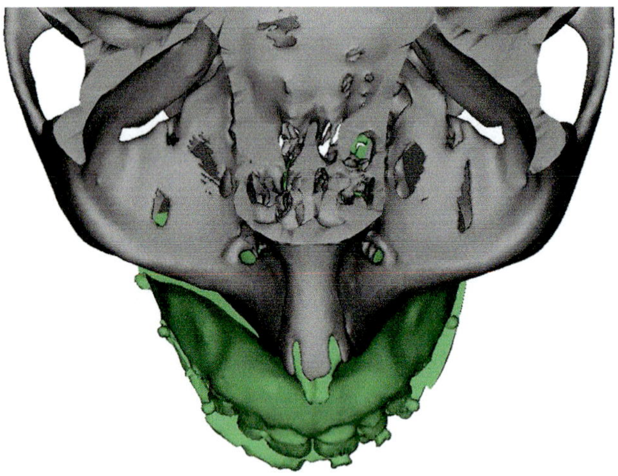

Fig. 6.89 VSP 3D LeFort I osteotomy final position superior view. (3D Systems Healthcare, Rock Hill, SC, USA)

Fig. 6.91 VSP 3D LeFort I osteotomy with bone removal measurements and 3D tooth roots frontal view. (3D Systems Healthcare, Rock Hill, SC, USA)

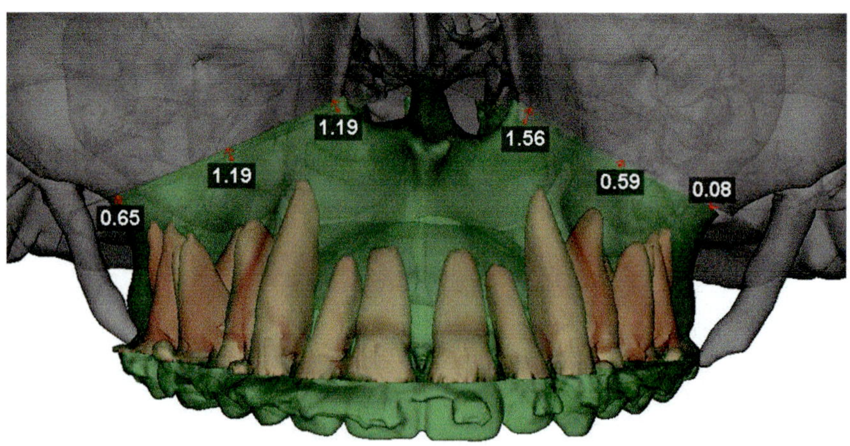

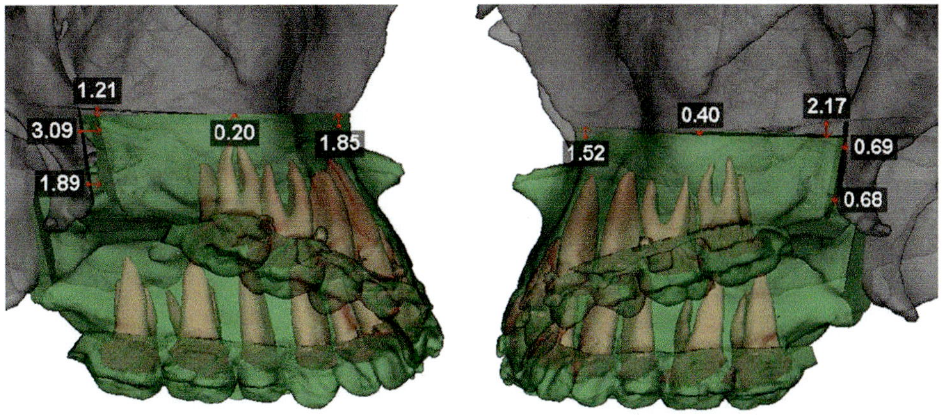

Fig. 6.92 VSP 3D LeFort I osteotomy with bone removal measurements and 3D tooth roots right and left lateral views. (3D Systems Healthcare, Rock Hill, SC, USA)

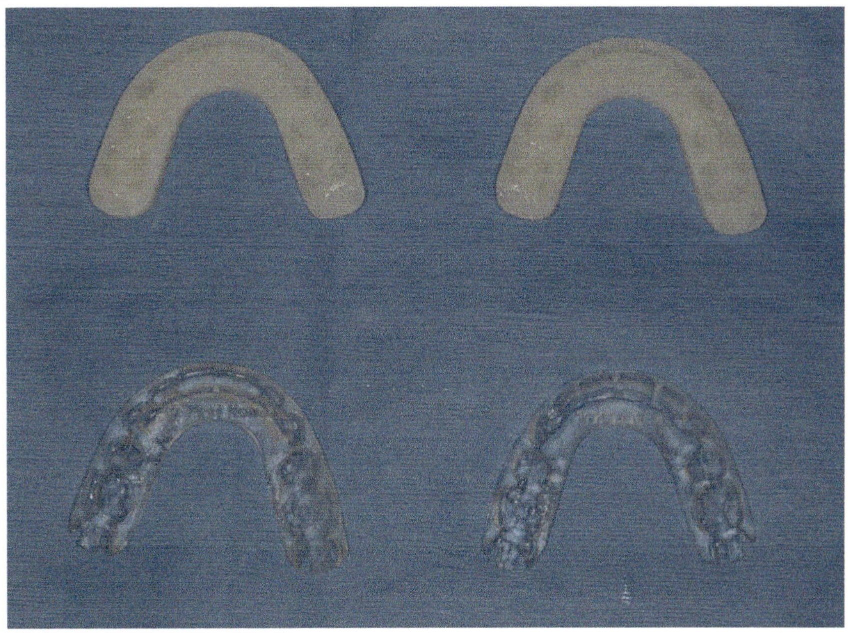

Fig. 6.93 Intermediate (opaque) and final (clear) rapid printed occlusal splints. (3D Systems Healthcare, Rock Hill, SC, USA)

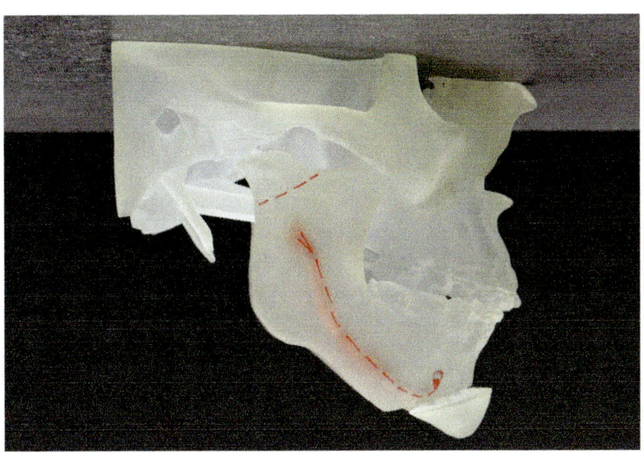

Fig. 6.94 3D stereolithographic model right lateral view with mandibular nerve and condylar resection osteotomy line, as well as the Lefort I osteotomy final position with Class I occlusion and planned genioplasty. (TMJ Concepts, Ventura, CA, USA)

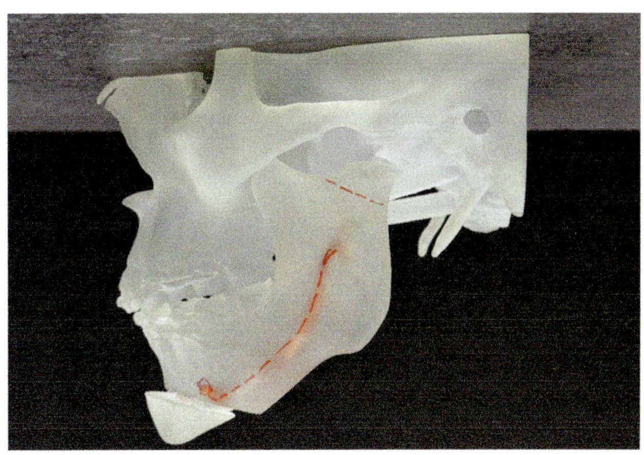

Fig. 6.95 3D stereolithographic model left lateral view with mandibular nerve and condylar resection osteotomy line, as well as the Lefort I osteotomy final position with Class I occlusion and planned genioplasty. (TMJ Concepts, Ventura, CA, USA)

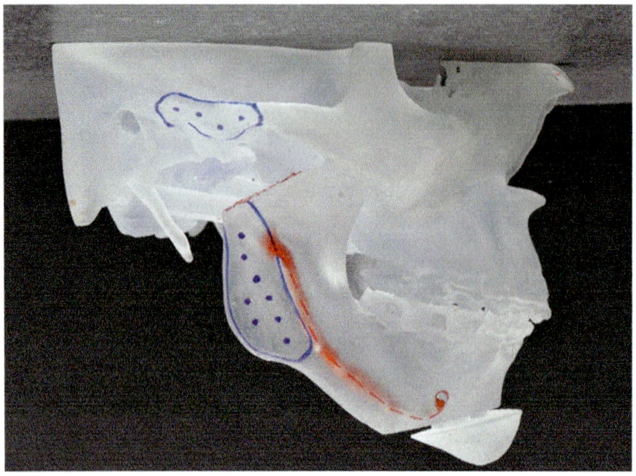

Fig. 6.96 3D stereolithographic mode right lateral view with mandibular nerve and post condylar resection and outlines for glenoid fossa and mandibular condylar prostheses, as well as the Lefort I osteotomy final position with Class I occlusion and planned genioplasty. (TMJ Concepts, Ventura, CA, USA)

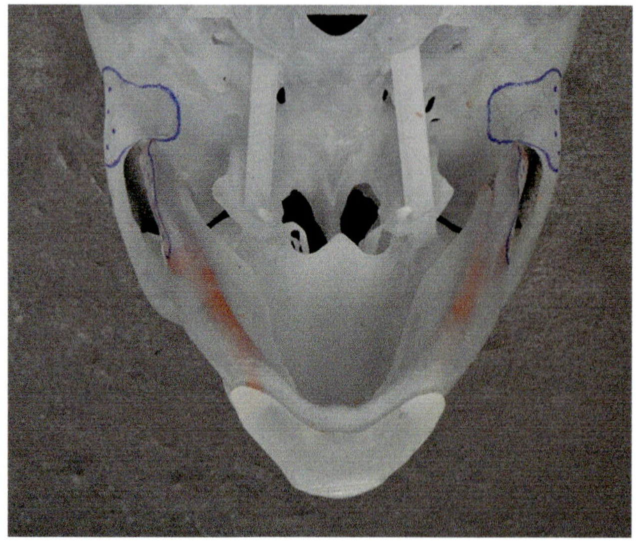

Fig. 6.98 3D stereolithographic model inferior submental view with mandibular nerve and post condylar resection and outlines for glenoid fossa prostheses and genioplasty, as well as the Lefort I osteotomy final position with Class I occlusion and planned genioplasty. (TMJ Concepts, Ventura, CA, USA)

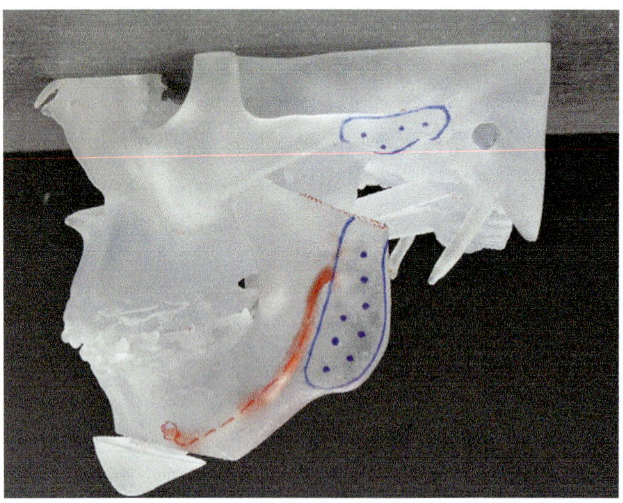

Fig. 6.97 3D stereolithographic model left lateral view with mandibular nerve and post condylar resection and outlines for glenoid fossa and mandibular condylar prostheses, as well as the Lefort I osteotomy final position with Class I occlusion and planned genioplasty. (TMJ Concepts, Ventura, CA, USA)

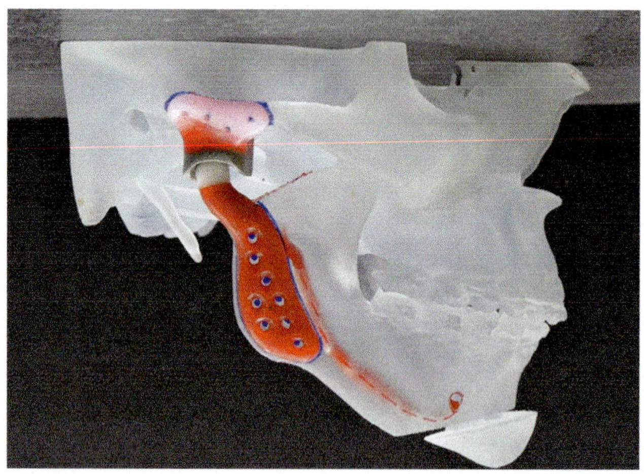

Fig. 6.99 3D stereolithographic model right lateral view with mandibular nerve and post condylar resection and wax up outlines for glenoid fossa and mandibular condylar prostheses, as well as the genioplasty. (TMJ Concepts, Ventura, CA, USA)

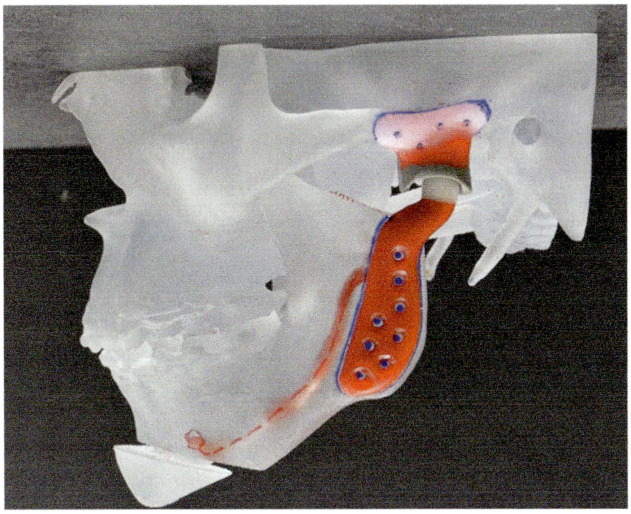

Fig. 6.100 3D stereolithographic model left lateral view with mandibular nerve and post condylar resection and wax up outlines for glenoid fossa and mandibular condylar prostheses, as well as the Lefort I osteotomy final position with Class I occlusion and planned genioplasty. (TMJ Concepts, Ventura, CA, USA)

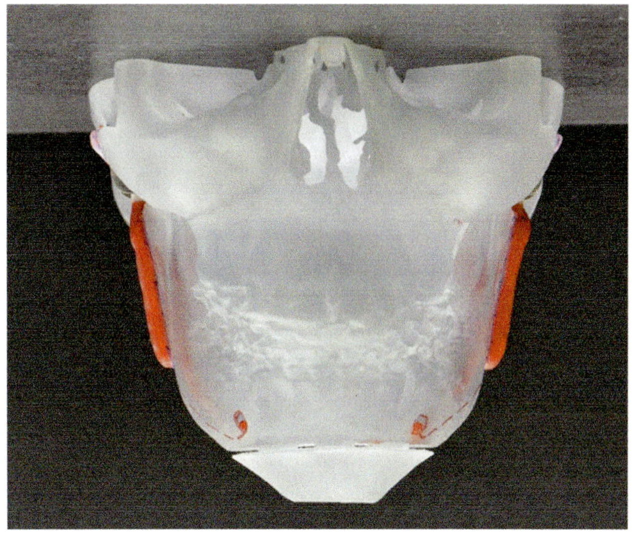

Fig. 6.102 3D stereolithographic model frontal view with mandibular nerve and post condylar resection and wax up outlines for glenoid fossa and mandibular condylar prostheses, as well as the Lefort I osteotomy final position with Class I occlusion and planned genioplasty. (TMJ Concepts, Ventura, CA, USA)

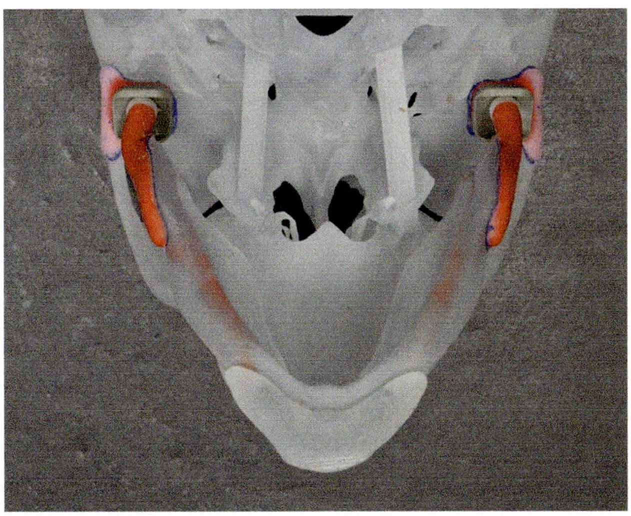

Fig. 6.101 3D stereolithographic model inferior view with mandibular nerve and post condylar resection and wax up outlines for glenoid fossa and mandibular condylar prostheses , as well as the Lefort I osteotomy final position with Class I occlusion and planned genioplasty. (TMJ Concepts, Ventura, CA, USA)

Fig. 6.103 Left and right stereolithographic condylar resection templates. (TMJ Concepts, Ventura, CA, USA)

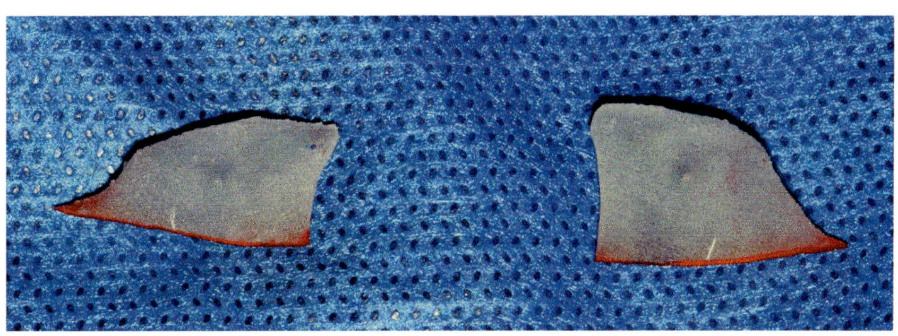

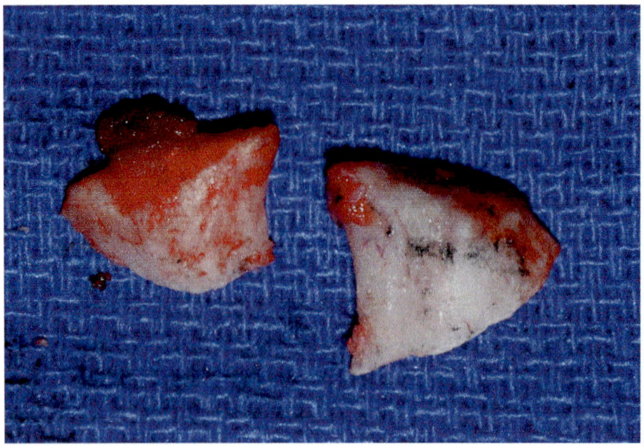

Fig. 6.104 Bilateral mandibular condylar resection specimens

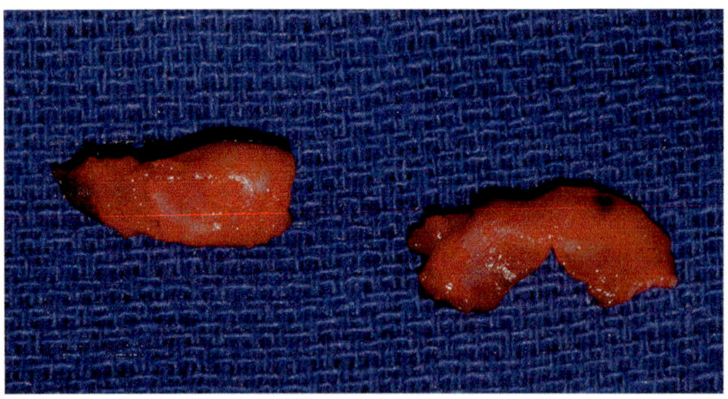

Fig. 6.105 Bilateral mandibular meniscectomy resection specimens

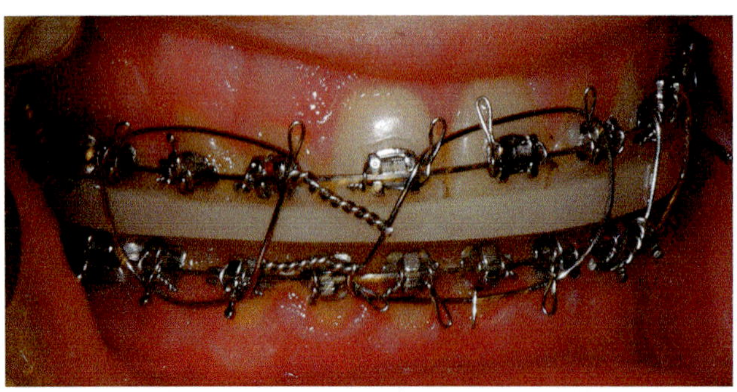

Fig. 6.106 Intraoperative view of intermediate splint with maxillomandibular fixation

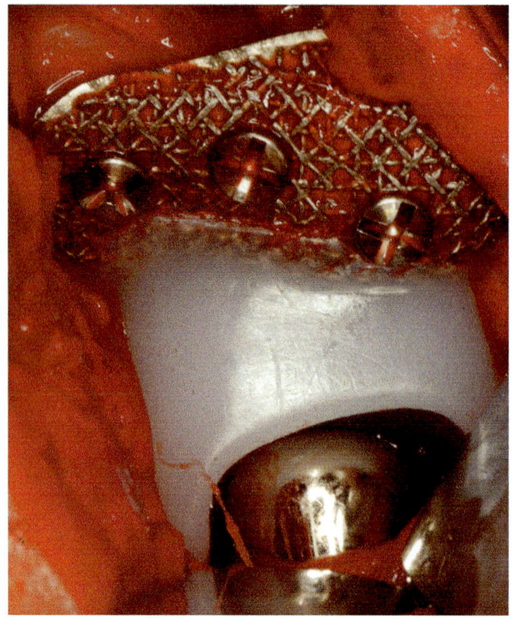

Fig. 6.107 Intraoperative view of right glenoid fossa and condylar prosthesis seating. (TMJ Concepts, Ventura, CA, USA)

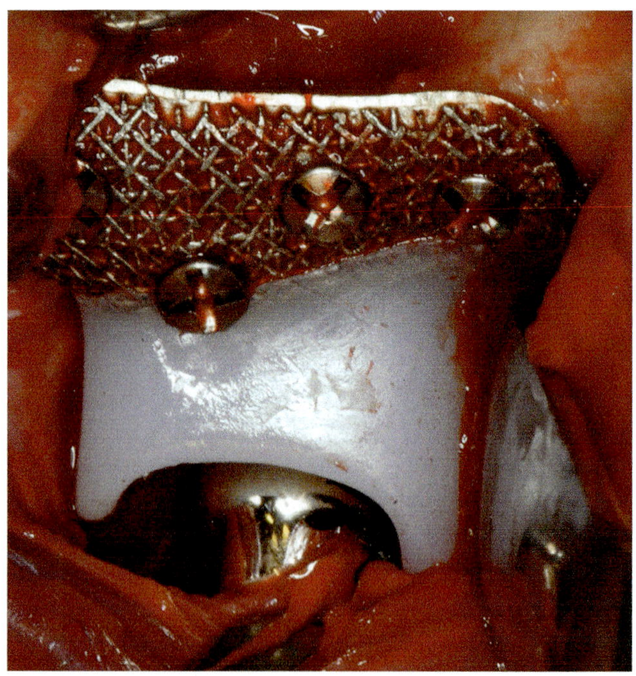

Fig. 6.108 Intraoperative view of left glenoid fossa and condylar prosthesis seating. (TMJ Concepts, Ventura, CA, USA)

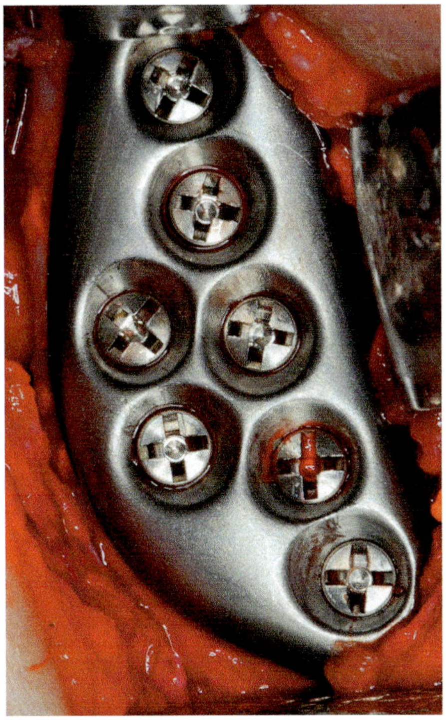

Fig. 6.109 Intraoperative view of right condylar prosthesis inferior aspect fixation. (TMJ Concepts, Ventura, CA, USA)

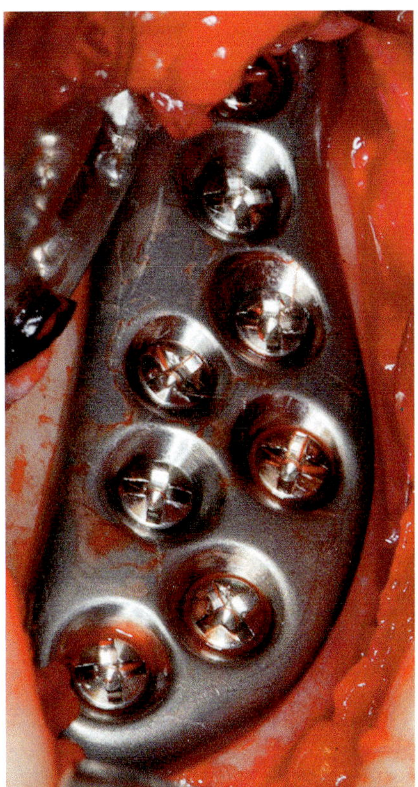

Fig. 6.110 Intraoperative view of left condylar prosthesis inferior aspect fixation. (TMJ Concepts, Ventura, CA, USA)

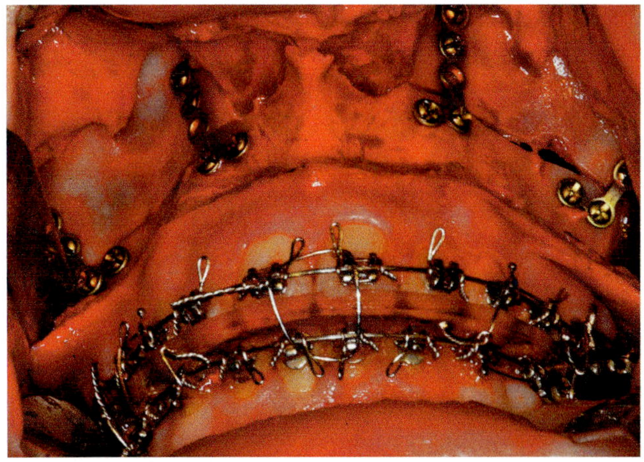

Fig. 6.111 Intraoperative view of LeFort I osteotomy with miniplate fixation and final splint following bilateral mandibular total condylar prostheses placement. (DuPuy Synthes Craniomaxillofacial, Paoli, PA)

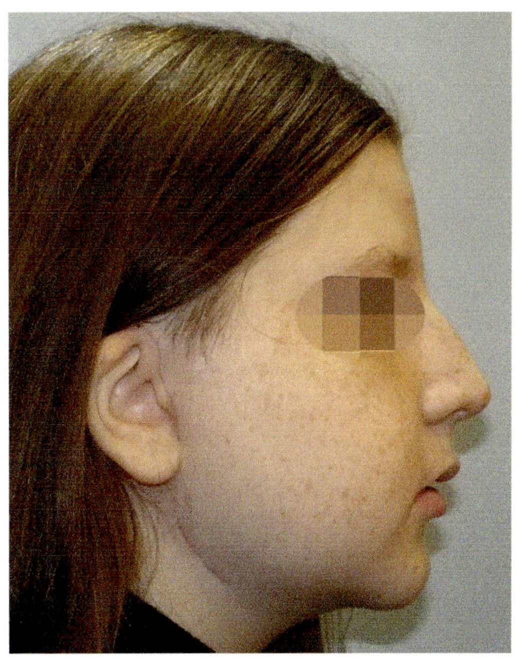

Fig. 6.112 Postoperative right lateral facial view (4 weeks)

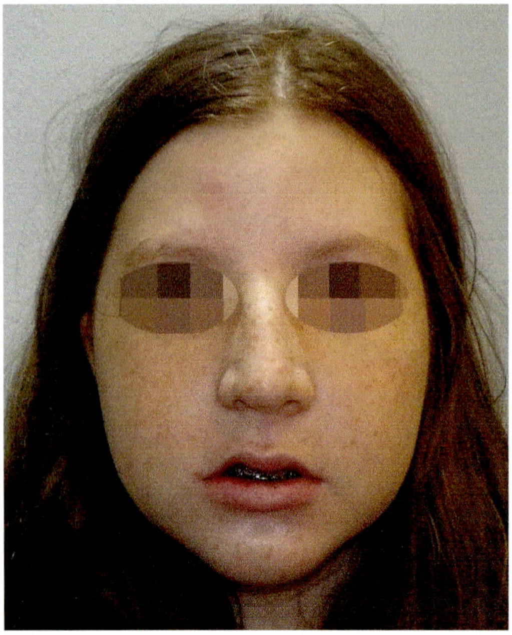

Fig. 6.113 Postoperative frontal facial view (4 weeks)

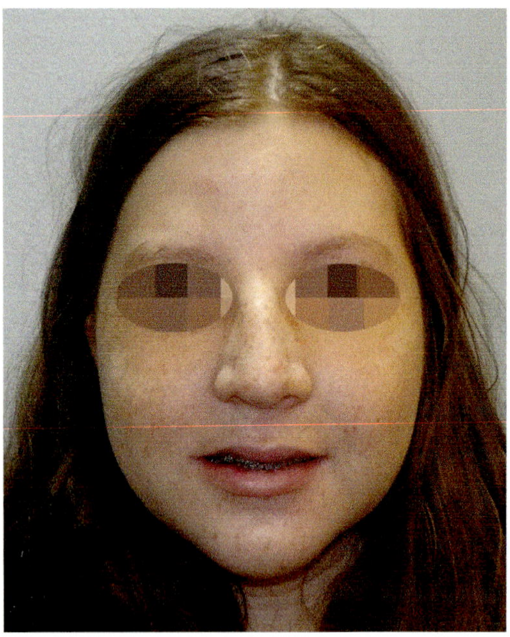

Fig. 6.114 Postoperative frontal facial view with smile (4 weeks)

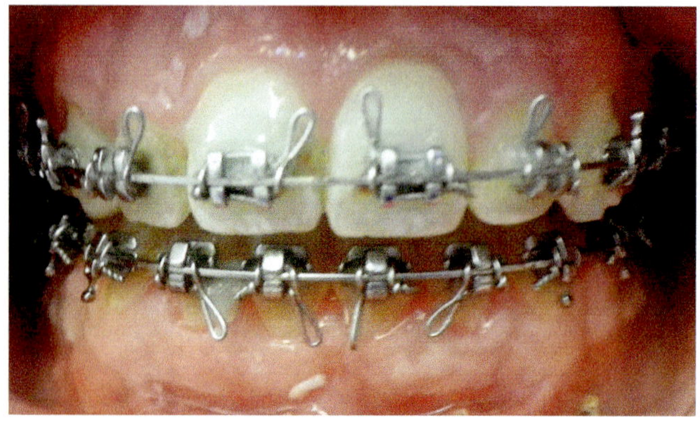

Fig. 6.115 Postoperative final occlusion frontal view (4 weeks)

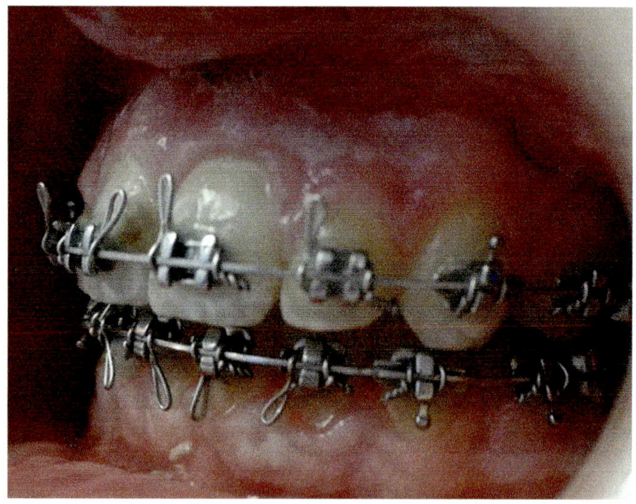

Fig. 6.116 Postoperative final occlusion left lateral view (4 weeks)

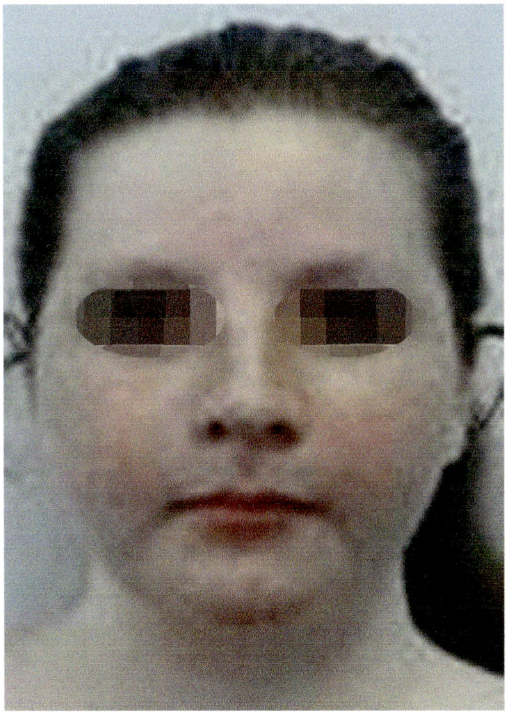

Fig. 6.117 Postoperative frontal facial view (1 year)

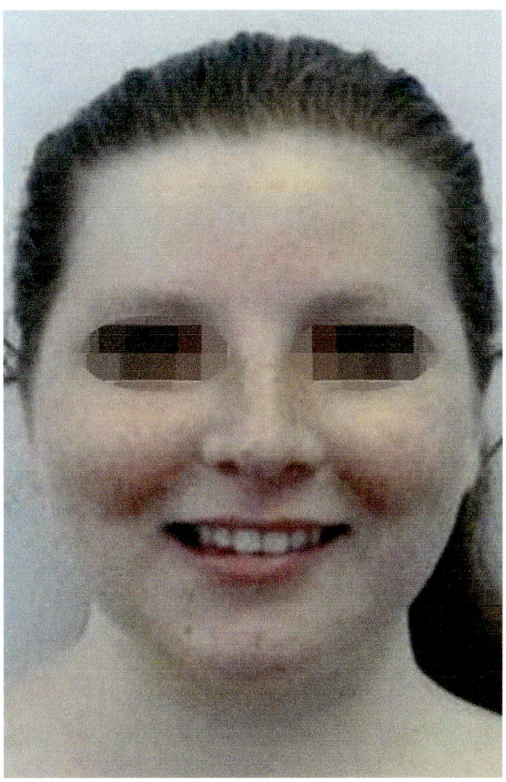

Fig. 6.118 Postoperative frontal facial view with smile (1 year)

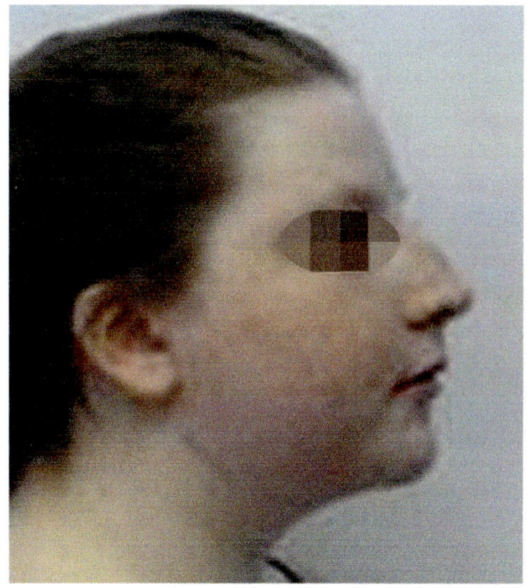

Fig. 6.119 Postoperative right lateral facial view (1 year)

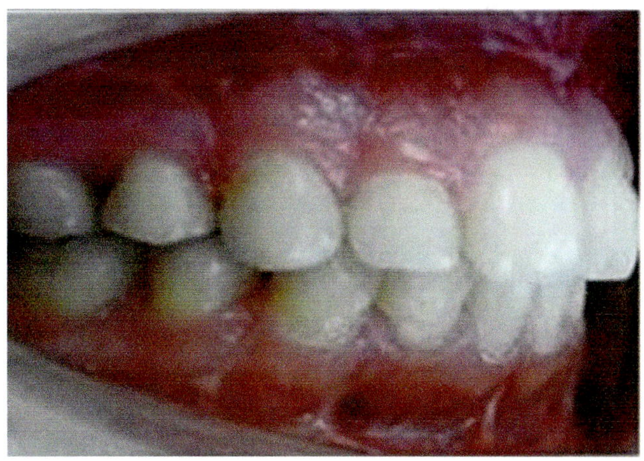

Fig. 6.120 Occlusal right lateral view (1 year)

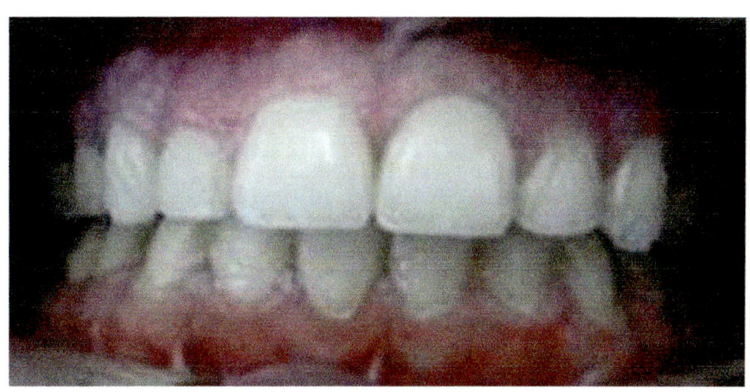

Fig. 6.121 Occlusal frontal view (1 year)

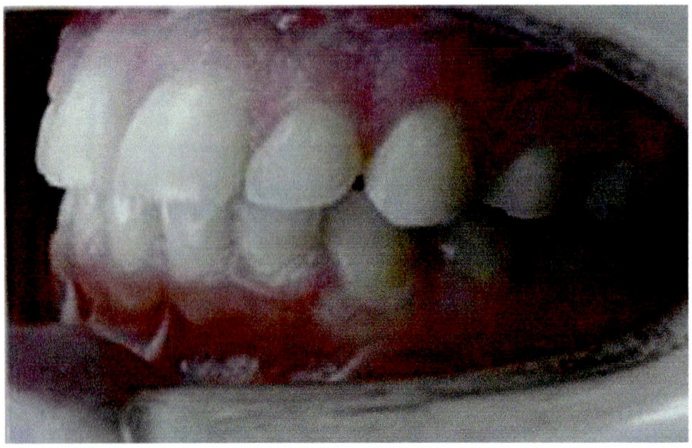

Fig. 6.122 Occlusal left lateral view (1 year)

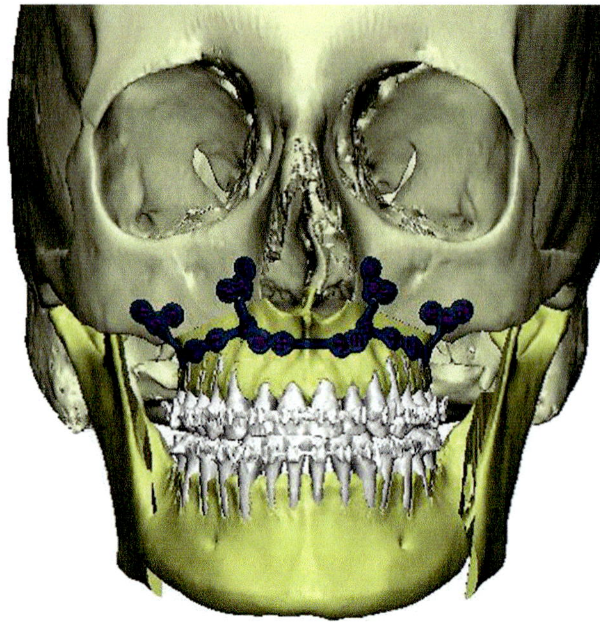

Fig. 6.124 Virtual orthognathic bimaxillary surgical planning of patient-specific custom bone plate for LeFort I osteotomy (Proplan and Trumatch, DePuy Synthes Craniomaxillofacial, Paoli, PA, USA). (Case courtesy of Prof. Dr. Dr. Alexander Schramm and PD Dr. Dr. Frank Wilde, Oral and Plastic Maxillofacial Surgery, University Hospital Ulm and Military Hospital Ulm, Ulm, Germany)

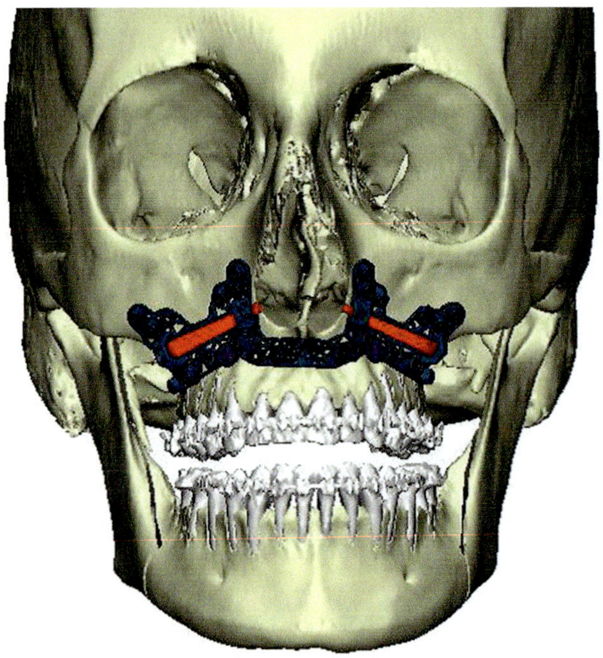

Fig. 6.123 Virtual orthognathic bimaxillary surgical planning of patient-specific custom surgical guide for LeFort I osteotomy and pre-drilling holes for custom bone plate (Proplan and Trumatch, DePuy Synthes Craniomaxillofacial, Paoli, PA, USA). (Case courtesy of Prof. Dr. Dr. Alexander Schramm and PD Dr. Dr. Frank Wilde, Oral and Plastic Maxillofacial Surgery, University Hospital Ulm and Military Hospital Ulm, Ulm, Germany)

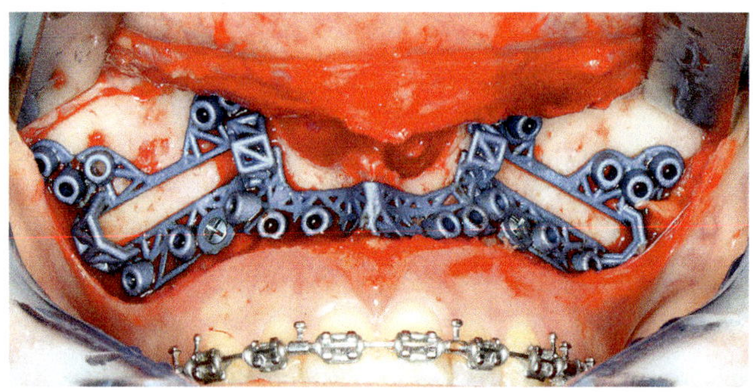

Fig. 6.125 Intraoperative view of patient-specific custom surgical guide fabricated from 3D printed Titanium Grade 2 using laser melting process for LeFort I osteotomy and predrilling holes for custom prebent bone plate (Proplan and Trumatch, DePuy Synthes Craniomaxillofacial, Paoli, PA, USA). (Case courtesy of Prof. Dr. Dr. Alexander Schramm and PD Dr. Dr. Frank Wilde, Oral and Plastic Maxillofacial Surgery, University Hospital Ulm and Military Hospital Ulm, Ulm, Germany)

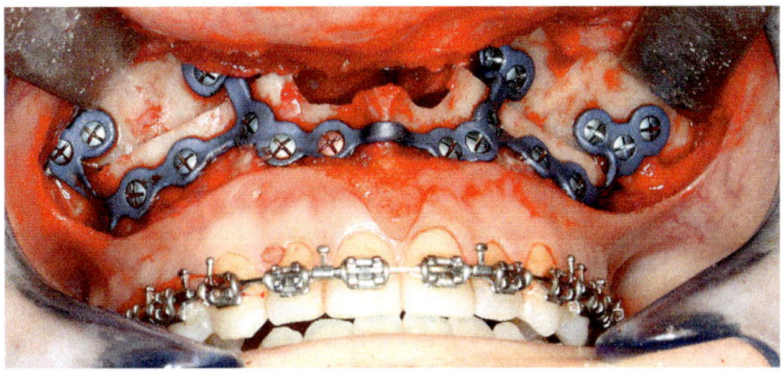

Fig. 6.126 Intraoperative view of patient-specific custom surgical guide for osteotomies and predrilling holes for custom bone plate from 3D printed Titanium Grade 2 using laser melting process (Proplan and Trumatch, DePuy Synthes Craniomaxillofacial, Paoli, PA, USA). (Case courtesy of Prof. Dr. Dr. Alexander Schramm and PD Dr. Dr. Frank Wilde, Oral and Plastic Maxillofacial Surgery, University Hospital Ulm and Military Hospital Ulm, Ulm, Germany)

Conclusion

As a result of advances in digital technologies such as VSP and rapid printing, orthognathic surgery has gone through an important evolution. Advances in surgical techniques, equipment, diagnostic tools, and planning software have changed how the surgery is currently being performed.

VSP is another adjunct to improve our surgical outcomes, save time and costs, and ultimately improve patient care. It has given us an accurate way to measure bone movements, supply rapid printed occlusal splints/surgical guides, and a 3D view of surgery that we have learned to trust. New 3D printed Titanium Grade 2 surgical guides for precision osteotomies and patient-specific bone plates are important developments.

As with all scientific advancements surgeons must always use good judgment and knowledge when incorporating new technologies into our treatment of patients.

References

1. Greenberg AM, Prein J, editors. Craniomaxillofacial Reconstructive and Corrective Bone Surgery: Principles of Internal Fixation Using the AO/ASIF Technique. New York: Springer Verlag; 2002. p. 581–622
2. Ellis E III, Tharanon W, Gambrell K. Accuracy of face-bow transfer effect on surgical prediction and postsurgical result. J Oral Maxillofac Surg. 1998;50:562.
3. Gribel B, Gribel M, Frazao D, McNamara J Jr, Manzi F. Accuracy and reliability of craniometric measurements on lateral cephalometry and 3D measurements on CBCT scans. Angle Orthod. 2011;81:26–35.
4. Bell R. Computer planning and intraoperative navigation in orthognathic surgery. J Oral Maxillofac Surg. 2011;69:592–605.
5. Barbenel J, Paul P, Khambay B, Walker F, Moos K, Ayoub A. Errors in orthognathic surgery planning: the effect of inaccurate study model orientation. Int J Oral Maxillofac Surg. 2010;39:1103–8.
6. Schramm A, Gellrich NC, Schmelzeisen R. Navigational surgery of the facial skeleton. Berlin: Springer; 2007.
7. Vannier M, Marsh J, Warren J. Three dimensional CT reconstruction images for craniofacial surgical planning and evaluation. Radiology. 1984;150:179.
8. Altobelli D, Kikinis R, Mulliken F, et al. Computer-assisted three-dimensional planning in craniofacial surgery. Plast Reconstr Surg. 1993;92:576.
9. Hohlweg-Majert B, Schon R, Schmelzeisen R, et al. Navigational maxillofacial surgery using virtual models. World J Surg. 2005;29:1530.
10. Luebbers H, Messmer P, Obwegeser J, et al. Comparison of different registration methods for surgical navigation in craniomaxillofacial surgery. J Craniomaxillofac Surg. 2008;36:109.

Computer Planning for Craniofacial Surgery

7

Oleh M. Antonyshyn, Glenn Edwards, and James G. Mainprize

Craniofacial Surgical Modeling

Virtual planning for surgery begins with high-quality, high-resolution 3D medical images. For bony structures, CT images are most commonly used [1], although MR may be beneficial for characterizing the soft tissue morphology near the affected sites. For planning, three-dimensional ultrasound is rarely used, but it has been demonstrated for surgical models of the nose and palate [2].

From the volumetric medical image data (i.e., 3D gridded array of volumetric elements or "voxels"), surfaces representing the bone structure are extracted by a variety of techniques. For CT, this is generally accomplished by finding the enclosing surface of voxels that exceed a threshold Hounsfield unit value corresponding to the bone. For high-quality surface extraction, there is a certain amount of user intervention to "paint" or delineate important structures that are less well defined or to remove structures that interfere with the model (e.g., surgical hardware).

Soft Tissue Deformation Models

Soft tissue changes following surgery are predicted. Computer simulations of soft tissue changes can be very powerful planning tools for the surgeon. The simulations generally rely on correspondence of the soft tissue contours that are dependent on the underlying bony surface.

O.M. Antonyshyn (✉)
Division of Plastic Surgery, Sunnybrook Health Sciences Centre, University of Toronto, Toronto, ON, Canada
e-mail: oantonyshyn@rogers.com

G. Edwards
Calavera Surgical Design, Toronto, ON, Canada

J.G. Mainprize
Department of Physical Sciences, Sunnybrook Research Institute, Toronto, ON, Canada

All soft tissue simulations divide the tissue compartment into many (~100–10,000) small components. In a "mass-spring model" (MSM), the tissue is represented as a set of points or nodes connected by springs. The MSM can be perturbed by applying forces such as that caused by displacement of the bone surface (such as following a genioplasty or a maxillary distraction). Numerical solution of the displacement of the MSM is performed by solving the network of differential equations for each node. MSM is computationally efficient, although not as accurate as other techniques. Because of its low computational overhead, MSM approaches can be incorporated into real-time simulation tools such as that used in 3dMD's (Atlanta, USA) soft tissue package in their "3dMDvultus" software package (http://www.3dmd.com/3dmd-software/ accessed 2014/03/15).

Alternatively, many simulation systems use finite element (FE) modeling that subdivides the soft tissue into many small, connected compartments which can be assigned mechanical properties of the tissue in that compartment [3]. These discretized compartments by virtue of being small have only a small number of degrees of freedom of motion compared to the numerous degrees of freedom the whole human head would have. Very simple equations of stress and strain on each of the finite elements can be calculated with very simple boundary conditions that ensure continuity can be solved numerically.

Surgical results following craniofacial reconstructive procedures are ultimately judged on the basis of the restoration of aesthetic form or proportion in facial surface morphology. Conceptually, it is therefore most appropriate to model the soft tissue surface of the face and then derive the skeletal modifications required to achieve that result. This is the guiding principle of all surgical simulation software for facial cosmetic procedures. Sculpt (Vectra 3D) is a very effective application which allows the surgeon to capture a 3D surface image of a patient, and then interactively simulate a wide variety of surgical options by manipulating the surface features. This has proven to be an extremely effective tool in communicating realistic options and expectations

A.M. Greenberg (ed.), *Digital Technologies in Craniomaxillofacial Surgery*, https://doi.org/10.1007/978-1-4939-1532-3_7

to patients, particularly for certain procedures such as rhinoplasties. Although it does not provide quantitative data to guide the manipulation of the osseocartilaginous framework of the nose, an experienced surgeon uses the surface simulation to estimate the degree of nasal augmentation or reduction, as well as to guide specific surgical steps (Fig. 7.1).

When surface anatomy is presented in conjunction with underlying skeletal anatomy, there is the possibility of interactively modeling the soft tissue surface and then deriving the skeletal alteration required to achieve that change in surface morphology. The 3D modeling relies on extracting both the skin surface and bone surface from a CT data set (which avoids image registration errors but provides a low-resolution skin surface image for manipulation) or alternatively, registration of a laser scan or surface image to a CT derived bone surface. Manipulation of the soft tissue surface can "suggest" the magnitude, direction, and shape of the underlying bony change (Fig. 7.2). Nevertheless, these models are only as accurate as the tissue parameters assigned to each element. In the above case, it was assumed that the soft tissue was generally homogeneous with approximate estimates of elasticity. Other approaches attempt to improve the model by incorporating muscle systems which constrains tissue motion preferentially along the muscle structures. Kim et al. [4] developed a facial atlas of the main muscle groups of the head and neck that could be morphed to the CT skull surface of the patient. Kim et al. use a mass-tensor method (MTM) that is described as a compromise between the computation efficiency of MSM and the accuracy of FEM. The MTM compartments of soft tissue are updated by setting directional properties of the elasticity of each compartment according to direction of the muscle fibers that intersected it.

Normative Skulls and Statistical Morphology

In many cases, correction of a defect relies on an understanding of what constitutes a "normal" contour.

This problem is easily solved when the defect or deformity is unilateral. Under these circumstances, the patient's own anatomy is generally sufficient to provide a normal contour. Mirroring the unaffected side provides an accurate representation of the missing geometry.

However, this approach is clearly not applicable when defects are bilateral or multicentric, when the midline is distorted, or when the craniofacial deformity is based on a more global disproportion which affects multiple bilateral anatomical sites. Having access to a large image dataset of reference skulls is helpful, but the variation in craniofacial morphology between individuals, even within ethnic or familial groups, is so large that identification of the best match contour for a specific patient is extremely difficult.

Conceptually, complex bilateral defects or disproportions are optimally reconstructed using a statistical average 3D

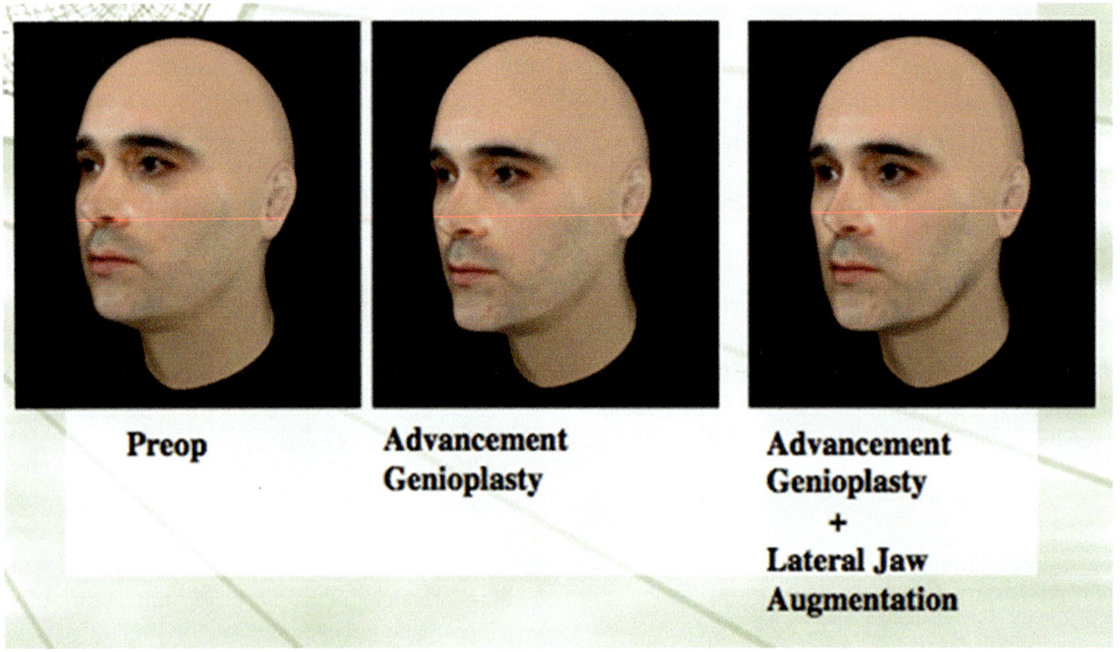

Fig. 7.1 The effectiveness of image manipulation as a tool for education and patient communication has previously been evaluated. Rhinoplasty patients as well as independent reviewers rated actual surgical results as good or better than computer predicted results (*Muhlbauer & Holm, PRS 115:2098, 2005; Agarwal A et al., PRS 119:1343,2007*). Patient satisfaction with the surgical result was significantly improved in those with preoperative image modeling, and patients reported clearer and more realistic informed consent (*Sharp HR et al., J Laryngol Otol 116:1009, 2002*) (FaceGen Modeller, Singular Inversions, Inc., Toronto, Canada)

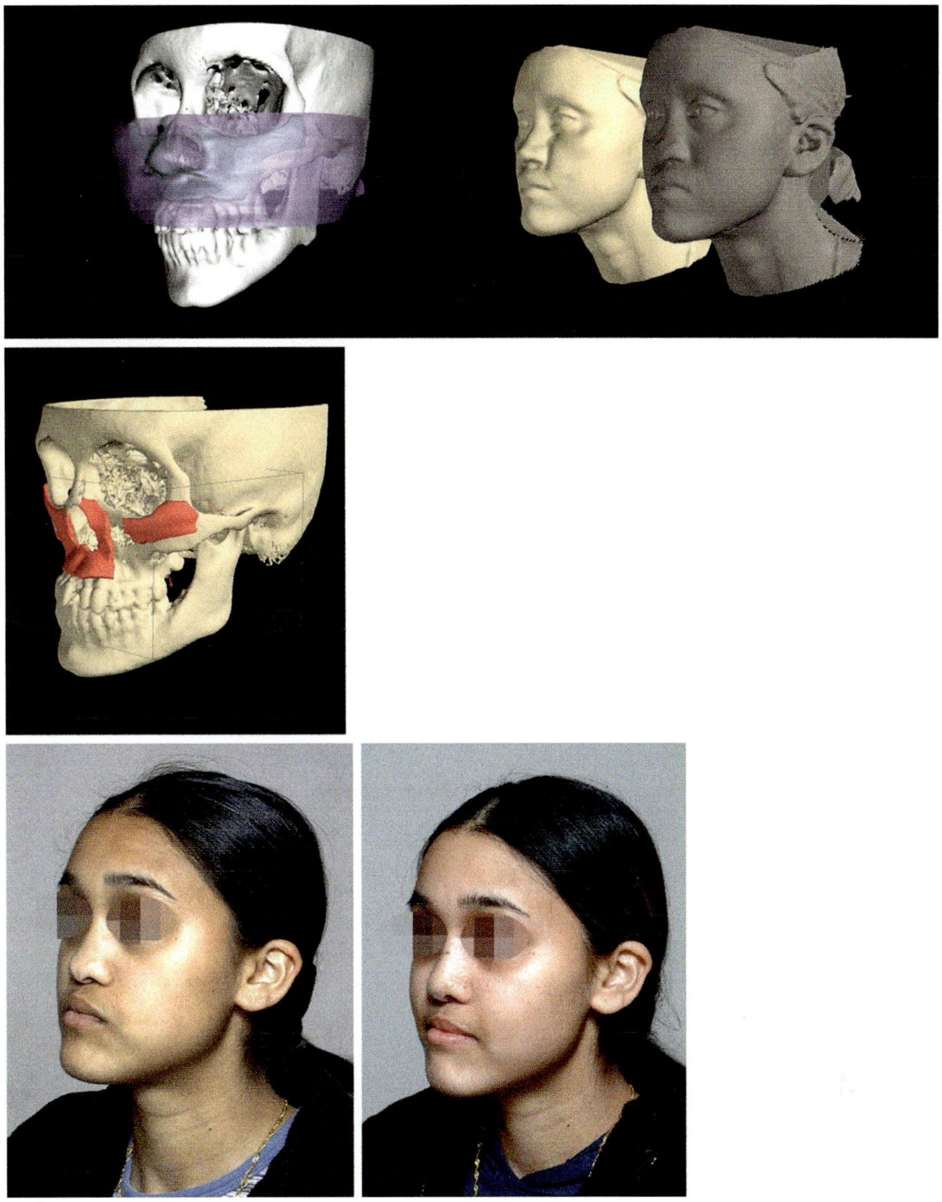

Fig. 7.2 When surface anatomy is presented in conjunction with underlying skeletal anatomy, there is the possibility of interactively modeling the soft tissue surface and then deriving the skeletal alteration required to achieve that change in surface morphology. The 3D modeling relies on extracting both the skin surface and bone surface from a CT data set (which avoids image registration errors but provides a low-resolution skin surface image for manipulation) or alternatively, registration of a laser scan or surface image to a CT derived bone surface. Manipulation of the soft tissue surface can "suggest" the magnitude, direction, and shape of the underlying bony change (Calavera Surgical Design, Toronto, Canada, and 3D Studiomax, Autodesk, San Raphael, CA, USA)

skull (based on a large sample of reference skulls) which is warped to the patient's residual anatomy to generate the missing geometry. This technique has previously been described as biometric morphing, and its application in modeling missing craniofacial anatomy has been demonstrated and validated [5] (Fig. 7.3).

The normative skull and its variations are analyzed in a variety of methods. First the shape correspondence between each skull dataset is identified. The simplest technique is by identifying corresponding landmarks (i.e., localized anatomic feature) on each skull [6]. However, landmarking is labor intensive, and there are only a small number of reliably identifiable landmarks on the skull surface, leading to poorly matched skulls with high user variability [7]. Increasing the number of points in the set is possible through the use of "semi-landmarks" that interpolate a number of points between landmarks that fall on some mathematically defined structure (i.e., points on a ridge or arranged on a smooth surface).

Alternatively, a high-density template in the form of a point cloud or mesh is registered to all of the skull surfaces in the training set. This imposes a one-to-one correspondence of all of the points on each skull. This template matching is a nonlinear registration process that can be computationally expensive. During this template matching step, or immediately following, all of the skull surfaces are registered (aligned) together and normalized to size. If there are a sufficient number of skulls, this may constitute a "library" of skulls from which a best match could be selected that matches the affected skull. Alternatively, there is a statistical reduction

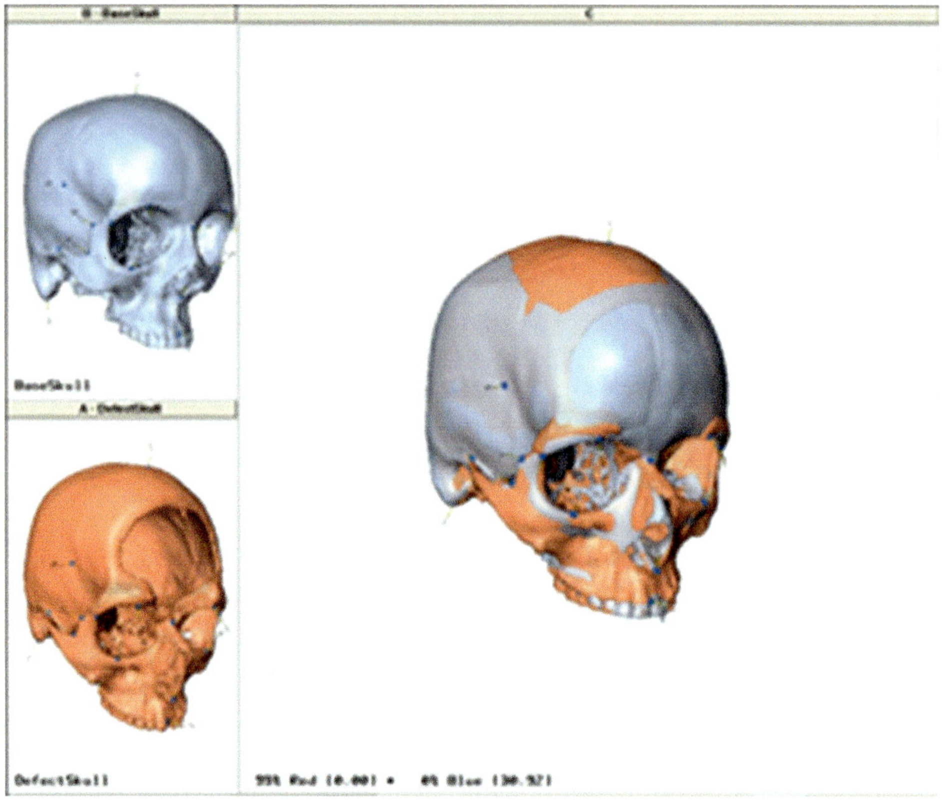

Fig. 7.3 Conceptually, complex bilateral defects or disproportions are optimally reconstructed using a statistical average 3D skull (based on a large sample of reference skulls) which is warped to the patient's residual anatomy to generate the missing geometry. This technique has previously been described as biometric morphing, and its application in modeling missing craniofacial anatomy has been demonstrated and validated ("Landmark", Institute for Data Analysis and Visualization, University of California, Davis, California, USA)

of the skull shape variations by principal component analysis [8] or similar data reduction techniques. In these approaches, principle components are extracted that represent a deformation or change in shape that explains a proportion of the shape variation seen in the population of skulls.

Thus, a normative skull defined for particular parameters (age, gender, ethnicity, height, weight) can potentially be a very powerful tool for surgical planning for incomplete skulls [9]. These libraries of skull shapes could be accessed for closest match for a particular individual both geometrically and by patient-specific parameters. Several groups have attempted to do this. For example, Saber et al. [10] have digitized the 103 pediatric skulls and created averaged the surfaces together at specific age groups (8–12 months) and manufactured templates of the normative infant head for bandeau plates used in fronto-orbital remodeling for treatment of unicoronal, bicoronal, or metopic synostosis.

Quantitative Analysis of Surface Morphology

Quantitative analysis of surface morphology can be of vital importance to surgical planning for specific cases or to the objective evaluation of surgical outcomes. This has previously been employed in the documentation of facial swelling, assessment of results of soft tissue augmentation with fillers or fat grafts, and the documentation of the morphological alterations resulting from cleft repair.

Quantitation of 3D surface area is extremely useful in predicting whether there is sufficient tissue to undertake a planned reconstruction. 3D surface scans are increasingly employed in precisely measuring defect size, the surface area of skin flaps, or the surface area of expanded tissues, to guide flap choice or design (Fig. 7.4).

Rapid Prototyping

- Rapid prototyping is a design and manufacturing methodology that encompasses both additive and subtractive manufacturing processes to shorten the time required for an end product (Fig. 7.5). For medical applications, this is advantageous and can be employed in a number of ways. The process is similar in all cases and starts with patient CT/MRI data that is converted into a 3D representation and then used to model a custom design solution with a variety of off-the-shelf software packages. This virtual model can then be used to make patient-specific surgical devices using rapid prototyping techniques. For example, it can be used to create surgical reference models, templates and cutting guides, custom forming tools, and even manufacture implants directly (Figs. 7.6–7.8).

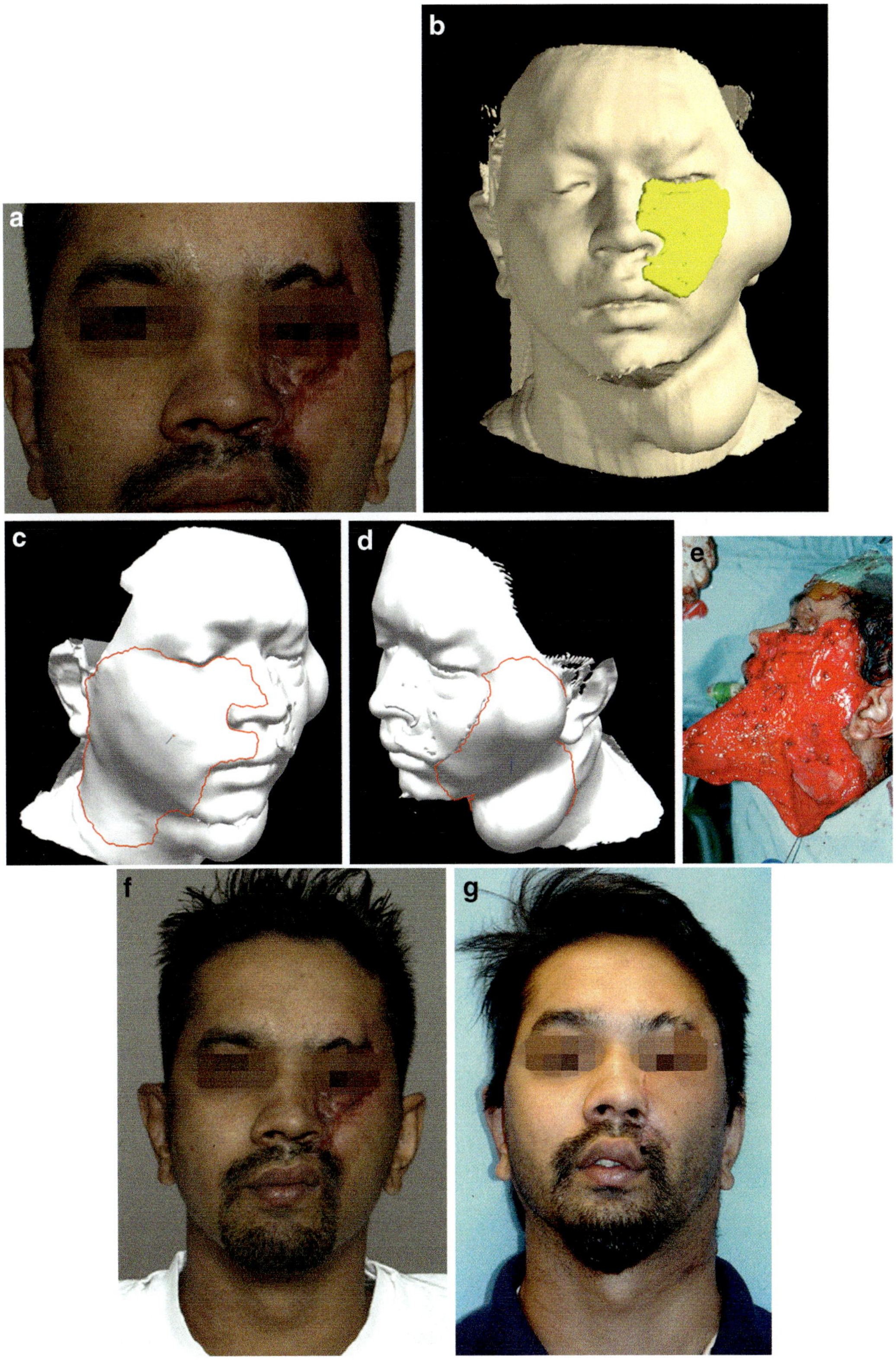

Fig. 7.4 Quantitation of 3D surface area is extremely useful in predicting whether there is sufficient tissue to undertake a planned reconstruction. 3D surface scans are increasingly employed in precisely measuring defect size, the surface area of skin flaps, or the surface area of expanded tissues, to guide flap choice or design. Patient with burn scar contracture left face (**a**). Two tissue expanders are inserted in the left neck and cheek, respectively, and the area to be resurfaced is quantitated (**b**). Comparative quantitative analysis of the normal right cheek (**c**) and the expanded left face and neck tissues (**d**) ensures adequate skin flap for resurfacing (**e**). The preoperative (**f**) and postoperative (**g**) appearance (Cyberware Inc., Monterey, CA, USA)

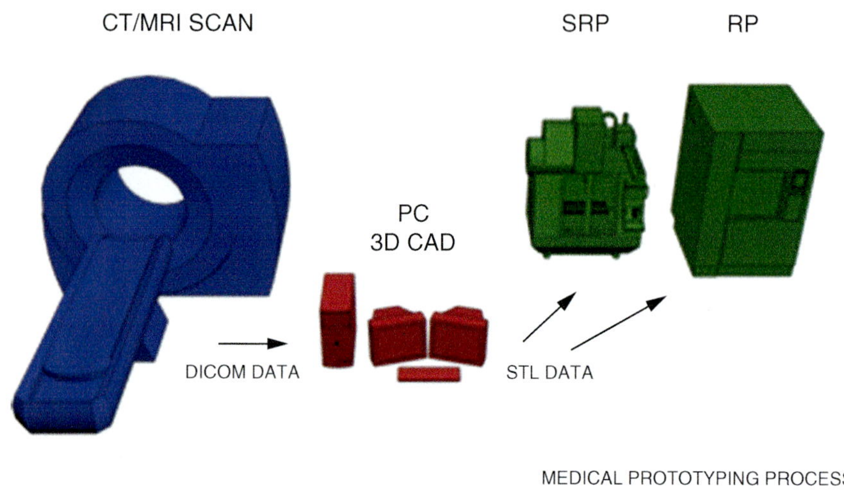

Fig. 7.5 CT or MRI image data is captured, exported to a workstation where all image processing and modeling is performed, and the completed virtual models are exported to RP machinery for manufacture of physical 3D models (Calavera Surgical Design, Toronto, Canada, and 510 3D Printer, Corp/3D Systems Healthcare, Rock Hill, SC, USA)

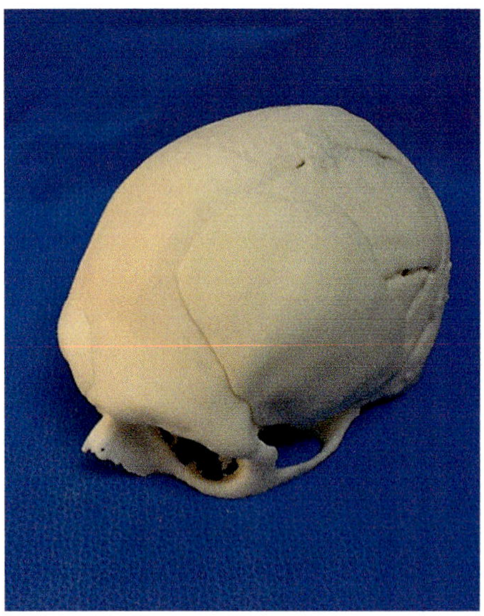

Fig. 7.6 Surgical reference models: implant planning and positioning (Calavera Surgical Design, Toronto, Canada)

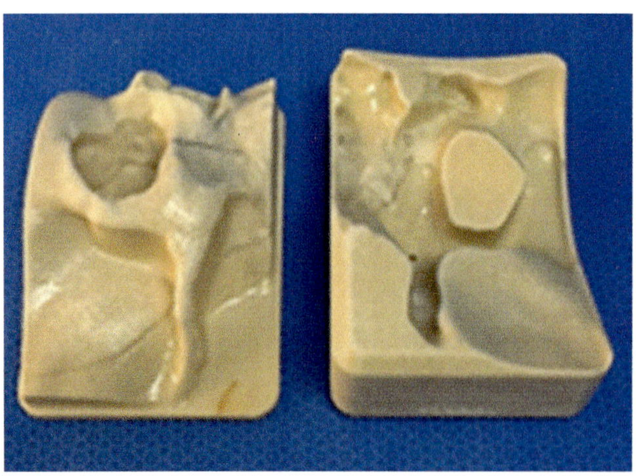

Fig. 7.7 Osteotomy templates: A positive (mold) and negative (forming tool) are generated to allow intraoperative shaping of a patient-specific implant (Calavera Surgical Design, Toronto, Canada)

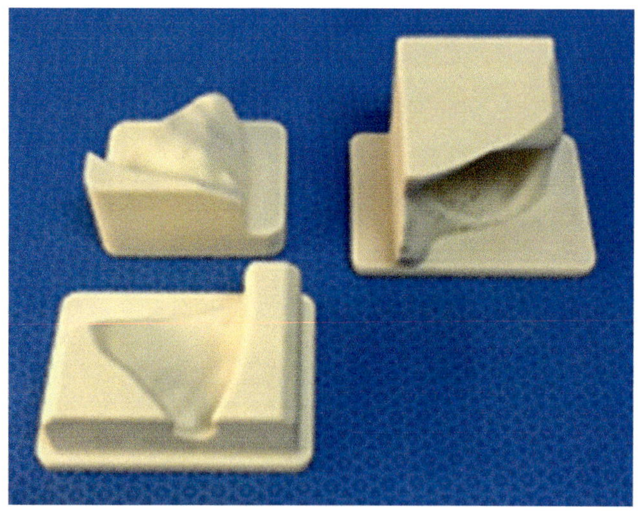

Fig. 7.8 Orbital mold and forming tool for intraoperative shaping of an orbital implant (Calavera Surgical Design, Toronto, Canada)

Cranial Vault Reconstruction

The goal of cranial vault reconstruction is to provide a permanent, stable, and structurally sound reconstruction which accurately reproduces the three-dimensional shape and surface contour of the skull. Accurate restoration of normal skull shape by manual shaping, however, is virtually impossible, particularly when defects are large or located in anatomical sites with complex surface topography. Computer-assisted design and manufacture of patient-specific alloplastic implants provides an obvious solution and was therefore pioneered in cranial vault reconstruction. Custom cranioplasty continues to lead the way in computer-generated implant technology, in terms of innovative materials, approaches and processes. Patient-specific implants restore normal anatomy with unprecedented precision and have been shown to decrease OR time, exposure time, and risk of contamination while resulting in improved cosmetic outcome and patient satisfaction [11, 12].

There are two principal approaches to custom cranioplasty:

1. The patient-specific skull implant can be prefabricated. This is currently the most commonly employed technique and has proven useful in elective reconstruction of established, stable defects of the cranium which will not be modified at the time of surgery
2. The patient-specific implant is manufactured intraoperatively by the surgeon. This is the technique of choice for defects which are unknown or undefined prior to surgery, i.e., benign and malignant skull tumors, and traumatic defects, where the size and shape of the defect will be determined at the time of surgery.

Prefabricated Implants for Known Defect

Prefabricated alloplastic implants are currently most commonly employed for the reconstruction of large, stable skull defects, where the margins of the defect are well defined and not likely to be altered at the time of surgery. A number of computer-assisted design/computer-assisted manufacturing (CAD/CAM) techniques for custom implant creation have been described [13–20]. The techniques used vary from "in-house" solutions performed by the surgeons themselves to commercially available, industry-manufactured implants. The most commonly used prosthetic cranioplasty materials include polymers (e.g., methyl methacrylate [21] and polyethylene), metals (e.g., titanium), and ceramics (e.g., hydroxyapatite). One of the most promising materials in current use is polyetheretherketone (PEEK), a thermoplastic material which is heat-stable and radiolucent and has modules of elasticity and density similar to that of the bone (Fig. 7.9).

Prefabricated implants have one major limitation. They are designed in advance to fit a specific defect. Any intraoperative modification of the size, shape, or bony margin of the defect renders the implant virtually useless. Clinically, this can occur under circumstances where a craniectomy is performed to remove bony tumors of the skull, osteoradionecrotic bone or osteomyelitic bone.

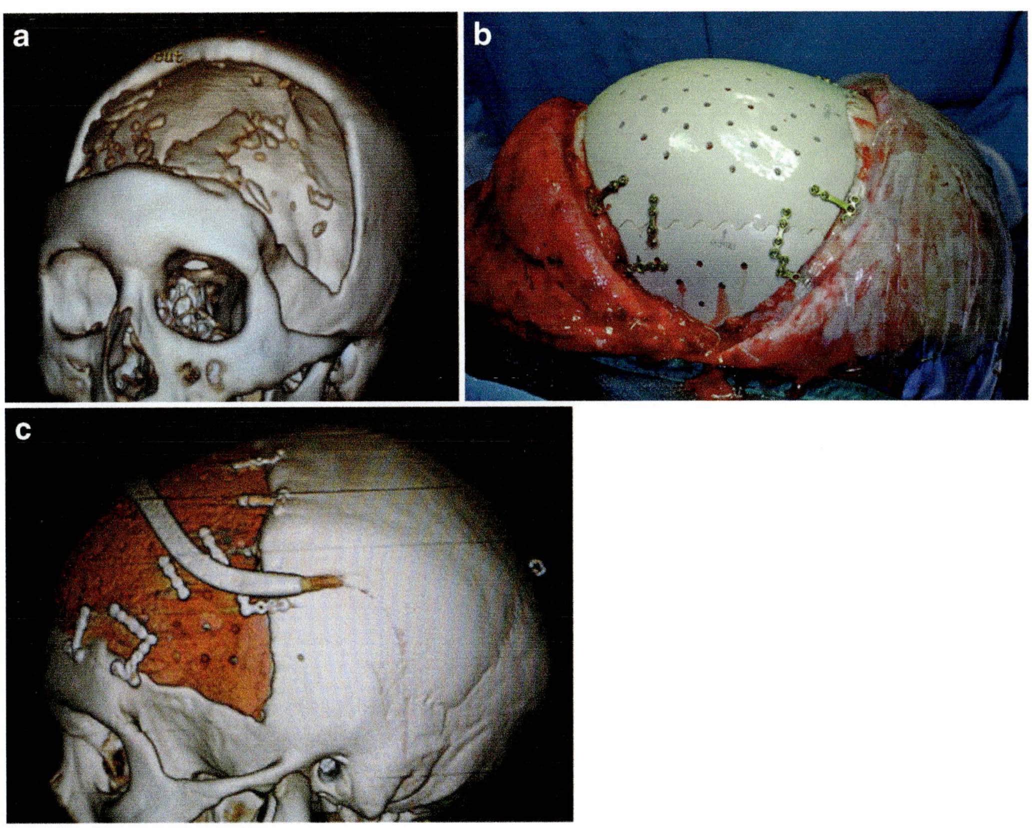

Fig. 7.9 A massive bilateral craniofrontal defect (**a**) is reconstructed with a prefabricated patient-specific PEEK implant (**b**) which is rigidly fixed to restore the premorbid skull shape (**c**) (DuPuy Synthes Craniomaxillofacial, Paoli, PA, USA)

Intraoperatively Manufactured Implants for Unknown Defect

Sunderland et al. [22] recently described a technique which allows intraoperative creation of a patient-specific titanium mesh implant. These implants have the unique capacity for intraoperative modification in the event that the size of the defect is unknown pre-operatively or if alteration of an existing skull defect is required. The technique relies on the computer modeling of optimal or desired postoperative skull morphology and preoperative fabrication of a patient-specific custom mold and forming tool. Intraoperatively, the surgeon employs the mold components in a custom pressing tool to shape titanium mesh that precisely restores skull contour and integrity (Fig. 7.10).

Orbital defects result from trauma or ablative tumor surgery. Precise restoration of the integrity as well as the three-dimensional configuration of the orbital cavity is critical to ensuring normal globe position and projection, as well as minimizing the possibility of functional complications such as diplopia, strabismus, and other visual disturbances. However, anatomical reconstruction of the orbit is a major technical challenge, due to the complex surface topography and the limited visualization offered by standard surgical approaches.

In an effort to improve restoration of the complex surface topography of the internal orbit, custom prefabricated orbital models [23] or implants [24, 25] have been described. Spatial orientation and precise placement of the implant through a limited access incision remain an issue, and some authors have advocated supplementing the technique with intraoperative navigation [26, 27].

Podolsky et al. [28] described a novel technique which incorporates both custom shaping of a patient-specific orbital implant to obliterate the orbital defect and utilizing the anatomy of the uninjured adjacent orbital bone to guide implant position and orientation. The surgeon is provided with a prefabricated custom mold and forming tool based on computer-assisted modeling of normal internal orbital shape. The mold is specifically designed to incorporate intact anatomy surrounding the defect. Intraoperatively, the surgeon utilizes a mechanical press to shape a sheet of orbital implant material (titanium, polyethylene, or composite). The resulting implant is "keyed" or registered to adjacent unaltered orbital rim or wall to ensure precise positioning and spatial orientation (Fig. 7.11).

Patient-Specific Autogenous Reconstruction

Despite the fact that alloplastic implants are being increasingly employed in craniofacial surgery, autogenous reconstruction remains the mainstay of treatment. Autogenous

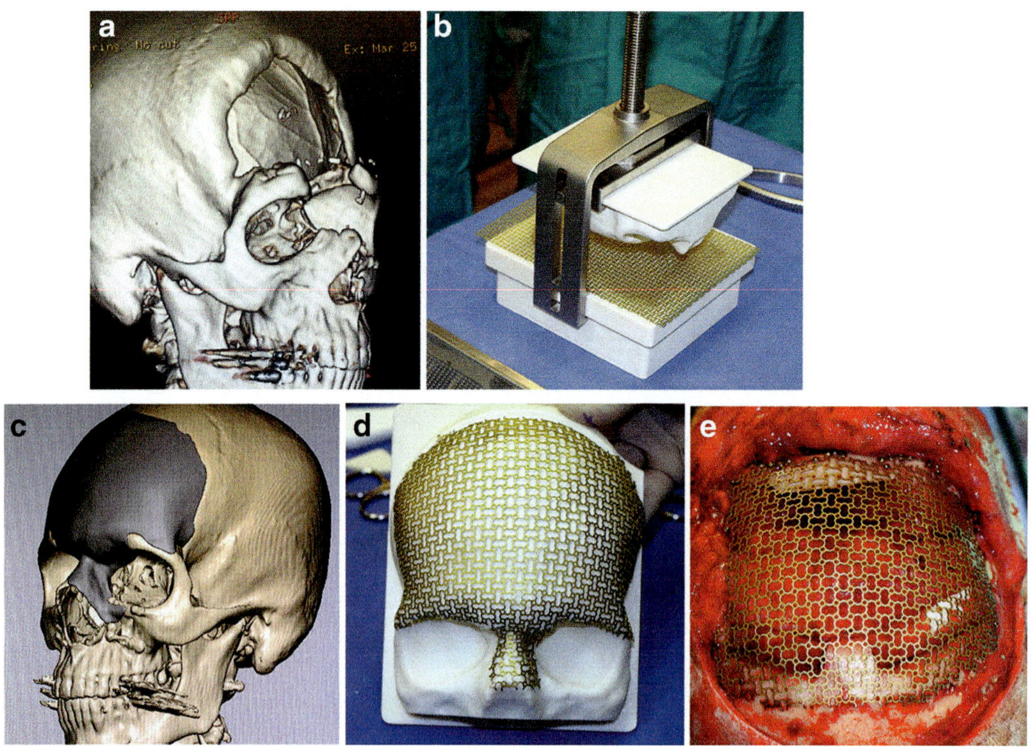

Fig. 7.10 Massive craniofrontal defect post tumor ablation complicated by infection (**a**). Further resection may be necessary, and prefabrication of a custom implant is therefore not possible. A custom mold and forming tool are employed intraoperatively (**b**) to compress a titanium mesh sheet into a custom implant which restores missing geometry (**c**) and beyond to overextended stable bony margins (**d**). The mesh provides an optimal shape regardless of intraoperative alterations to the margins (**e**) (Calavera Surgical Design, Toronto, Canada and Freeform, Sensable Technologies/Geomagic/3D Systems, Rock Hill, SC, USA DuPuy Synthes Craniomaxillofacial, Paoli, PA, USA)

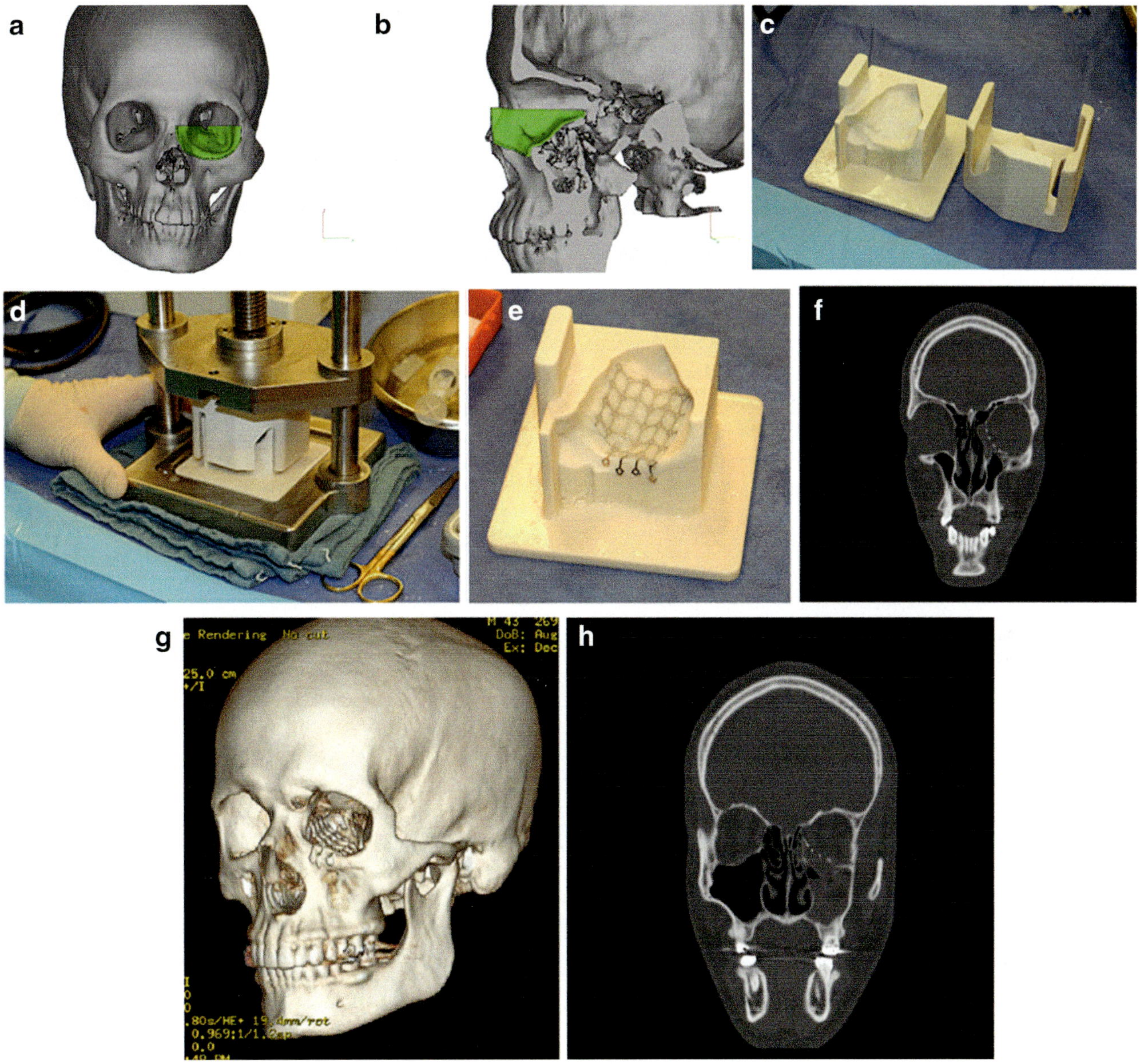

Fig. 7.11 The orbital reconstruction is modelled, and the desired shape is illustrated in *green* (**a** and **b**). A mold of the desired implant shape (**c**) is registered to the forming tool and compressed intraoperatively (**d**) to shape a custom implant (**e**) which restores the anatomy precisely and accurately (**f**, **g**, **h**) (Calavera Surgical Design, Toronto, Canada and Magics, Materialise, Leuven, Belgium, DuPuy Synthes Craniomaxillofacial, Paoli, PA, USA)

bone differs from alloplastic materials in its potential for revascularization, consolidation, and repair. Autogenous reconstructions are therefore preferred in circumstances where further skeletal growth is anticipated, where complex skeletal segments are malpositioned, or where there is a risk of contamination or exposure. Autogenous craniofacial reconstructions can be broadly categorized as:

1. Osteotomy, where a facial skeletal segment is mobilized, reshaped, and translocated
2. Bone transplant, where bone harvested from a remote site is transferred to a craniofacial site for obliteration of a cavity, for restoration of a defect, or to speed up consolidation or repair

Computer-assisted design and manufacture can be very effectively employed in both of these situations to assist in the planning and execution of autogenous reconstruction.

Modeling Craniofacial Osteotomies

Upper facial osteotomies can be extremely complex. They rely not only on a transposition of a major anatomical segment, but frequently a reshaping or reconfiguration of the osteotomy segment itself. This generally necessitates multiple simultaneous osteotomies. Modeling these osteotomies is therefore a challenge, and reliably implementing them in the operating room is particularly difficult.

A simpler and more effective approach is to model the final desired morphological result only and then to manufacture an intraoperative template of this ultimate contour. All of the intervening steps (i.e., specific placement of osteotomies, the number of osteotomy segments, the direction and degree of transposition of individual segments) are all performed manually by the surgeon at the time of surgery. The surgeon's objective is to cut and mobilize osteotomy segments to fit the computer-generated template.

This technique was previously described by D. J. Murray et al. [29] and has been very effectively employed in the reconstruction of congenital and posttraumatic deformities.

References

1. Papadopoulos MA, Christou PK, Christou PK, et al. Three-dimensional craniofacial reconstruction imaging. Oral Surg Oral Med Oral Pathol Oral Radiol Endod. 2002;93(4):382–93.
2. Zeilhofer H-F, Sader R, Kliegis U, et al. Models by 3D-ultrasound. Phidias Rapid Prototyp Med. 2000;5:1–4.
3. Yue X, Wang L, Wang R. Tissue modeling and analyzing with finite element method: a review for cranium brain imaging. Int J Biomed Imaging. 2013;2013:781603.
4. Kim H, Jürgens P, Weber S, Nolte L-P, Reyes M. A new soft-tissue simulation strategy for cranio-maxillofacial surgery using facial muscle template model. Prog Biophys Mol Biol. 2010;103(2–3):284–91.
5. Teshima TL, Patel V, Mainprize JG, Edwards G, Antonyshyn OM. A three-dimensional statistical average skull: Application of biometric morphing in generating missing anatomy. J Craniofac Surg. 2015;26(5):1634–8.
6. Bookstein FL. Principal warps: thin-plate splines and the decomposition of deformations. IEEE Trans Patt Anal. 1989;11(6):567–85.
7. Heimann T, Meinzer H-P. Statistical shape models for 3D medical image segmentation: a review. Med Image Anal. 2009;13(4):543–63.
8. Rohlf FJ, Marcus LF. A revolution in morphometrics. Trends Ecol Evol. 1993;8:129.
9. Dean D, Bookstein F, Koneru S, et al. Average African American three-dimensional computed tomography skull images: the potential clinical importance of ethnicity and sex. J Craniofac Surg. 1998;9(4):348–58.
10. Saber NR, Phillips J, Looi T, et al. Generation of normative pediatric skull models for use in cranial vault remodeling procedures. Childs Nerv Syst. 2012;28(3):405–10.
11. Spetzger U, Vougiokas V, Schipper J. Materials and techniques for osseus skull reconstruction. Minim Invasive Ther Allied Technol. 2010;19:110–21.
12. Lee SC, Wu CT, Lee ST, Chen PJ. Cranioplasty using polymethyl methacrylate prostheses. J Clin Neurosci. 2009;16:56–63.
13. Cabraja M, Klein M, Lehmann TN. Long-term results following titanium cranioplasty of large skull defects. Neurosurg Focus. 2009;26:E10.
14. Goh RCW, Chang CN, Lin CL, Lo LJ. Customised fabricated implants after previous failed cranioplasty. J Plast Reconstr Aesthet Surg. 2010;63:1479–84.
15. Dean D, Min KJ, Bond A. Computer aided design of large-format prefabricated cranial plates. J Craniofac Surg. 2003;14:819–32.
16. Eufinger H, Wehmoller M, Harders A, Heuser L. Prefabricated prostheses for the reconstruction of skull defects. Int J Oral Maxillofac Surg. 1995;24:104–10.
17. Wulf J, Busch LC, Golz T, et al. CAD generated mold for preoperative implant fabrication in cranioplasty, Medicine meets virtual reality, vol. 13. Amsterdam: IOS Press; 2005. p. 608–10.
18. Solaro P, Pierangeli E, Pizzoni C, Boffi P, Scalese G. From computerized tomography data processing to rapid manufacturing of custom-made prostheses for cranioplasty. J Neurosurg Sci. 2008;52:113–6.
19. Chiarini L, Figurelli S, Pollastri G, et al. Cranioplasty using acrylic material: a new technical procedure. J Craniomaxillofac Surg. 2004;32:5–9.
20. Eschbach L. Nonresorbable polymers in bone surgery. Injury. 2000;31(Suppl 4):22–7.
21. Gerber N, Stieglitz L, Peterhans M, Nolte LP, Raabe A, Weber S. Using rapid prototyping molds to create patient specific polymethylmethacrylate implants in cranioplasty. Conf Proc IEEE Eng Med Biol Soc. 2010;2010:3357–60.
22. Sunderland IRP, Edwards G, Mainprize J, Antonyshyn O. A technique for intra-operative creation of patient-specific titanium mesh implants for cranioplasty where the size of the skull defect is unknown pre-operatively. Plast Surg (Oakv). 2015 Summer;23(2):95–9.
23. Mustafa SF, Evans PL, Bocca A, Patton DW, Sugar AW, Baxter PW. Customized titanium reconstruction of post-traumatic orbital wall defects: a review of 22 cases. Int J Oral Maxillofac Surg. 2011 Dec;40(12):1357–62.
24. Hoffmann J, Cornelius CP, Groten M, Probster L, Pfannenberg C, Schwenzer N. Orbital reconstruction with individually copy-milled ceramic implants. Plast Reconstr Surg. 1998 Mar;101(3):604–12.
25. Metzger MC, Schon R, Zizelmann C, Weyer N, Gutwald R, Schmelzeisen R. Semiautomatic procedure for individual preforming of titanium meshes for orbital fractures. Plast Reconstr Surg. 2007 Mar;119(3):969–76.
26. Schmelzeisen R, Gellrich NC, Schoen R, Gutwald R, Zizelmann C, Schramm A. Navigation-aided reconstruction of medial orbital wall and floor contour in cranio-maxillofacial reconstruction. Injury. 2004 Oct;35(10):955–62.
27. Schmelzeisen R, Schramm A. Computer-assisted reconstruction of the facial skeleton. Arch Facial Plast Surg. 2003 Sept–Oct;5(5):437.
28. Podolsky DJ, Mainprize J, Edwards G, Antonyshyn O. Patient-specific orbital implants: development and implementation of technology for more accurate orbital reconstruction. J Craniofac Surg. 2016 Jan;27(1):131–3.
29. Murray DJ, Edwards G, Mainprize JG, Antonyshyn O. Optimizing craniofacial osteotomies: applications of haptic and rapid prototyping technology. J Oral Maxillofac Surg. 2008;66(8):1766–72.

Craniomaxillofacial Implants Based on 3D Modeling

8

Marc C. Metzger and Rainer Schmelzeisen

Introduction

A new era of surgical reconstruction began in the early 1990s with the introduction of computer-assisted surgery [1–10]. In the year 1994, the application of this technology for craniomaxillofacial surgery was introduced by Haßfeld et al. who presented the removal of skull base tumors, followed by other application areas such as foreign body removal, implantology, and orthognathic surgery [11–15]. By further development of planning software, it was possible to merge different image modalities, to segment anatomical fragments, to mirror the unaffected to the affected side, to import virtual implants and dental splints, and to export the virtual reconstructions for the creation of models [16–33]. In parallel, new printing and milling technologies allowed the manufacturing of patient-specific models and implants on the basis of CT data [20, 25, 34–43].

Since the introduction of the cone beam computer tomography (CBCT) technique in 1997, smaller devices have been available for three-dimensional image data acquisition [44–46]. The introduction of mobile CBCT devices in the operating room has offered the intraoperative radiological control option, which has led the surgical outcome also to a higher-quality step [47–51] [29, 47–50, 52–60]. An implementation of this technology into existing virtual planning and navigation methods is simple through the standardized DICOM data format and allows the development of new possibilities with regard to patient registration and simulation [52, 54, 55, 61–64].

Considering the large amount of these three-dimensional DICOM data, which are produced and stored every day, cephalometric analysis of anatomical mean shapes is now found another way. Besides this, mathematical algorithims such as the principal component analysis (PCA) allows the analysis not only of cephalometric points but also whole surface shapes and sizes. Recently, these techniques have been used to generate standardized anatomical forms, clustered by different sizes to produce osteosynthesis plates and implants presenting better fitting and biomechanical properties [39, 41, 65–68].

With regard to the craniomaxillofacial area, both kinds of properties mentioned above are well represented at the orbital cavity. Within the orbital cavity, the three-dimensional shape is of great importance for precise reconstruction.

Anatomical Preformed Orbital Implant

Orbital reconstructions are seen to be one of the most challenging procedures. Orbital floor fractures are frequently associated with medial wall fractures. The orbital floor has an initial shallow convex section behind the rim, then inclines upward behind the globe, and inclines upward to meet the medial wall, creating a distinct bulge behind the globe. These convex curves of the medial wall and floor create a "postbulbar constriction" of the orbital cavity, which must be reconstructed when the orbit is rebuilt following fractures. Treatment is directed at the precise anatomical reconstruction of orbital shape and volume in order to restore the correct position of the eye.

The three-dimensional reconstruction of the orbital walls, the repositioning of the prolapsed soft tissue, and the restoration of the ligament are necessary conditions of correct positioning and functionality of the eyeball [19, 69–74]. A review of the literature reveals the use of multiple approaches and multiple implant materials for orbital reconstruction [75–78]. Titanium fan plates have shown to be biocompatible and available and offer rigid support in larger defects [79]. However, accurate bending for precise reconstruction of the bony orbit is technique dependent and time-consuming [19]. To address this issue, some surgeons use sterilized skull

M.C. Metzger (✉) • R. Schmelzeisen
Department of Maxillofacial and Oral Surgery, University of Freiburg, Freiburg, Germany
e-mail: marc.metzger@uniklinik-freiburg.de

A.M. Greenberg (ed.), *Digital Technologies in Craniomaxillofacial Surgery*, https://doi.org/10.1007/978-1-4939-1532-3_8

models to assist with accurate intraoperative bending. More recently, computed tomography (CT) scans have been used to evaluate the premorbid shape of the contralateral orbit and mirror the data to the injured side. This data can be used to fabricate stereolithographic models or alloplastic implants for reconstruction [80–84]. These techniques, in combination with intraoperative navigation, can improve the precision of surgical repair [19, 82, 83, 85–93]. However, they are costly and not available at all institutions. Therefore, the intention was to design an anatomical preshaped orbital implant covering the orbital floor and medial wall which would be available at once without additional efforts and fitting for most individuals.

By using CT data of unaffected orbital cavities, topographical analysis could be performed, and mean shapes of the orbital floor and medial wall were calculated [68]. The evaluation of the fitting accuracy was tested in a cadaver study with 16 orbits, resulting in a mean distance of 0.81 ± 0.74 mm [94]. Further clinical studies have shown the practicability of these standardized anatomical preformed orbital implants [66, 95].

Implant Design

The preformed mesh implants are available in two sizes (small and large) for the left and right eyes. The posterior edge and medial wall of the implant can be trimmed to optimize the implant to the fracture size. In a central part, the implant has a stiff s-shape design following the common anatomical form of the orbital floor. Intersection bars guarantee a fast cutting to size resulting in smooth edges. At the anterior aspect of the implant, two arms can be used for screw fixation at the anterior inferior orbital rim (Figs. 8.1 and 8.2).

Placement

Preformed orbital mesh implants are commonly inserted through a transconjunctival incision for floor defects or a combined transconjunctival and transcaruncular approach for two wall defects. The entire bony defect should be exposed and the bony margins visualized. During preparation typical orbital landmarks should be exposed to guarantee the accurate placement (Fig. 8.3). At the anterior aspect, the infraorbital rim, the inferior orbital fissure, and the lacrimal fossa are important. After removing the displaced orbital soft tissue out of the maxillary sinus, the posterior orbital edge, which is commonly not fractured, has to be found. Onto this region the orbital implant has to be placed to offer bony support (Fig. 8.4). The optical nerve will be at least 10 mm away from the preparation and will be out of the danger zone.

Clinical Case

A 61-year-old male sustained blunt trauma to right orbit. The ophthalmological exam presented severe soft tissue swelling, bruising, and diplopia. The CT imaging demonstrated severe displacement of the orbital floor, putting the patient at risk for late enophthalmos and dystopia as well as strabismus (Fig. 8.5).

Preoperative planning was performed using a common 3D modeling software (iPLan, Brainlab, Munich, Germany).

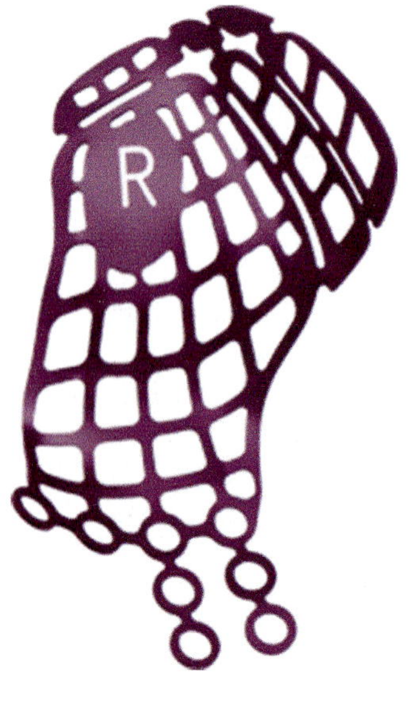

Fig. 8.1 Design and functional areas of the preformed orbital implant (DePuy Synthes Craniomaxillofacial, Padi, PA, USA)

After importing the CT data, autosegmentation was performed automatically including this step in the data preprocessing during data import. The segmented unaffected left orbital cavity was mirrored to the affected side presenting the virtual reconstruction. In a second step, the virtual implant was implemented and placed at the correct position including the criteria mentioned above (Fig. 8.6).

The preformed orbital mesh implant was inserted through a transconjunctival incision for the floor defect. The implant was fixed to the inferior orbital rim with two screws. During the operation, intraoperative navigation and imaging were performed. Acquiring CBCT data after inserting and placing the implant demonstrated that the implant was in the correct position. Image fusion allowed the comparison of the actual achieved reconstruction with the preoperative planned reconstruction (Fig. 8.7). A forced duction test was performed to ensure unrestricted movement of the globe.

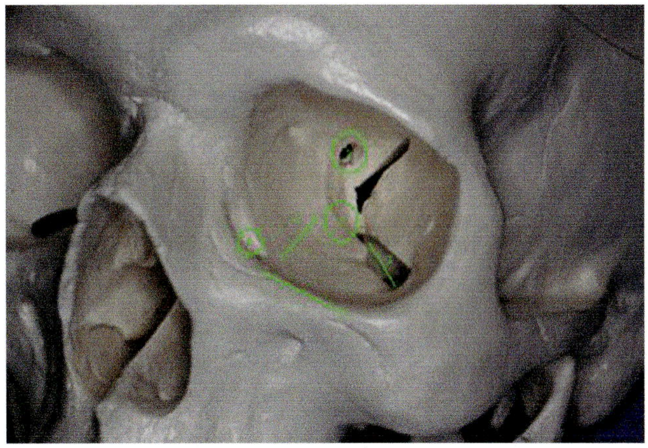

Fig. 8.3 Important anatomical structures for placing the implant: (1) orbital rim, (2) inferior orbital fissure, (3) posterior orbital ledge, (4) junction between orbital floor and medial wall, (5) lacrimal fossa

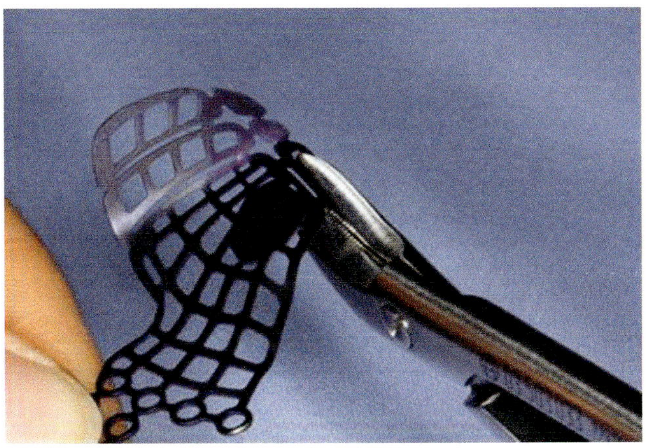

Fig. 8.2 Cutting to size can easily be performed by reducing the intersection bars (DuPuy Synthes Craniomaxillofacial, Paoli, PA, USA)

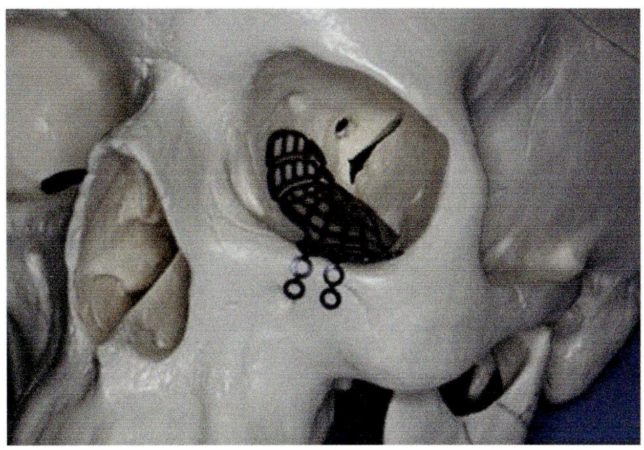

Fig. 8.4 Placement of the implant in an artificial skull. At the anterior aspect of the orbital rim, the fixation with one or two screws is possible (DuPuy Synthes Craniomaxillofacial, Paoli, PA, USA)

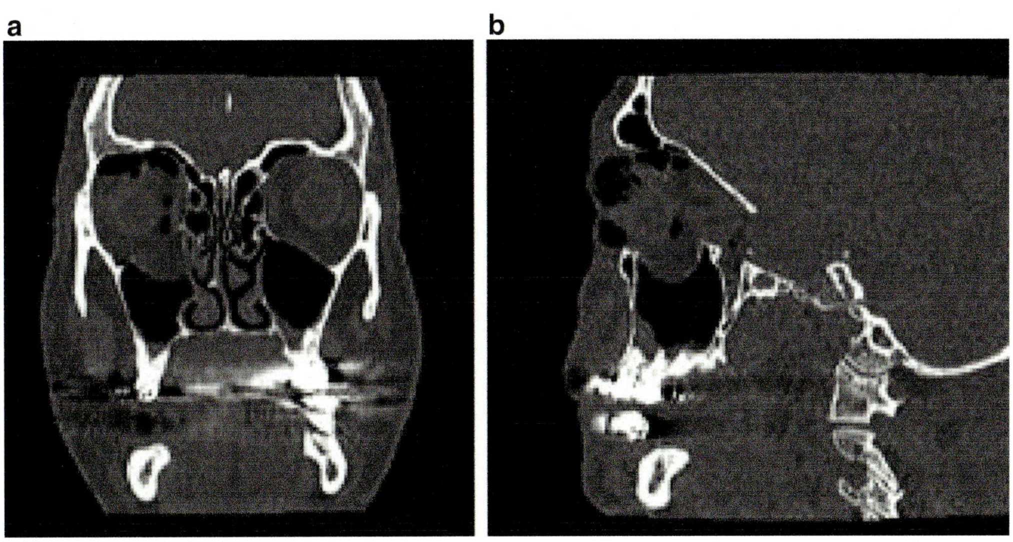

Fig. 8.5 CT scan of a patient presenting with a right orbital floor fracture (**a**) coronal view, (**b**) sagittal view

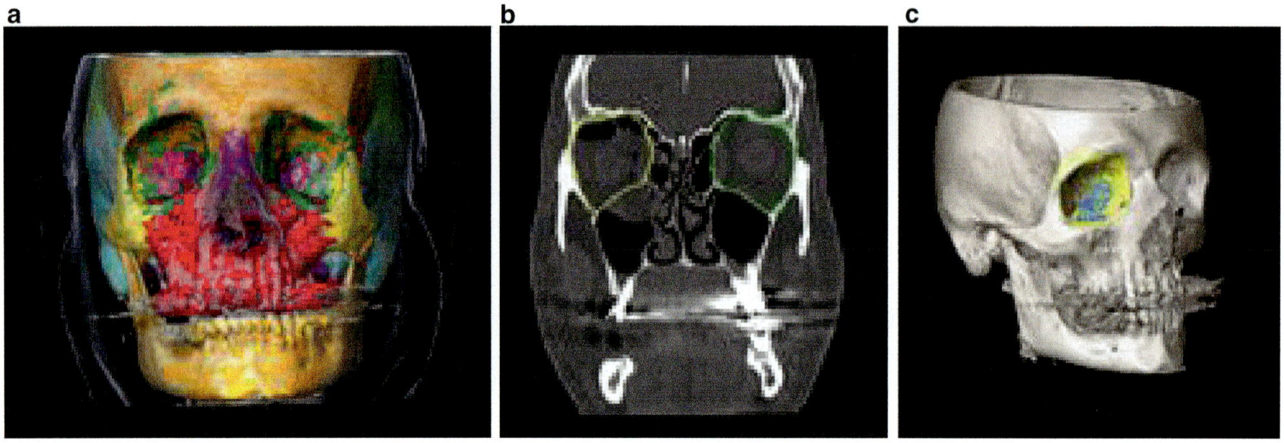

Fig. 8.6 Preoperative planning steps: (**a**) autosegmentation as a data preprocessing step performing the segmentation automatically during the data import, (**b**) mirroring the unaffected left orbital cavity (*green*) to the affected side (*yellow*), (**c**) placement of a virtual preformed orbital implant to cover the defect (iPlan, Brainlab, Munich, Germany)

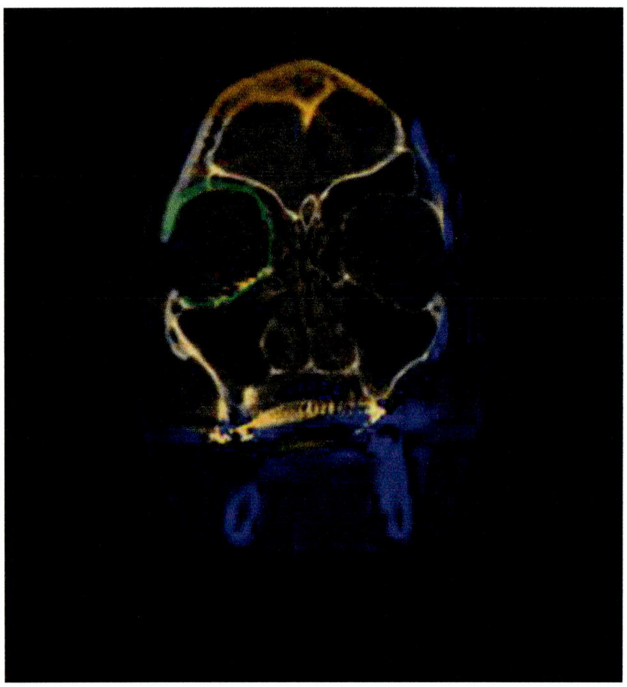

Fig. 8.7 Intraoperative image fusion of the preoperative planning dataset and the acquired CBCT dataset comparing the achieved reconstruction and the preoperative planning (iPlan, Brainlab, Munich, Germany)

References

1. Watanabe E, Watanabe T, Manaka S, Mayanagi Y, Takakura K. Three-dimensional digitizer (neuronavigator): new equipment for computed tomography-guided stereotaxic surgery. Surg Neurol. 1987 Jun;27(6):543–7.
2. Burm JS, Chung CH, Oh SJ. Pure orbital blowout fracture: new concepts and importance of medial orbital blowout fracture. Plast Reconstr Surg. 1999 Jun;103(7):1839–49.
3. Salvolini U. Traumatic injuries: imaging of facial injuries. Eur Radiol. 2002 Jun;12(6):1253–61.
4. Marsh JL, Gado M. The longitudinal orbital CT projection: a versatile image for orbital assessment. Plast Reconstr Surg. 1983 Mar;71(3):308–17.
5. Waitzman AA, Posnick JC, Armstrong DC, Pron GE. Craniofacial skeletal measurements based on computed tomography: part I. Accuracy and reproducibility. Cleft Palate Craniofac J. 1992 Mar;29(2):112–7.
6. Farkas LG, Katic MJ, Forrest CR, Alt KW, Bagic I, Baltadjiev G, et al. International anthropometric study of facial morphology in various ethnic groups/races. J Craniofac Surg. 2005 Jul;16(4):615–46.
7. Chau A, Fung K, Yip L, Yap M. Orbital development in Hong Kong Chinese subjects. Ophthalmic Physiol Opt. 2004 Sep;24(5):436–9.
8. Furuta M. Measurement of orbital volume by computed tomography: especially on the growth of the orbit. Jpn J Ophthalmol. 2001 Nov–Dec;45(6):600–6.
9. Bentley RP, Sgouros S, Natarajan K, Dover MS, Hockley AD. Normal changes in orbital volume during childhood. J Neurosurg. 2002 Apr;96(4):742–6.
10. Converse JM, Smith B, Obear MF, Wood-Smith D. Orbital blowout fractures: a ten-year survey. Plast Reconstr Surg. 1967 Jan;39(1):20–36.
11. Hassfeld S, Muhling J, Zoller J. Intraoperative navigation in oral and maxillofacial surgery. Int J Oral Maxillofac Surg. 1995 Feb;24(1 Pt 2):111–9.
12. Frodel JL Jr, Pacheco E. The use of intraoperative image-guided surgical techniques for reconstruction of orbital and zygomatic deformities. Facial Plast Surg. 1999;15(1):83–9.
13. Ploder O, Wagner A, Enislidis G, Ewers R. Computer-assisted intraoperative visualization of dental implants. Augmented reality in medicine. Radiologe. 1995 Sep;35(9):569–72.
14. Wagner A, Ploder O, Enislidis G, Truppe M, Ewers R. Virtual image guided navigation in tumor surgery—technical innovation. J Craniomaxillofac Surg. 1995 Oct;23(5):217–3.
15. Marmulla R, Hilbert M, Niederdellmann H. Inherent precision of mechanical, infrared and laser-guided navigation systems for computer-assisted surgery. J Craniomaxillofac Surg. 1997 Aug;25(4):192–7.
16. Hill DL, Hawkes DJ, Hussain Z, Green SE, Ruff CF, Robinson GP. Accurate combination of CT and MR data of the head: validation and applications in surgical and therapy planning. Comput Med Imaging Graph. 1993 Jul–Oct;17(4–5):357–63.
17. Woods RP, Mazziotta JC, Cherry SR. MRI-PET registration with automated algorithm. J Comput Assist Tomogr. 1993 Jul-Aug;17(4):536–46.

18. Hill DL, Hawkes DJ, Gleeson MJ, Cox TC, Strong AJ, Wong WL, et al. Accurate frameless registration of MR and CT images of the head: applications in planning surgery and radiation therapy. Radiology. 1994 May;191(2):447–54.
19. Gellrich NC, Schramm A, Hammer B, Rojas S, Cufi D, Lagreze W, et al. Computer-assisted secondary reconstruction of unilateral posttraumatic orbital deformity. Plast Reconstr Surg. 2002 Nov;110(6):1417–29.
20. Bell RB, Markiewicz MR. Computer-assisted planning, stereolithographic Modeling, and intraoperative navigation for complex orbital reconstruction: a descriptive study in a preliminary cohort. J Oral Maxillofac Surg. 2009 Dec;67(12):2559–70.
21. De Rosa V, Ionna F, Mozzillo N, Parascandolo S, Ziviello M. 3D spiral computerized tomography in the reconstructive treatment of malignant maxillofacial tumors. Radiol Med. 2000 Dec;100(6):424–8.
22. Gripp S, Doeker R, Glag M, Vogelsang P, Pape H. Conventional and virtual simulation in retrobulbar irradiation. Strahlenther Onkol. 2000 Mar;176(3):131–4.
23. Hassfeld S, Zoller J, Albert FK, Wirtz CR, Knauth M, Muhling J. Preoperative planning and intraoperative navigation in skull base surgery. J Craniomaxillofac Surg. 1998 Aug;26(4):220–5.
24. Hohlweg-Majert B, Schon R, Schmelzeisen R, Gellrich NC, Schramm A. Navigational maxillofacial surgery using virtual models. World J Surg. 2005 Dec;29(12):1530–8.
25. Metzger MC, Hohlweg-Majert B, Schon R, Teschner M, Gellrich NC, Schmelzeisen R, et al. Verification of clinical precision after computer-aided reconstruction in craniomaxillofacial surgery. Oral Surg Oral Med Oral Pathol Oral Radiol Endod. 2007 Oct;104(4):e1–10.
26. Meyer U, Stamm T, Meier N, Joos U. First experience with a public domain computer-aided surgical system. Br J Oral Maxillofac Surg. 2002 Apr;40(2):96–104.
27. Pham AM, Rafii AA, Metzger MC, Jamali A, Strong EB. Computer modeling and intraoperative navigation in maxillofacial surgery. Otolaryngol Head Neck Surg. 2007 Oct;137(4):624–31.
28. Westendorff C, Gulicher D, Dammann F, Reinert S, Hoffmann J. Computer-assisted surgical treatment of orbitozygomatic fractures. J Craniofac Surg. 2006 Sep;17(5):837–42.
29. Zizelmann C, Gellrich NC, Metzger MC, Schoen R, Schmelzeisen R, Schramm A. Computer-assisted reconstruction of orbital floor based on cone beam tomography. Br J Oral Maxillofac Surg. 2007 Jan;45(1):79–80.
30. Zizelmann C, Schramm A, Schon R, Ridder GJ, Maier W, Schipper J, et al. Computer assisted methods in reconstructive and function-preserving orbital surgery. New capabilities of computer assisted preoperative surgical planning (CAPP) and computer assisted surgery (CAS). HNO. 2005 May;53(5):428–38.
31. Metzger MC, Schon R, Weyer N, Gutwald R, Schmelzeisen R. Computer-assisted extracorporeal orbital reconstruction after optic nerve decompression by removal of sphenoid bone. Ann Plast Surg. 2006 Aug;57(2):223–7.
32. Metzger MC, Hohlweg-Majert B, Schwarz U, Teschner M, Hammer B, Schmelzeisen R. Manufacturing splints for orthognathic surgery using a three-dimensional printer. Oral Surg Oral Med Oral Pathol Oral Radiol Endod. 2008 Feb;105(2):e1–7.
33. Metzger MC, Bittermann G, Dannenberg L, Schmelzeisen R, Gellrich NC, Hohlweg-Majert B, et al. Design and development of a virtual anatomic atlas of the human skull for automatic segmentation in computer-assisted surgery, preoperative planning, and navigation. Int J Comput Assist Radiol Surg. 2013;8(5):691–702.
34. Hemmy DC, David DJ, Herman GT. Three-dimensional reconstruction of craniofacial deformity using computed tomography. Neurosurgery. 1983 Nov;13(5):534–41.
35. Eufinger H, Wehmoller M, Harders A, Heuser L. Prefabricated prostheses for the reconstruction of skull defects. Int J Oral Maxillofac Surg. 1995 Feb;24(1 Pt 2):104–10.
36. Vannier MW, Marsh JL, Warren JO. Three dimensional CT reconstruction images for craniofacial surgical planning and evaluation. Radiology. 1984 Jan;150(1):179–84.
37. Sader R, Zeilhofer HF, Kliegis U, Deppe H, Horch HH. Precision of 3D-assisted surgical planning with rapid prototype techniques. Mund Kiefer Gesichtschir. 1997 May;1(Suppl 1):S61–4.
38. Petzold R, Zeilhofer HF, Kalender WA. Rapid prototyping technology in medicine—basics and applications. Comput Med Imaging Graph. 1999 Sep-Oct;23(5):277–84.
39. Metzger MC, Schon R, Schmelzeisen R. Preformed titanium meshes: a new standard? Skull Base. 2007 Jul;17(4):269–72.
40. Metzger MC, Schon R, Schulze D, Carvalho C, Gutwald R, Schmelzeisen R. Individual preformed titanium meshes for orbital fractures. Oral Surg Oral Med Oral Pathol Oral Radiol Endod. 2006 Oct;102(4):442–7.
41. Metzger MC, Schon R, Zizelmann C, Weyer N, Gutwald R, Schmelzeisen R. Semiautomatic procedure for individual preforming of titanium meshes for orbital fractures. Plast Reconstr Surg. 2007 Mar;119(3):969–76.
42. Schon R, Metzger MC, Zizelmann C, Weyer N, Schmelzeisen R. Individually preformed titanium mesh implants for a true-to-original repair of orbital fractures. Int J Oral Maxillofac Surg. 2006 Nov;35(11):990–5.
43. Hughes CW, Page K, Bibb R, Taylor J, Revington P. The custom-made titanium orbital floor prosthesis in reconstruction for orbital floor fractures. Br J Oral Maxillofac Surg. 2003 Feb;41(1):50–3.
44. Mozzo P, Procacci C, Tacconi A, Martini PT, Andreis IA. A new volumetric CT machine for dental imaging based on the cone-beam technique: preliminary results. Eur Radiol. 1998;8(9):1558–64.
45. Ng P, Chu C, Young N, Soo M. Imaging of orbital floor fractures. Australas Radiol. 1996 Aug;40(3):264–8.
46. Hohlweg-Majert B, Metzger MC, Kummer T, Schulze D. Morphometric analysis – cone beam computed tomography to predict bone quality and quantity. J Craniomaxillofac Surg. 2011 Jul;39(5):330–4.
47. Heiland M, Schmelzle R, Hebecker A, Schulze D. Intraoperative 3D imaging of the facial skeleton using the SIREMOBIL Iso-C3D. Dentomaxillofac Radiol. 2004 Mar;33(2):130–2.
48. Heiland M, Schulze D, Blake F, Schmelzle R. Intraoperative imaging of zygomaticomaxillary complex fractures using a 3D C-arm system. Int J Oral Maxillofac Surg. 2005 Jun;34(4):369–75.
49. Siewerdsen JH, Moseley DJ, Burch S, Bisland SK, Bogaards A, Wilson BC, et al. Volume CT with a flat-panel detector on a mobile, isocentric C-arm: pre-clinical investigation in guidance of minimally invasive surgery. Med Phys. 2005 Jan;32(1):241–54.
50. Pohlenz P, Blessmann M, Blake F, Gbara A, Schmelzle R, Heiland M. Major mandibular surgical procedures as an indication for intraoperative imaging. J Oral Maxillofac Surg. 2008 Feb;66(2):324–9.
51. Korbmacher H, Kahl-Nieke B, Schollchen M, Heiland M. Value of two cone-beam computed tomography systems from an orthodontic point of view. J Orofac Orthop. 2007 Jul;68(4):278–89.
52. Barker E, Trimble K, Chan H, Ramsden J, Nithiananthan S, James A, et al. Intraoperative use of cone-beam computed tomography in a cadaveric ossified cochlea model. Otolaryngol Head Neck Surg. 2009 May;140(5):697–702.
53. Blake FA, Blessmann M, Pohlenz P, Heiland M. A new imaging modality for intraoperative evaluation of sinus floor augmentation. Int J Oral Maxillofac Surg. 2008 Feb;37(2):183–5.
54. Grobe A, Weber C, Schmelzle R, Heiland M, Klatt J, Pohlenz P. The use of navigation (BrainLAB vector vision(2)) and intraoperative 3D imaging system (Siemens Arcadis Orbic 3D) in the treatment of gunshot wounds of the maxillofacial region. Oral Maxillofac Surg. 2009 Sep;13(3):153–8.
55. Hamming NM, Daly MJ, Irish JC, Siewerdsen JH. Effect of fiducial configuration on target registration error in intraoperative cone-beam CT guidance of head and neck surgery. Conf Proc IEEE Eng Med Biol Soc. 2008;2008:3643–8.

56. Mischkowski RA, Zinser MJ, Ritter L, Neugebauer J, Keeve E, Zoller JE. Intraoperative navigation in the maxillofacial area based on 3D imaging obtained by a cone-beam device. Int J Oral Maxillofac Surg. 2007 Aug;36(8):687–94.
57. Pohlenz P, Blake F, Blessmann M, Smeets R, Habermann C, Begemann P, et al. Intraoperative cone-beam computed tomography in oral and maxillofacial surgery using a C-arm prototype: first clinical experiences after treatment of zygomaticomaxillary complex fractures. J Oral Maxillofac Surg. 2009 Mar;67(3):515–21.
58. Pohlenz P, Blessmann M, Blake F, Heinrich S, Schmelzle R, Heiland M. Clinical indications and perspectives for intraoperative cone-beam computed tomography in oral and maxillofacial surgery. Oral Surg Oral Med Oral Pathol Oral Radiol Endod. 2007 Mar;103(3):412–7.
59. Rafferty MA, Siewerdsen JH, Chan Y, Daly MJ, Moseley DJ, Jaffray DA, et al. Intraoperative cone-beam CT for guidance of temporal bone surgery. Otolaryngol Head Neck Surg. 2006 May;134(5):801–8.
60. Rafferty MA, Siewerdsen JH, Chan Y, Moseley DJ, Daly MJ, Jaffray DA, et al. Investigation of C-arm cone-beam CT-guided surgery of the frontal recess. Laryngoscope. 2005 Dec;115(12):2138–43.
61. Feuerstein M, Mussack T, Heining SM, Navab N. Intraoperative laparoscope augmentation for port placement and resection planning in minimally invasive liver resection. IEEE Trans Med Imaging. 2008 Mar;27(3):355–69.
62. Hamming NM, Daly MJ, Irish JC, Siewerdsen JH. Automatic image-to-world registration based on x-ray projections in cone-beam CT-guided interventions. Med Phys. 2009 May;36(5):1800–12.
63. Teber D, Guven S, Simpfendorfer T, Baumhauer M, Guven EO, Yencilek F, et al. Augmented reality: a new tool to improve surgical accuracy during laparoscopic partial nephrectomy? Preliminary in vitro and in vivo results. Eur Urol. 2009 Aug;56(2):332–8.
64. Aschendorff A, Maier W, Jaekel K, Wesarg T, Arndt S, Laszig R, et al. Radiologically assisted navigation in cochlear implantation for X-linked deafness malformation. Cochlear Implants Int. 2009;10(Suppl 1):14–8.
65. Probst FA, Mast G, Ermer M, Gutwald R, Schmelzeisen R, Pautke C, et al. MatrixMANDIBLE preformed reconstruction plates—a two-year two-institution experience in 71 patients. J Oral Maxillofac Surg. 2012 Nov;70(11):e657–66.
66. Strong EB, Fuller SC, Wiley DF, Zumbansen J, Wilson MD, Metzger MC. Preformed vs intraoperative bending of titanium mesh for orbital reconstruction. Otolaryngol Head Neck Surg. 2013 Jul;149(1):60–6.
67. Metzger MC, Vogel M, Hohlweg-Majert B, Mast H, Fan X, Rudell A, et al. Anatomical shape analysis of the mandible in Caucasian and Chinese for the production of preformed mandible reconstruction plates. J Craniomaxillofac Surg. 2011 Sep;39(6):393–400.
68. Metzger MC, Schon R, Tetzlaf R, Weyer N, Rafii A, Gellrich NC, et al. Topographical CT-data analysis of the human orbital floor. Int J Oral Maxillofac Surg. 2007 Jan;36(1):45–53.
69. Farkas LG. Accuracy of anthropometric measurements: past, present, and future. Cleft Palate Craniofac J. 1996 Jan;33(1):10–8; discussion 9–22.
70. Schramm A, Gellrich N-C, Naumann S, Bühner U, Schön R, Schmelzeisen R. Non-invasive referencing in computer assisted surgery. Med Biol Eng Comp Suppl. 1999;37:644.
71. Guo L, Tian W, Feng F, Long J, Li P, Tang W. Reconstruction of orbital floor fractures: comparison of individual prefabricated titanium implants and calvarial bone grafts. Ann Plast Surg. 2009;63(6):624–31.
72. Mazock JB, Schow SR, Triplett RG. Evaluation of ocular changes secondary to blowout fractures. J Oral Maxillofac Surg. 2004 Oct;62(10):1298–302.
73. Clauser L, Galie M, Pagliaro F, Tieghi R. Posttraumatic enophthalmos: etiology, principles of reconstruction, and correction. J Craniofac Surg. 2008 Mar;19(2):351–9.
74. Mustarde JC. The role of Lockwood's suspensory ligament in preventing downward displacement of the eye. Br J Plast Surg. 1968 Jan;21(1):73–81.
75. Potter JK, Ellis E. Biomaterials for reconstruction of the internal orbit. J Oral Maxillofac Surg. 2004 Oct;62(10):1280–97.
76. Burm JS. Internal fixation in trapdoor-type orbital blowout fracture. Plast Reconstr Surg. 2005 Sep 15;116(4):962–70.
77. Buchel P, Rahal A, Seto I, Iizuka T. Reconstruction of orbital floor fracture with polyglactin 910/polydioxanon patch (ethisorb): a retrospective study. J Oral Maxillofac Surg. 2005 May;63(5):646–50.
78. Burnstine MA. Clinical recommendations for repair of orbital facial fractures. Curr Opin Ophthalmol. 2003 Oct;14(5):236–40.
79. Ellis E 3rd, Tan Y. Assessment of internal orbital reconstructions for pure blowout fractures: cranial bone grafts versus titanium mesh. J Oral Maxillofac Surg. 2003 Apr;61(4):442–53.
80. Schipper J, Ridder GJ, Spetzger U, Teszler CB, Fradis M, Maier W. Individual prefabricated titanium implants and titanium mesh in skull base reconstructive surgery. A report of cases. Eur Arch Otorhinolaryngol. 2004 May;261(5):282–90.
81. Hoffmann J, Cornelius CP, Groten M, Probster L, Pfannenberg C, Schwenzer N. Orbital reconstruction with individually copy-milled ceramic implants. Plast Reconstr Surg. 1998 Mar;101(3):604–12.
82. Hoffmann J, Cornelius CP, Groten M, Probster L, Schwenzer N. Using individually designed ceramic implants for secondary reconstruction of the bony orbit. Mund Kiefer Gesichtschir. 1998 May;2(Suppl 1):S98–101.
83. Holck DE, Boyd EM Jr, Ng J, Mauffray RO. Benefits of stereolithography in orbital reconstruction. Ophthalmology. 1999 Jun;106(6):1214–8.
84. Metzger MC, Schön R, Zizelmann C, Weyer N, Gutwald R, Schmelzeisen R. Semi-automatic procedure for individual preforming of titanium meshes for orbital fractures. Plast Reconstr Surg. 2007;119(3):969–76.
85. Schmelzeisen R, Gellrich NC, Schoen R, Gutwald R, Zizelmann C, Schramm A. Navigation-aided reconstruction of medial orbital wall and floor contour in cranio-maxillofacial reconstruction. Injury. 2004 Oct;35(10):955–62.
86. Schmelzeisen R, Schramm A. Computer-assisted reconstruction of the facial skeleton. Arch Facial Plast Surg. 2003 Sep-Oct;5(5):437.
87. Bite U, Jackson IT, Forbes GS, Gehring DG. Orbital volume measurements in enophthalmos using three-dimensional CT imaging. Plast Reconstr Surg. 1985 Apr;75(4):502–8.
88. Eufinger H, Wittkampf AR, Wehmoller M, Zonneveld FW. Single-step fronto-orbital resection and reconstruction with individual resection template and corresponding titanium implant: a new method of computer-aided surgery. J Craniomaxillofac Surg. 1998 Dec;26(6):373–8.
89. Heissler E, Fischer FS, Bolouri S, Lehmann T, Mathar W, Gebhardt A, et al. Custom-made cast titanium implants produced with CAD/CAM for the reconstruction of cranium defects. Int J Oral Maxillofac Surg. 1998 Oct;27(5):334–8.
90. Perry M, Banks P, Richards R, Friedman EP, Shaw P. The use of computer-generated three-dimensional models in orbital reconstruction. Br J Oral Maxillofac Surg. 1998 Aug;36(4):275–84.
91. Chang PS, Parker TH, Patrick CW Jr, Miller MJ. The accuracy of stereolithography in planning craniofacial bone replacement. J Craniofac Surg. 2003 Mar;14(2):164–70.
92. Kermer C, Lindner A, Friede I, Wagner A, Millesi W. Preoperative stereolithographic model planning for primary reconstruction in craniomaxillofacial trauma surgery. J Craniomaxillofac Surg. 1998 Jun;26(3):136–9.

93. Zizelmann C, Metzger MC, Gellrich NC, Schoen R, Schmelzeisen R. Minimal invasive computer-assisted reconstruction of orbital floor based on cone beam tomography. Br J Oral Maxillofac Surg. 2005;45:79–80.
94. Metzger MC, Schon R, Weyer N, Rafii A, Gellrich NC, Schmelzeisen R, et al. Anatomical 3-dimensional pre-bent titanium implant for orbital floor fractures. Ophthalmology. 2006 Oct;113(10):1863–8.
95. Scolozzi P, Jaques B. Computer-aided volume measurement of posttraumatic orbits reconstructed with AO titanium mesh plates: accuracy and reliability. Ophthal Plast Reconstr Surg. 2008 Sep–Oct;24(5):383–9.

9 Facial Implant Cosmetic Augmentation Using Digital Technologies

Alex M. Greenberg and Barry Eppley

The perception of facial beauty is based on personal, societal, and professional concepts of esthetics and ideal human form. Facial beauty has been studied since ancient times through mathematics, philosophy, and art [1–3]. With the scientific advances of modern medicine and surgery, this has allowed a deeper understanding of human anatomy, pathology, and their influences on facial beauty. Recent technological advances have increased the tools available to surgeons of the facial region to achieve improvements in their techniques and results [4]. Facial augmentation is an important aspect of cosmetic and reconstructive surgery that can benefit from new advances in digital radiology and rapid prototyping technologies. This chapter will demonstrate the use of 3-D stereolithographic models to adapt stock implants and virtual planning to create patient-specific solid silicone implants for facial implant fabrication. Facial augmentation for esthetic, acquired, facial rejuvenation, and congenital deformities has been performed using a variety of autogenous materials since the early work of Gillies and Aufricht [5–7]. Facial implants have become commonly performed procedures for augmentation of the chin, mandibular angles, zygomas, nasal, and forehead regions using a variety of alloplastic materials and need to be in harmony and proportion with the major esthetic zones of the face and the other anatomic structures. Alloplastic stock implants with standard shapes and sizes have been successfully used for more than 50 years since the first report of Rubin [8]. Solid silicone, polyethylene, HTR, and ePTFE have been the most commonly used materials which are available as both stock implants and blocks for hand carving [9–11]. Stock implants have been successfully used but can have limitations in their use because of the small number of sizes and great variations of patient anatomy and cosmetic considerations (Fig. 9.1a–x). Stock implants can be better selected and customized by hand carving through the use of 3-D stereolithographic models. This chapter will review methods for the fabrication of custom facial implants based on stereolithographic models and virtual planning to create patient-specific solid silicone implants. Although there are additional costs of a stereolithographic model, time for creation of the implant(s), and costs for implant fabrication, patient-specific implants can provide significant advantages over stock implants. For the method of hand fabricated custom facial implants, wax is utilized to form prototypes of these implants on 3-D stereolithographic anatomically accurate models which are carved to the desired contours. The wax prototype is then converted to the final solid silicone implant by an experienced laboratory. The style of implant custom prepared depends on the indications for its use, whether for primary or secondary genioplasty, mandibular angle augmentation, or zygomatic augmentation. It is especially helpful in cases of revision genioplasty when osteotomies have had relapse, contour irregularities, step defects, or an undesirable result. Satisfactory capsule formation around the implants permits smooth soft tissue contours. These implants are placed only using an intraoral incision.

A.M. Greenberg (✉)
Division of Oral and Maxillofacial Surgery, Columbia University College of Dental Medicine, 18 East 48th Street Suite 1702, New York, NY 10017, USA
e-mail: nycimplant@aol.com

Patient Evaluation and Anthropometric Measurements

The perception of facial beauty is based on many factors which includes sex, ethnicity, size, facial proportions, and cultural attitudes. It can be difficult to determine in a society exactly what the current concept of beauty may be. We can look at the historical record since ancient times and there are many references in both art and literature (Fig. 9.1y). Patients need to be evaluated for hard and soft tissue aspects of their deformity. Hard tissue analysis includes bony anatomy and dental occlusion. Patient anthropometric analysis includes a clinical examination with a facial proportions analysis as defined by Farkas [12, 13] and others. For chin augmentation, this should include lateral cephalometric radiographic analyses of Burstone [14–16], Ricketts [17]

A.M. Greenberg (ed.), *Digital Technologies in Craniomaxillofacial Surgery*, https://doi.org/10.1007/978-1-4939-1532-3_9

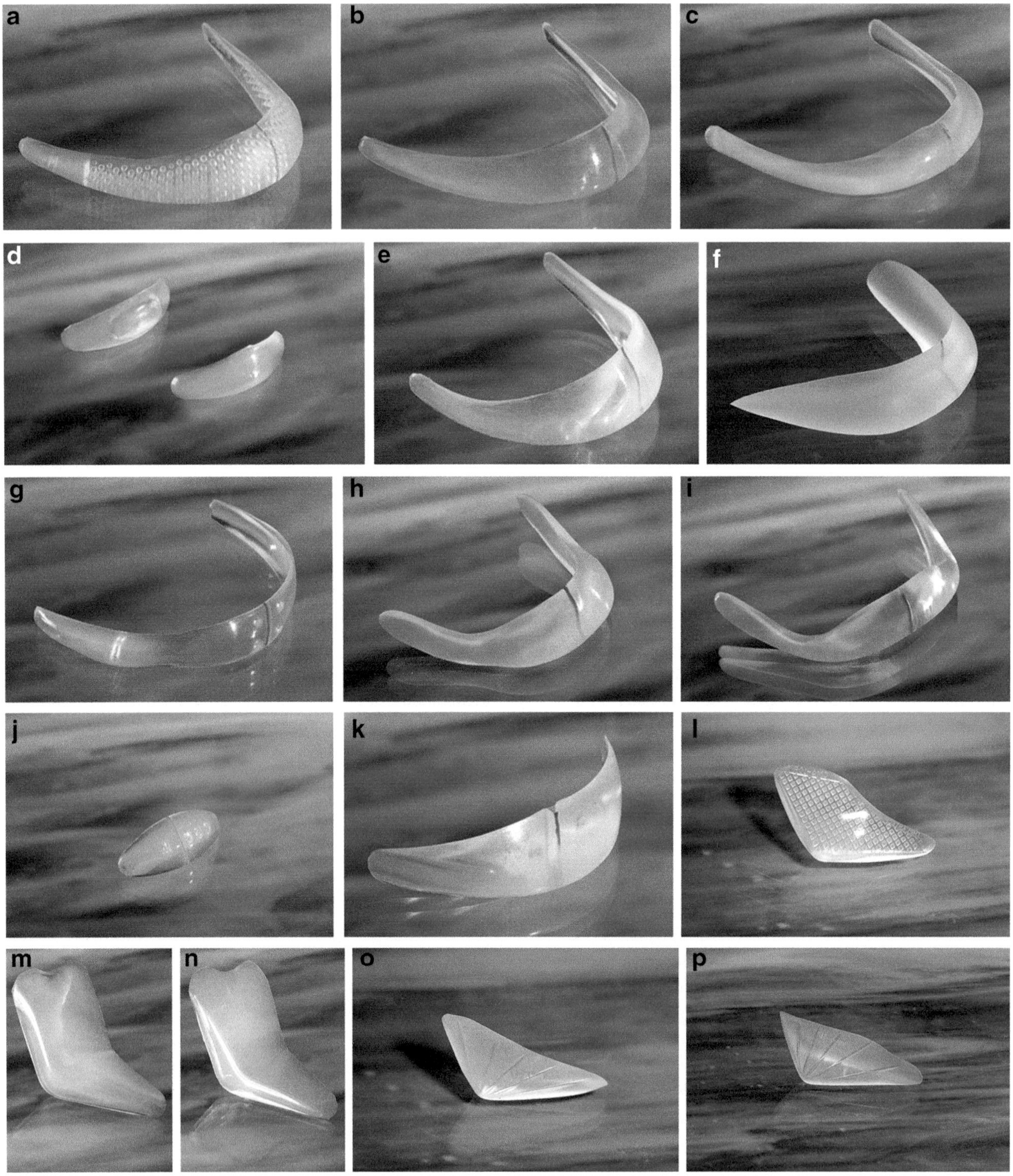

Fig. 9.1 Examples of various stock silicone chin, mandibular angle, and malar implants. (**a**) Conform™ Extended Anatomical Chin Implant (Implantech, Ventura, CA, USA). (**b**) Extended Anatomical Chin Implant (Implantech, Ventura, CA, USA). (**c**) Terino Extended Anatomical™ Chin Implant (Implantech, Ventura, CA, USA). (**d**) Glasgold Wafer™ for the Extended Anatomical Chin and Glasgold Wafer™ for the Pre-Jowl Chin (Implantech, Ventura, CA, USA). (**e**) Flowers Mandibular Glove® (Implantech, Ventura, CA, USA). (**f**) Vertical Lengthening Chin (Implantech, Ventura, CA, USA). (**g**) Mittelman Pre-Jowl® (Implantech, Ventura, CA, USA). (**h**) Terino Square Chin – Style I (Implantech, Ventura, CA, USA). (**i**) Terino Square Chin – Style II (Implantech, Ventura, CA, USA). (**j**) Curvilinear Silicone Chin (Implantech, Ventura, CA, USA). (**k**) Anatomical Chin (Implantech, Ventura, CA, USA). (**l**) Conform™ Mandibular Angle implant (Implantech, Ventura, CA, USA). (**m**) Lateral Mandibular Angle™ implant (Implantech, Ventura, CA, USA). (**n**) Posterior Mandibular Angle™ implant (Implantech, Ventura, CA, USA). (**o**) Widening mandibular angle implant (Implantech, Ventura, CA, USA). (**p**) Vertical mandibular angle implant (Implantech, Ventura, CA, USA). (**q**) Binder Submalar ® implant (Implantech, Ventura, CA, USA). (**r**) Binder Submalar II ® implant (Implantech, Ventura, CA, USA). (**s**) Conform Binder Submalar ® implant (Implantech, Ventura, CA, USA). (**t**) Conform Terino Malar Shell® (Implantech, Ventura, CA, USA).

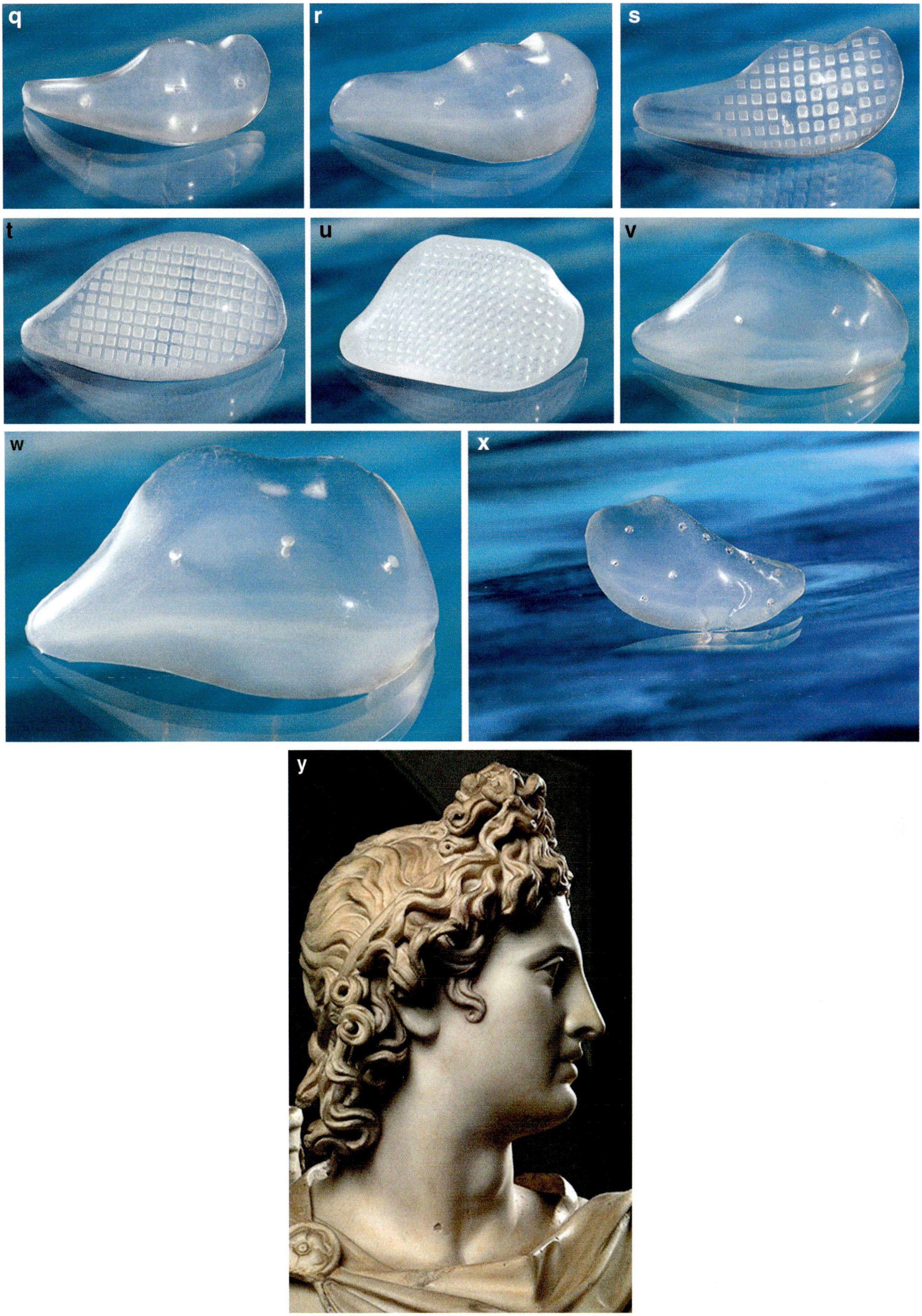

Fig. 9.1 (continued) (**u**) Conform™ Midfacial (Implantech, Ventura, CA, USA). (**v**) Terino Malar Shell® (Implantech, Ventura, CA, USA). (**w**) Combined Submalar Shell™ (Implantech, Ventura, CA, USA). (**x**) Flowers Tear Trough® (Implantech, Ventura, CA, USA). (**y**) Classic sculpture representing golden ratio (By permission, Apollo Belvedere, Vatican Museum, Rome, Italy)

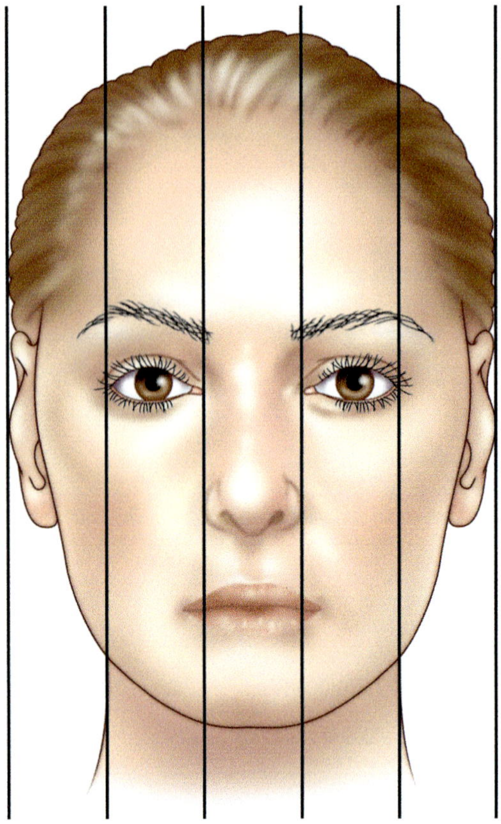

Fig. 9.2 Frontal facial view in vertical fifth divisions

and Steiner [18, 19], and Gonzalez-Ulloa [20–22], as well as the soft tissue evaluation of neck-throat angle. The mandibular form is classified as low, medium, and high plane. Lip posture and competence, as well as the presence of mentalis strain need to be evaluated. 3-D imaging also provides possibilities for the evaluation of the facial bones and overlying soft tissues.

Facial proportions take into consideration the relationship between the esthetic zones of the chin, eyes, nose, cheekbones, maxilla, mandible, and frontal region. For a face to be considered esthetically pleasing, a balance and harmony between these esthetic zones needs to exist [23]. The face can be divided horizontally and vertically from a frontal perspective. The vertical evaluation begins with a midline from which the face is then divided into five zones (Fig. 9.2), the central zone being the medial canthi/nasal alar base, in equal units until the lateral external ear boundaries. In the lateral view, the "Zero Meridian" of Gonzalez-Ulloa [20–22] is utilized from soft tissue nasion vertically perpendicular to the Frankfort plane or cephalometrically to SN (corrected in COGS) (Fig. 9.3) [14, 15].

The face is also divided into vertical thirds: uppermost (hairline to glabella (G)), middle (glabella (G)) to subnasale (Sn), and lower (subnasale (Sn)) to menton (Mn) [23] (Fig. 9.4a, b). The neck is considered a separate anatomic region that can have influence on the perception of the facial

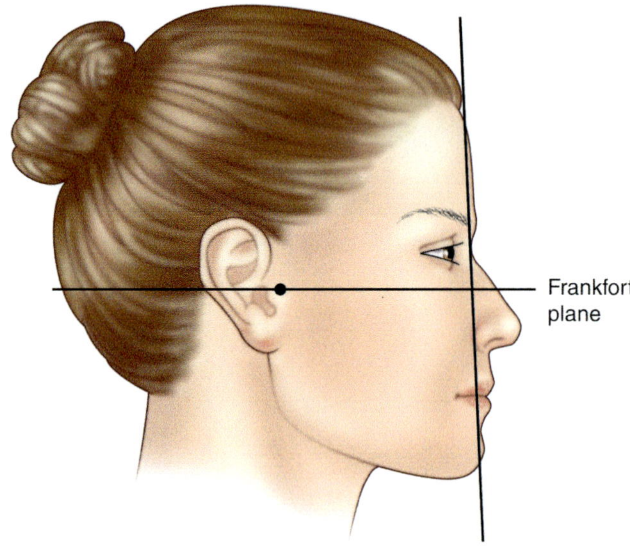

Fig. 9.3 Frankfort Horizontal with Gonzalez-Ulloa Zero Meridian

form and age of the patient. Skin texture, presence of rhytids, and support are of special importance in the older patient [24]. Facial shapes are classified as round, oval, square, and diamond/pear/tapered ovoid (Fig. 9.5) [23].

Custom Alloplastic Genioplasty

Chin Evaluation

The chin is one of the major esthetic units structures of the face (chin, nose, eyes, cheekbones, mandibular angles, and forehead). Different facial proportions are used to determine the ideal chin esthetics, with various clinical and radiographic analyses utilized. The chin is the most important structure of the facial skeletal framework of the lower facial third, and its ideal esthetic is in balance with the lower lip and the labiomental fold as the dividing boundary. The upper/midface and lower face proportions represent an esthetic balance of facial harmony based on the golden ratio of 1: 1.618 [25–27] which has been described since ancient times (Fig. 9.6). The lower facial third consists of a horizontal line drawn from subnasale (Sn). The chin has both vertical, horizontal, and width aspects that contribute to its appearance. The chin can be evaluated separate from the mandible and both structures are closely related based on occlusion. The classical proportion utilized for chin evaluation is the "Zero Meridian" (Gonzalez-Ulloa Line) [20–22] of classical Greek sculpture, as a vertical line drawn from soft tissue nasion perpendicular to the Frankfort horizontal or corrected SNA of the COGS analysis [20–22, 27]. Soft tissue pogonion (Pg) should be coincident with the "Zero Meridian" [20–22]. The mentolabial sulcus should be

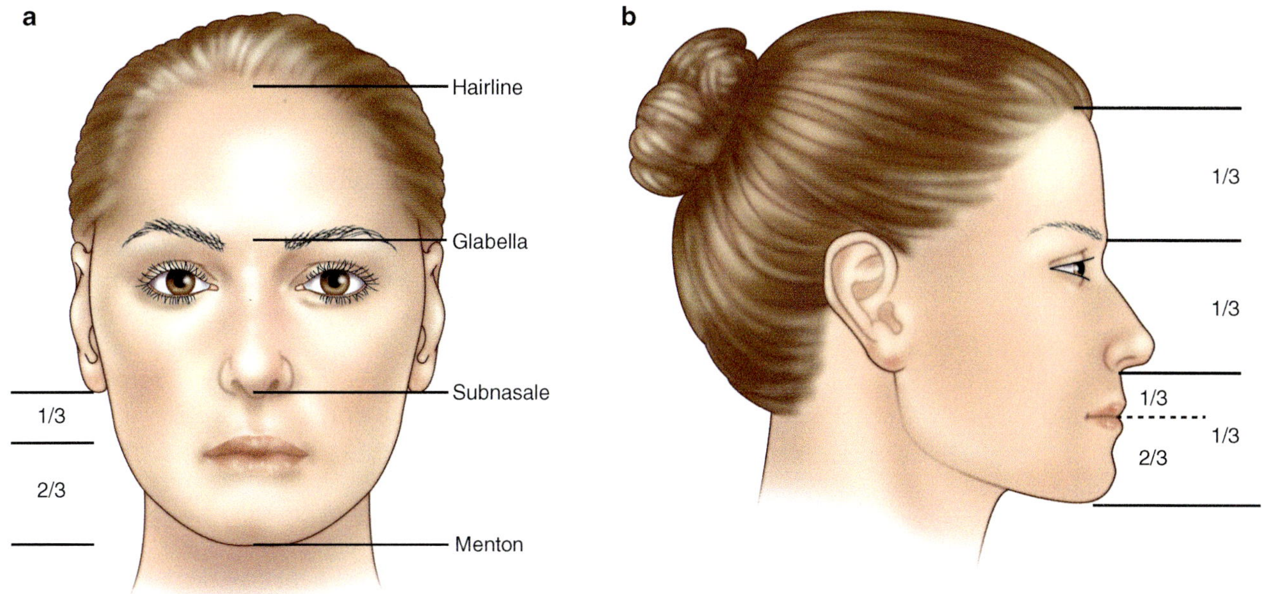

Fig. 9.4 (**a**) Frontal facial view in vertical thirds. Subnasale to stomion superioris one third to stomion superioris to menton two thirds ratio. (**b**) Lateral facial view in vertical thirds. Subnasale to stomion superioris 1/3 to stomion superioris to menton 2/3 ratio

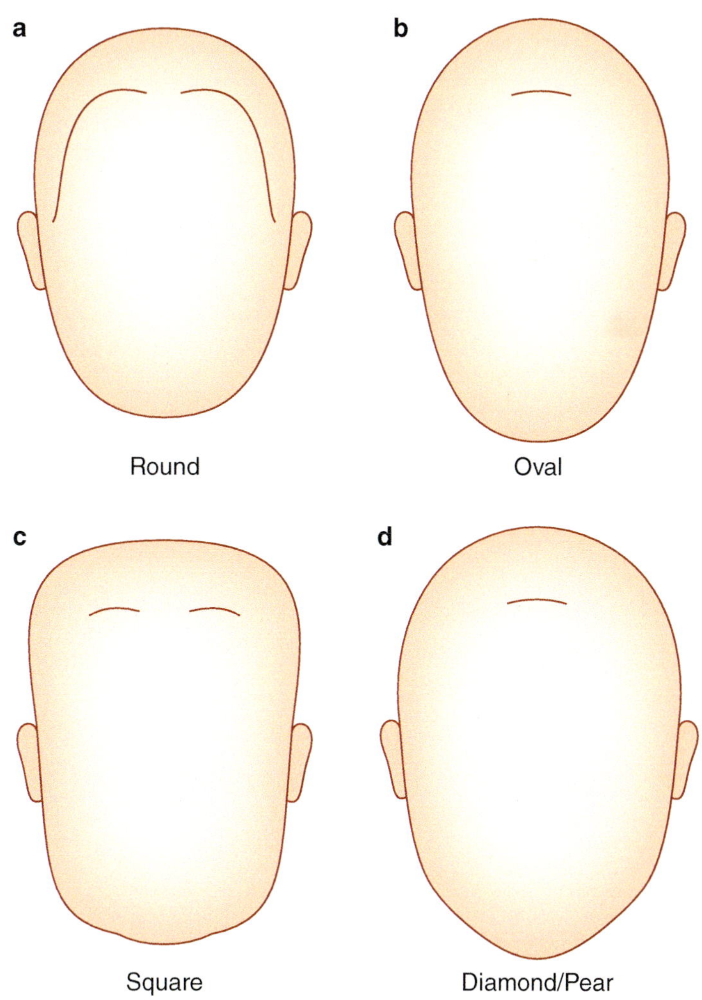

Fig. 9.5 Four basic facial types: (**a**) round, (**b**) oval, (**c**) square, (**d**) diamond/pear/tapered ovoid

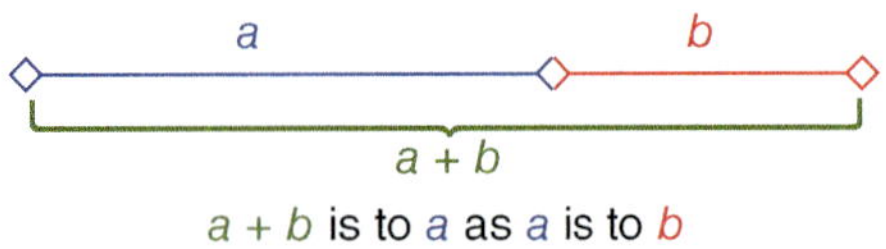

Fig. 9.6 The golden ratio 1:1.618

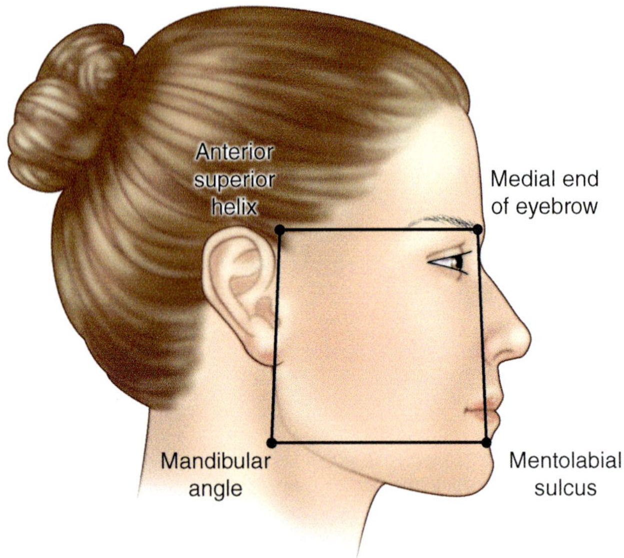

Fig. 9.7 Leonardo's square

Table 9.1 Classification of dental occlusion

Class I
Class II
Class III with mandibular prognathism
Class III with maxillary hypoplasia and normal mandible

3–4 mm posterior to Sn-Pg [23]. The chin can also be defined by Leonardo's square from the mentolabial sulcus to the mandibular angle (Gn-Me) to the anterior superior helix and the medial end of the eyebrow [23] (Fig. 9.7). The proportion of the upper to the lower lip should be in a ratio of Sn-Stm(s) to Stm(i)-Me 1/3–2/3. This provides a ratio of Sn-Stm(s)/Stm(i)-Me = 1:2 or 0.5. A ratio of >0.5 represents vertical chin excess, while <0.5 will be a vertical deficiency [23].

There are also different considerations between the youthful and the aging face with respect to the chin. In the young the elastic properties of the soft tissues allow a more direct correlation between the underlying bony structure and the overlying soft tissues in terms of an osteotomy or implant. In the aging face, the ptosis or laxity of the submental tissues can include lipodystrophy and platysma herniation. In the young the reconstruction of the chin relates to combined orthognathic surgery or individual chin procedures specific to proportionate balance with the face. In the aging population, a pre-existing chin deformity and bony contour deficiency often correlate to laxity of soft tissues for which chin augmentation alone in certain cases can also significantly improve the neck-throat angle and skin laxity [24]. Drape of the middle facial third can also provide significant rejuvenation from chin augmentation even without a facelift. In other circumstances chin implants may be combined with other facelifting procedures to manage the geniomandibular notch, jowling, and marionette lines. The neck-throat angle can range from perpendicular to obtuse. In some patients there is no definition with a straight line from the chin to the neck.

Dental occlusion is also readily evaluated on visual inspection and is important to evaluate in a systematic fashion (Table 9.1) [23] (Fig. 9.8); many patients with chin deficiency will have a Class II dentofacial deformity.

Fig. 9.8 Angle's classification of occlusion and facial types. (**a**) Class I. (**b**) Class II. (**c**) Class III

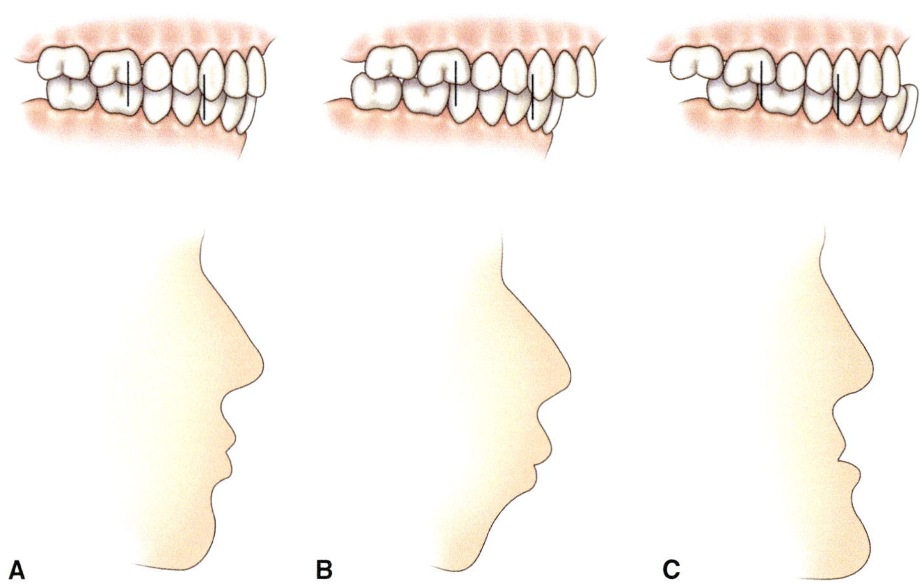

CT Scanning for Evaluation and Creation of a Stereolithographic Model

In addition to the clinical evaluation of the patient, it is also necessary to obtain a CT or CBCT of the patient with a 3-D image generated. Bony anatomy is best evaluated using a lateral cephalometric radiograph (Fig. 9.9) or other 3-D CT imaging modalities [28, 29] (Fig. 9.10a, b). The advantage of CBCT with a full FOV is that in addition to the CT data, it also provides a lateral cephalometric view. To obtain an accurate image, the patient's upper and lower lips should be at rest [14] and the head in a natural position relative to Frankfort Horizontal when performing the CBCT. The DICOM data is then transferred to a service provider either on a disk or uploaded via a website in order to then fabricate a stereolithographic model. Stereolithographic models are highly accurate anatomically correct representations of the mandible with an accuracy within 0.3 mm and can be color printed with the position of the mandibular nerve and the mental foramen (Fig. 9.11). All models for this article were fabricated by 3D Systems Healthcare (Rock Hill, SC, USA) and Biomedical Modeling (Boston, MA, USA). These models are also accurate for the position of the mandibular nerve and the mental foramen [28, 29]. Stereolithographic models for purely alloplastic genioplasty do not have to include the condylar portion which is less expensive.

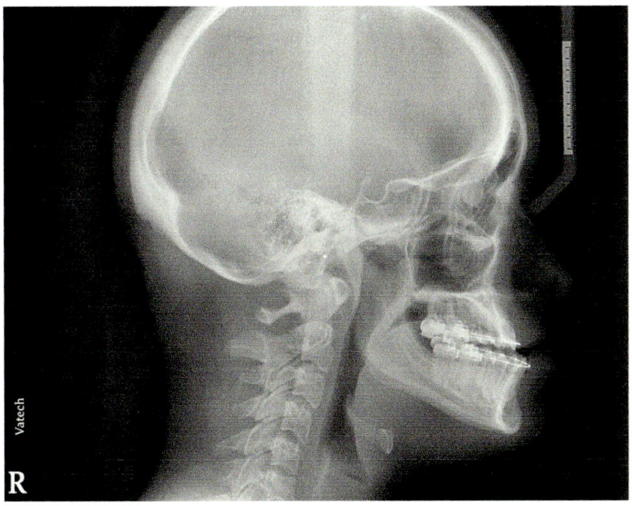

Fig. 9.9 Lateral cephalometric radiograph

A lateral cephalometric radiograph allows the chin to be evaluated in the sagittal and vertical dimensions. A PA cephalometric radiograph allows the chin to be evaluated in the vertical and lateral dimensions (Fig. 9.12).

Facial Moulage

The use of facial moulage can be essential in the analysis and preparation of custom facial implants, as it provides a 3-D representation for reference and wax application for implant simulation. It is obtained by either the application of either polyether or alginate impression materials directly to the face with nasal straws in place to allow breathing. Bent paper clips are placed into the preset material to allow retention of plaster of Paris strips for support of the moulage for removal

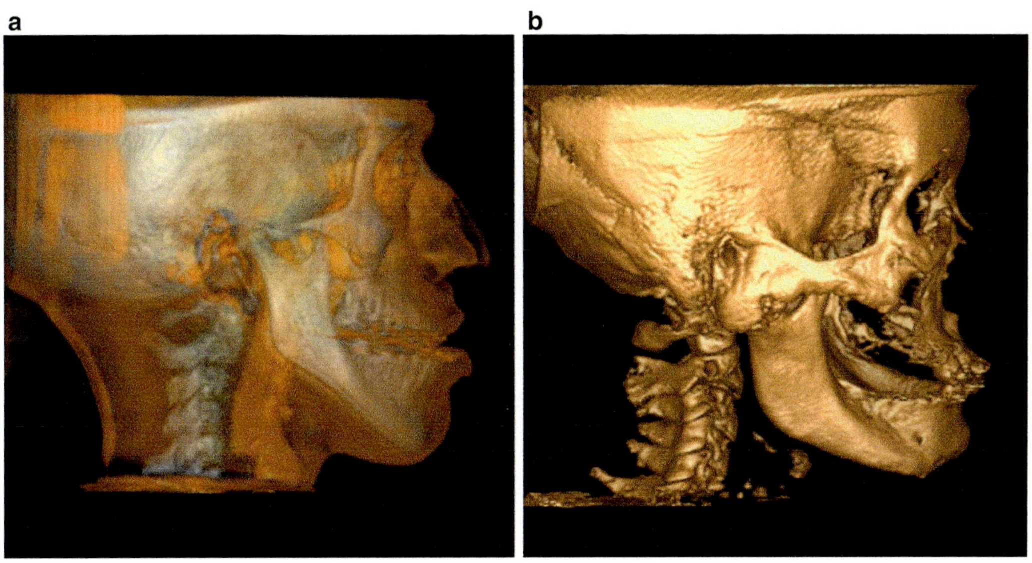

Fig. 9.10 CBCT 3-D images. (**a**) 3-D skin and bone window. (**b**) Bone window

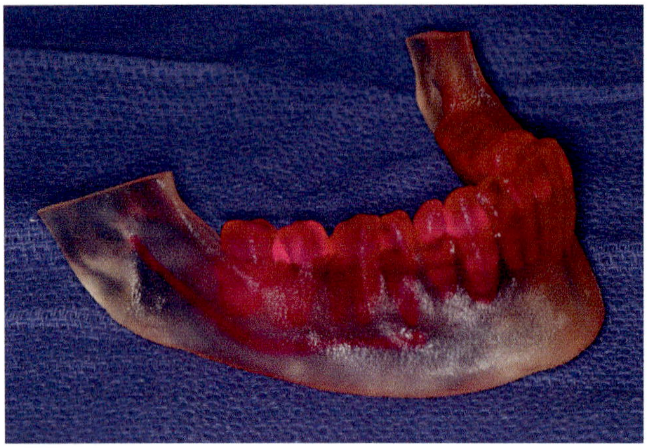

Fig. 9.11 Stereolithographic mandible model

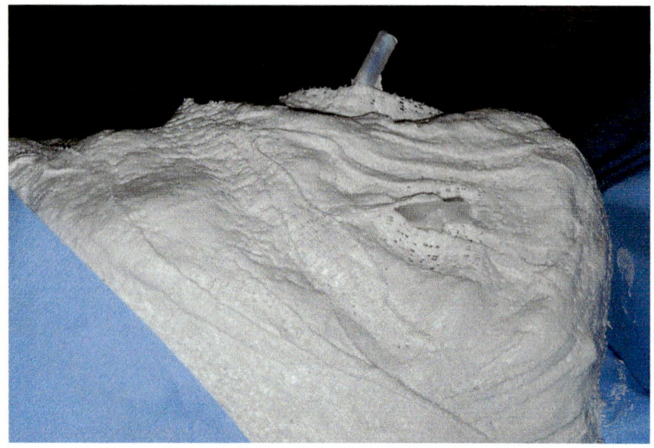

Fig. 9.13 Facial moulage with plaster of Paris covering and nasal straws

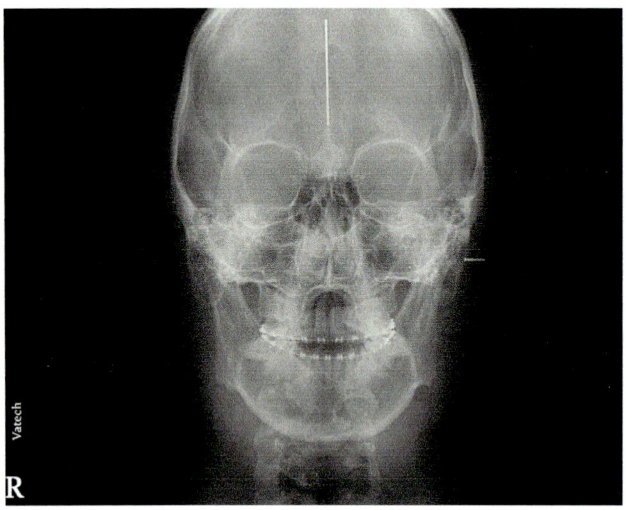

Fig. 9.12 PA cephalometric radiograph

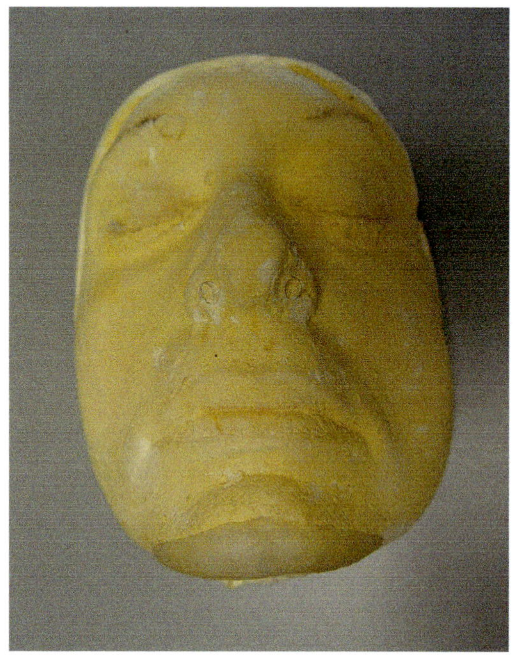

Fig. 9.14 Stone facial moulage model

and pouring of stone (Fig. 9.13). Once the moulage is complete, it is removed and stone is poured into the mold creating the positive model (Fig. 9.14). Patients need to be told to maintain facial expression in a relaxed position and not to animate when the impression material is applied in order to obtain an accurate mold.

The chin morphology and its proportions to the other major facial esthetic units will determine the surgical approach. The chin should be considered as a single structure, even though it has developed embryologically by fusion in the facial midline of the two mandibular halves [30]. This can be seen in many patients when there is radiographic evidence of a symphyseal midline suture. The chin is anatomically defined as the region of the anterior mandible bounded by the mental foramina, the inferior border up to the apices of the first and second premolar teeth, and the midline mental protuberance (Fig. 9.15). Laterally positioned mental tubercles may be prominent and represent muscle attachments and help provide support for the soft tissue drape of the chin. The mental nerves are of great clinical importance as they provide sensation of the lower lip and chin as well as the buccal mucosa and gingiva. Soft tissue dissection must take into careful consideration the mental nerves and their identification, preservation, and avoidance of injury. The mental nerve often extends as a loop anterior to the foramen with the incisive nerve branches that are of little clinical significance [31].

In planning the alloplastic genioplasty, there are other important anatomic structures and clinical landmarks which include the mentalis, depressor anguli oris, depressor labii inferioris, levator labii inferioris, digastric muscles, and the apices of the mandibular incisors, canines, and premolars.

Chin morphology can vary considerably in relation to dental occlusion in the sagittal, vertical, and lateral dimensions but will follow certain general patterns based on dental occlusion. Patients can have a normal Class I occlusion with retrogenia and vertical hyperplasia or hypoplasia. A Class III dental occlusion secondary to mandibular prognathism will usually have a prominent chin (Fig. 9.16a). Class II secondary to maxillary hyperplasia with a normal or retrognathic mandible is often associated with retrogenia (Fig. 9.16b). Soft tissue evaluation includes the lips, mentalis activity, labiomental fold, and neck. The lips can vary in their morphology in close correlation with the dental occlusion and any associated dentofacial deformity.

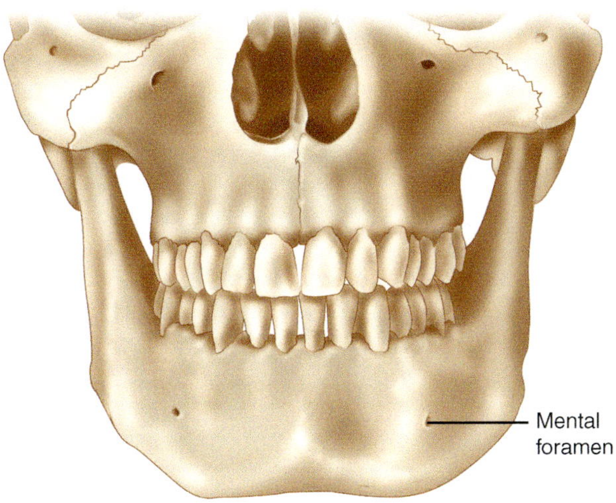

Fig. 9.15 Chin regional anatomy

Analysis of the chin should then include the following:

1. Lips and labiomental fold
2. Neck to mandible relationship
3. Nasal anatomy
4. Chin position
5. Dental occlusion

Zide developed the QUAC analysis for the chin (Quick Analysis of the Chin) to include (1) lip eversion, (2) anterior teeth, (3) chin pad thickness, (4) labiomental fold depth, and (5) dynamic chin pad motion with smile [32].

The essential elements of analyzing the chin involve the other related structures of the lips, nose, and neck. The lips by themselves have specific contours. The lower lip can have a high, middle, or low labiomental fold with an average depth of 4 mm with long (Fig. 9.17) or short superior lip form [32] (Fig. 9.18). This can also be considered as a high or low position of the labiomental fold. Position of the superior portion of the lip also be influenced by the occlusion with a rolled over lower lip seen in Class II malocclusion (Fig. 9.19a) and a lack of neck-throat definition (Fig. 9.19b). Depending on the occlusion, lip competence and animation will play an important role in analysis as well. A retruded chin in the presence of lip incompetence will create a flattened appearance of the chin pad and lengthening of the

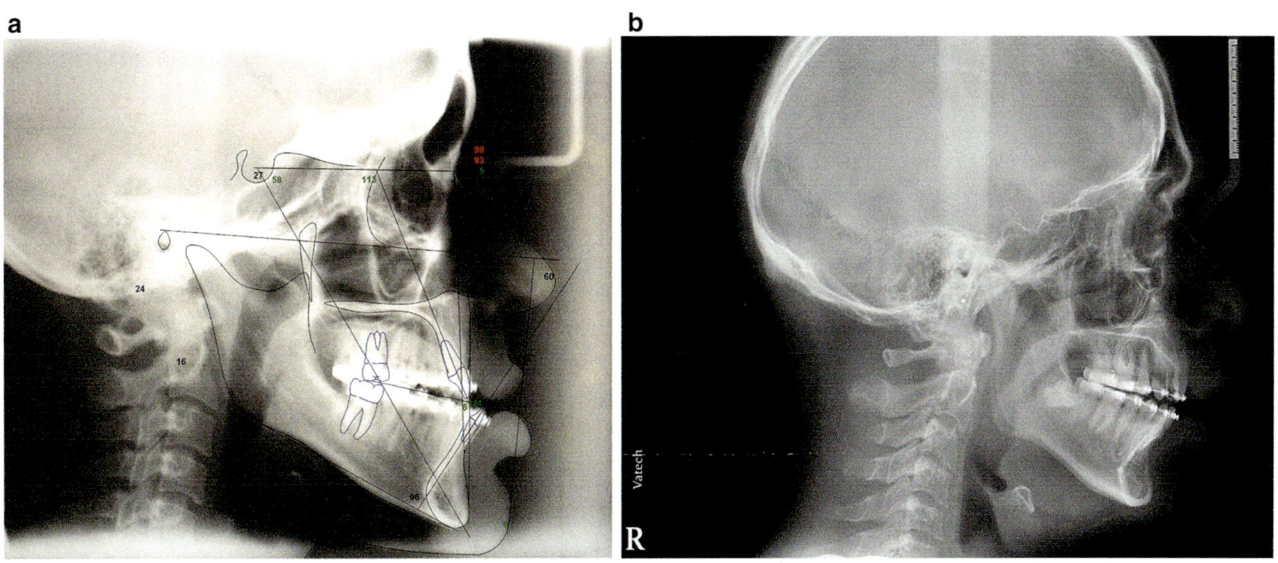

Fig. 9.16 (**a**) Lateral cephalometric radiograph of Class III mandibular prognathism. (**b**) Lateral cephalometric radiograph of Class II skeletal malocclusion with retrognathia and retrognathia

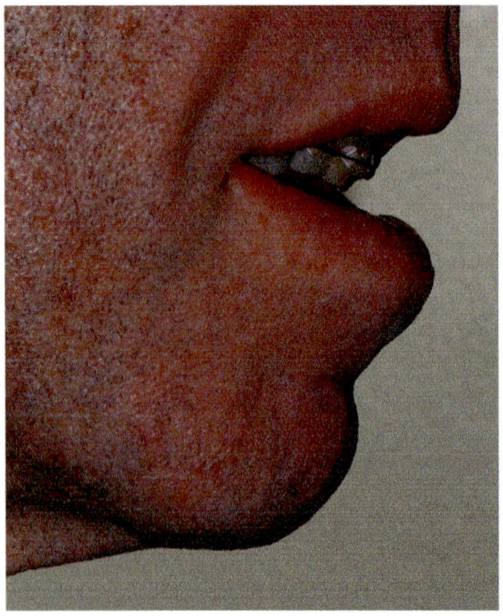

Fig. 9.17 Long lower lip

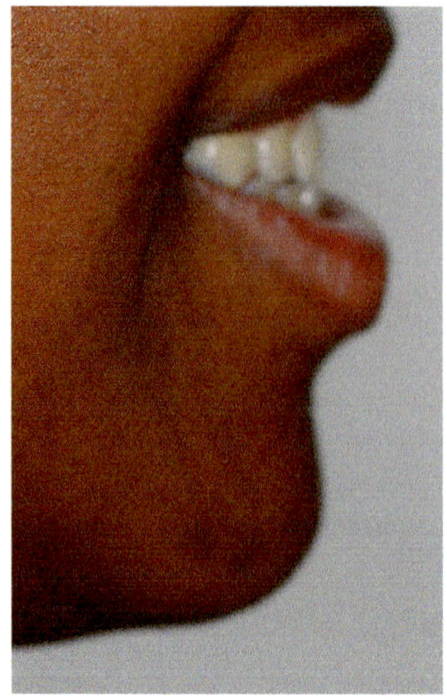

Fig. 9.18 Short superior lower lip

Fig. 9.19 (**a**) Class II malocclusion with everted lower lip. (**b**) Class II malocclusion with everted lower lip and lack of neck-throat angle definition

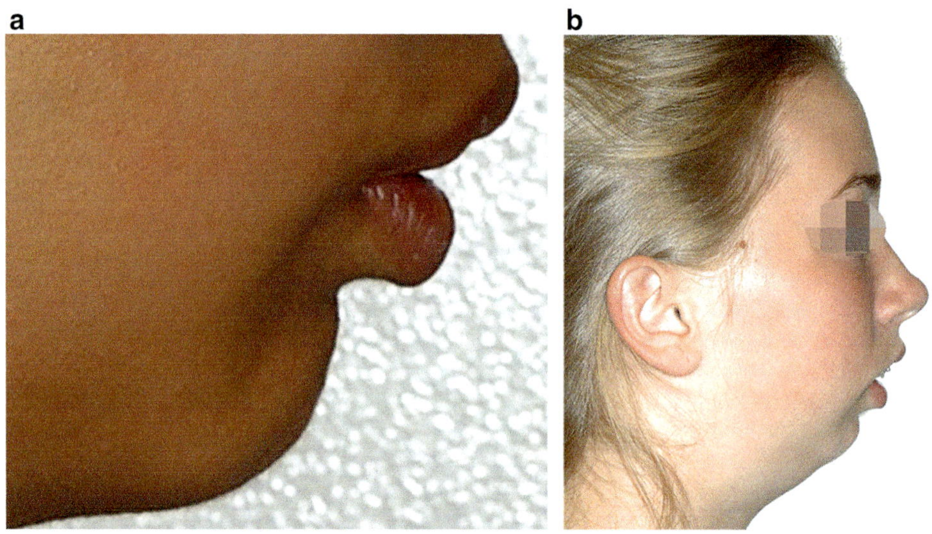

lower lip and chin with "mentalis strain" and loss of the labiomental sulcus (Fig. 9.20). It is essential in the clinical evaluation that the chin be evaluated both in repose and animation. In repose the chin will appear in its true anatomic form, while in animation in closure of the lips or puckering, functional appearance becomes evident such as mentalis strain or fasciculations [17]. Fasciculations and irregularities in the chin pad appearance will add to the appearance of a deformity and are often increased in previously operated chins, whether by implant or osteotomy (Fig. 9.21). Vertical height of the lip to chin dimension is also important with respect to the classical facial proportions of the "golden ratio" also referred to as Rickett's divine proportion [25, 26] and other anthropometric norms such as the work of Farkas and others [12–14]. Proportions of the face in vertical dimension should be 43%:57% from N-Sn to Sn-Me [23] (Fig. 9.22a, b). The nasal tip also influences perception of the chin with a large nose creating the appearance of a retruded chin and a small nose creating a more balanced or large chin [32] (Fig. 9.23a, b). The neck is also an important factor depending on whether there is a distinct jaw throat angle that is acute or obtuse. If lipodystrophy is present, the chin also loses its definition (Fig. 9.24). In the aging patient, lipodystrophy and platysma disruption or ptosis is more common and it is important to determine if liposuction or platysma repair is needed. This will influence the inferior aspect of the chin and whether a distinct jaw line is present. Jowling with loss of the geniomanibular definition and midfacial loss of lip support are also aspects of the aging chin and need to be noted if present. The neck-throat angle of cervical point (C)

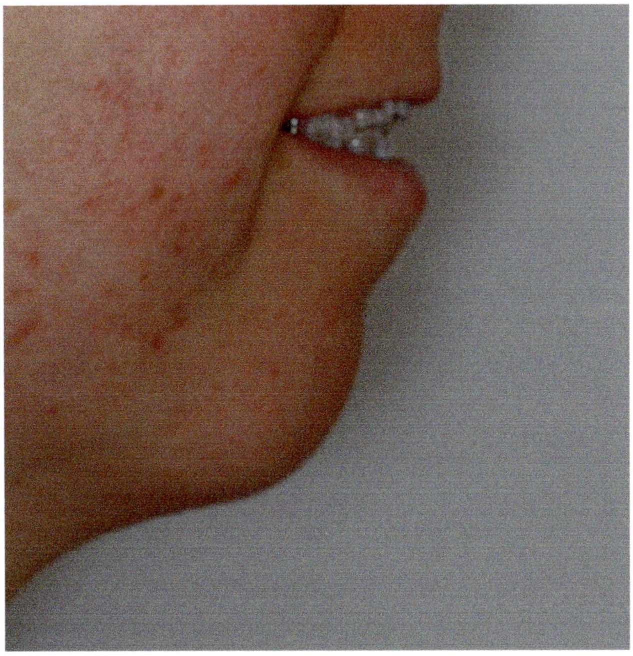

Fig. 9.20 Lower lip and chin mentalis strain

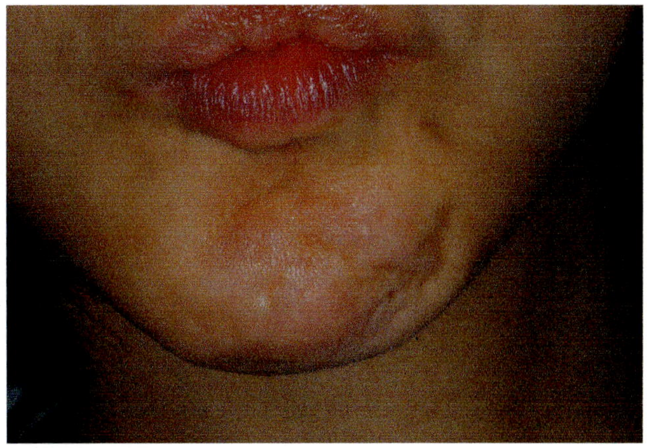

Fig. 9.21 Soft tissue fasciculations of chin also demonstrates loss of depressor labia inferioris inferior insertion

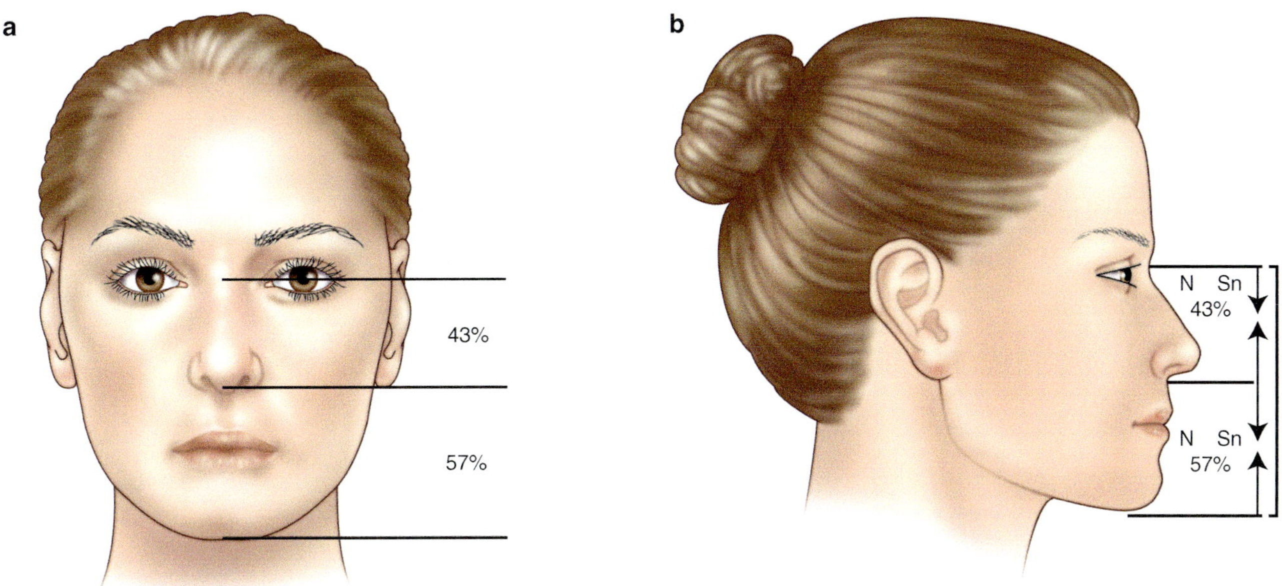

Fig. 9.22 (a) Frontal facial view of proportions from nasion to menton. (b) Lateral facial of proportions from nasion to menton

to mandibular angle (Gn) ideal is = 100 degrees. The mento-cervical angle of Powell G-Pg/Me-C = 85 degrees [23] (Fig. 9.25). Use of radiographic, photographic, and clinical objective analysis is critical to the complete understanding of the chin morphology. Other adjuncts such as photographs, facial moulage, and software programs such as Dolphin using 3-D CT data (Dolphin Imaging, Chatsworth, CA, USA) can also be very useful. Evaluation of the patient can include both numerical analysis of a lateral cephalometric radiograph using certain established evaluative methods. Prediction tracings whether from acetate drawings or software create should be utilized. While facial proportion measurements can be an important planning aid, it is still the surgeon's visual evaluation of the patient and discussions with the patient to establish the diagnosis of the facial deformity, patient desires, and surgical plan.

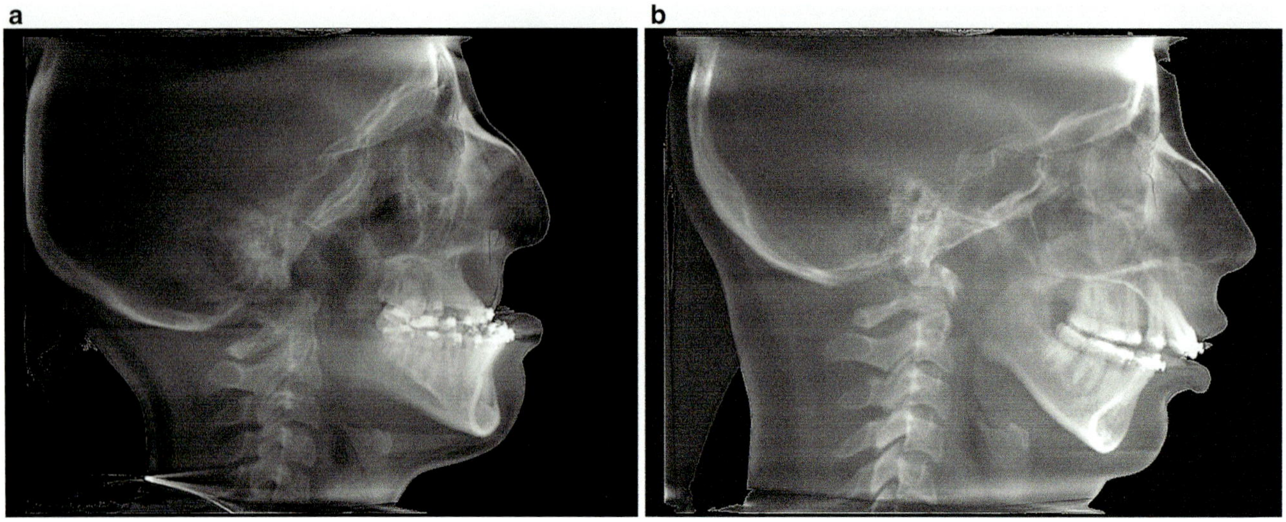

Fig. 9.23 (**a**) Large nose creating greater appearance of retrogenia in a cleft palate patient with Class III malocclusion. (**b**) Large nose creating greater appearance of retrogenia in a patient with Class II malocclusion

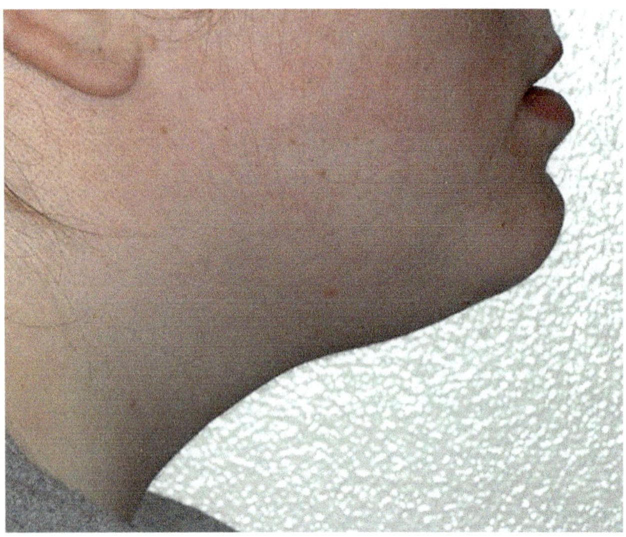

Fig. 9.24 Submental lipodystrophy and obtuse neck-throat angle

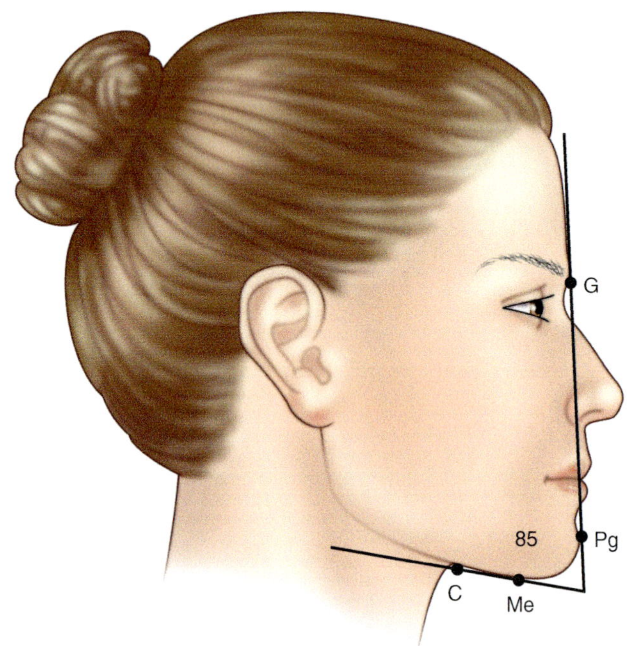

Fig. 9.25 The mentocervical angle of Powell

Surgical Planning for Custom Alloplastic Genioplasty

Patients who are being considered for custom alloplastic genioplasty need to be categorized as to whether they have a dentofacial deformity related to skeletal malocclusion or a pure dysmorphology of the chin or normal findings. The final result will depend on both the hard and soft tissues that will be affected by the possible orthognathic surgical procedures that can have both active and passive effects on chin morphology. Orthognathic surgery can result in the passive reduction or augmentation of the chin depending on whether a mandibular advancement or setback procedure is being performed [33, 34] (Fig. 9.26a–d). This can also affect asymmetry of the mandible as well. Patients who need chin augmentation may have had orthognathic surgery or as a simultaneous procedure. Consultation with the orthodontist for planned orthognathic surgery and chin augmentation is an essential communication in establishing the treatment plan.

In treatment planning it is helpful to classify chin morphology for alloplastic genioplasty. This should be based on

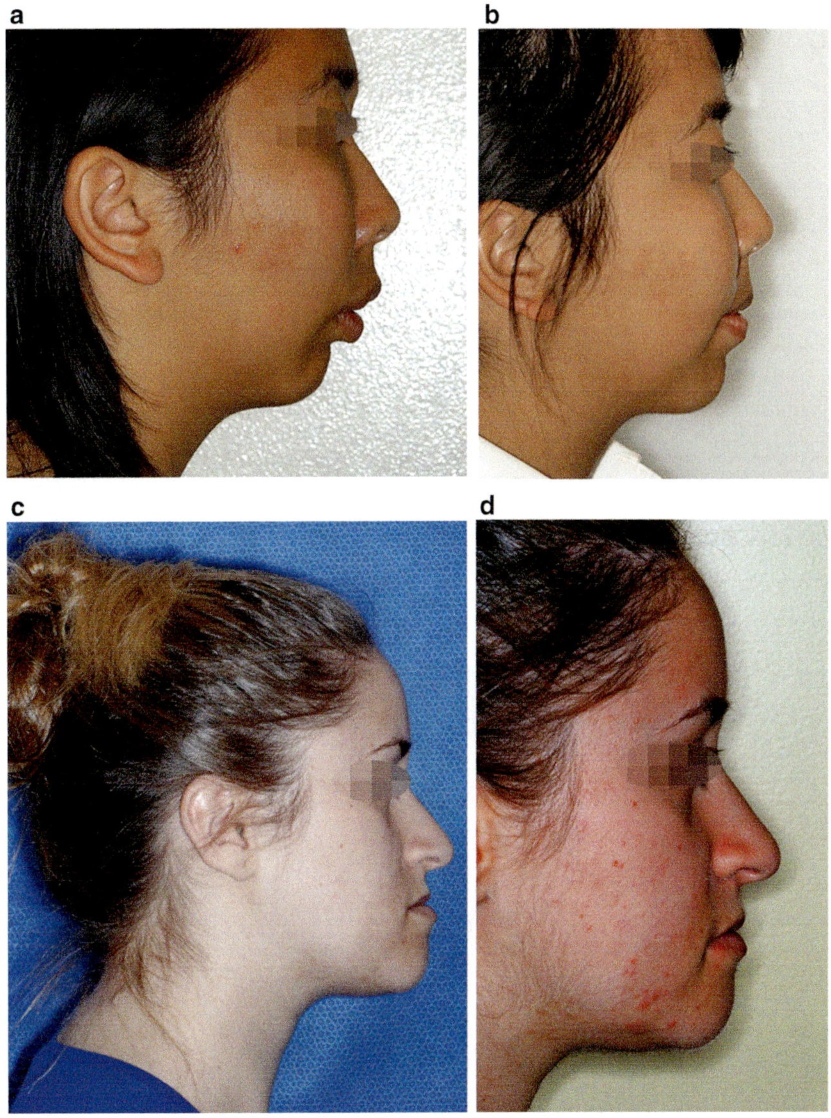

Fig. 9.26 (**a**) Preoperative lateral facial view Class II skeletal malocclusion. (**b**) Lateral facial view postoperative bilateral mandibular sagittal ramus osteotomies with passive chin advancement. (**c**) Lateral facial view Class III skeletal malocclusion with mandibular prognathism. (d) Lateral facial view postoperative bilateral mandibular vertical ramus osteotomies with passive chin retropositioning

the vertical, horizontal, and transverse (frontal) dimensions, as well as the presence of any asymmetry. Evaluation of the skeletal and soft tissue landmarks in the chin should be observed for coincidence with the facial and dental midlines. Chin retrusion or asymmetry can occur as the result of previous fractures or traumatic injuries to the mandibular condyle and meniscus, TMJ pathology, or congenital or developmental malformations. Hemimaxillary-hemimandibular hyperplasia [35] and vertical maxillary hyperplasia with clockwise mandibular autorotation usually as a Class II skeletal malocclusion with retrogenia should be identified correctly. Analyses of the nose and neck are essential in the evaluation of the chin. The nose is the central prominent projection of the face, and its size and form can change the harmony of the chin to the face. The ideal nasal length is 1/3 of facial height with a normal nasal tilt angle of 95 degrees which can depend on chin position [23]. The nasofrontal angle will be 30–40 degrees [23]. Having the patient protrude the mandible can allow the surgeon to gain an understanding of how augmentation can change the appearance of the chin. [16]. Depending on the plan of alloplastic augmentation, the effects of profile changes in the chin area can be significantly different in the horizontal and vertical position depending on the chin width desired. The mean ratio of soft tissue to hard tissue augmentation is generally 1:1 at pogonion [36–38]. Classification of chin types is important to diagnosis and should include the hard and soft tissue aspects of chin morphology (see Table 9.2).

Soft tissue considerations include lip incompetence with mentalis strain, lip morphology, asymmetry [39], fasciculations, aging changes such as marionette lines and rhytids, skin texture, neck/chin drape, submental crease, submental lipodystrophy, scarring, and hardware effects from prior surgery, and geniomandibular notches, or a superior perpendicular edge from prior anterior horizontal mandibular osteotomy [24, 32] (Fig. 9.27a–c). Old hardware can

Table 9.2 Classification of chin types

Horizontal-lateral
(a) Flat
(b) S-shaped
(c) Retruded
Horizontal-frontal
(a) Wide
(b) Narrow or pointed
(c) Symmetry
Vertical-lateral
(a) Vertical hyperplasia
(b) Vertical hypoplasia
Vertical frontal
(a) Short
(b) Normal
(c) Long
(d) Symmetry

often be left in place if they are miniplates, but larger plates from fractures should be removed. Implants can be, designed so that screw fixation holes are located to avoid retained hardware. Patients may also present with completely normal chins in proportion and in harmony with the face that they would like to augment as their own personal preference. Men have a preference for strong chins and may also request the creation of a midline cleft.

As with any cosmetic procedure, successful outcomes are highly dependent on good communication between the surgeon and the patient with regard to the surgical plan and expectation of the result. Patients with unrealistic expectations or a mismatch between their physical appearance and a desired facial change may need psychological counseling. Failure of the surgeon to correctly diagnose the deformity, incorrect fabrication of the implant, or a combination of the two can lead to a patient displeased with the result. Guyuron

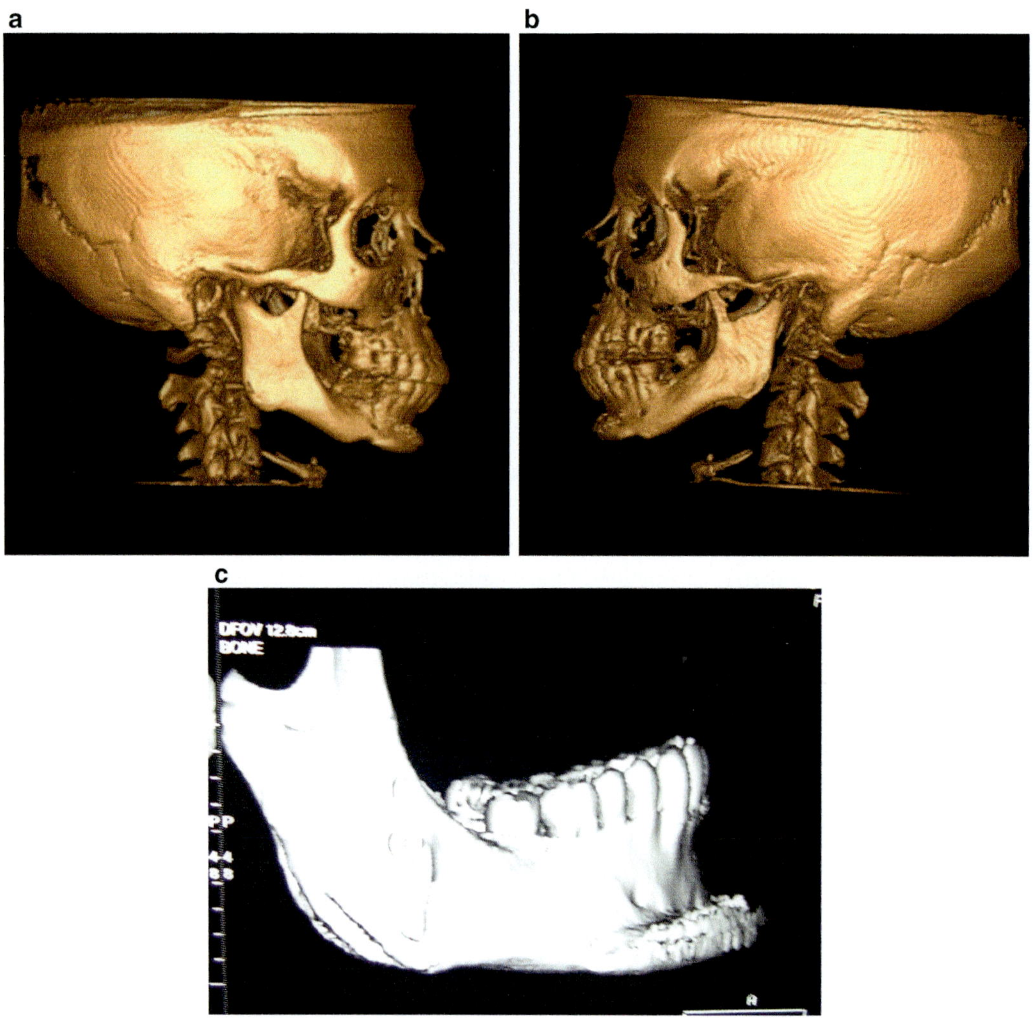

Fig. 9.27 (**a**) Right lateral view CBCT with mandibular inferior notch following anterior horizontal mandibular osteotomy. (**b**) Left lateral view CBCT with mandibular inferior notch following anterior horizontal mandibular osteotomy. (**c**) Superior aspect of inferior osteotomy segment with perpendicular ledge

et al. have reviewed the advantages and disadvantages of genioplasty by either alloplastic implant or osteotomy [40]. Thomson designed a sagittal genioplasty to reduce the geniomandibular notches in 1985, but it has not gained widespread use. Alloplastic chin implants are better for small augmentation, pointed chin, reoperation, in office procedures, and combined chin/angle procedures.

Lateral Cephalometric Prediction Tracing

Lateral cephalometric prediction is highly accurate, can be helpful for the planning of custom alloplastic genioplasty, and can be done manually by acetate paper tracings or with the use of simulation software. While software for 3-D computerized hard and soft tissue prediction programs have made virtual treatment planning of orthognathic surgery and genioplasty by anterior horizontal mandibular osteotomy possible, they are less developed for alloplastic augmentation. Completely accurate 3-D soft tissue changes associated with the bony movements cannot yet be predicted.

There are several cephalometric analysis and planning methods for chin evaluation for esthetic chin position prediction. Examples would include COGS [14–16], Ricketts [17, 26], and Steiner [18, 19]. Other frequently used profile reference lines are Riedel's plane, Rickett's "E" esthetic line, and Gonzalez-Ulloa's "Zero Meridian" line [20–22] for evaluating and planning the ideal chin position and contour.

Rickett's "E" line is drawn from the nasal tip (pronasale Pn) to soft tissue pogonion (Pg(s)). The lower lip Stomion (Sto(i)) should be 2.0 mm posterior to Rickett's "E" line with a standard deviation of +/−3.0 mm as an esthetic ideal [23] (Fig. 9.28). The Gonzalez-Ulloa "Zero Meridian" [20–22] line is a vertical line drawn from nasion perpendicular to the Frankfort Horizontal plane. The ideal chin position in profile should have the soft tissue pogonion on average coincident to or +/−2 mm in relation to this line. Esthetic chin projection can also be determined by creating a vertical line through subnasale perpendicular to Frankfort Horizontal plane (Fig. 9.29) with the soft tissue pogonion 3 mm +/−3 mm behind this line [32]. The posterior-anterior cephalometric x-ray can be helpful in the assessment of mandibular asymmetry and for planning the lateral movement, setting the midline or cant correction.

The triangle analysis of Powell et al. [23] allows all of the different profile angles to be put together in the evaluation and then plan the ideal proportions of an esthetic face. In this analysis the nasofrontal (NFr), nasofacial (NFa), nasomental line, and nasomental angle mentocervical (MC) are all included [23] (Fig. 9.30).

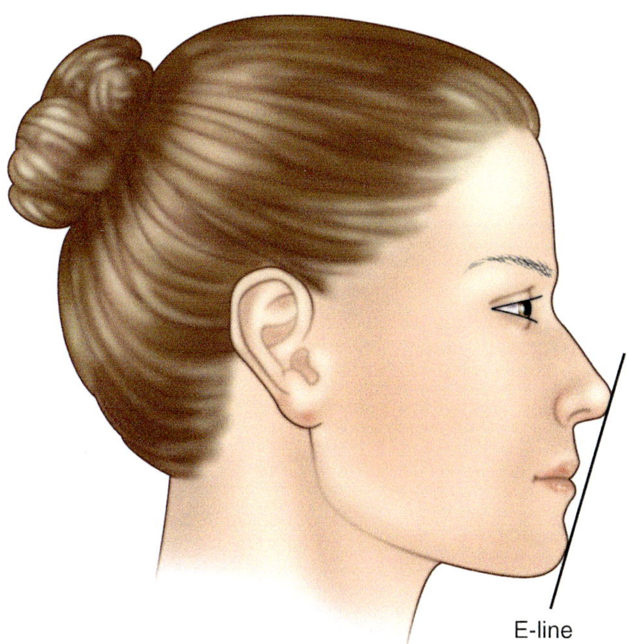

Fig. 9.28 Rickett's E-line

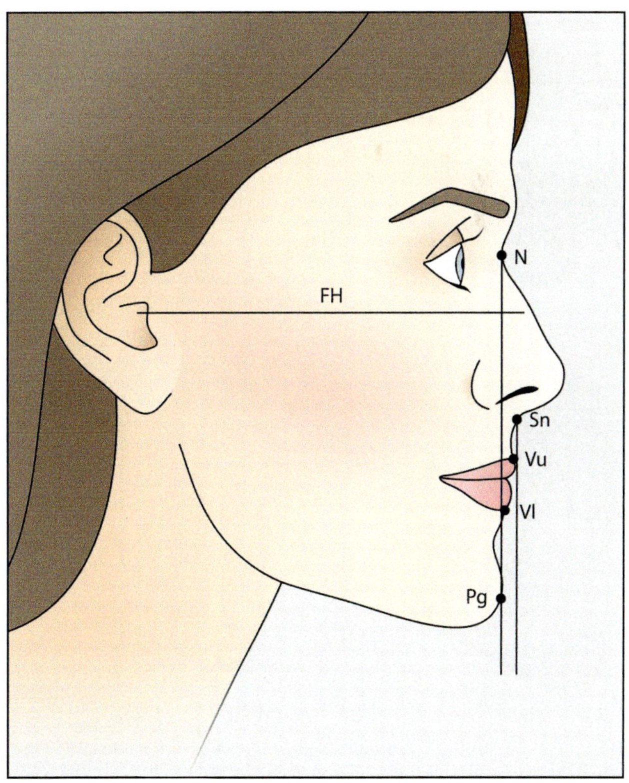

Fig. 9.29 Gonzalez-Ulloa line from nasion through Frankfort Horizontal and subnasale *vertical line* from subnasale perpendicular to Frankfort Horizontal

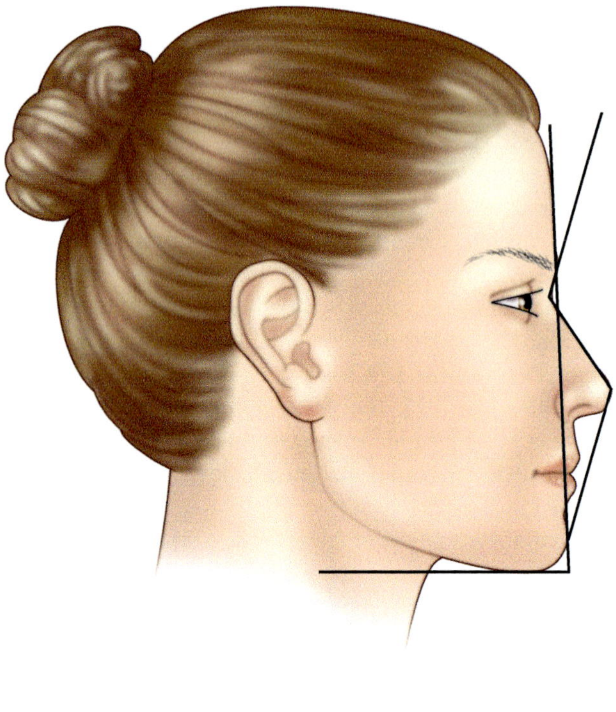

Fig. 9.30 The triangle analysis of Powell

Alloplastic Genioplasty with Custom Chin Implants

Genioplasty is commonly performed for reduction, augmentation, and symmetry. It has had limitations based on an individual's bone anatomy and morphology and commercially available stock alloplastic implants (Figs. 9.1a–k). Limitations of stock implants relate to trying to fit a variety of patients to a small number of standard sizes, even with adaption [41]. Genioplasty can be achieved by the anterior horizontal mandibular osteotomy for vertical reduction or augmentation with and without grafting [42, 43] (Fig. 9.31a–d). A narrow pointed chin is usually associated with a Class II malocclusion and is often a poor candidate for an osteotomy unless a midline split or other bone graft/alloplast augmentation is utilized. A chin implant is able to provide a better result by providing width to the chin. The chin point may be acceptable with lateral augmentation provided in those circumstances.

Custom and stock alloplastic genioplasty have included the use of solid silicone [41], PEFE [9, 44], HTR [11], and Mersilene [45]. Genioplasty has been extensively reviewed with respect to diagnosis, treatment planning, and technique [32, 36–39, 45–49].

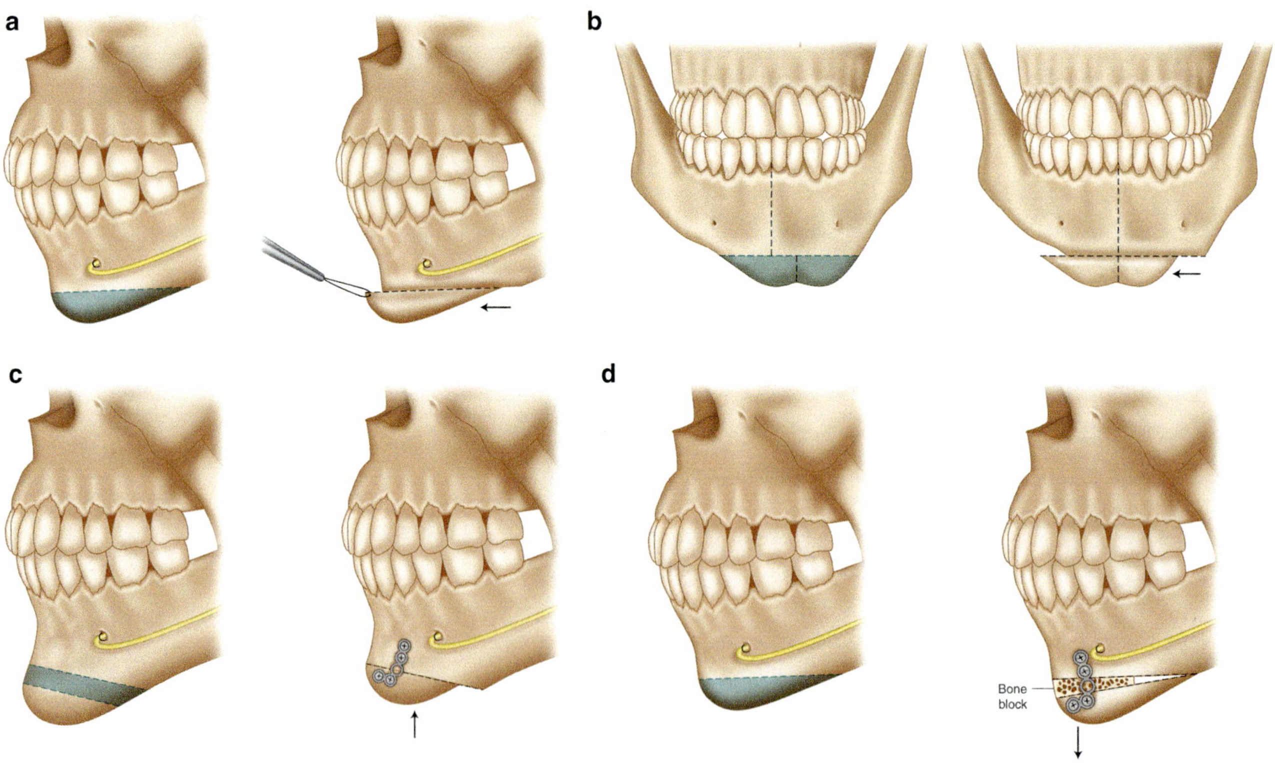

Fig. 9.31 (a) Anterior horizontal mandibular osteotomy (sliding genioplasty). (b) Anterior horizontal mandibular osteotomy (sliding genioplasty) with midline correction. (c) Anterior horizontal mandibular osteotomy (sliding genioplasty) with vertical reduction via wedge resection. (d) Anterior horizontal mandibular osteotomy (sliding genioplasty) with vertical augmentation via bone grafting

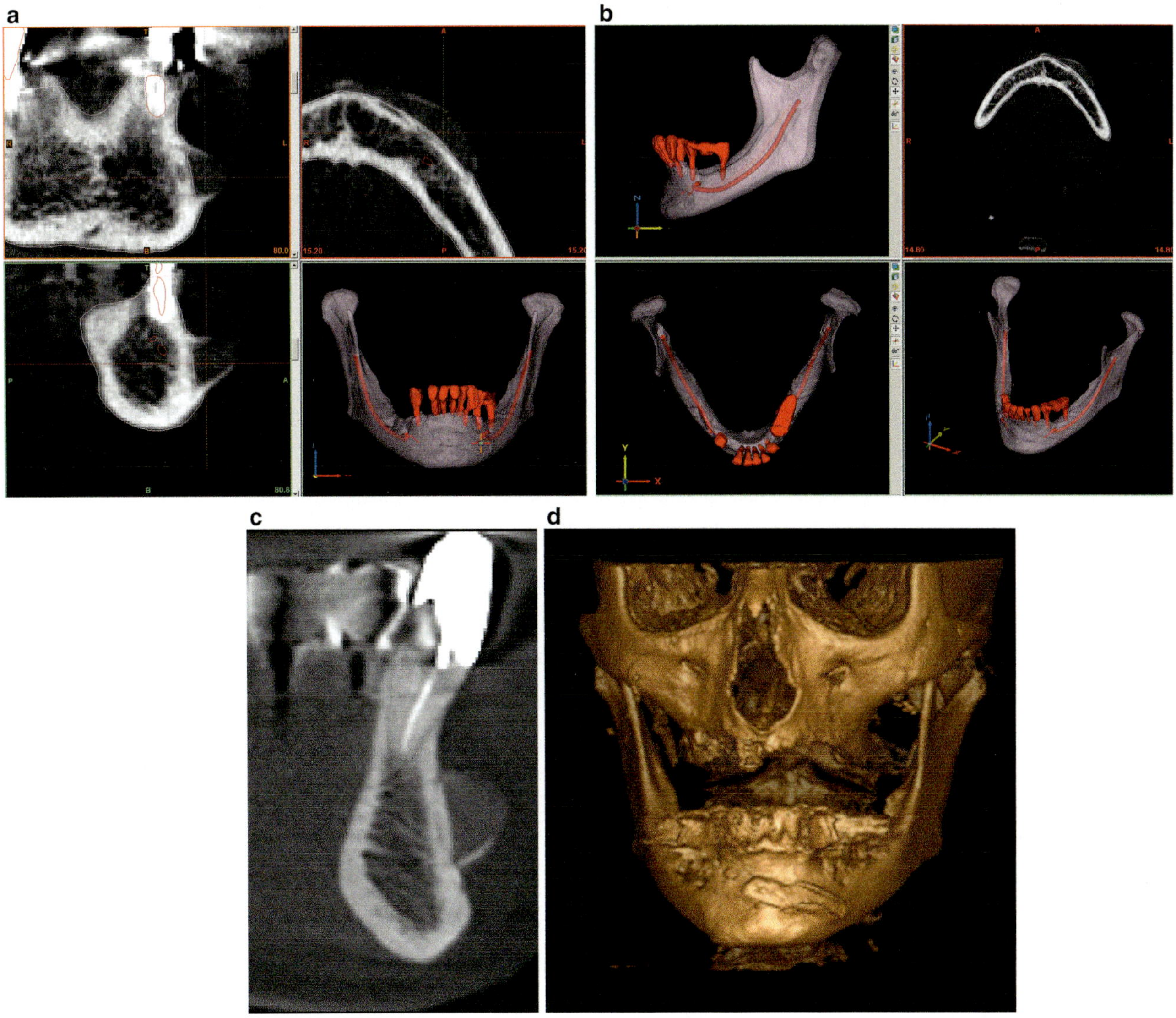

Fig. 9.32 Alloplastic stock button chin implant with migration and underlying bone resorption with calcification of implant capsule. (**a**) Sagittal, axial, and 3-D views. (**b**) Axial and 3-D views. (**c**) Oblique sagittal view. (**d**) 3-D frontal view

As a result of the development of hardware for internal fixation, this has allowed for improvements in orthognathic surgery and in the anterior horizontal mandibular osteotomy [50]. In some cases patients will undergo initial osteotomies of the chin that will be followed by simultaneous or staged alloplastic augmentation either for the management of residual osteotomy irregular contours or for increased augmentation. Custom chin solid silicone implants can address augmentation in the sagittal, lateral, and vertical dimensions in a predictable manner which has been noted by Zide et al. as a desirable outcome [32]. Many surgeons have placed small oval "button" chin implants without screw fixation, which will migrate over time secondary to mentalis muscular activity [47–49, 51] (Figs. 9.32 and 9.33).

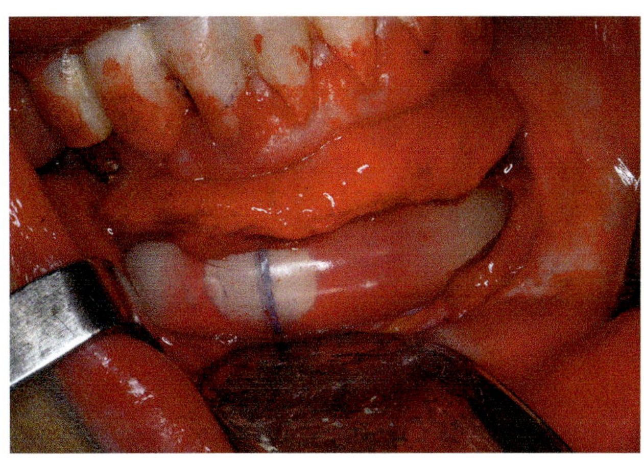

Fig. 9.33 Alloplastic stock button chin implant with superior migration and advanced bone resorption (same patient as 9.32 **a–d**)

The style of custom solid silicone implant presented here is a variation of the anatomical implant (shelf type) in which there is a wrap around the inferior anterior mandible so as to create the anterior projection and horizontal inferior portion that blends with the lateral border of the mandible to provide a smooth jaw line with the geniomandibular regions [47, 50, 52, 53]. The anatomical (shelf type) implant will be more stable with less chance to move as a result of mentalis muscle activity and displacement with potential for erosion [32, 47, 50]. Screw fixation of alloplastic implants allows precise positioning, maintenance of implant position, and prevention of mobility with associated bone resorption [50, 51]. Familiarity with various internal fixation systems is essential for surgeons performing genioplasty procedures. Screw fixation of these implants provides further stability and prevention of displacement and resorption [50–53]. A smooth transition from the superior to the inferior portion of the chin enhances the esthetic outcome and also creates a better jaw line for the soft tissues of the neck and labiomental fold. This is an advantage over the anterior horizontal mandibular osteotomy technique of genioplasty whereby there is a perpendicular edge or notching of the mandible and the inferior segment which increases with greater degrees of advancement. Through the use of custom implants with feathered edges, there is the avoidance of irregular edges along the posterior inferior border of the chin segment at the junction with the intact mandible. The labiomental sulcus can have a smoother contour with a chin implant compared to the ledge at the superior aspect of the anterior horizontal mandibular osteotomy inferior segment. The use of the 3D sterolithographic model also allows advanced knowledge of the position of the mental foramen which should be avoided in the custom chin implant design.

Technique for Wax Application and Carving of the Implant

The method to create a wax block outline for the chin implant is to first analyze the dimension which is desired to augment. The creation of the chin implant wax prototype begins with the lateral cephalometric analysis to determine the desired AP dimension to advance soft tissue pogonion relative to the "Zero Meridian" line [20–22, 54] and Ricketts "E" line [17, 23, 26]. The ratio of hard to soft tissue augmentation of an implant is approximately 1:1 which is similar to the anterior horizontal mandibular osteotomy [36–38]. Once AP augmentation is determined, attention is paid to the width issues and how much the chin should be widened which should blend the AP augmentation to the width. Finally height is assessed to decide on the morphology of the chin and where augmentation needs to be added in a vertical dimension. This relates to both the degree of vertical deficiency and the labiomental fold. It also depends on the clinical problem being treated and whether the chin is unoperated or operated. Unoperated chins have pristine anatomy to which augmentation is being performed for the first time. The operated chin can present with much more difficult problems to solve besides the deficiency. Often there are scarring of tissues, presence of hardware, implants to be removed, and severe bone contour deformities that make the dissection more difficult and the creation of the implant more time consuming.

The unoperated bony chin with clinical retrogenia will present with several common variations:

1. Narrow width and height with normal sized pointed tip
2. Normal width with short tip
3. Vertical deficiency with normal width and tip
4. Anterior chin vertical deficiency with "bowing" with midline cleft
5. Midline cleft
6. Prominent geniomandibular notches
7. Lipodystrophy with obtuse neck-throat angle
8. Microgenia

The operated bony chin with clinical retrogenia or deformity will present with several common variations:

1. Geniomandibular notches increased at the junction of the osteotomy segments
2. Malposition of the inferior osteotomy chin segment with asymmetry
3. Protruding hardware from bone resorption
4. Excessively advanced chin with deep labiomental fold ("witch's chin")
5. Relapse of a BSSO symmetric or asymmetric
6. Excessive wedge excision with flattening of the chin and square appearance
7. Inappropriate simultaneous use of an alloplastic implant over a bony genioplasty
8. Bone resorption with migration of stock chin implant into bone
9. Stock implant malposition with asymmetry

Clefting of the chin is usually a soft tissue definition. It is rare to see a cleft in the mental region of the mandible [32]. It is due to the binding of the soft tissue as a result of embryonic facial formation with midline fusion of the facial halves. Clefting may be soft tissue only, and upon dissection and placement of the implant, it may not be maintained. This is an important aspect to discuss with patients, especially males and whether the cleft should be maintained in the implant design and soft tissue closure.

Wax Prototype Design

The creation of the implant begins with the application of Vaseline to the stereolithographic model as a light film so that the wax will not stick. Ropes of wax (Modern Materials

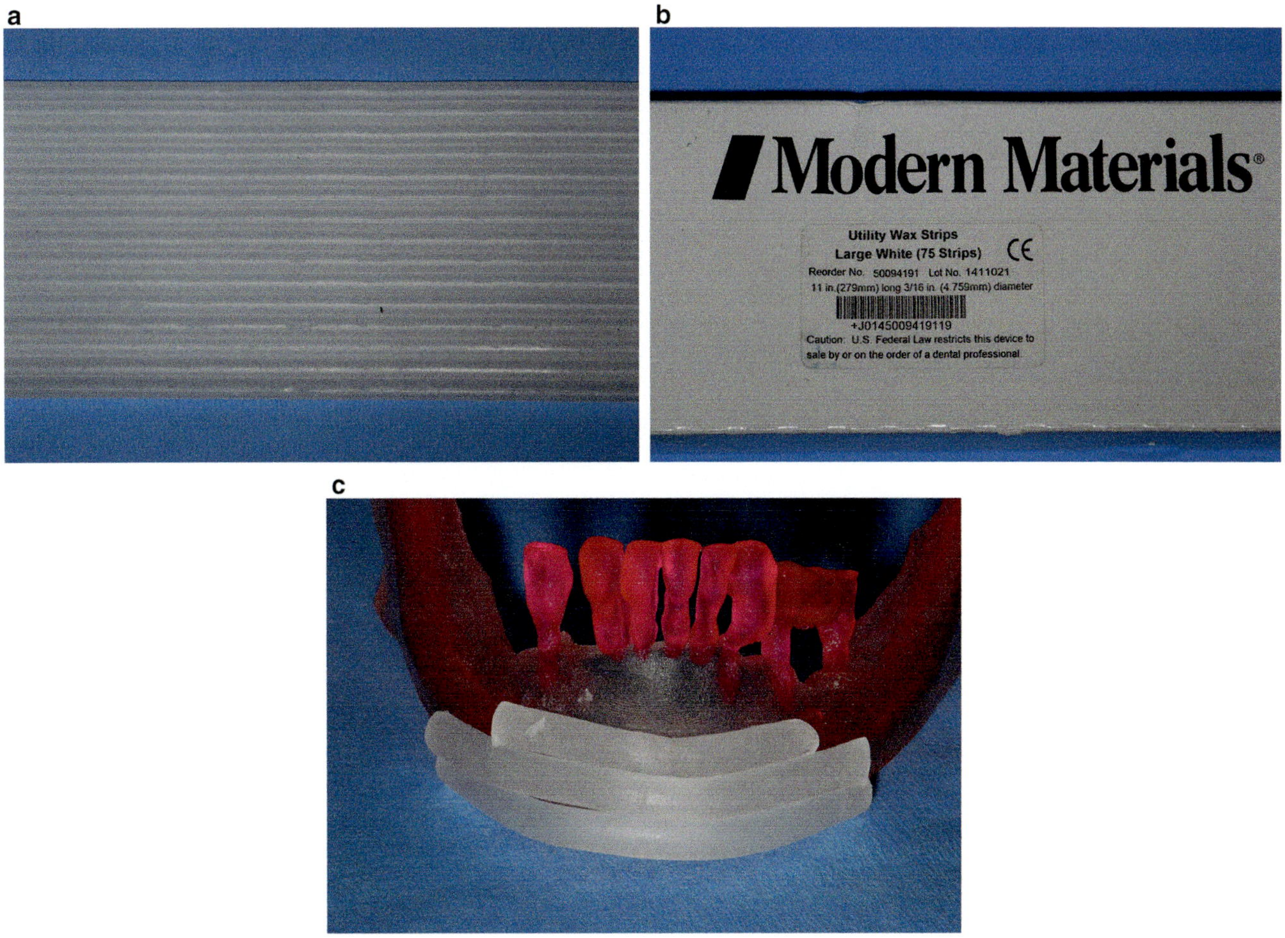

Fig. 9.34 (**a**) UtilityWax Strips Large White. (**b**) Modern Materials Utility Wax Strips Large White, Heraeus Kulzer, South Bend, IN, USA (With Permission). (**c**) Application of wax to 3-D stereolithographic model for custom chin implant

Utility Wax Strips Large White, Heraeus Kulzer, South Bend, IN, USA with permission) are then hand rolled for softening and then pressed onto the model to begin to form the implant (Fig. 9.34a–c). The wax can begin to be shaped with the carving knife by the cutting away of excess. The edge of the blade can then be used to carve away thin layers of wax to shape it (Fig. 9.35a–c). Irregular surfaces can be filled in with small pieces of wax pressed onto the wax form. Smoothing with the side of the knife or by finger pressure or rubbing is then performed. Edging of the implant with the sharp edge of the knife then takes place to define the borders, and then removal of wax within 5 mm of the mental foramina and creation of a superior labial border 5 mm below the apices of teeth which are easily visualized on the model. Feathering of edges to ensure a smooth contour from the implant to the bony margins is then performed. Once the implant has achieved a basic shape, it can be removed from the model, and with a Boley gauge, the thickness of the implant can be measured and determined to be satisfactory or if addition or subtraction needs to be performed by further carving (Fig. 9.35d). It can be helpful to hold the model and implant against a lateral cephalometric prediction tracing to see if the augmentation is correct. Facial moulage with wax chin prototypes applied can also be helpful at this stage of implant prototype development. Often the clinician will find that the stereolithographic model helps to define the implant size and shape as it represents the anatomic deformity. The presence of retained hardware is taken into consideration for the edges of the labial anterior form and positions planned for placement of screw fixation holes. The final implant design can be shown to the patient as part of the consultation process and can even be removed and placed on the patient's skin to estimate the augmentation. The stereolithographic model needs to be periodically lubricated with Vaseline to ensure that the wax prototype can be removed without damage. If the wax prototype is difficult to remove, the model can be placed in a freezer to harden the wax which makes it easier to carefully remove. The wax prototype is left on the stereolithographic model and carefully wrapped and shipped to the implant manufacturer. The manufacturer will be advised as to the hardness of the silicone to be used from very soft, soft, medium, and hard. Medium is the usually pre-

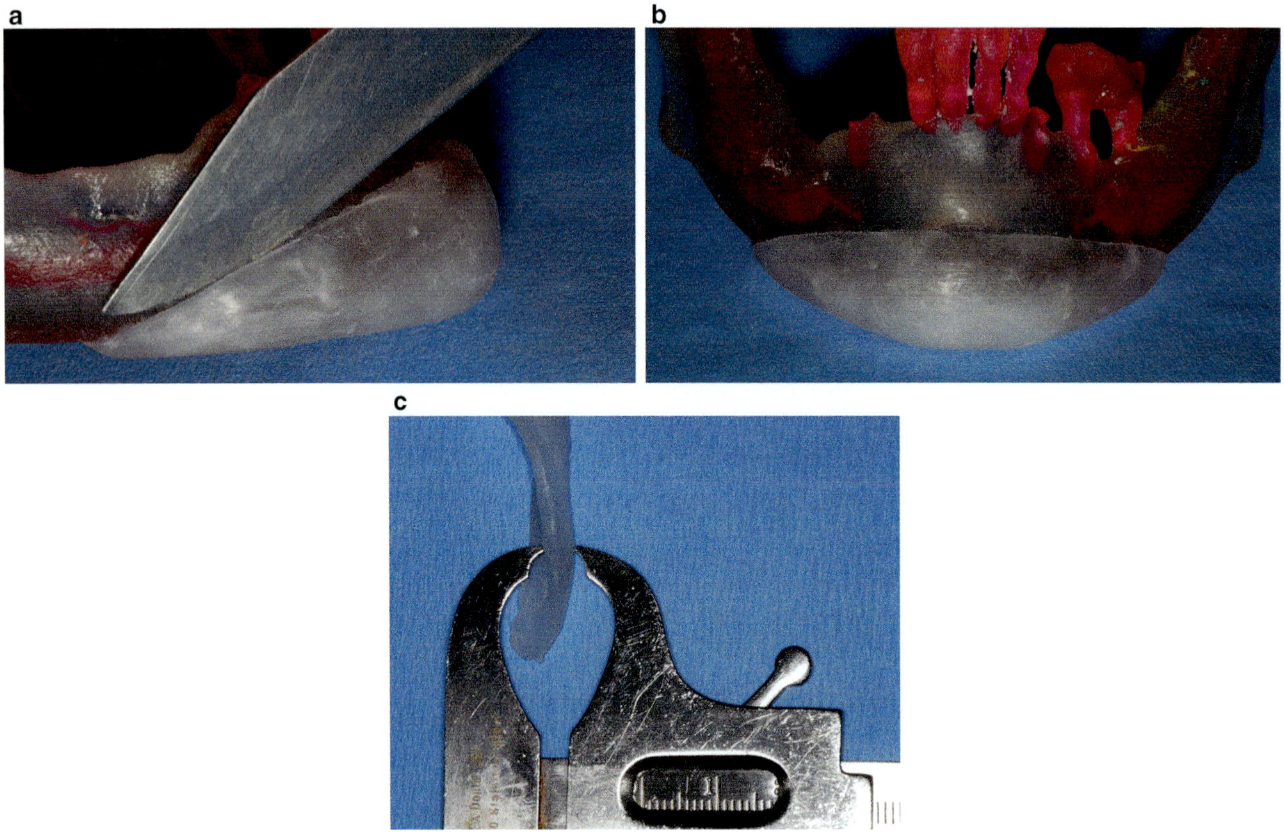

Fig. 9.35 (**a**) Carving of wax prototype for custom chin implant. (**b**) Wax prototype for custom chin implant. (**c**) Use of Boley gauge to determine thickness of wax prototype

ferred gauge as it provides rigidity yet feels natural to the patient because it has some depressability like skin. It also allows flexibility for ease of insertion into the surgical site. When the implant is placed, it will become encapsulated which helps to further develop the smooth contour of the implant, binds the implant closer to the bone, and prevents its displacement. All of the implants in this series were fabricated by Implantech, Ventura, CA, USA.

Difficult Retreatment Cases

Patients who have had unsatisfactory genioplasty results following previous chin implants and anterior horizontal mandibular osteotomy will present with a wide range of deformities [51, 55–57]. These deformities can be related to relapse after an anterior horizontal mandibular osteotomy combined with bilateral mandibular ramus sagittal split osteotomies [34], parasymphysis notches, incorrect segment positioning, contour irregularities, improperly placed hardware, and bone resorption around hardware, and relapse of mandibular sagittal ramus osteotomies with or without anterior horizontal mandibular osteotomy can be managed well if treated with custom implants. Custom implants allow correction of the chin contours and postsurgical defects. Chin reoperation poses several concerns with respect to both hard and soft tissues. The bony issues can be readily addressed by the chin implant. Soft tissue issues relate to scar tissue formation, including failure to repair of the mentalis muscle or its inadequate resuspension. In severe cases of mentalis muscle injury or failure to repair it correctly, this can result in significant ptosis of the lower lip and excessive display of mandibular incisors and lip incompetence. Retreatment of these cases is achieved by the resuspension of mentalis muscle to the bone with direct muscle repair by bilateral direct bone anchorage of the superior aspect of the mentalis muscle which is sutured into superiorly placed holes in the bone below the incisor apices and was first reported by Zide and McCarthy [58]. A fascia lata sling may be needed as well to resuspend the lower lip through a bilateral facelift incision (Fig. 9.36a–d) [59]. Lower lip ptosis is a common complication of Anterior Horizontal Mandibular Osteotomy when only the mucosa is closed without care to reattach the cut ends of the bilateral mentalis muscles. Adequate soft tissue redraping with or without other soft tissue procedures such as liposuction, neck lift, or platysma repair, in combination with the implant, can rejuvenate the chin and neck.

Retreatment of failed chin implants can pose similar concerns as there are invariably both hard and soft tissue issues [51, 60–63]. Failure includes migration of the implant usually in a superior direction secondary to mentalis activity. Bone resorption can occur as well as bone formation in the foreign body capsule surrounding the implant. Removal of the implant without replacement can be problematic and lead

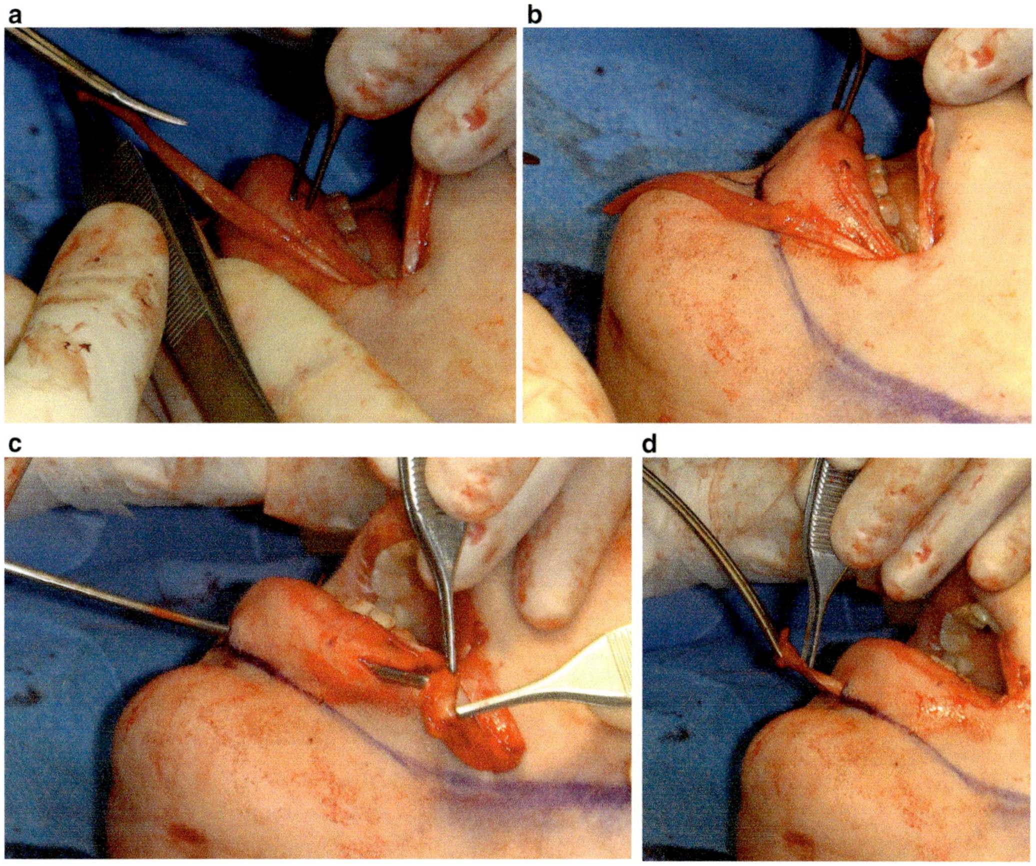

Fig. 9.36 (**a**) Fascia lata sling graft following insertion through the midface and brought through the lateral aspect of the lower lip. (**b**) Fascia lata sling graft following insertion through the lateral aspect of the lower lip. (**c**) Fascia lata graft following insertion through the lateral aspect of the lower left lip and about to be pulled through midline lower lip incision. (**d**) Fascia lata graft following insertion through the lateral aspect of the lower left lip and pulled through midline lower lip incision. (Elliot Rose, M.D., Plastic and Reconstructive Surgeon, The Mount Sinai Hospital, New York, NY, USA)

to unsatisfactory scarring and wrinkling of the chin soft tissue with dimpling, bunching, and ptosis [32]. Immediate reconstruction with custom chin implants fabricated from 3-D models can avoid the soft tissue deformity of a staged approach. Sometimes this can be necessary in the case of dehiscence or the presence of infection. When a chin implant is present and planned for removal and immediate replacement, the mandible can be delineated from the implant in a stereolithographic model created to allow the fabrication of an anatomically correct custom chin implant.

Prejowl Lateral Augmentation

There are many circumstances in which a narrow pointed chin has adequate projection, and it is preferable to augment the lateral aspect of the chin more than the anterior aspect, which was described by Mittelman [46]. In these cases the anterior aspect of the chin implant is thin with thickening at the lateral aspects. This technique is especially helpful for the aging face in which there is a prejowl ptosis which can be recontoured and resuspended in combination with a combined facelift and custom chin implant.

Table 9.3 Manufacturer's specifications for implant sterilization (Implantech, Ventura, CA, USA)

Clean the implant with hot water, soap, and soft brush using gloved hands, and rinse the implant with distilled water. A gravity displacement autoclaving cycle machine should be used. Do not use prevacuum or flash cycle. The sterilization regime should be 30 minutes minimum at 250 degrees F, 15 PSI (121 degrees C, 1 kg/cm2), or 15 minutes minimum at 270 degrees F, 30 psi (132 degrees, 2 kg/cm^2)

Preoperative Implant Inspection and Preparation

The implant when received from the manufacturer should be fitted on the 3-D model to ensure correct fabrication, fit, and screw hole position. As the implant is made from silicone, it can still be modified, and if not satisfactory, a new wax prototype can be sent to the manufacturer for refabrication of the implant. The 3-D model should be thoroughly cleaned of any Vaseline prior to the fitting of the implant. The implant should be autoclave sterilized according to the manufacturer's specifications (Table 9.3).

a

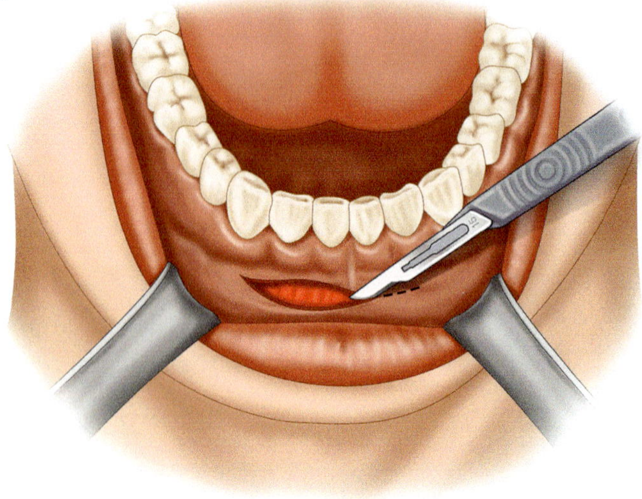

b

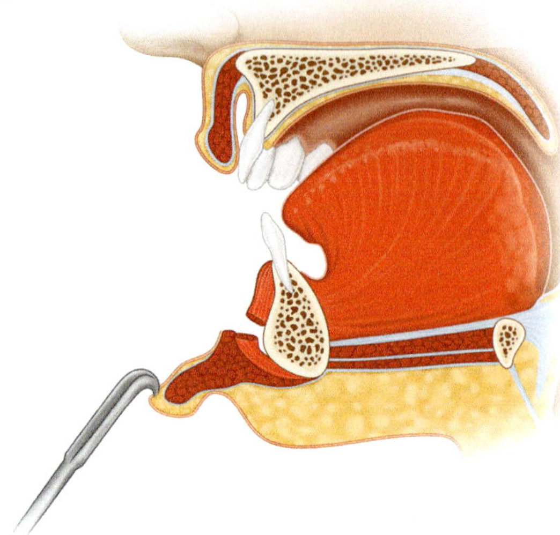

Fig. 9.37 (**a**) Anterior mandibular buccal vestibular incision. (**b**) Lateral view of anterior mandibular buccal vestibular incision with superior muscle cuff

Surgical Procedure

The alloplastic genioplasty procedure is performed via a transoral anterior buccal vestibular incision (Fig. 9.37a). An alternative approach can be through a submental transcutaneous incision. These procedures can be performed both in the hospital and office settings under full general anesthesia or moderate sedation. Prior to the anterior buccal vestibular incision, local anesthesia with epinephrine is infiltrated into the anterior mandibular vestibule and lingual tissues via cutaneous and intraoral routes. The initial incision starts perpendicular to the mucosa with the lower lip retracted outward, preferably using a #15 scalpel blade, from the region of the left mandibular first premolar across the midline to the right mandibular first premolar. Electrocautery should be avoided for the intraoral approach as it can cause damage to the soft tissues and there is an increased risk of wound dehiscence and implant exposure. The incision should be 5mm below the mucogingival junction so as to preserve adequate tissue for closure. The dissection continues through mucosa, submucosa, perimandibular, and mentalis musculature. The surgeon must be careful to ensure that the plane of the incision does not perforate the skin. Once the mucosa and submucosal tissues are incised, the direction of the incision then changes to become perpendicular to the anterior chin and continues through the mentalis muscle and periosteum down to the bone (Fig. 9.37b). A thick cuff of the mentalis should be left along the superior aspect of incision so that reapproximation of mentalis muscles resuspends the soft tissues upon closure of the incision. This thick superior muscle of mentalis also provides coverage of the implant. The dissection is accomplished to the right and left of the midline via a curved freer or #9 periosteal elevator with completion of the subperiosteal dissection and elevation of the soft tissues with careful exposure of the bilateral mental nerves that are identified and preserved throughout the procedure. The inferior border should be completely exposed anteriorly and posteriorly to the mental foramina so as to create a space for the insertion of the implant (Fig. 9.38a). Care should be taken to avoid perforation of the periosteum as skin dimpling and contractions can occur. The wound should be irrigated with normal saline solution and the implant inserted (Fig. 9.38b). An advantage of solid silicone implants is that they can be bent to allow insertion, unlike the stiff polyethylene types that can only be inserted in two parts divided in the midline.

The implant margin should be placed at least 5 mm below the position of mental foramina to avoid injury to the inferior alveolar nerve. There are limitations in terms of the dimensions for which a chin implant can be placed via an intraoral incision which is approximately 1 cm in anterior thickness. Larger implants will require a submental incision. Vertical reference marks can be helpful to help ensure the correct positioning of the implant. The anatomic fit of patient-specific implants helps to ensure that correct placement is achieved. The implant should be aligned with the dental midline, and the midline screw fixation hole can provide such a reference. The wound is then closed in layers with care to reapproximate the mentalis muscles (Fig. 9.39).

Nerve Damage

Temporary hypoesthesia is expected in nearly all of the patients in the early postoperative period. The best way to

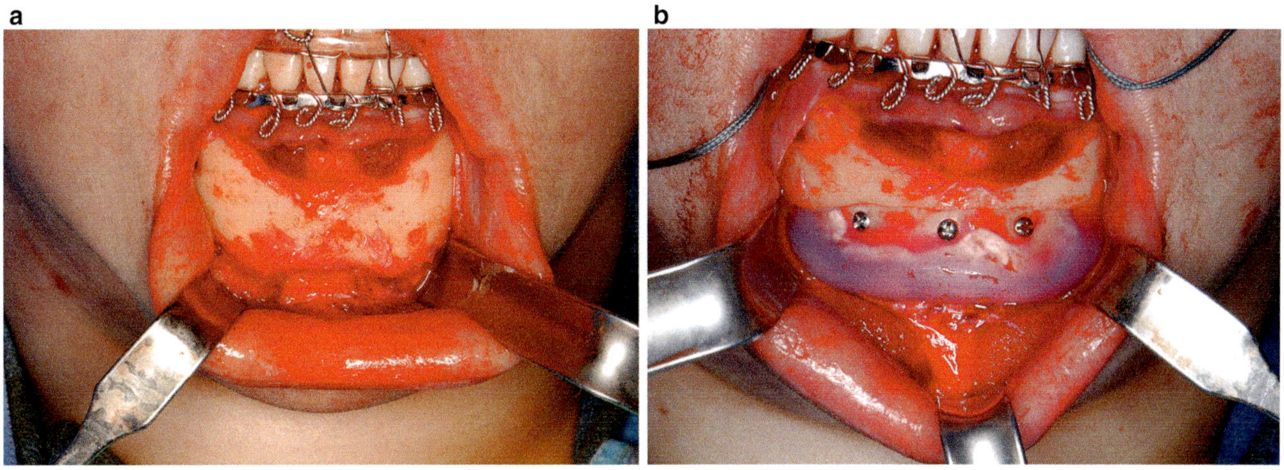

Fig. 9.38 (**a**) Exposure of anterior mandible with complete inferior border elevation of periosteum. (**b**) Insertion of custom chin implant

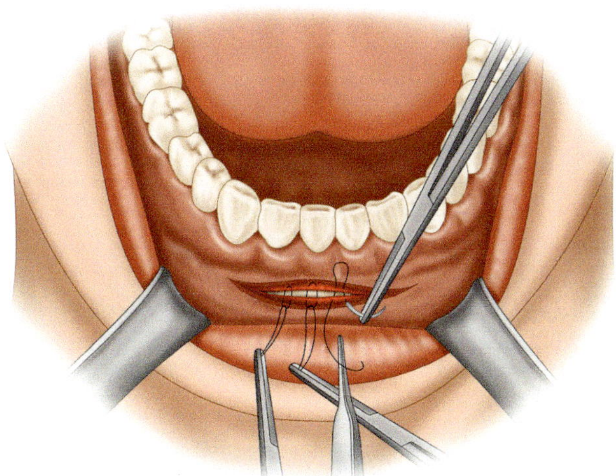

Fig. 9.39 Reapproximation of mentalis muscle prior to closure of mucosal incision

avoid permanent nerve injury is through careful soft tissue dissection, identification and preservation of the bilateral mental nerves, and implant design. The mucosal incision should be placed superior to the mental foramen to avoid injury to the mental nerve. Return of sensation of damaged mental nerves can be difficult to predict, and patients need to be informed of this risk of the procedure.

Case Examples

Case 1

A 30-year-old female was dissatisfied with her chin and felt that it was small. A CBCT was obtained and a 3-D model fabricated with custom wax up of the chin implant and a prototype and final solid silicone custom implant fabricated (Implantech, Ventura, CA, USA). Surgery was performed in an office ambulatory setting under local anesthesia and IV sedation with placement of the implant through a buccal sulcular incision and fixation with three 1.5 mm screws (DuPuy Synthes Craniomaxillofacial, Paoli, PA, USA). Postoperative result was highly satisfactory (Figs. 9.40–9.51) (Alex M. Greenberg, DDS, Oral and Maxillofacial Surgeon, New York, NY, USA).

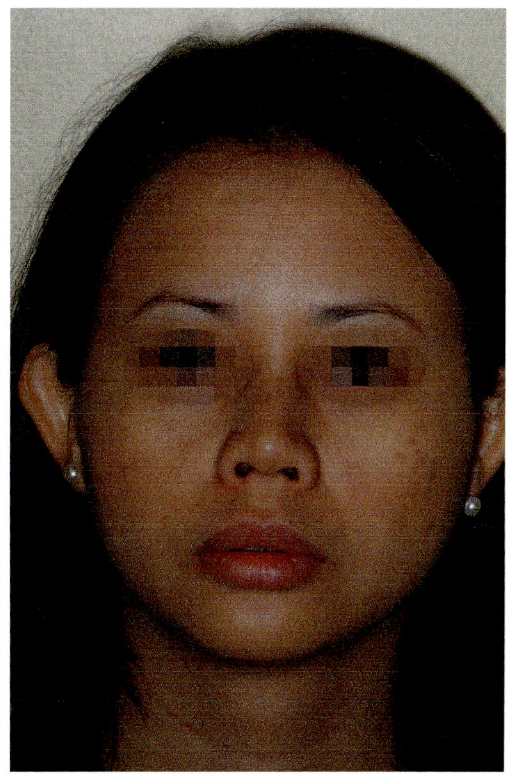

Fig. 9.40 Frontal facial preoperative view chin hypoplasia

Case 2

An 18-year-old male was unhappy with the lack of projection of his chin and felt self-conscious of this deformity (Figs. 9.52 and 9.53). A CBCT was obtained and a 3-D model fabricated

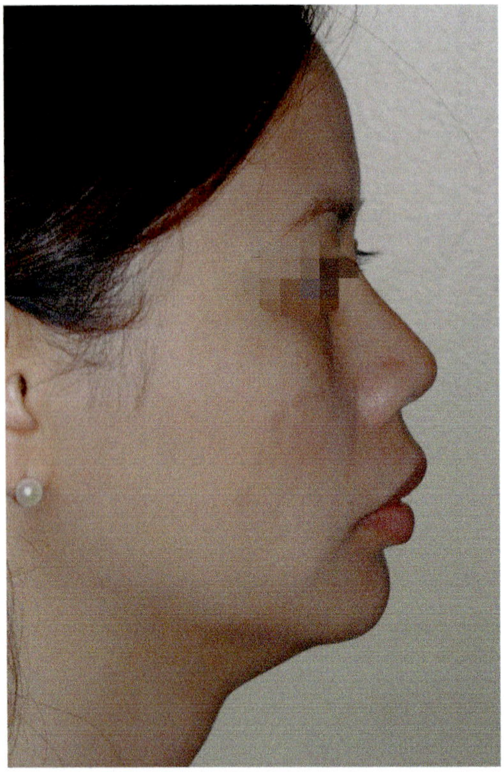

Fig. 9.41 Lateral facial preoperative view chin hypoplasia

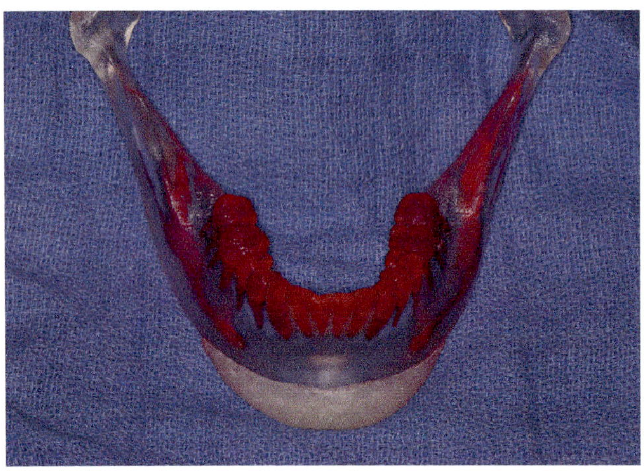

Fig. 9.42 Frontal view of custom wax chin implant prototype

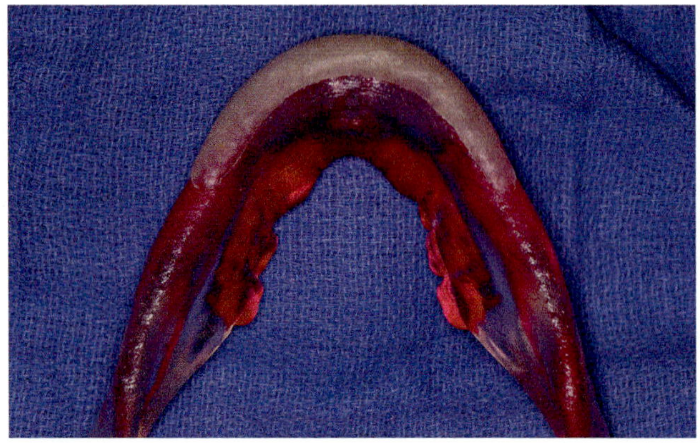

Fig. 9.43 Inferior view of custom wax chin implant prototype fitted to 3-D model

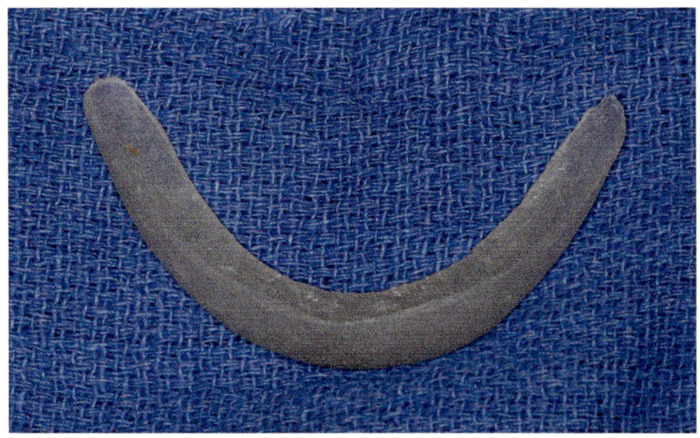

Fig. 9.44 Superior view of custom wax chin implant prototype fitted to 3-D model

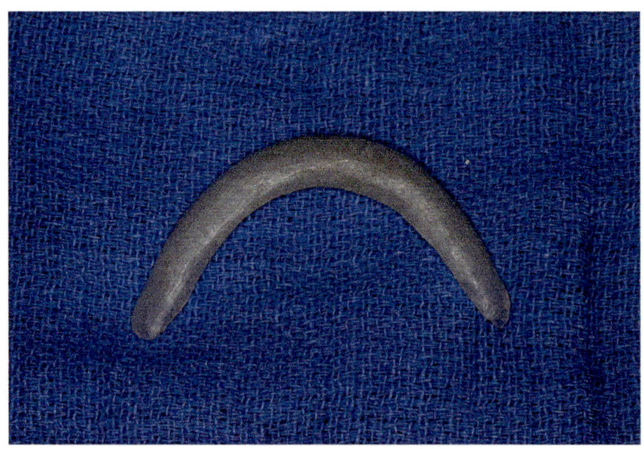

Fig. 9.45 Inferior view custom wax chin implant prototype

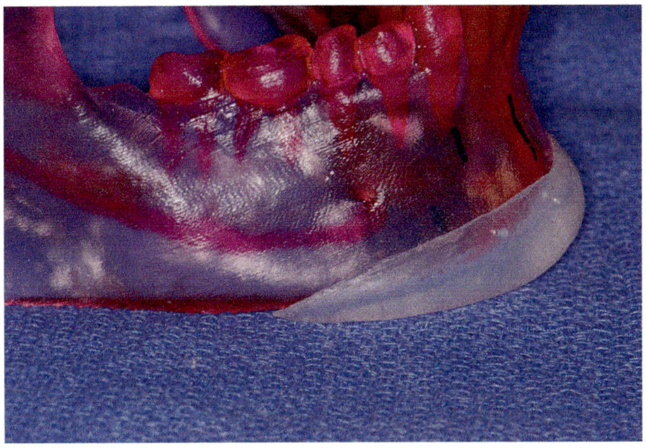

Fig. 9.46 Anterior lateral view of custom chin solid silicone implant fitted to stereolithographic 3-D model. Note: 5 mm distance between superior lateral implant edge and mental nerve

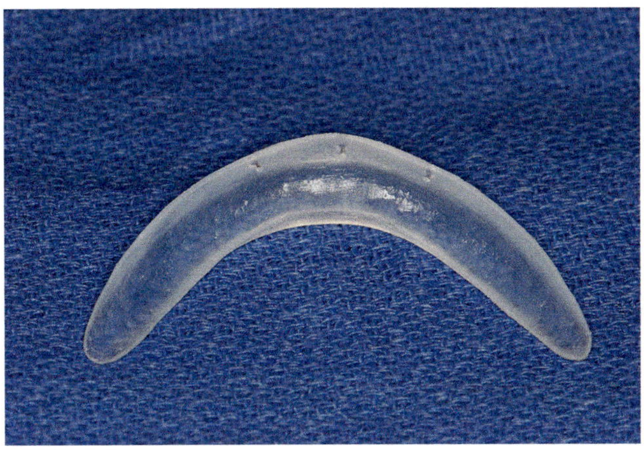

Fig. 9.47 Superior view of custom chin solid silicone implant. Note: Screw holes for screw fixation superior implant edge including the midline to orient the implant to the midline

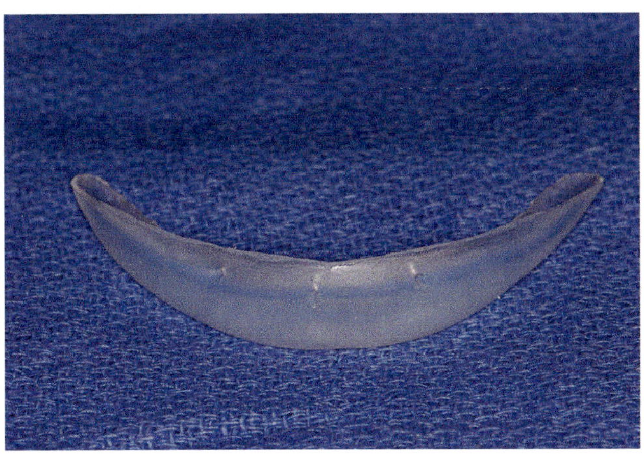

Fig. 9.48 Anterior superior view of custom chin solid silicone implant

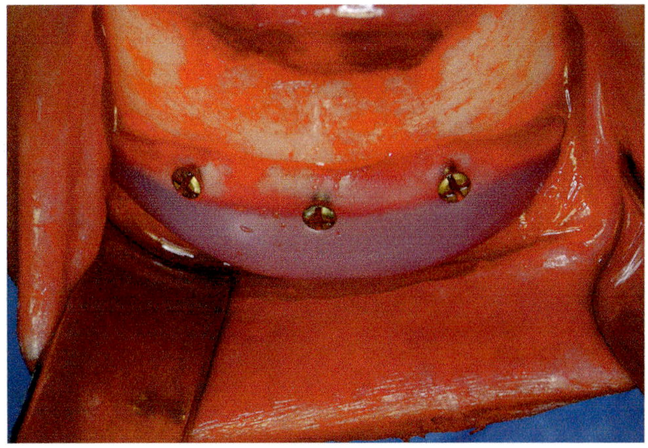

Fig. 9.49 Intraoperative view of insertion of custom chin solid silicone implant with three fixation screws

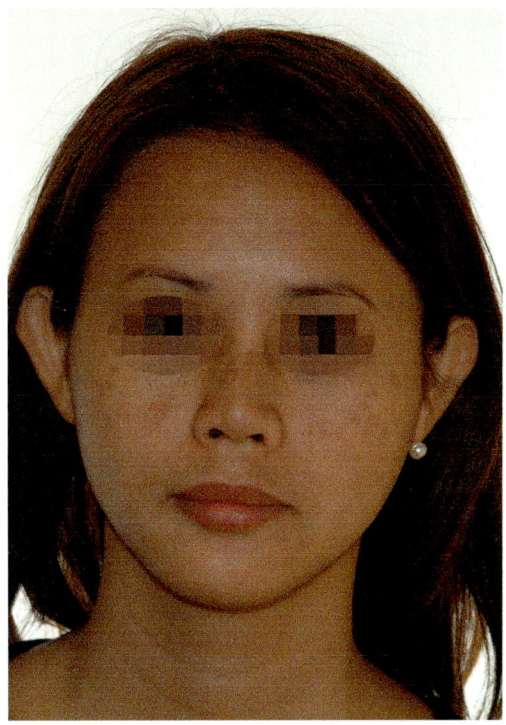

Fig. 9.50 Postoperative frontal view of custom chin solid silicone implant

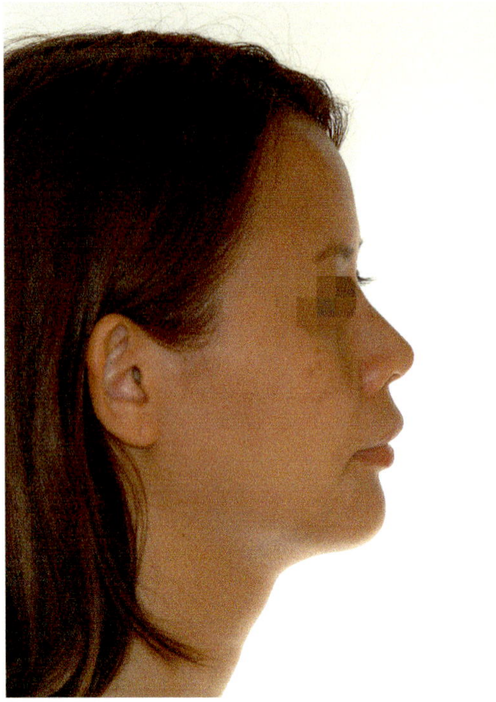

Fig. 9.51 Postoperative lateral view of custom chin solid silicone implant

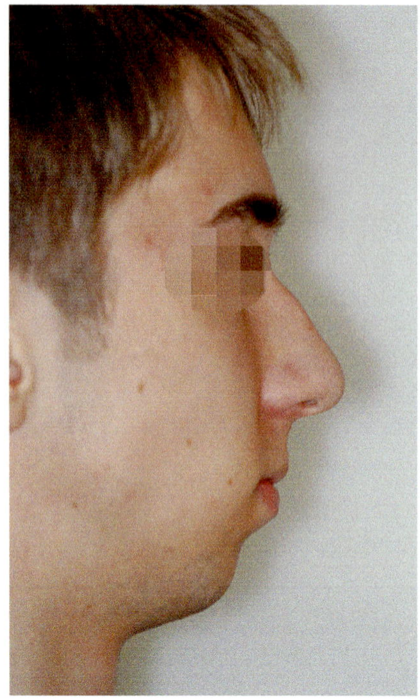

Fig. 9.53 Preoperative lateral facial view

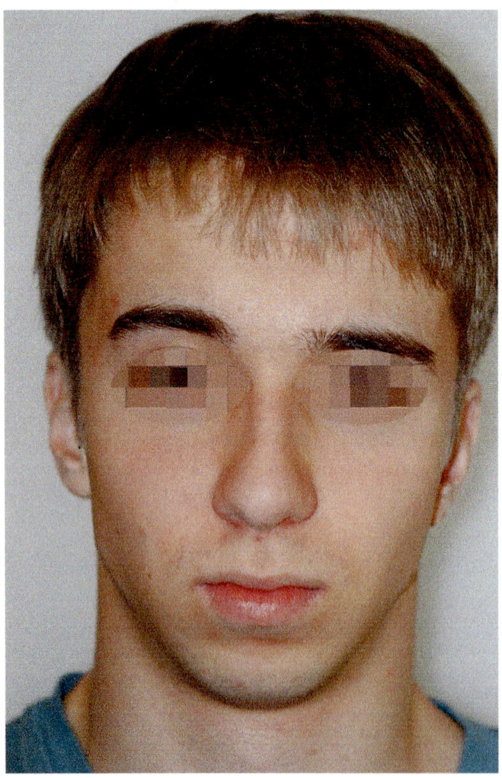

Fig. 9.52 Preoperative frontal facial view

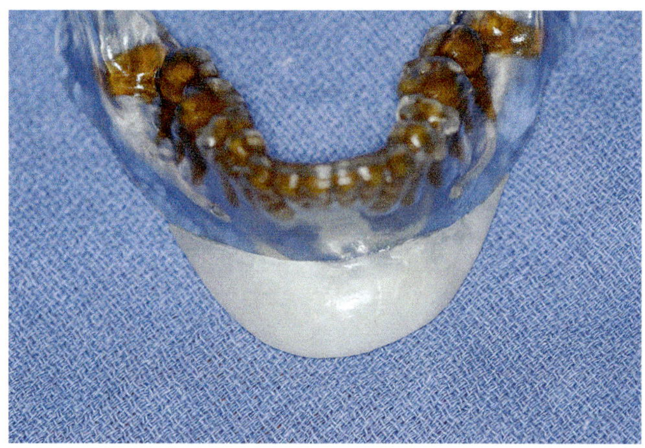

Fig. 9.54 Frontal view of custom wax chin implant prototype fitted to 3-D model

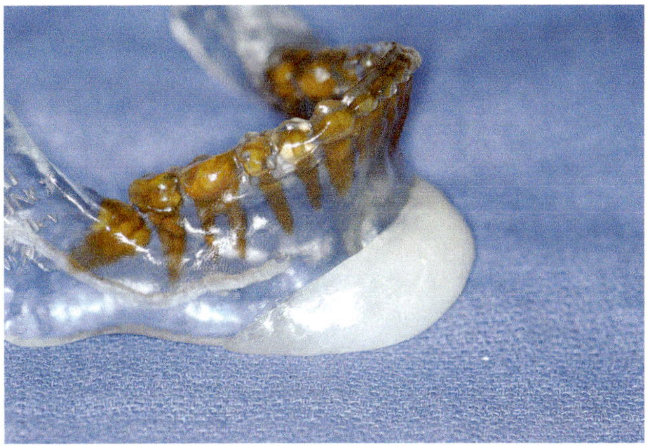

Fig. 9.55 Anterior lateral view of custom wax chin implant prototype fitted to 3-D model

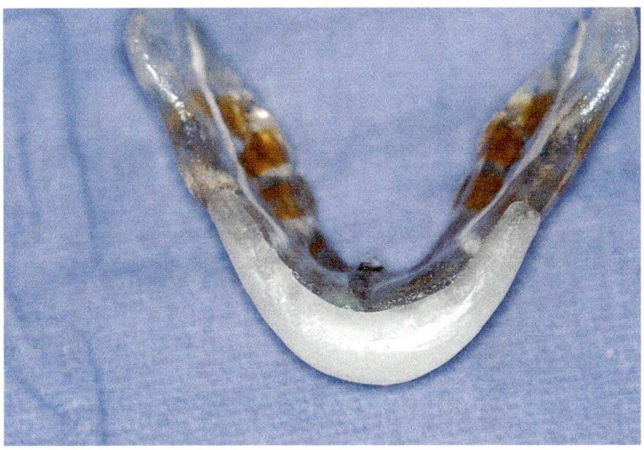

Fig. 9.56 Inferior view of custom wax chin implant prototype fitted on 3-D model

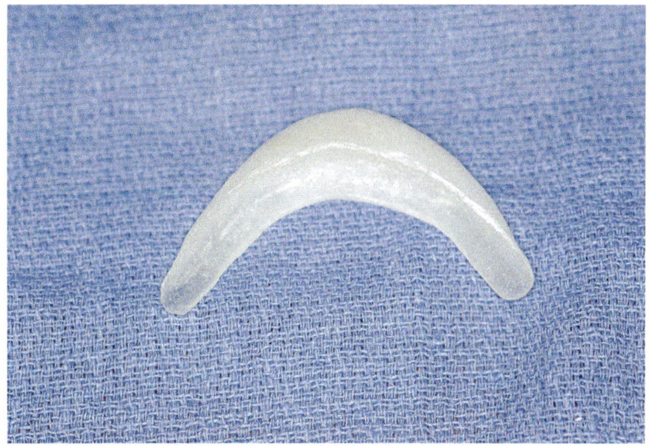

Fig. 9.57 Superior view of custom chin implant wax prototype

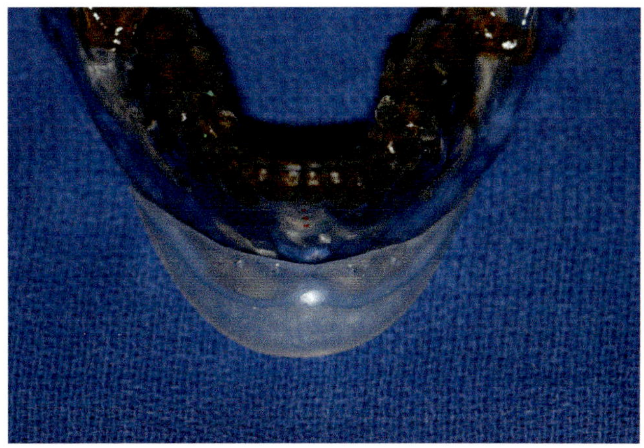

Fig. 9.58 Anterior superior view of custom chin solid silicone implant fitted to 3-D model

with custom wax up of the chin implant (Figs. 9.54–9.57) and a prototype and final solid silicone custom implant fabricated (Implantech, Ventura, CA, USA) (Figs. 9.58–9.61). Surgery was performed in an office ambulatory setting under local anesthesia and IV sedation with placement of the implant through a buccal sulcular incision and fixation with 4 1.5 mm screws (DuPuy Synthes Craniomaxillofacial, Paoli, PA, USA) (Fig. 9.62). This large implant with 9 mm in AP augmentation was at the limit of the size of an implant that can be inserted through an intraoral incision. Postoperative result was highly satisfactory (Figs 9.63 and 9.64). (Alex M. Greenberg, DDS, Oral and Maxillofacial Surgeon, New York, NY, USA).

Case 3

A 30-year-old female presented following prior bilateral mandibular ramus sagittal split osteotomies and anterior horizontal mandibular osteotomy with relapse and retrogenia. She did not want to undergo further orthognathic surgery and preferred chin augmentation. As there were bilateral genio-mandibular notches and retained hardware, a solid silicone custom chin implant genioplasty was performed with retained hardware left in place (Figs. 9.65–9.83). This case demonstrates the advantages of alloplastic genioplasty in reoperation cases. (Alex M. Greenberg, DDS, Oral and Maxillofacial Surgeon, New York, NY, USA).

Conclusion

Custom solid silicone chin implants based on stereolithographic 3-D models have highly accurate fit and can provide improved results over stock chin implants that are currently available from other manufacturers. Advantages are improved contours, feathered edges with less obvious implant outlines, decreased operating time, ease of insertion, and greater choices of material hardness. Disadvantages are cost of CT scan, 3-D models, facial moulage, and time and ability to carve these implants from wax. As an artistic endeavor, for the surgeon willing to spend the time to create these types of patient-specific implants, the results and patient satisfaction are well worth the additional effort.

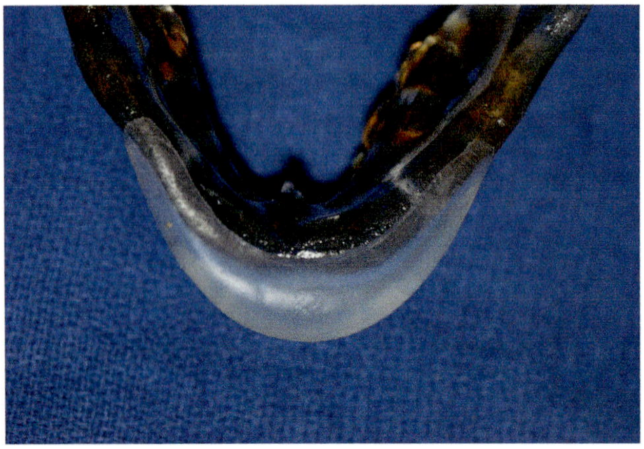

Fig. 9.59 Inferior superior view of custom chin solid silicone implant fitted to 3-D model

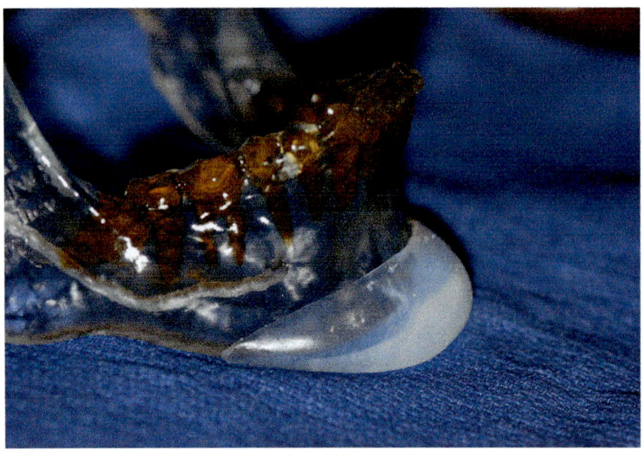

Fig. 9.60 Anterior lateral view of custom chin solid silicone implant fitted to stereolithographic 3-D model

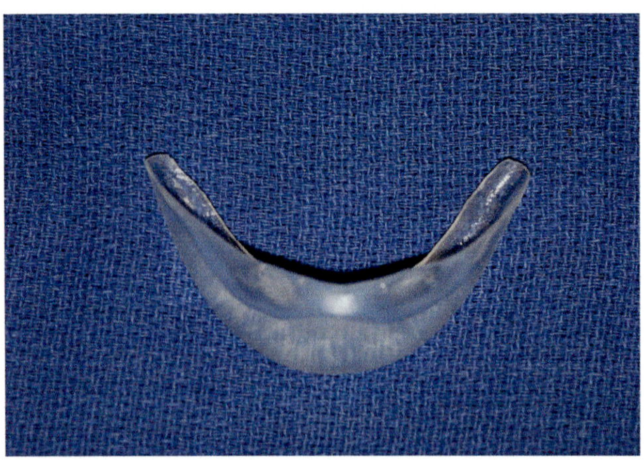

Fig. 9.61 Superior view of custom chin solid silicone implant

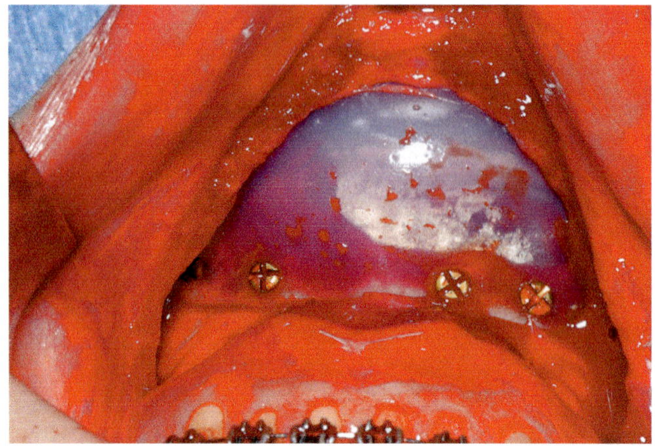

Fig. 9.62 Intraoperative view of insertion of custom chin solid silicone implant with four fixation screws

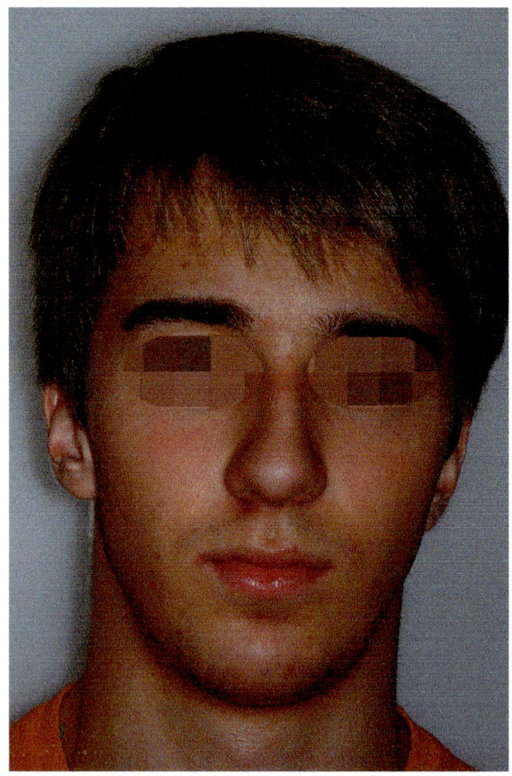

Fig. 9.63 Postoperative frontal view of custom chin solid silicone implant

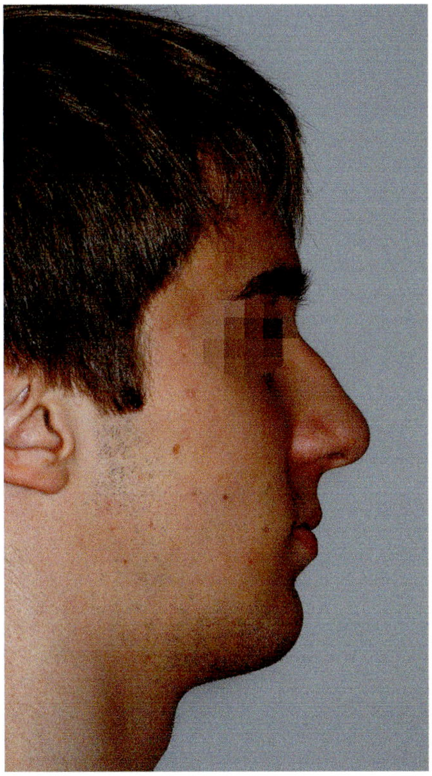

Fig. 9.64 Postoperative lateral view of custom chin solid silicone implant

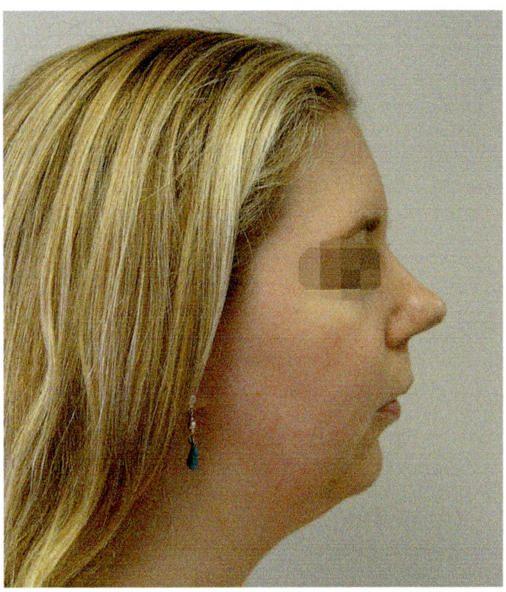

Fig. 9.65 Preoperative lateral facial view

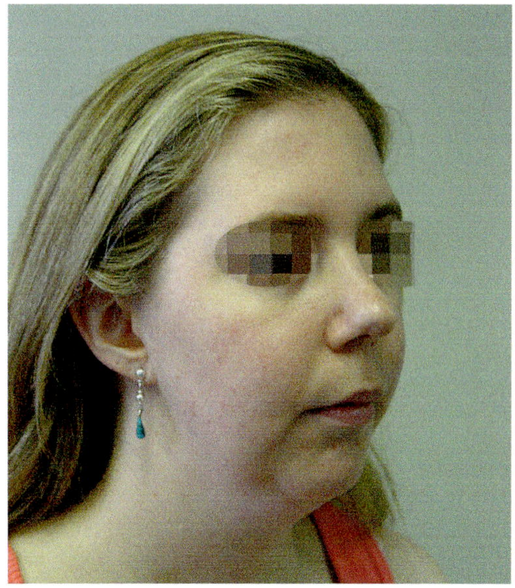

Fig. 9.66 Preoperative right 3/4 facial view

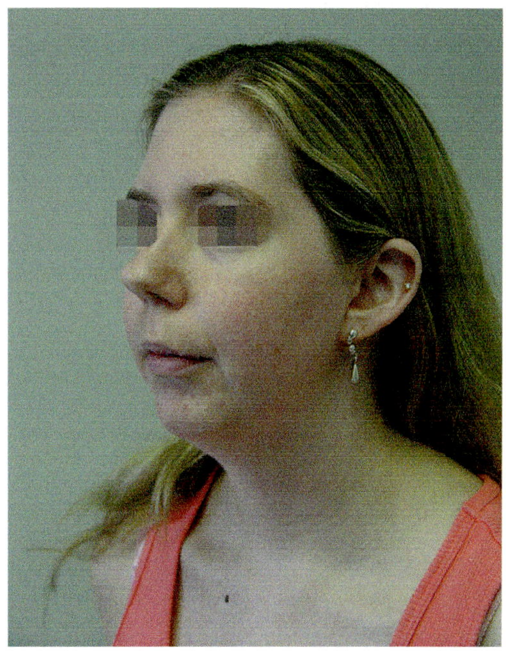

Fig. 9.67 Preoperative left 3/4 Facial view

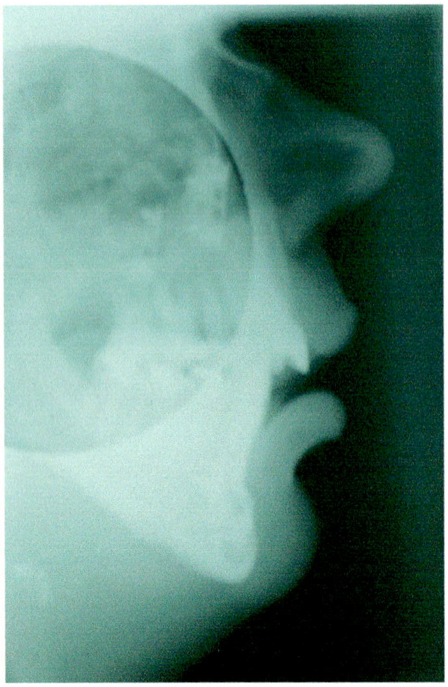

Fig. 9.68 Preoperative lateral cephalometric radiograph of bilateral mandibular sagittal split ramus osteotomies and genioplasty relapse with retrogenia

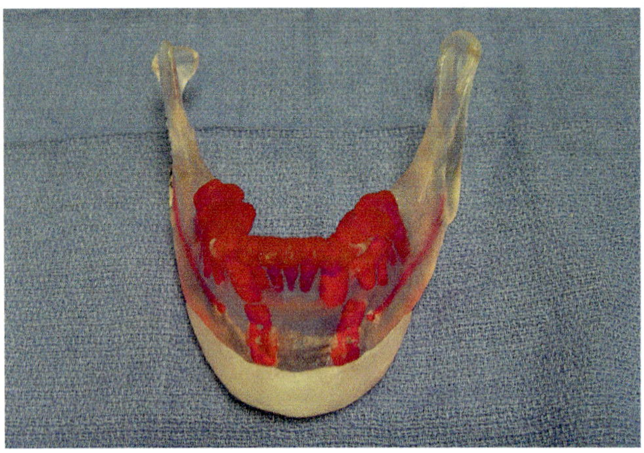

Fig. 9.69 Frontal view of custom wax chin implant prototype. Note retained chin mini plates

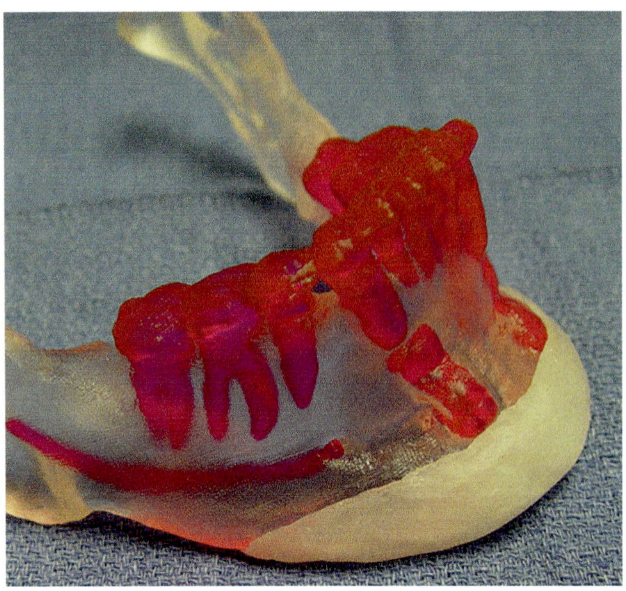

Fig. 9.70 Right anterior lateral view of custom wax chin implant prototype fitted to 3-D model

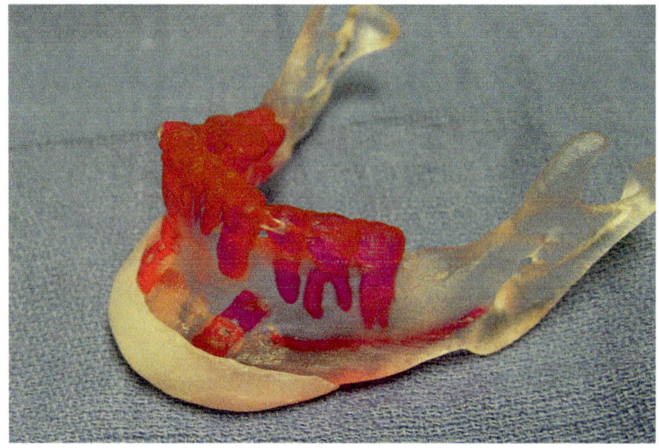

Fig. 9.71 Left anterior lateral view of custom wax implant prototype fitted to 3-D model

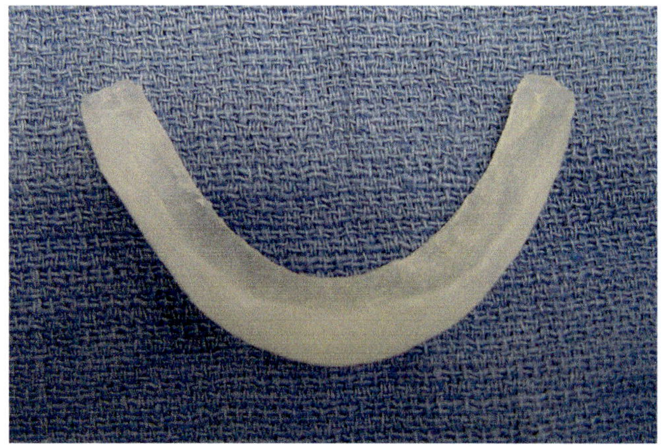

Fig. 9.72 Frontal superior view of custom wax chin implant prototype

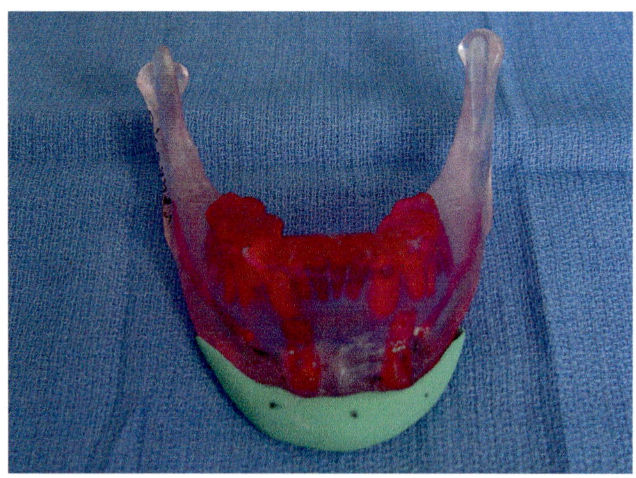

Fig. 9.73 Frontal superior view of silicone chin implant prototype fitted to 3-D model. Note: Markings for holes for fixation with 3 screws. The center hole is coincident with the facial midline

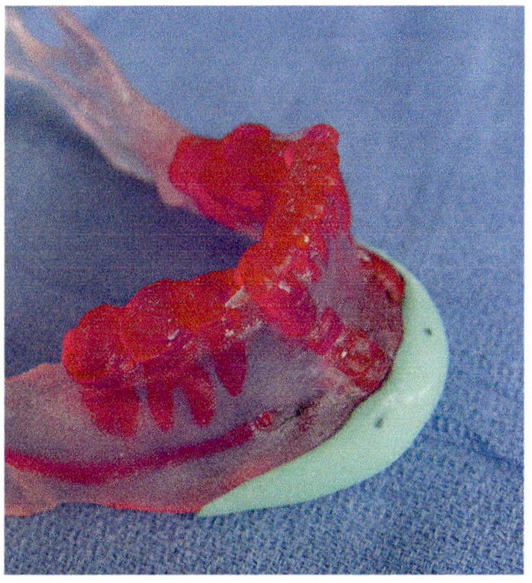

Fig. 9.74 Right anterior lateral view of silicone custom chin implant prototype fitted to 3-D model

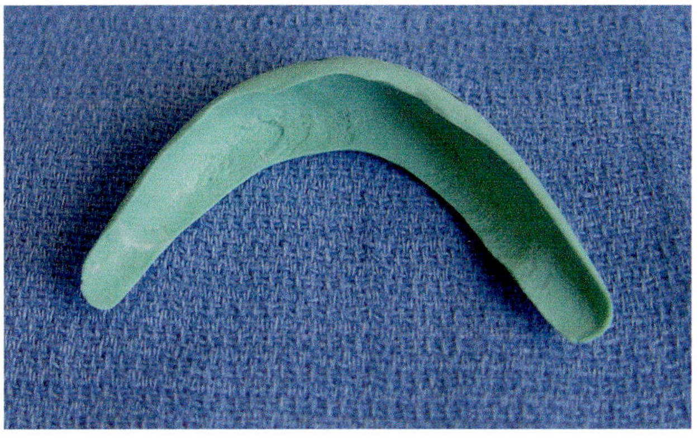

Fig. 9.75 Superior interior view of custom silicone chin implant prototype

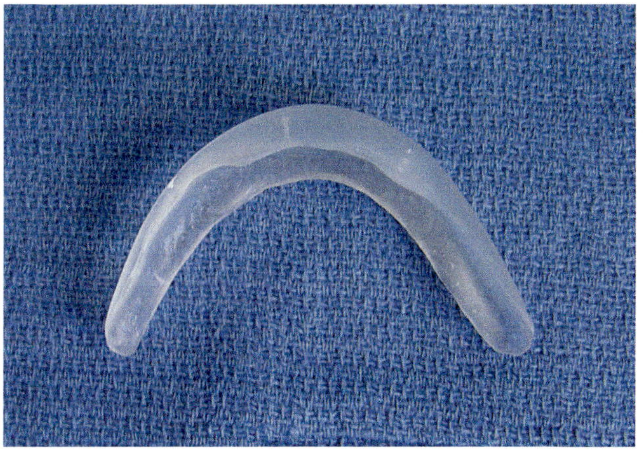

Fig. 9.76 Superior interior view of final silicone chin implant

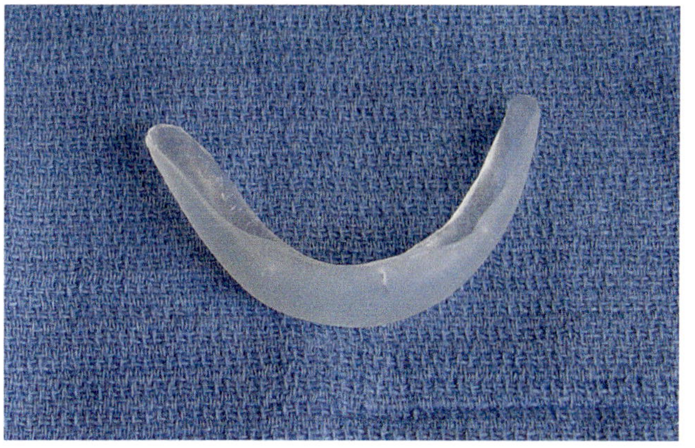

Fig. 9.77 Superior exterior view of final silicone chin implant

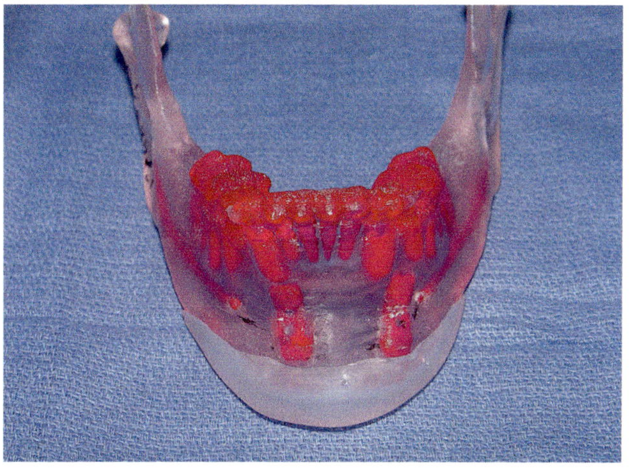

Fig. 9.78 Frontal superior view of final solid silicone chin implant prototype fitted to 3-D model

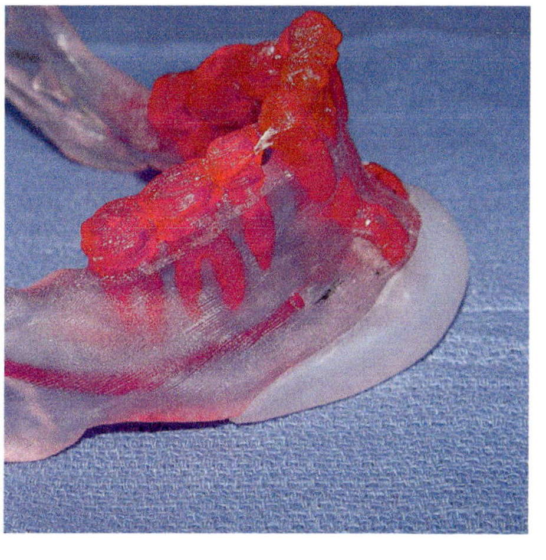

Fig. 9.79 Right lateral superior view of final silicone chin implant fitted to 3-D model

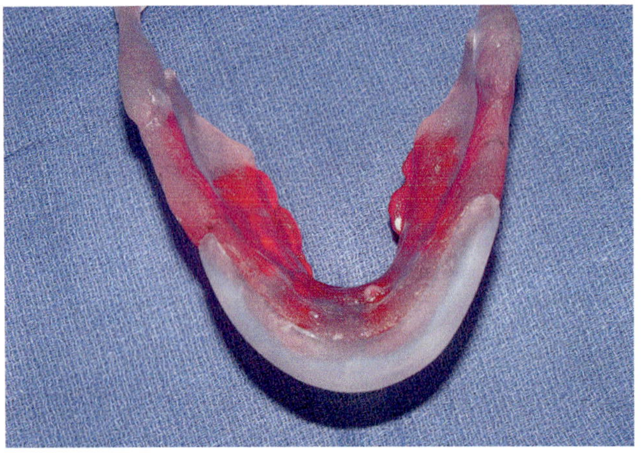

Fig. 9.80 Inferior view of solid silicone chin implant prototype fitted to 3-D model

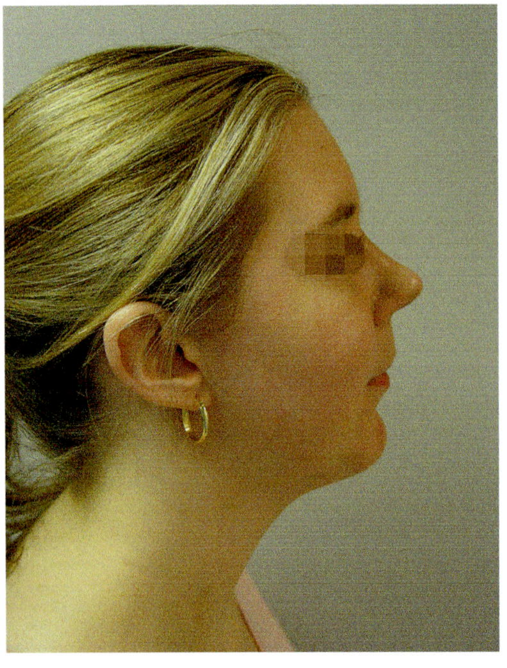

Fig. 9.81 Postoperative right lateral facial view

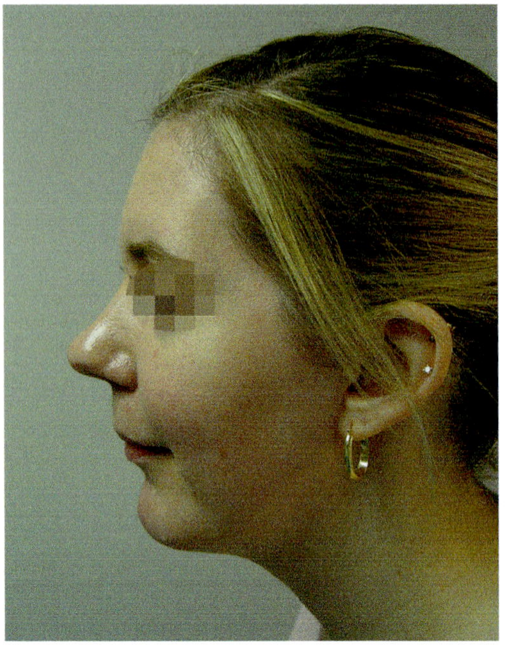

Fig. 9.82 Postoperative left lateral facial view

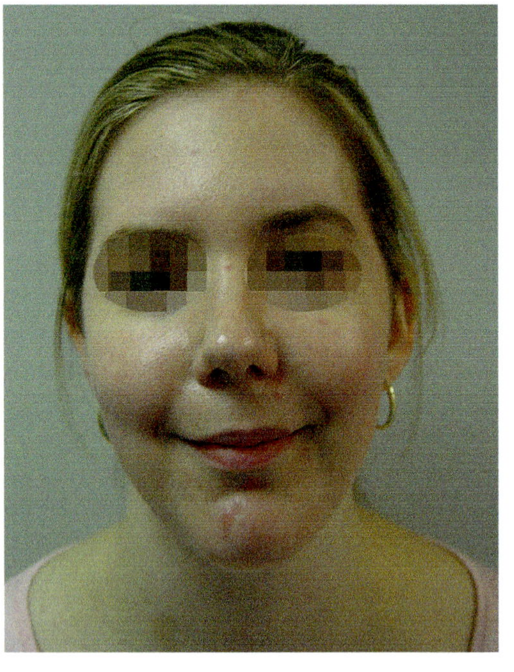

Fig. 9.83 Postoperative frontal facial view

Mandibular Angle Alloplastic Augmentation

The mandibular angle is an esthetic aspect of the face that is less commonly addressed (Fig. 9.84). However, it has its own particular clinical presentation, deformities, and contribution to overall facial esthetics [64–66]. The mandibular angle can present with normal contours, masseter hypertrophy [67–69], hypoplasia, and acquired deformities with loss of angle definition (Table 9.4) [47].

These deformities of the mandibular angle can be unilateral or bilateral. The mandibular angles can be classified based on a total lack of definition with either a concavity or straight plane in which there is no differentiation between the neck and mandibular inferior border and angle.

Mandibular angle augmentation has been performed with various methods including bone grafting, fat transplantation, fillers, and alloplastic materials (Figs. 9.1m–p) [4, 9, 64–66]. Alloplasts have included the use of solid silicone, polyethylene, HTR, and PEFE. Custom-designed implants have been reported using 3-D models as a template [4, 9, 70]. A total of 11

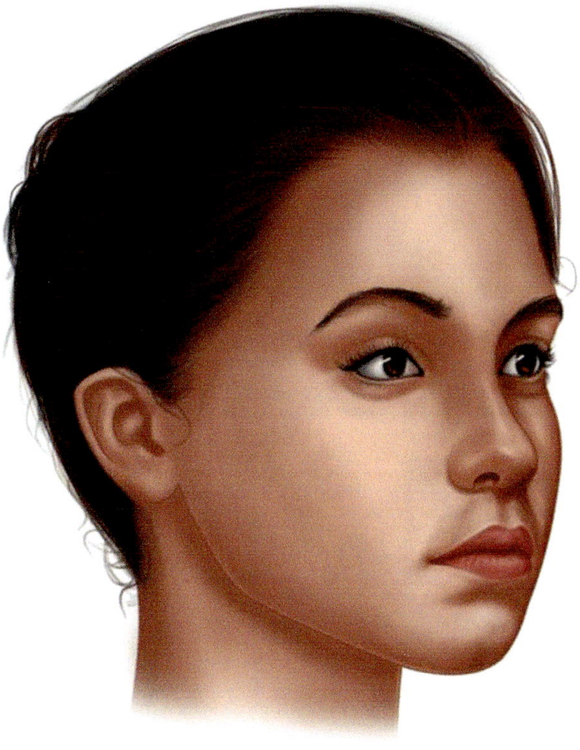

Fig. 9.84 Ideal right mandibular angle with rounded jaw line and distinct definition from the neck

Table 9.4 Mandibular angle deformity classification

I. Masseter hypertrophy
II. Normal masseter and bone contour
III A. Masseter hypoplasia
III B. Bone hypoplasia
III C. Combined masseter and bone hypoplasia
IV A. Acquired deformities: sagittal osteotomies
IV B. Acquired deformities: vertical osteotomies
IV C. Acquired deformities: trauma
IV D. Acquired deformities: tumor

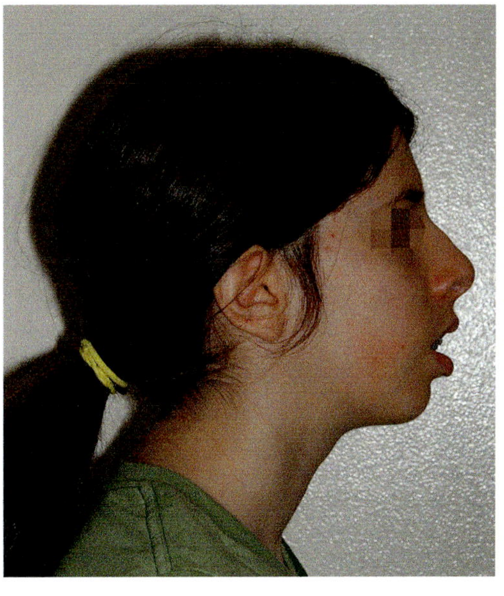

Fig. 9.85 Dolichocephaly (long face syndrome) facial type

patients had 21 custom mandibular angle solid silicone implants placed. Two implants was removed due to infection. One implant was a hand-carved polyethylene implant using a stereolithographic model as a template at the time of operation. One implant was removed because as an early case a buccal vestibular incision was utilized with wound dehiscence, and a second case 7 years after placement with cutaneous dehiscence following pharyngitis and necrosis of an adjacent lymph node.

A method for custom fabrication of mandibular angle implants from solid silicone utilizing 3-D stereolithographic models is described. Wax is utilized to form the mandibular angle implant and it is carved to the desired contours. The style of custom implant to be prepared depends on the indications for its use, whether for purely esthetic or reconstructive methods. For purely esthetic indications, these are patients with mandibular angle hypoplasia with indistinct definition between the mandibular angle and the neck. For females, this will be a subtle rounded augmentation, while in males, it will be larger and more square-like appearance. Differences between dolichocephaly (long face syndrome) [71] (Fig. 9.85) and brachycephaly (short face syndrome) [71] (Fig. 9.86) will be seen in the mandibular plane angle and clockwise rotation of the mandible in Class II and vertical maxillary hyperplasia patients. Patients can develop asymmetric ramus length and loss of angle as a result of trauma whether from a condylar fracture, incorrect setting of

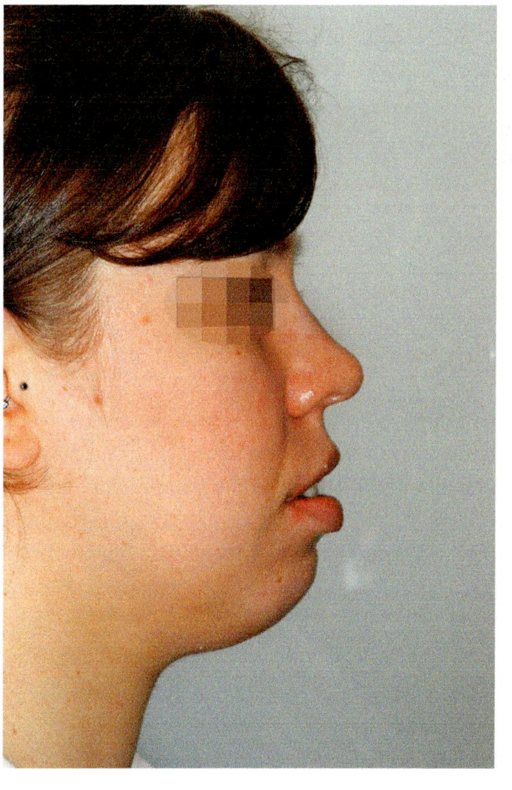

Fig. 9.86 Brachycephaly (short face syndrome) facial type

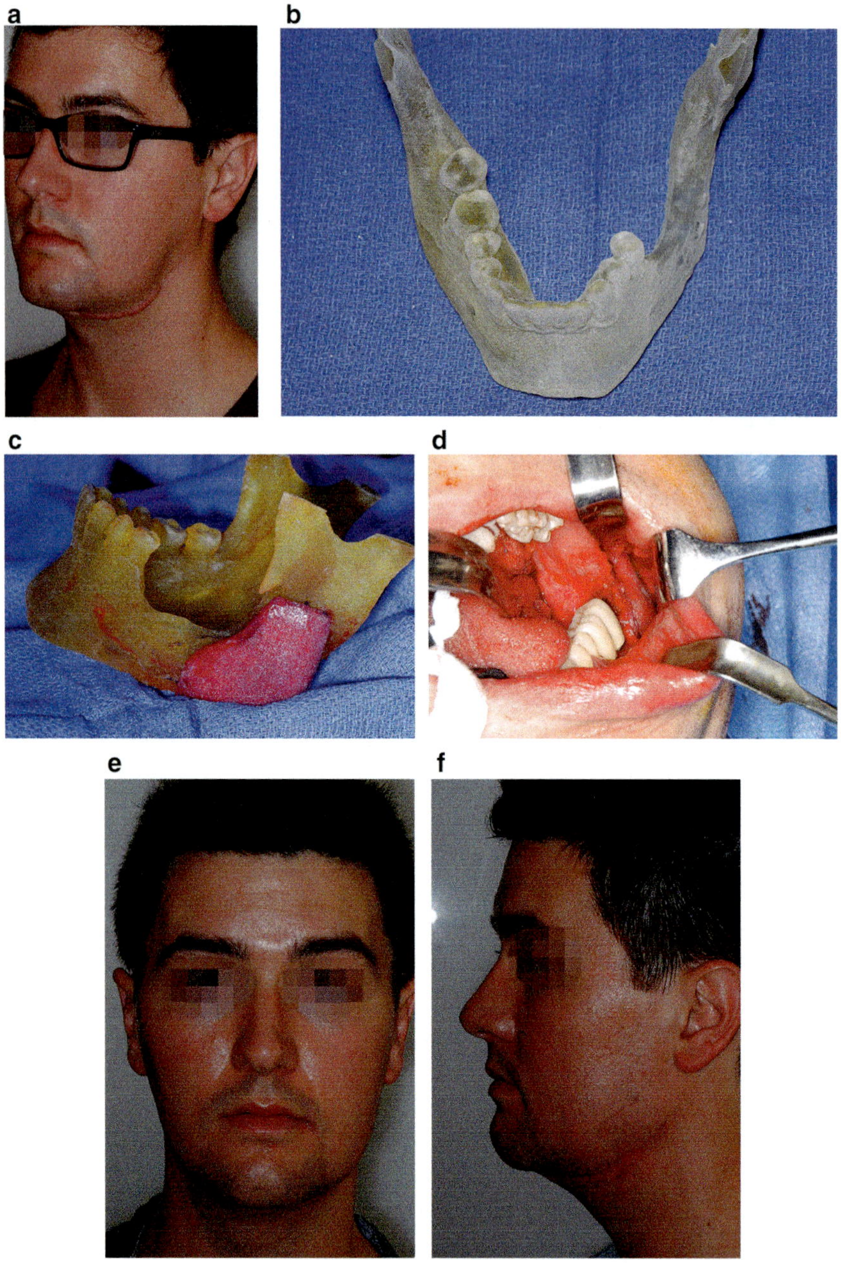

Fig. 9.87 (**a**) Left 3/4 facial view of left mandibular angle postsurgical deformity following partial mandibulectomy of ameloblastic fibroma and immediate free iliac crest bone graft. (**b**) Rapid printed 3-D mandible model. (**c**) Intraoperative custom hand-carved PEFE left mandibular angle implant. The implant fills in the step between the proximal segment and bone graft, re-establishes the jaw line at the inferior border. (**d**) Intraoperative intraoral placement of custom hand-carved PEFE left mandibular angle implant with screw fixation via transbuccal trocar. (**e**) Postoperative frontal facial view. (**f**) Postoperative left lateral facial view

body, symphysis, or parasymphysis fractures, in which the mandibular angle acquires a reduced intergonial dimension. Patients with tumors involving the mandibular angle can also benefit from custom implants (Fig. 9.87). Custom mandibular angle implants are indicated for reconstruction of previously operated patients. It is especially helpful in cases of revision of contour deformities secondary to mandibular osteotomies. Mandibular vertical ramus osteotomy contour irregularities can occur as a result of large or asymmetric movements, patients with thicker bone segments, or malposed segments Fig. 9.88a–g). For mandibular sagittal ramus osteotomies, there can be a loss of mandibular angle because of a stepped defect that results from large advancements with narrowing of the intergonial dimension and an inferior movement of the distal segment with loss of alignment of at the inferior border between the proximal and distal segments (Fig. 9.88h–j). In mandibular advancements with maxillary impaction for the correction of vertical maxillary excess, there is a superior movement of the distal segment which results in a narrowing of the intergonial dimension and a step defect. Rotational movements of bilateral mandibular sagittal ramus osteotomies for asymmetry can have a combination of inferior and superior placed distal segments with step deformities. Patients who have undergone excessive reduction of the mandibular angle by masseter reduction with or without bone recontouring may be suitable for restoration of

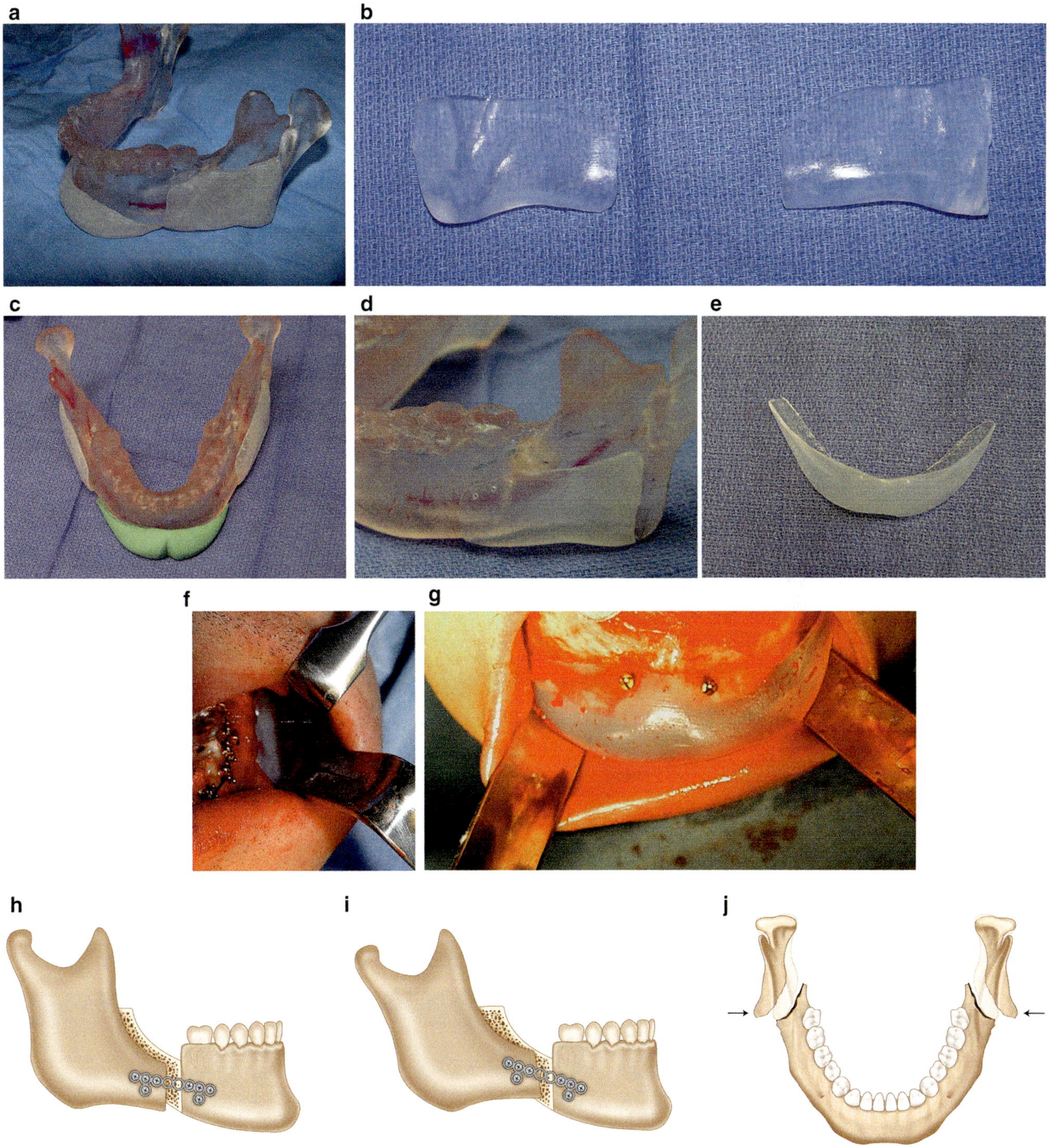

Fig. 9.88 (**a**) Lateral view of mandibular ramus vertical osteotomy with malposition of segments and resultant deformity of the angle and wax prototypes for custom left mandibular angle and chin implants. (**b**). Bilateral custom solid silicone implant created for correction of mandibular angle deformities secondary to vertical ramus osteotomies. (**c**) Superior frontal view of bilateral mandibular angle custom solid silicone implants and prototype of custom chin implant fitted to 3-D stereolithographic model. Note cleft in chin. (**d**) Lateral view of left mandibular angle custom solid silicone implant fitted to 3-D stereolithographic model. (**e**) Superior anterior view of custom solid silicone chin implant with midline cleft. (**f**) Intraoperative view placement of left mandibular angle custom solid silicone implant with screw fixation. (**g**) Intraoperative view placement of custom solid silicone chin implant with screw fixation. (**h**) Lateral view of mandibular ramus sagittal split osteotomy with advancement correct position of segments. (**i**) Lateral view of mandibular ramus sagittal split osteotomy with advancement incorrect position of segments with inferior and anterior positioning of distal segment and superior rotation of proximal segment resulting in loss of angle definition with step deformity. (**j**) Superior view of mandibular ramus sagittal split osteotomy with advancement and narrowing of intergonial distance resulting in loss of angle prominence with deformity

contour with the use of implants. The loss of masseter attachment creates a separate problem, because on animation when the masseter contracts the muscle bulge can be seen superior to its original location because of disruption of the pterygomasseteric sling (Fig. 9.89). This can be a difficult problem to solve and can require a combination of an implant with masseter reattachment or other soft tissue procedures [72].

These implants are placed only using an intraoral incision, and after early experience with a single case of wound dehiscence and loss of implant, the placement of the incision has been modified from a buccal sulcus incision similar to vertical ramus or sagittal split osteotomies to a buccal gingival sulcus incision with distal molar "hockey stick" and anterior vertical release (Fig. 9.90). This allows better coverage of the implant with the flap and has eliminated implant wound dehiscence. Satisfactory capsule formation permits smooth soft tissue contours. The most commonly used solid silicone implant texture has been "medium" which allows flexibility for insertion of the implant and adaption to the mandible during capsule formation.

This method of custom mandibular angle solid silicone implant fabrication includes an improvement in the design of the mandibular angle implant compared to previous "stock" implant designs with a change from the "S" curve [73] (Fig. 9.91a) at the inferior anterior aspect to a "trapezoid" that runs along the inferior aspect of the external oblique ridge of the mandible to permit improved intraoral screw fixation (Fig. 9.91b, c). It is also unnecessary to extend the implants beyond the midportion of the ramus as many "stock" implants do, to allow greater maintenance of masseter attachment to the bone. Most of the augmentation that is needed for the mandibular angle is in the inferior 1/3 of the

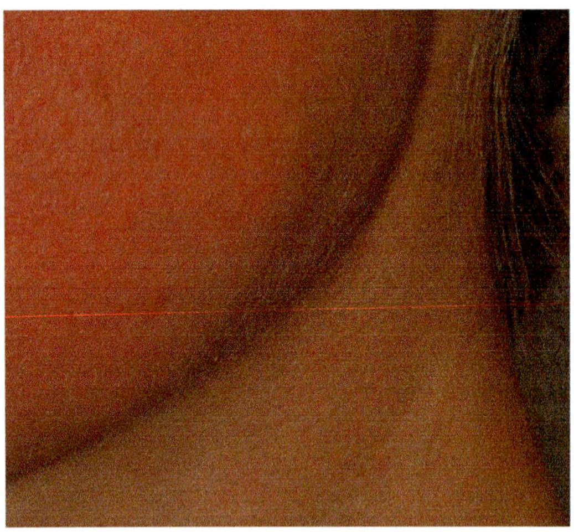

Fig. 9.89 Left mandibular angle loss of masseter or attachment following reduction procedure with superior bulge of masseter edge on clenching

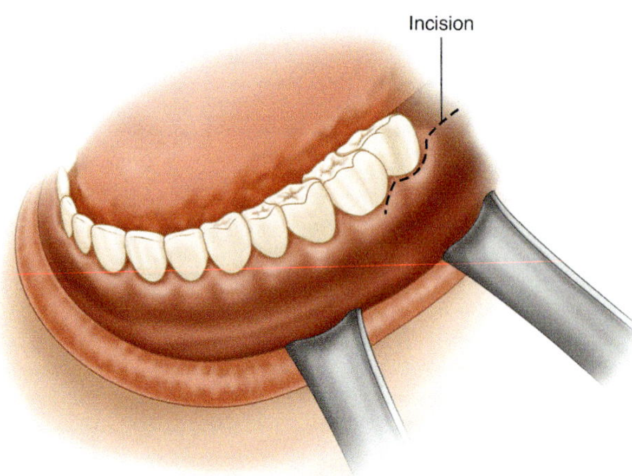

Fig. 9.90 Example of intraoral posterior buccal crestal incision with anterior vertical release for mandibular angle implant placement

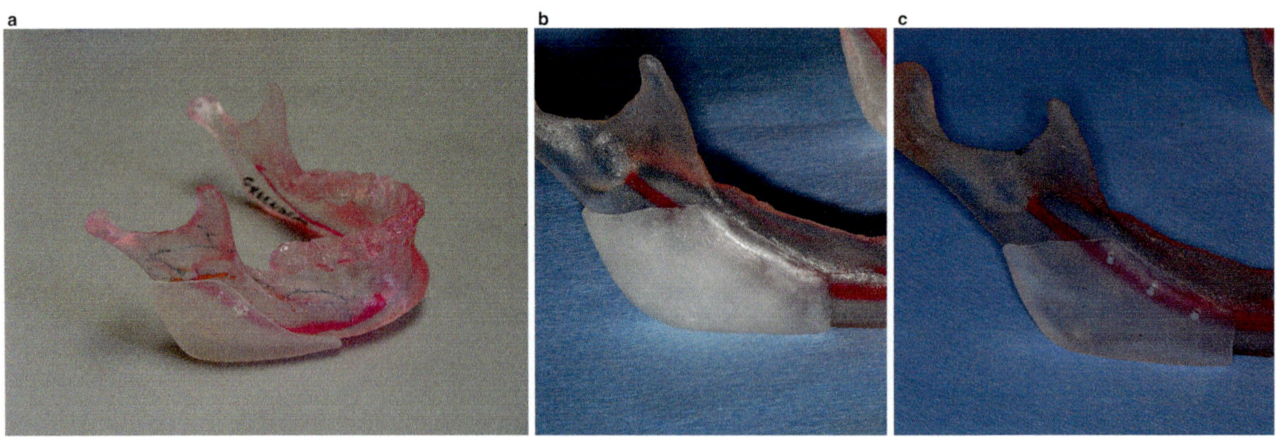

Fig. 9.91 (**a**) Example of earlier S shaped mandibular angle implant for which it was difficult to achieve fixation through an intraoral approach. (**b**) Improved design with pentagon shaped implant with anterior superior extension to allow intraoral screw hole placement as wax prototype. (**c**) Final solid silicone angle implant with screw holes along the anterior superior border to allow intraoral screw placement and the avoidance of the mandibular nerve

ramus, and therefore superior extension is not necessary. In creating these implants, there is consideration of the shape for inferior masseter contours. Some patients will have a greater rounded definition of the masseter on contraction along the inferior third, while others will be less distinct. Implants can be more smoothly rounded or have a "bulge" to create a greater simulation of masseter contraction.

Screw fixation of these implants provides further stability and prevention of displacement and resorption. Screws can be inserted into preplanned holes along the superior aspect of the implant via an intraoral approach. The implants are designed with a thin extended superior and anterior border along the external oblique crest without crossing its superior border.

Patient Evaluation and Anthropometric Measurements

Patients need to be evaluated for hard and soft tissue aspects of their deformity. There will be significant differences between unoperated patients with developmental deformities and operated patients with alterations in the bony anatomy and scar formation. Symmetry is a very important aspect to evaluate. Patients who have had orthognathic mandibular surgery will often have differences between the two sides. Unoperated patients may have developmental or acquired differences in their facial symmetry. Dental occlusion must be evaluated as many of these patients are Class II. It would be rare for a Class III mandibular prognathism patient to have mandibular angle hypoplasia, even in a high angle case. Occlusal cant is often associated with differences in ramus heights, shorter on the side rotated upward and longer on the side rotated downward. Notches at the junction of the body and angle, lateral spurs, and masseter muscle variations need to be noted. Soft tissue of the neck is critical, especially if there is an obtuse neck-throat angle. Lipodystrophy must also be evaluated to determine if liposuction or platysma repair is needed. Patient ¾ view black-and-white and colored photos, clinical examination, and 2-D and 3-D images are essential for treatment planning.

CT Scanning for Evaluation and Creation of a Stereolithographic Model

The patient will need to undergo CT or CBCT with the head in a natural position relative to Frankfort Horizontal. The DICOM data is then transferred to a service provider either on a disk or uploaded via a website in order to then fabricate a stereolithographic model. Stereolithographic models for mandibular angles must include the full condyle for mandibular angle custom implant fabrication.

Patient Anthropometric Analysis

The mandibular angle has several variations that are not harmonious. Benign masseteric hypertrophy can be an excessive contour due to bone or muscle or a combination of both, and often the mandibular angles will be curved with a lateral flare [66–69] (Fig. 9.92a, b). There have been various analyses proposed for the evaluation of benign masseteric hypertrophy, but there do not appear to be specific analysis for classification of other deformities of the mandibular angle. Patients with benign masseteric hypertrophy can be managed with nonsurgical Botox injections or surgical procedures to reduce muscle and bone excess [69]. The risorius muscle will overlie the mid portion of the anterior aspect of the masseter and will sometimes be affected by Botox injections. Patients can be classified according to certain facial types such as dolichocephalic and brachyocephalic which can be pertinent to the mandibular angle. Dolichocephalic patients can present with long face syndrome [71] with or without anterior open bite and can present with mandibular angle hypoplasia. Brachyocephalic [71] facial types will have masseter hyperplasia that can still have a lack of mandibular angle to neck

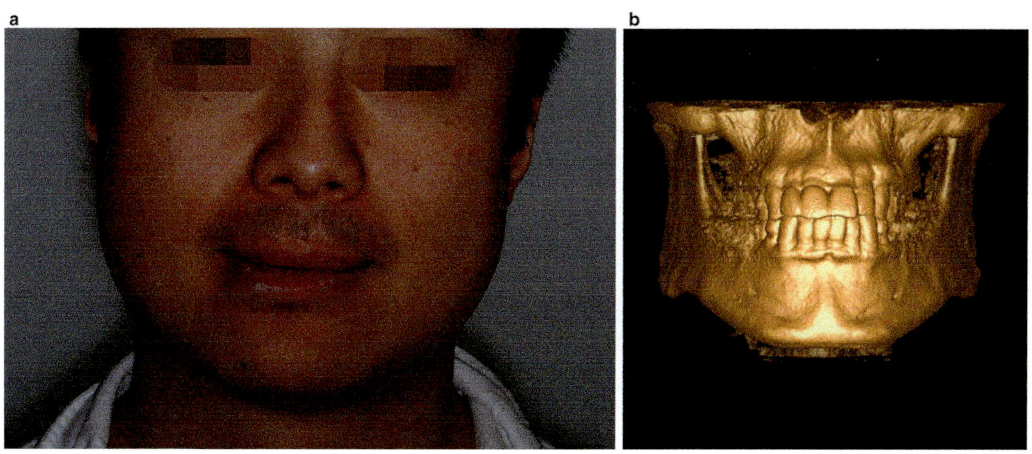

Fig. 9.92 (**a**) Bilateral masseter hypertrophy. (**b**) 3-D CBCT frontal view of bilateral mandibular angle bony hyperplasia with flaring

definition. Clinical examination includes a facial proportions analysis which should include the comparison to the proportions and contours of the malar eminences, zygomas, submalar, chin, and mandibular width/jaw line.

Mandibular angle deficiency is the result of:

1. Sagittal ramus osteotomies.
2. Inverted L osteotomies.
3. Disharmony secondary to hemimandibular hyperplasia on the unaffected side resulting in imbalance, treated and untreated mandibular condylar fractures, incorrectly treated mandibular body, parasymphysis, symphysis, and multiple fractures with inadequate correction and resultant narrowing of the intergonial angle which can be unilateral and bilateral.
4. Acquired mandibular angle deficiencies can be soft or hard tissue or both following procedures to reduce benign masseteric hypertrophy or for jaw slimming procedures.
5. Vertical ramus osteotomies.

Patients may also present with preangle notching of the inferior border which can be treated with an implant or removal of the mandibular angle (Fig. 9.93a). Patients who have undergone radiation therapy of the head and neck can present with parotid-masseteric atrophy which can reveal an underlying skeletal deformity (Fig. 9.93b, c). Head and neck cancer, parotidectomy, and mandibular resection with or without reconstruction can all have associated deformities of the mandibular angle.

Achieving Balance with Chin with or without an Implant

Many patients with an ill-defined mandibular angle seek to have a more prominent angle. Men prefer to have large prominent angles to project masculinity and strength, while women like to have defined jaw line with less skin laxity. For women, a more prominent mandibular angle will also help to accentuate the submalar concavity which is considered to be esthetically pleasing and a sign of beauty. Women should have a more delicate mandibular angle than men.

The mandibular angle needs to be balanced with the zygoma and the zygomatic arch. Frequently these patients have strong malar eminences but lack definition of the angles. Mandibular angle esthetics are also determined by the mandibular plane angle. It is in the high plane Class II cases that are usually more deficient compared to patients with horizontal mandibular planes which have better jaw line definition. Straightening of a high plane mandibular angle can be achieved with a custom angle implant. Using Leonardo's square [23], it is possible to analyze the mandibular angle and determine if it needs to be moved inferiorly. The mandibular angle can range from being almost a straight line to a 90 degree junction between the ascending ramus and the horizontal body. Ideal ranges include NF = 115–13 degrees, NFa = 30–40 degrees, NMe 120–132 degrees, and MC 80–95 degrees. Unless there is a very high angle with the mandible setback with mandibular bilateral vertical ramus osteotomies, it will widen; with sagittal split osteotomies, it may stay the same.

Technique for Wax Application and Carving of the Implant

The method to create a wax block outline for the mandibular angle implant is to analyze the dimension which is desired to augment. This is often helped by the structure of the stereolithographic model and its inherent bony deficiency. This is also where the art of being able to assess the patient's esthetic

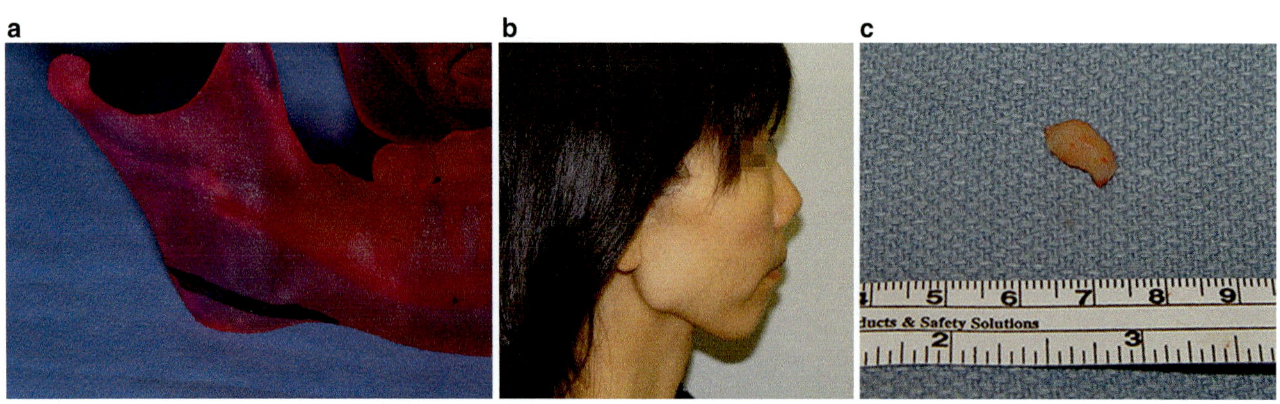

Fig. 9.93 (**a**) 3-D stereolithographic model with preangular notch demonstrating osteotomy line for removal of bony angle. (**b**) Right mandibular preangle notch and the patient following full course radiation therapy with atrophy of the parotid muscle. (**c**) Bony angle removed via intraoral approach using an oscillating saw

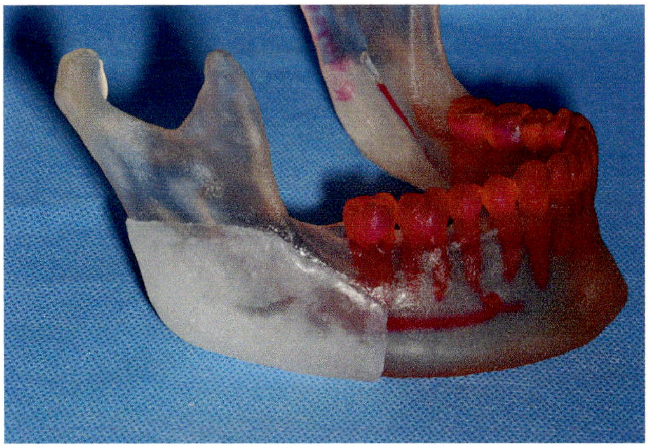

Fig. 9.94 Right lateral view of mandibular angle custom implant wax initial form of prototype fitted to 3-D model

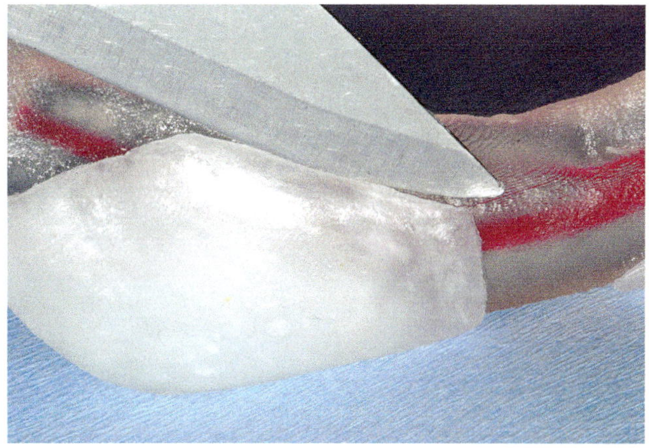

Fig. 9.95 Feathering of superior edge of mandibular angle custom implant wax prototype with knife

features and desired contours comes into play, and requires the complete review of clinical examination, facial photographs, facial moulage and PA cephalometric and CT radiographs. It is important for the mandibular angle implant to "wrap around the inferior border" so as to create a smooth contour and straightening of the jaw line to provide better definition and extension of the patient's jaw line. This inferior augmentation also helps to create a "defining line" or boundary between the mandibular angle and the neck, which is often indistinct in these patients, and augmentation at the site of the thickened masseter muscle insertion and contraction "bulge." Increments of between 5–10 mm are typically the thicknesses of these implants at the point of maximum augmentation which corresponds to the insertion of the masseter and the raised muscle mass that is prominent at the mandibular angle. Superiorly above the midportion of the implant, it should be thin to blend by feather edging along the middle of the ascending ramus where augmentation is less necessary.

The 3-D stereolithographic model is coated with Vaseline to prevent sticking of the wax. Ropes of wax (Modern Materials Utility Wax Strips Large White, Heraeus Kulzer, South Bend, IN, USA) are then hand rolled for softening and then pressed onto the model to begin to form the implant along the mandibular angle region as a block that should curve around the inferior border and posterior borders (Fig. 9.94). A laboratory knife is then used to begin to carve the wax to the desired form (Fig. 9.95). The main augmentation is on the lateral aspect of the mandibular ramus and inferior border. It has been found that a modification of the earlier Epker [73] style of mandibular angle has been developed so as to provide the ability of the implant to have ease of intraoral screw fixation. This is achieved by extending the anterior portion of the implant from the inferior border to a superior direction along the lateral oblique ridge of the mandible which is superior to the mandibular nerve which can be marked on the model. This is important from a fixation point of view, and screw holes for the implant should be placed along the superior margins to allow intraoral placement of the screws with the avoidance of a skin incision and use of a trocar.

Once the general outline has been achieved, the implant needs to be removed from the model so as to begin to measure the thickness with a Boley gauge. Depending on the amount of augmentation desired, it is important to have equal symmetry between each angle in its thickness and condyle head to gonion length. Greater definition of the mandibular angle can be achieved by thickening the wax and defining the mandibular posterior border, whether in unilateral or bilateral cases. The edges of the implant need to be feathered along the anterior aspects so that the implant is extremely thin and blends with the inferior and lateral borders so as to prevent a step in the skin which is unesthetic.

The model with the completed wax implant prototypes (Figs. 9.95 and 9.96) is then sent to a laboratory to be fabricated into solid silicone (Figs. 9.97 and 9.98). Various hardnesses of silicone are available ranging from hard, medium, soft, and extra soft. All implants that I have utilized to date have been medium in hardness as it provides a firm yet resilient sensation that is pleasing to the patient as it provides a more natural feeling on palpation. The medium texture implant is also easier to insert around the inferior and posterior border due to its flexibility. The implant when received from the manufacturer should be checked on the 3-D model to ensure correct fabrication, fit, and screw hole placement (Figs. 9.99 and 9.100). The 3-D model should be thoroughly cleaned of Vaseline prior to the fitting of the implant. The implant is then autoclave sterilized according to the manufacturer's specifications (Table 9.3). Once placed on the operating table, the implant can be kept in a basin containing normal saline solution.

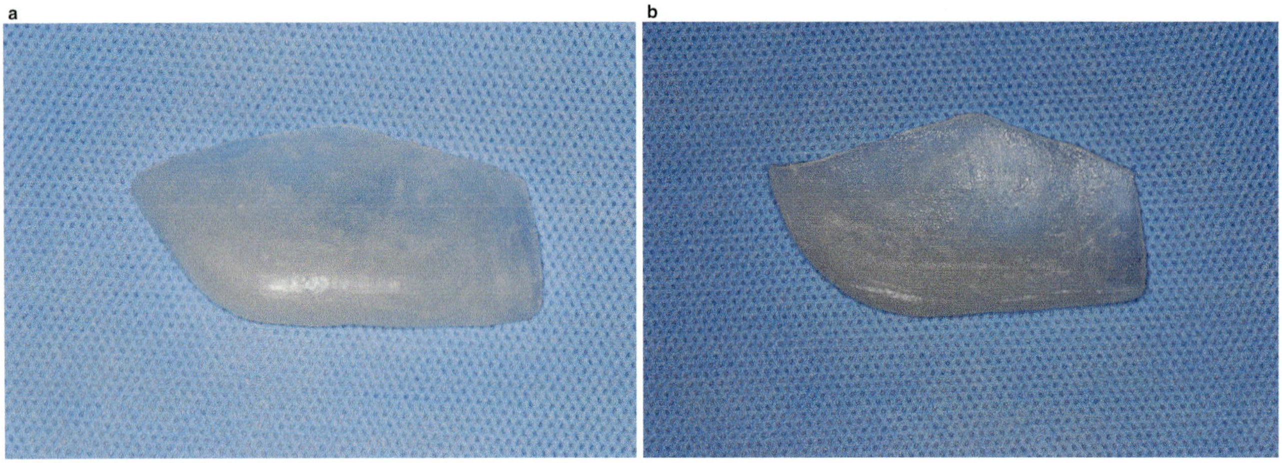

Fig. 9.96 (**a**) Right mandibular angle custom implant works prototype exterior view. (**b**) Right mandibular angle custom implant wax prototype interior view

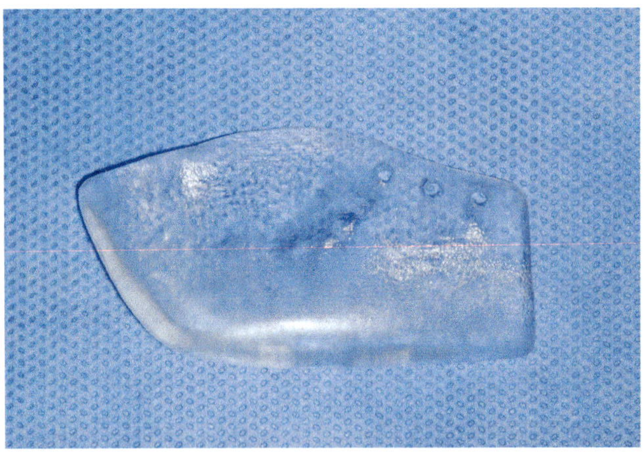

Fig. 9.97 Right mandibular angle custom solid silicone implant exterior view

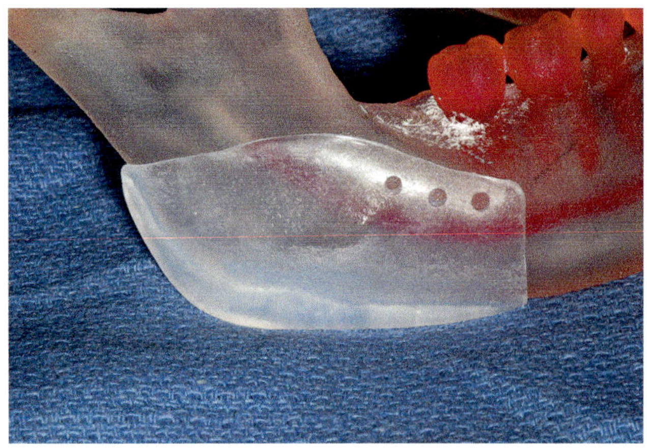

Fig. 9.99 Right mandibular angle custom solid silicone implant fitted to 3-D model lateral view. Note screw holes along superior anterior border will be placed along the external oblique ridge

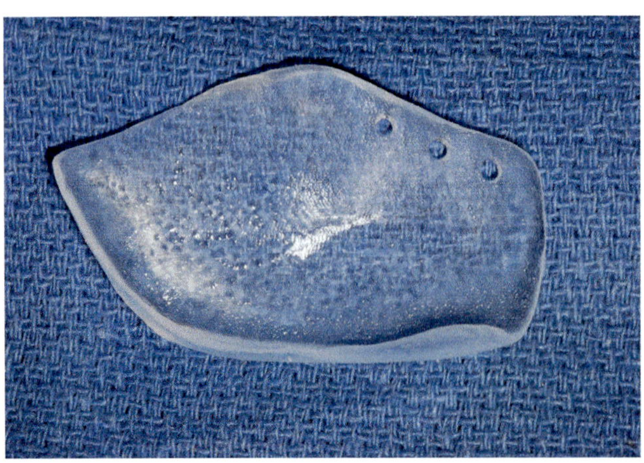

Fig. 9.98 Right mandibular angle custom solid silicone implant interior view with screw holes

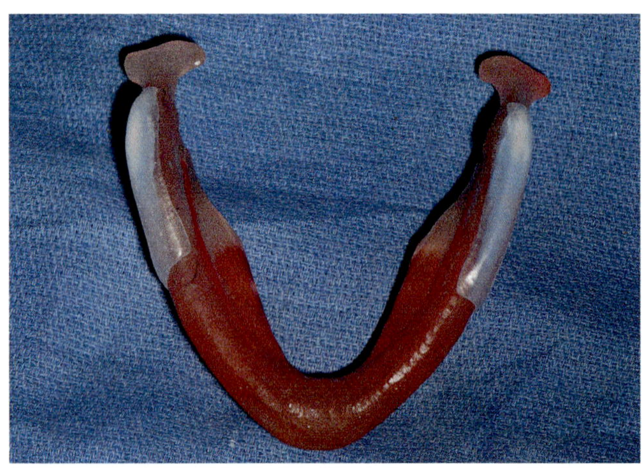

Fig. 9.100 Bilateral mandibular angle custom solid silicone implants fitted to 3-D model interior view note for the feathering of edges along the inferior border margins

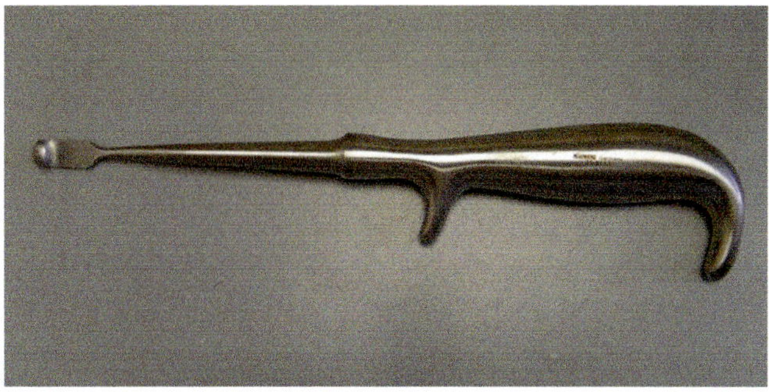

Fig. 9.101 Hargis sling stripper ("J stripper") instrument (Lorenz, Zimmer Biomet Microfixation, Jacksonville, FL, USA)

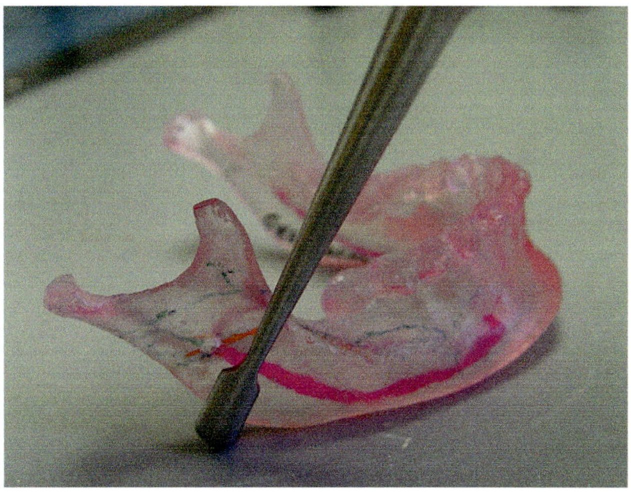

Fig. 9.102 Hargis sling stripper ("J stripper"), Lorenz, Zimmer Biomet Microfixation, Jacksonville, FL, USA applied to lateral aspect of right mandibular angle and ramus

Surgical Technique

These procedures can be performed both in the hospital and office settings under full general anesthesia or moderate sedation. After local anesthetic has been given as local infiltration via intraoral and transcutaneous approaches (mandibular blocks for in office moderate sedation), a posterior buccal incision preferably using a #15 scalpel blade is created at a 45 degree angle through mucosa, submucosa, and perimandibular musculature and extends along the gingival buccal sulcular attached gingiva of the molars with an anterior vertical releasing along the retromolar pad and through the buccal gingival sulcus so as to create a full-thickness mucoperiosteal flap that provides maximal coverage of the implant (Fig. 9.90). An earlier lateral buccal vestibular incision similar to the approach for a vertical ramus ostetomy has been discontinued due to the complications experienced from dehiscence of the wound overlying the superior aspect of the implant and its exposure, infection, and subsequent need for removal. The anterior vertical releasing incision should be anterior to the planned position of the anterior edge of the implant (Fig. 9.90). Utilizing a freer or #9 periosteal elevator, a full-thickness mucoperiosteal flap is reflected. A V-notched ramus retractor is then used to dissect the temporalis muscles free from the ascending ramus, and the subperiosteal dissection continues laterally to elevate the masseter attachments from the underlying mandible with care to avoid perforation of the periosteum.

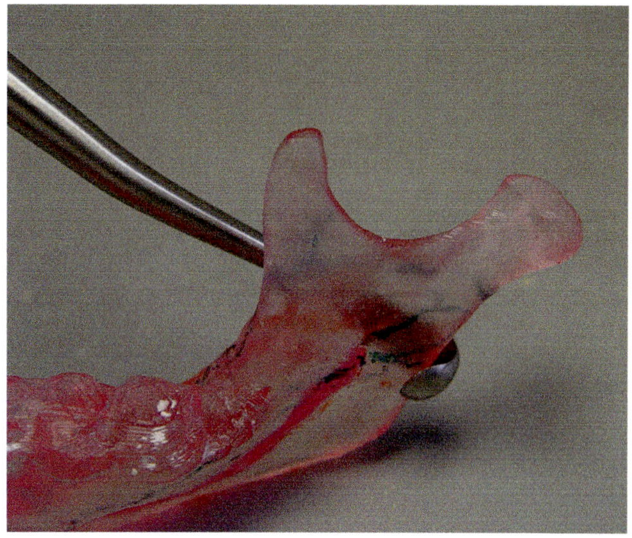

Fig. 9.103 Medial aspect view of Hargis sling stripper ("J stripper"), Lorenz, Zimmer Biomet Microfixation, Jacksonville, FL, USA applied along the posterior border of the right mandibular ramus

A curved periosteal freer (Obwegeser type) is utilized to reflect the periosteum to the level of the inferior border. A Hargis sling stripper ("J stripper"), Lorenz, Zimmer Biomet Microfixation, Jacksonville, FL, USA is then inserted along the inferior border so as to complete the subperiosteal dissection, elevation, and exposure of the mandibular angle and ramus (Figs. 9.101, 9.102, and 9.103). Care should be taken when using the Hargis sling stripper ("J stripper"), Lorenz, Zimmer Biomet Microfixation, Jacksonville, FL, USA as it can lacerate the masseter, and the curved periosteal elevator may be less traumatic. At this time the wound is irrigated and the implant is inserted and the desired positon is confirmed. The curved end of the curved freer can be used against the inferior edge of the implant to help ensure that it is correctly seated. Because of the anatomic fit of these implants once inserted, they are easily seated and the superior edge along the external oblique ridge can also provide a reference to correct seating. Once verification of the implant position has been achieved, then the transoral monocortical screw fixation is performed with two or three 1.3 or 1.5 mm bone screws (DuPuy Synthes Craniomaxillofacial, Paoli, PA, USA). The wound is then copiously irrigated and closed with 4–0 vicryl sutures.

Case Reports

Case 4

A 34-year-old male patient presented with severe Class II anterior open bite and bilateral mandibular angle hypoplasia with retrogenia as a type of long face syndrome. A LeFort I osteotomy was performed with bilateral mandibular angle custom solid silicone implants and an anterior horizontal mandibular osteotomy (Figs. 9.104–9.139). (Alex M. Greenberg, DDS, Oral and Maxillofacial Surgeon, New York, NY, USA).

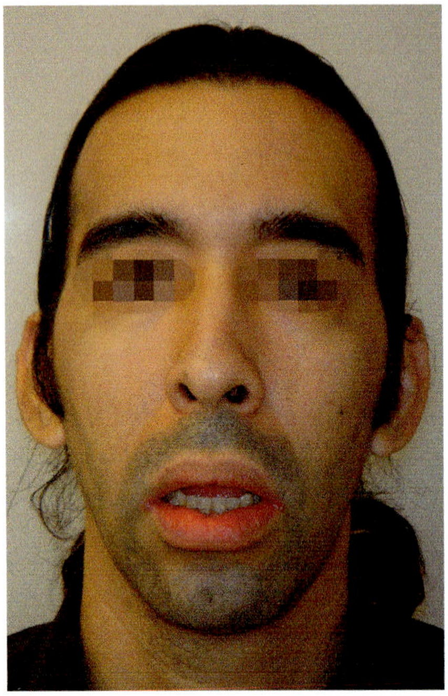

Fig. 9.104 Preoperative frontal facial view of patient with severe anterior open bite, bilateral mandibular angle lack of definition, and retrognathia

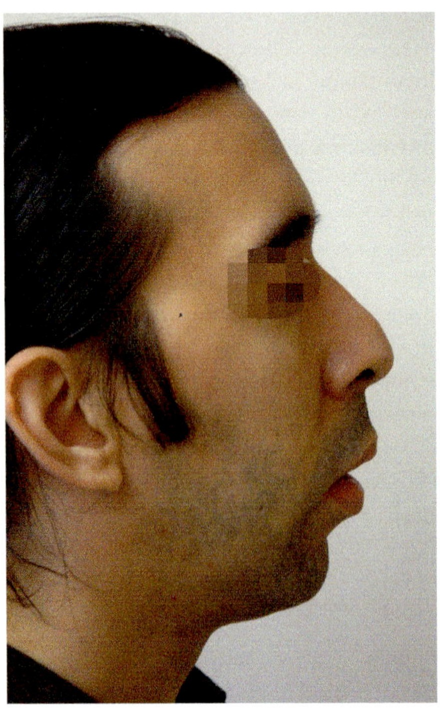

Fig. 9.105 Preoperative lateral right facial view

Case 5

A 19-year-old female patient presented with a cleft soft palate and mild Class II malocclusion that was orthodontically treated and bilateral mandibular angle hypoplasia and retrogenia. A combined plastic and maxillofacial surgical procedure was performed with placement of bilateral mandibular angle custom solid silicone implants and anterior horizontal mandibular osteotomy with simultaneous liposuction of the neck (Richard Skolnick, Plastic Surgeon, NY, NY) to improve the definition of the bone and implant contours. (Figs. 9.140–9.158). (Alex M. Greenberg, DDS, Oral and Maxillofacial Surgeon, New York, NY, USA)

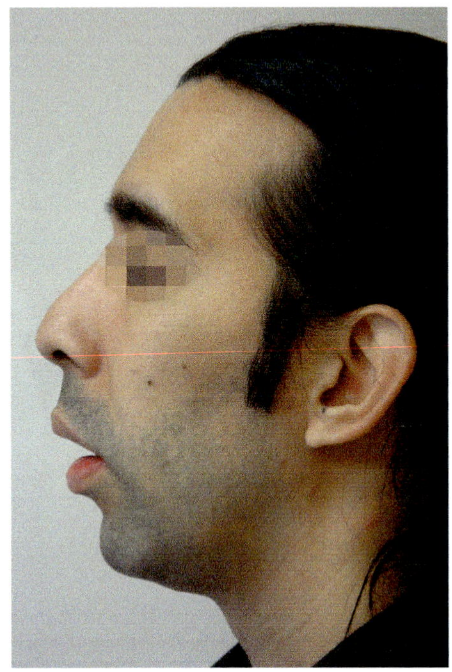

Fig. 9.106 Preoperative lateral left facial view

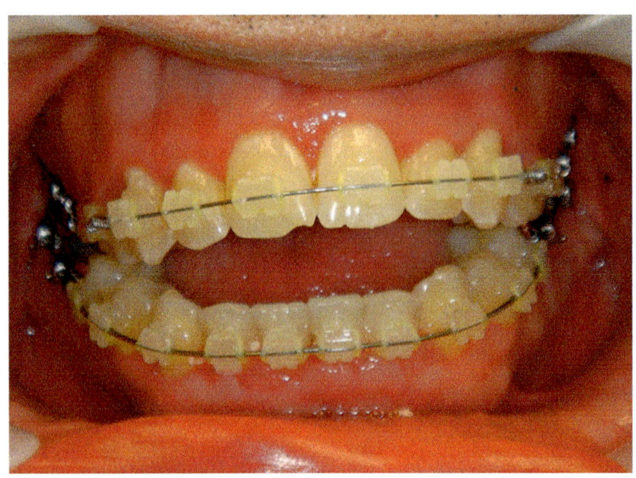

Fig. 9.107 Preoperative frontal view of skeletal Class II malocclusion

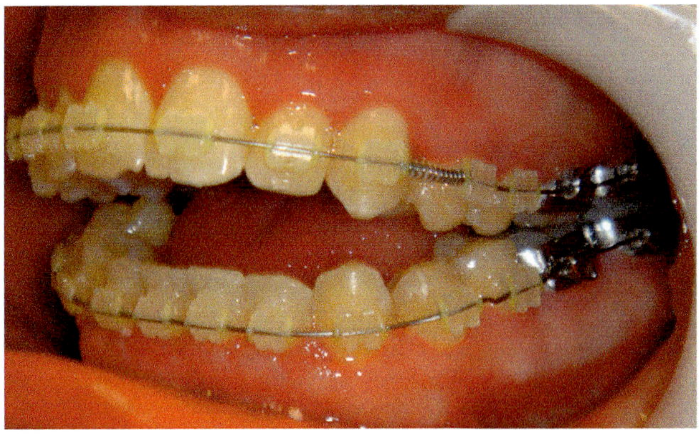

Fig. 9.108 Preoperative left frontal view of Class II skeletal malocclusion

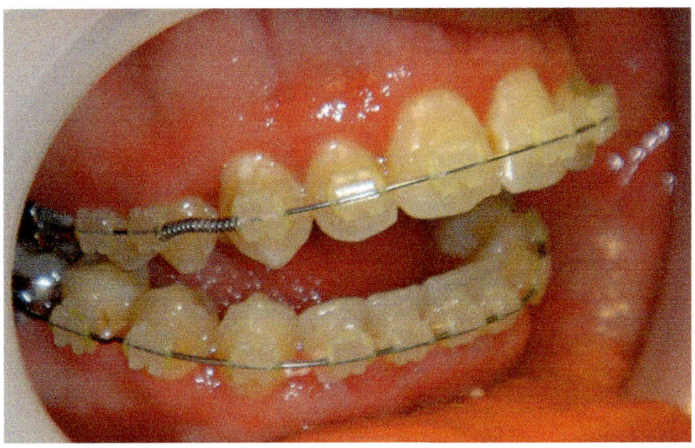

Fig. 9.109 Preoperative right frontal view of Class II skeletal malocclusion

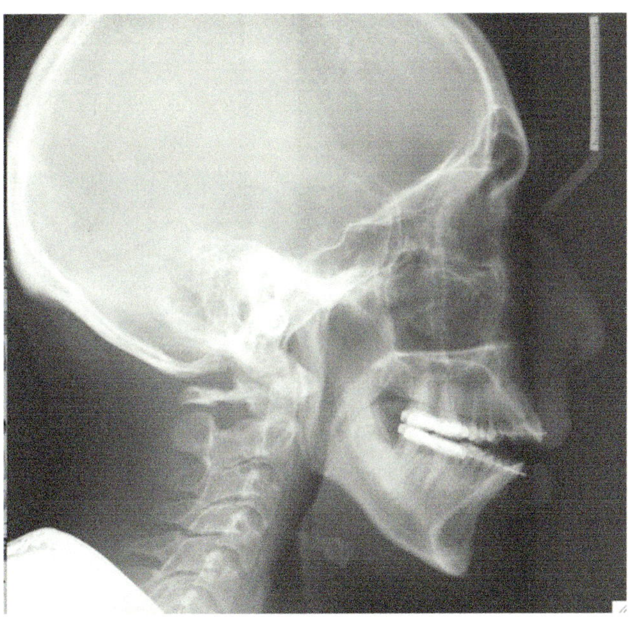

Fig. 9.110 Preoperative right lateral cephalometric radiograph view

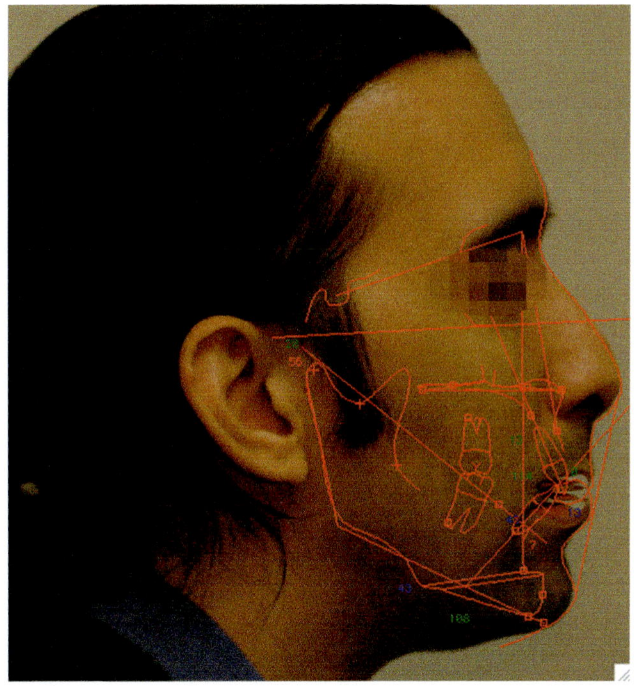

Fig. 9.111 Simulation LeFort I osteotomy with sliding genioplasty advancement right lateral view

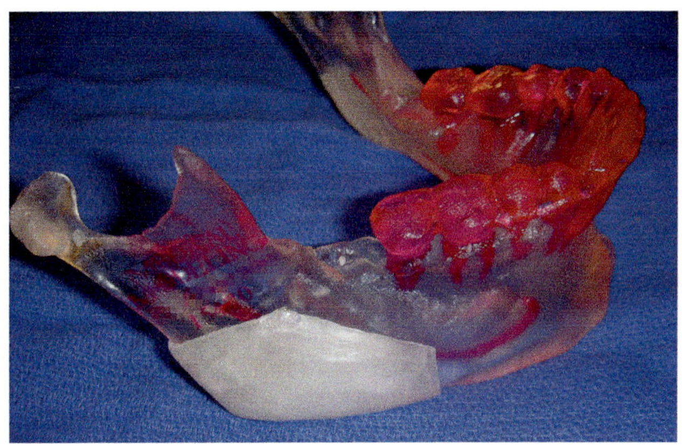

Fig. 9.112 Right mandibular implant wax prototype fitted to 3-D model

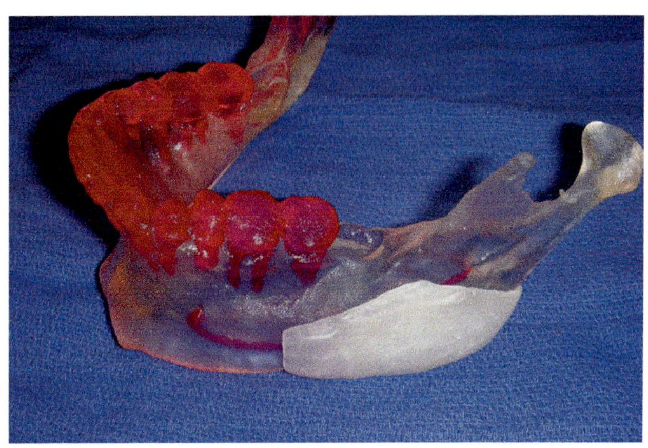

Fig. 9.113 Left mandibular implant wax prototype fitted to 3-D model

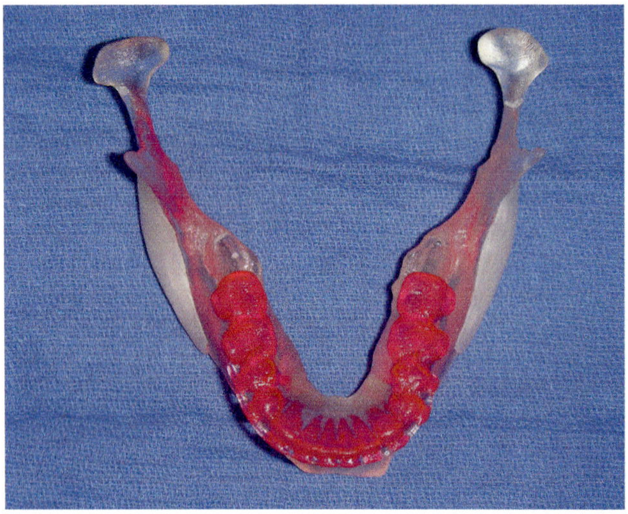

Fig. 9.114 Bilateral mandibular custom angle implant wax prototypes fitted to 3-D model superior view

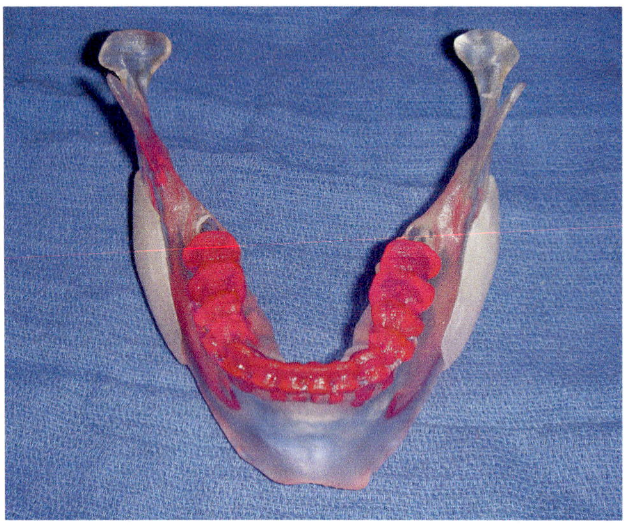

Fig. 9.115 Bilateral mandibular custom angle implant wax prototypes fitted to 3-D model anterior superior view

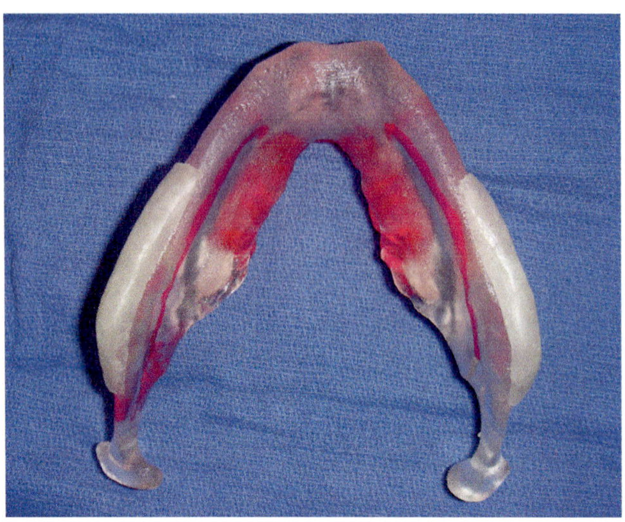

Fig. 9.116 Bilateral mandibular custom angle implant wax prototypes fitted to 3-D model inferior view

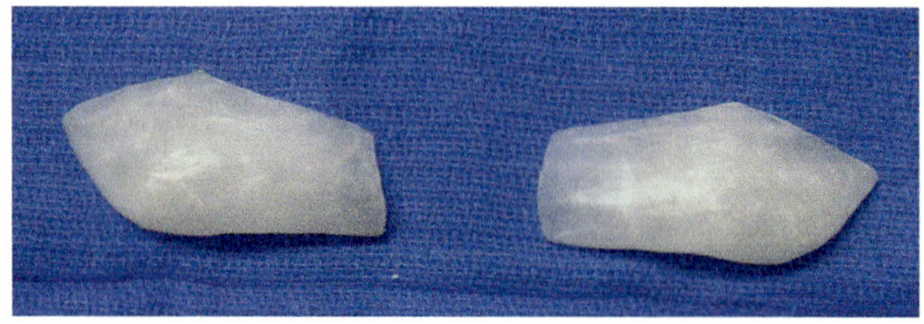

Fig. 9.117 Bilateral mandibular custom angle implant wax prototypes exterior view

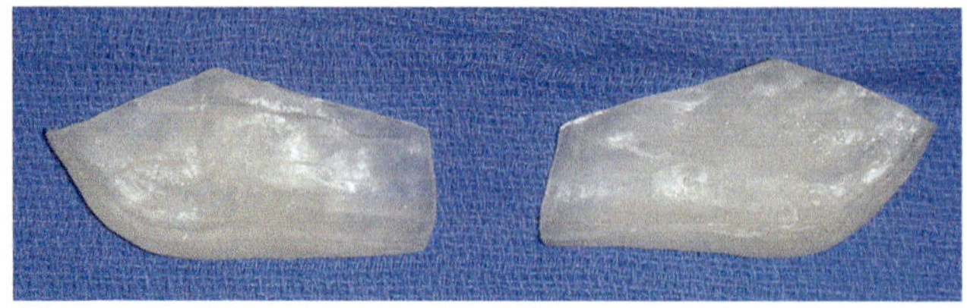

Fig. 9.118 Bilateral mandibular custom angle implant wax prototypes interior view

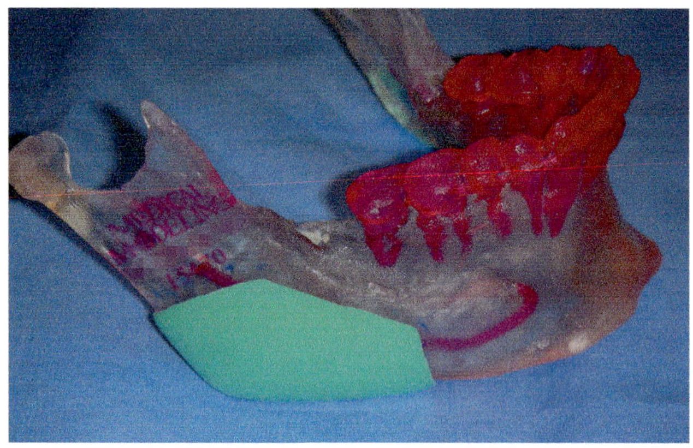

Fig. 9.119 Right mandibular angle custom implant silicone prototype fitted to 3-D model

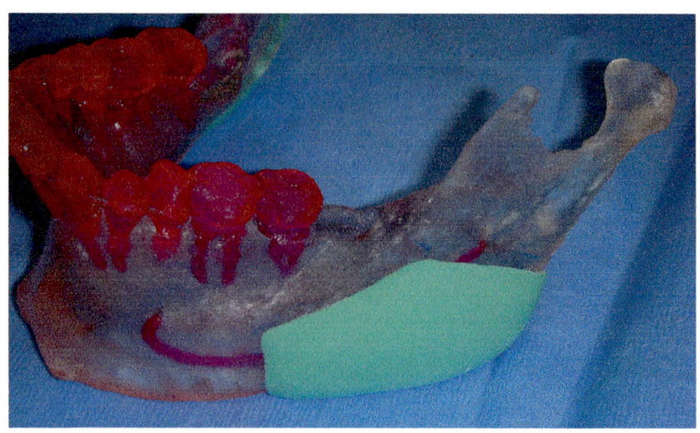

Fig. 9.120 Left mandibular angle custom implant silicone prototype fitted to 3-D model

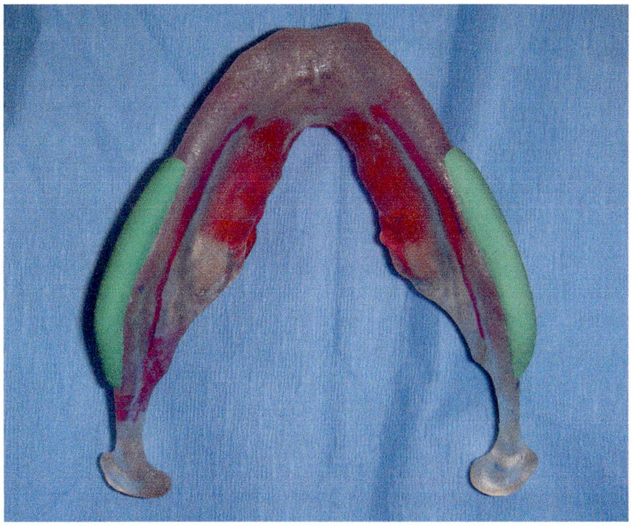

Fig. 9.121 Bilateral mandibular custom angle implant silicone prototypes fitted to 3-D model inferior view

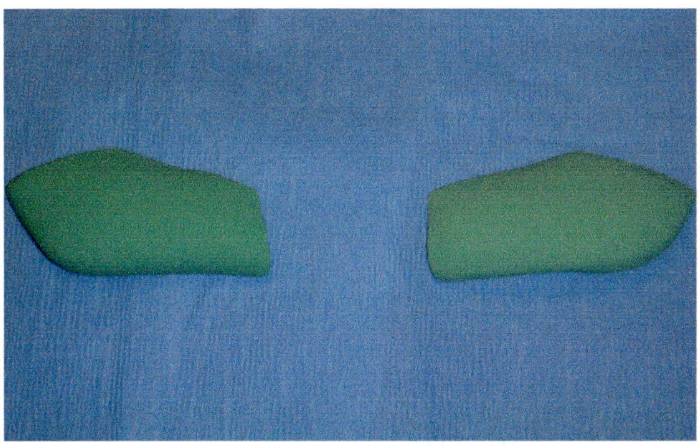

Fig. 9.122 Bilateral mandibular custom angle implant silicone prototypes exterior view

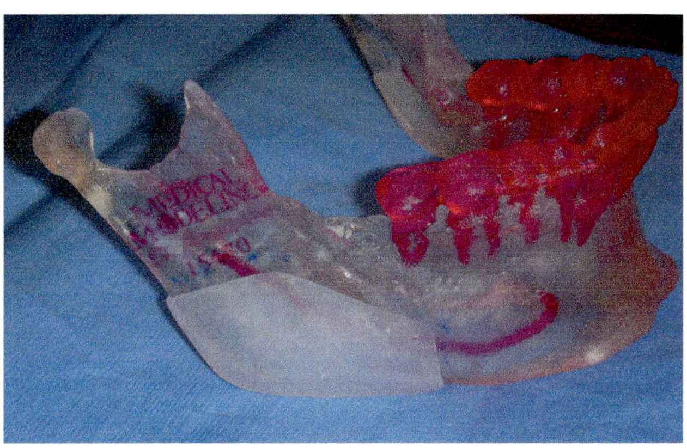

Fig. 9.123 Right mandibular angle final custom solid silicone implant fitted to 3-D model. Note: 3 screw holes along the anterior superior border

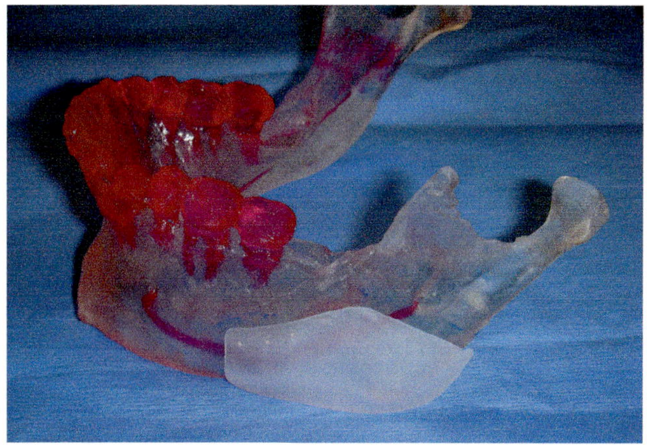

Fig. 9.124 Left mandibular angle final custom solid silicone implant fitted to 3-D model

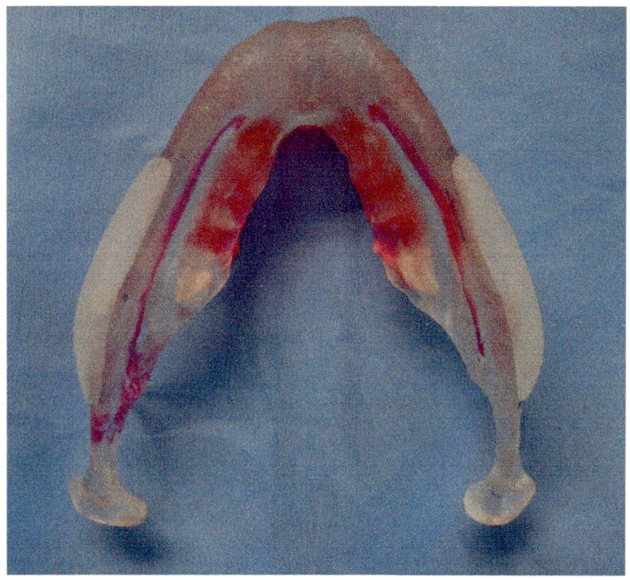

Fig. 9.125 Bilateral mandibular angle custom solid silicone implants fitted to 3-D model inferior view

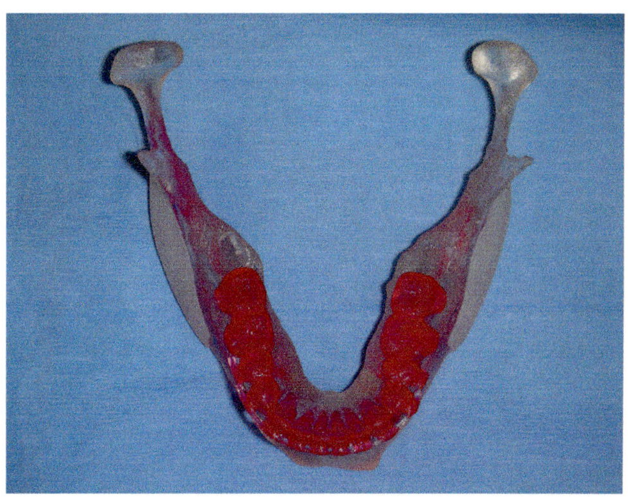

Fig. 9.126 Bilateral mandibular angle custom solid silicone implants fitted to 3-D model superior view

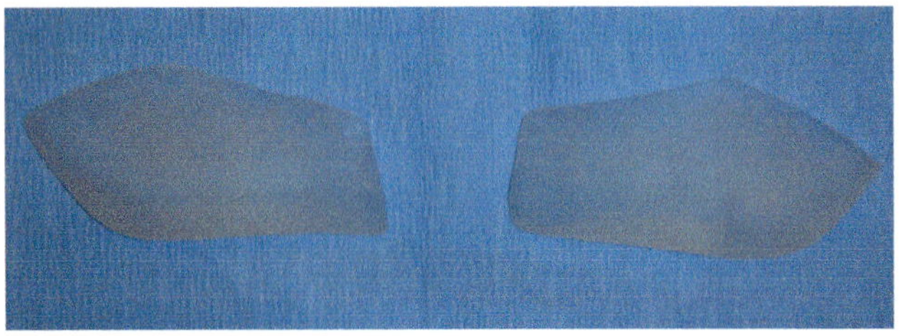

Fig. 9.127 Bilateral mandibular angle custom solid silicone implants exterior view

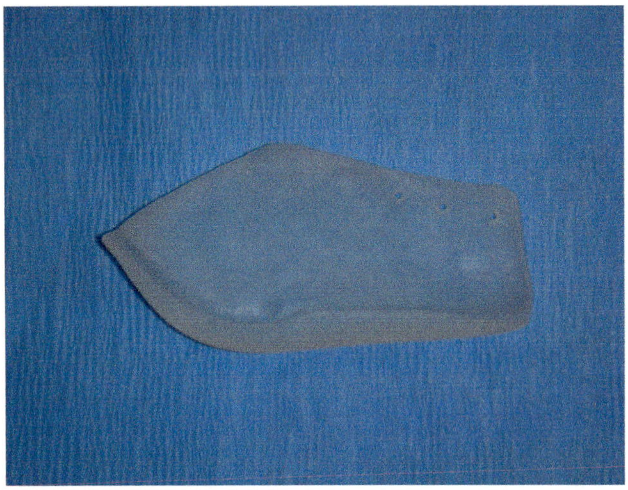

Fig. 9.128 Left mandibular angle custom solid silicone implant interior view. Note: 3 screw holes anterior superior border

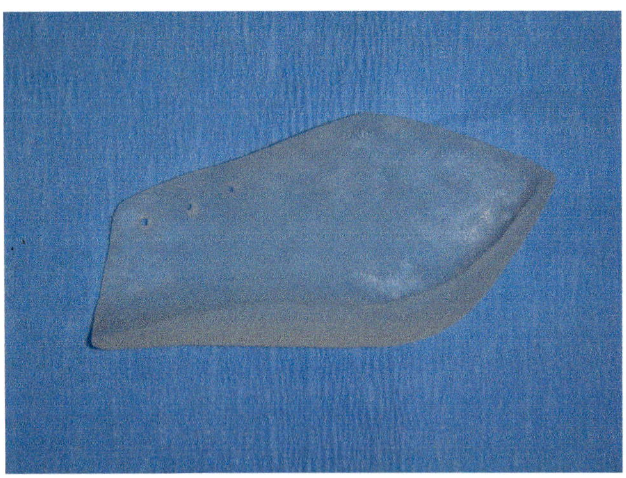

Fig. 9.129 Right mandibular angle final custom solid silicone implant interior view. Note: 3 screw holes anterior superior border

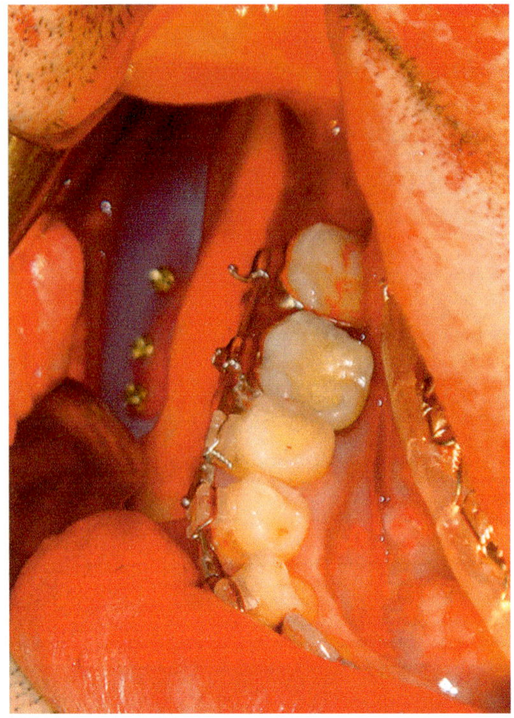

Fig. 9.130 Intraoperative view right mandibular angle custom solid silicone implant with screw fixation (DuPuy Synthes Craniomaxillofacial, Paoli, PA, USA)

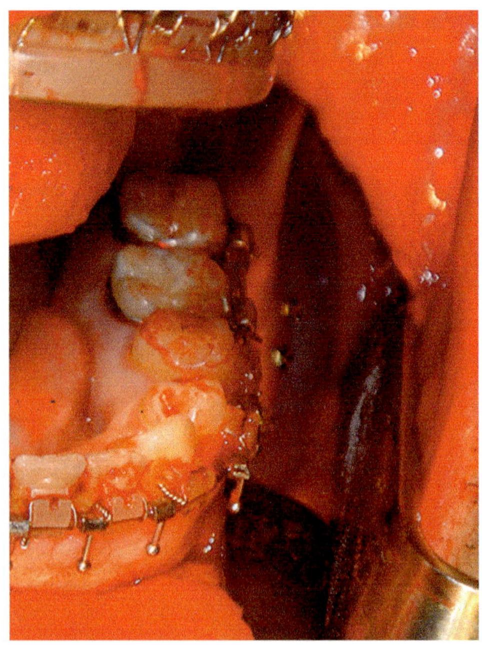

Fig. 9.131 Intraoperative view left mandibular angle custom solid silicone implant with screw fixation (DuPuy Synthes Craniomaxillofacial, Paoli, PA, USA)

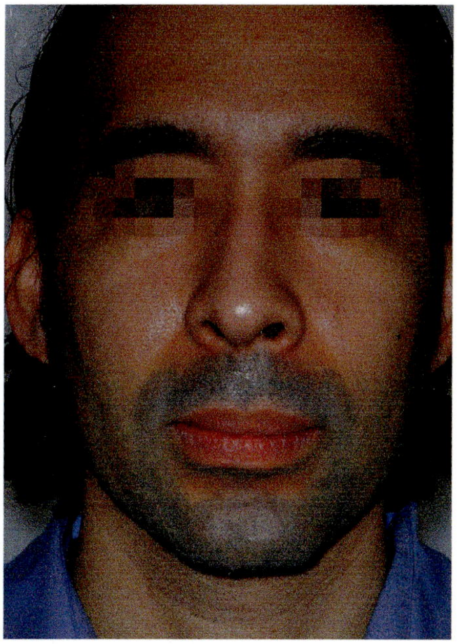

Fig. 9.132 Postoperative frontal facial view

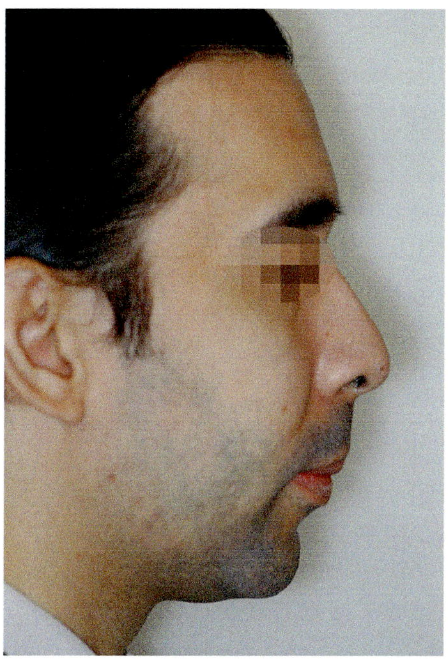

Fig. 9.133 Postoperative right lateral facial view

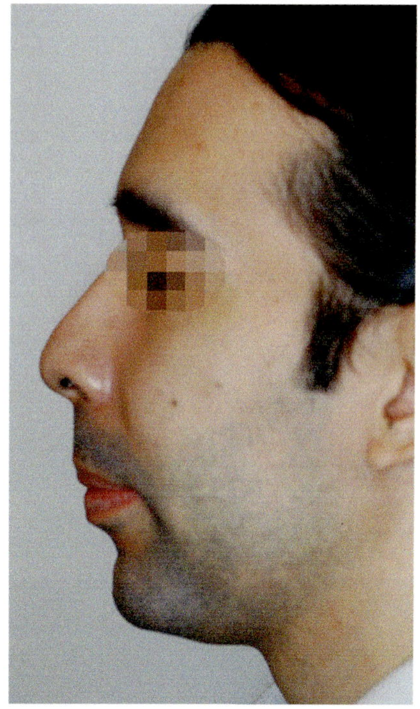

Fig. 9.134 Postoperative left lateral facial view

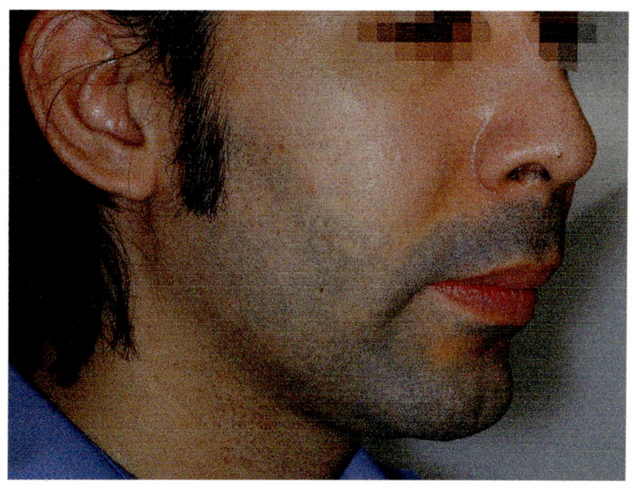

Fig. 9.135 Postoperative right 3/4 facial view

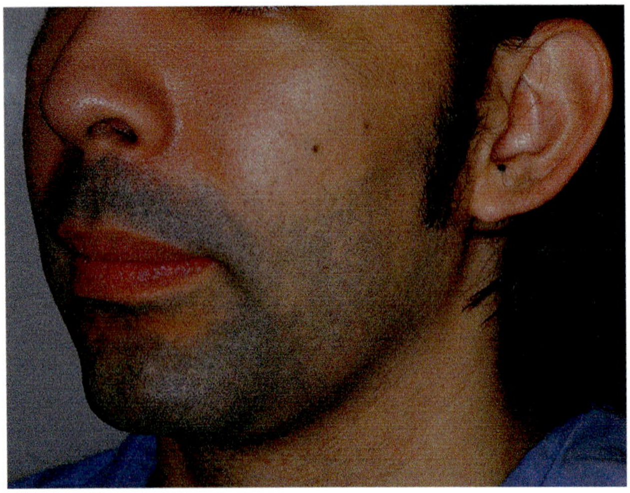

Fig. 9.136 Postoperative left 3/4 facial view

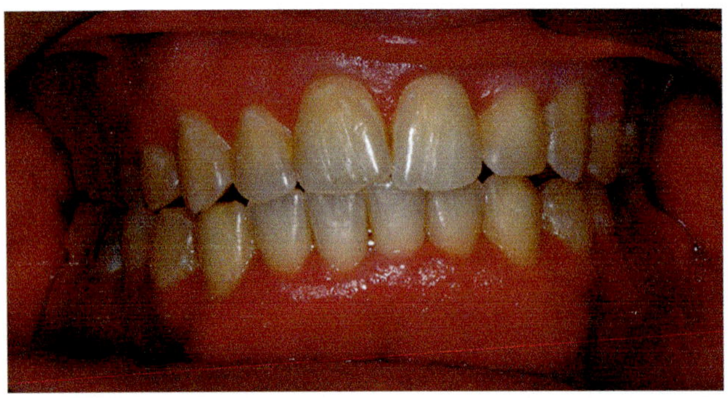

Fig. 9.137 Postoperative frontal occlusal view

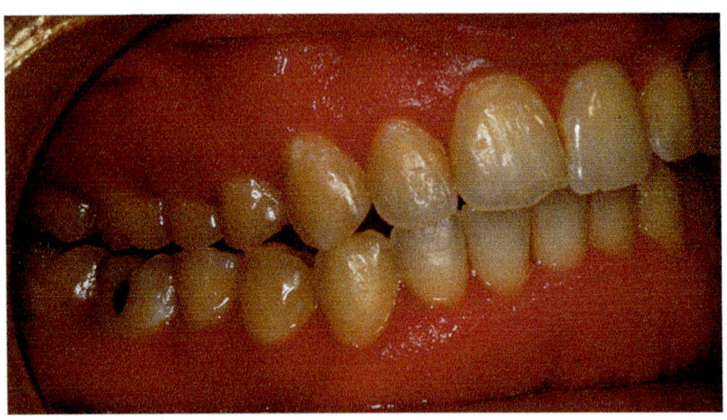

Fig. 9.138 Postoperative right lateral occlusal view

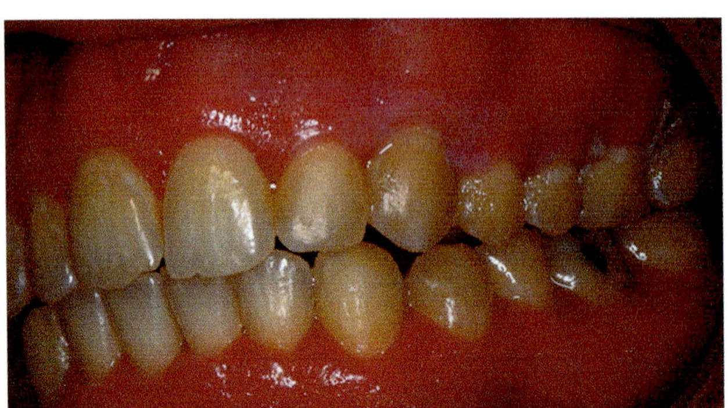

Fig. 9.139 Postoperative left lateral occlusal view

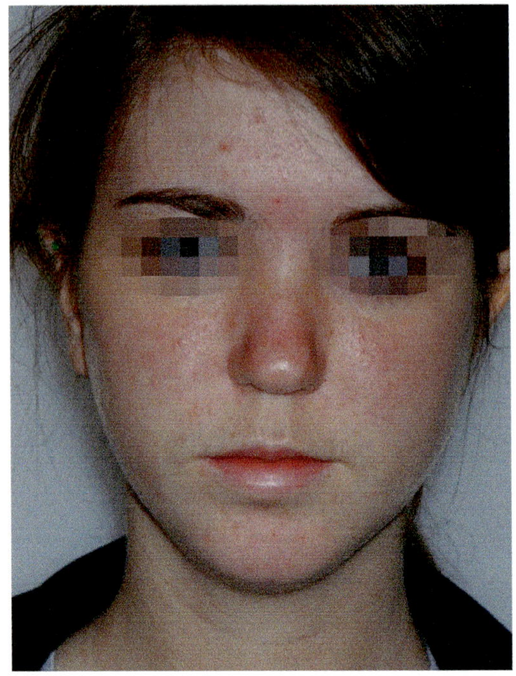

Fig. 9.140 Preoperative frontal facial view bilateral mandible angle hypoplasia and retrogenia

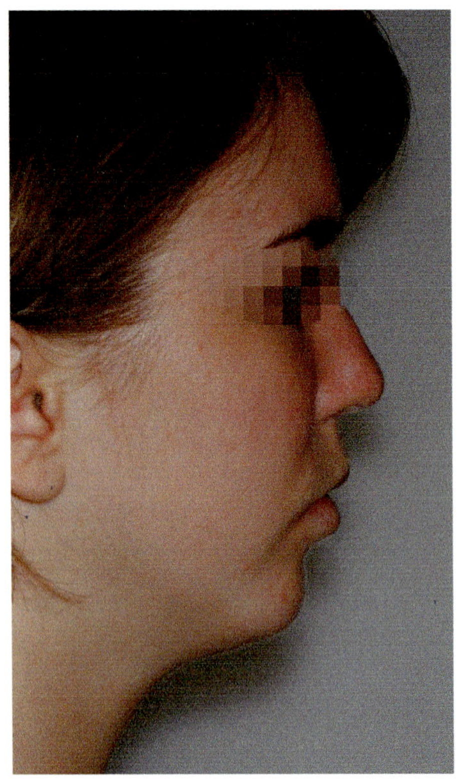

Fig. 9.141 Preoperative right lateral facial view

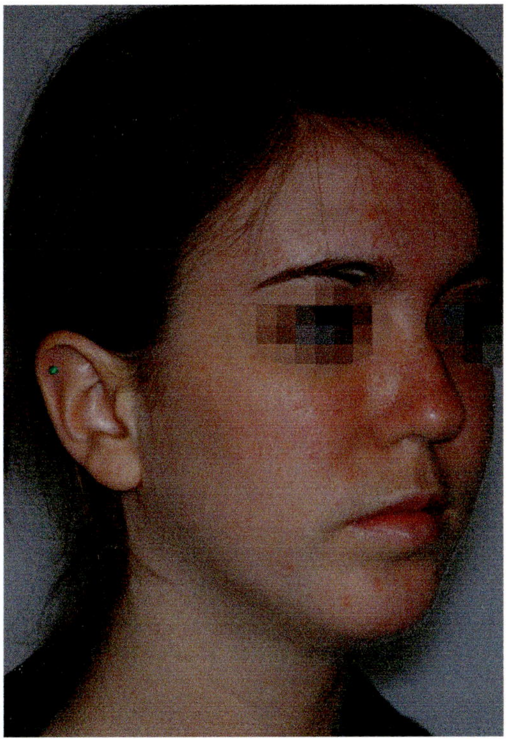

Fig. 9.142 Preoperative right 3/4 facial view

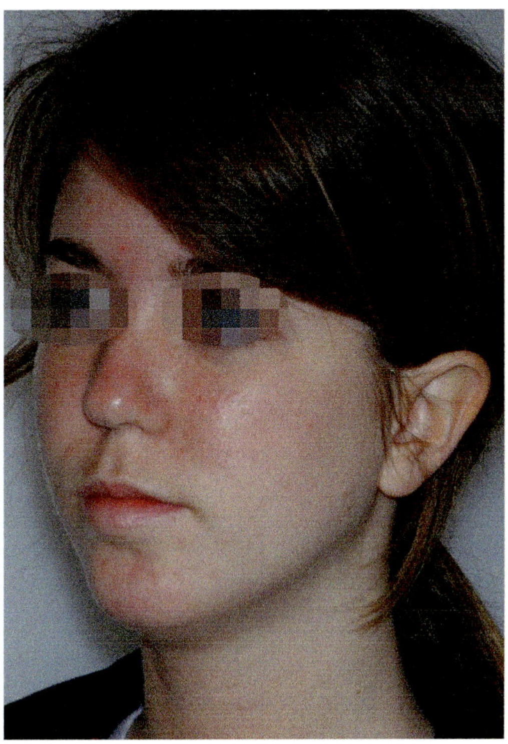

Fig. 9.143 Preoperative left 3/4 facial view

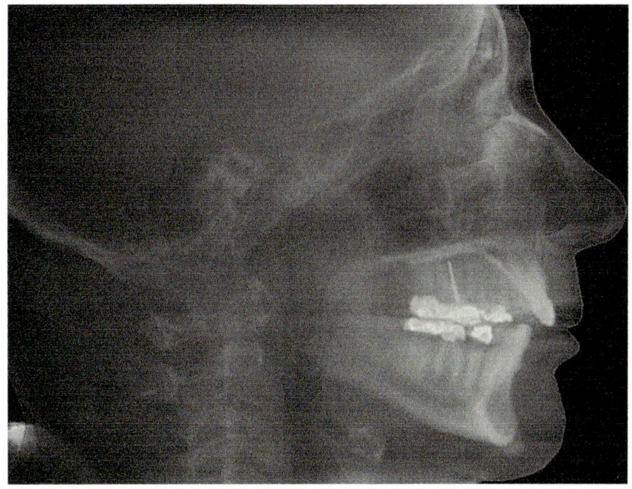

Fig. 9.144 Lateral cephalometric radiograph

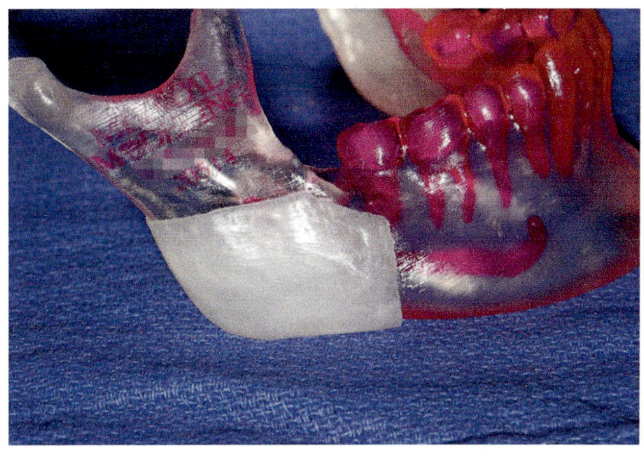

Fig. 9.145 Right mandibular custom angle implant wax prototype fitted to 3D model

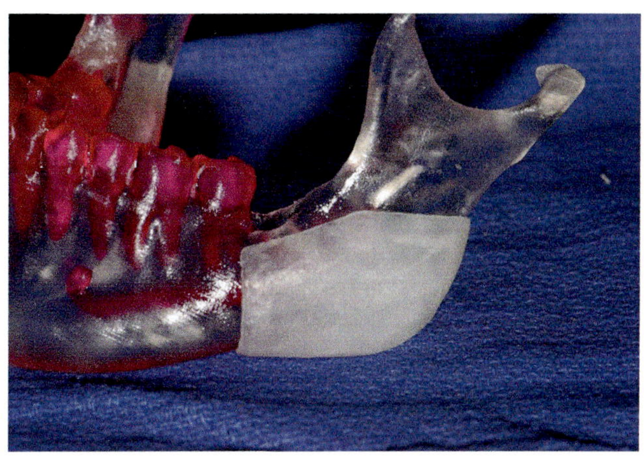

Fig. 9.146 Left mandibular custom angle implant wax prototype fitted to 3D model

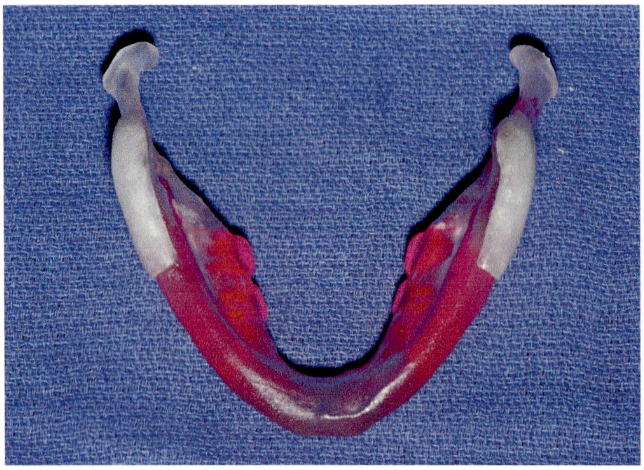

Fig. 9.147 Bilateral mandibular custom angle implant wax prototypes fitted to 3-D model inferior view

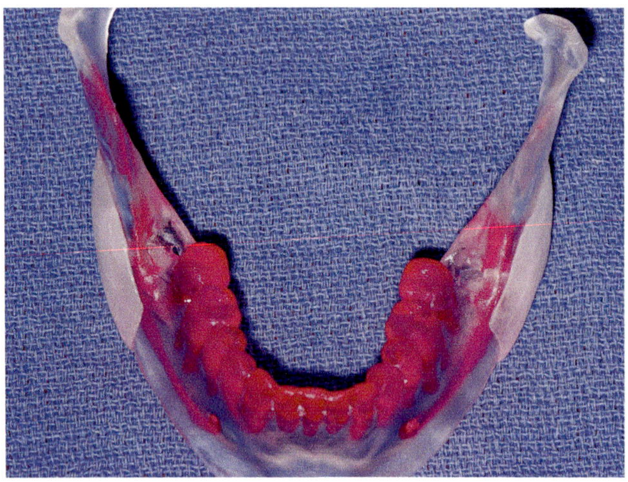

Fig. 9.148 Bilateral mandibular custom angle implant wax prototypes fitted to 3-D model superior anterior view

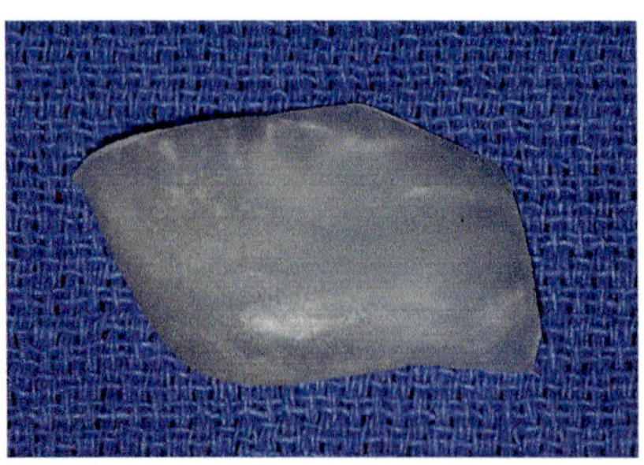

Fig. 9.149 Right mandibular custom angle implant wax prototype exterior view

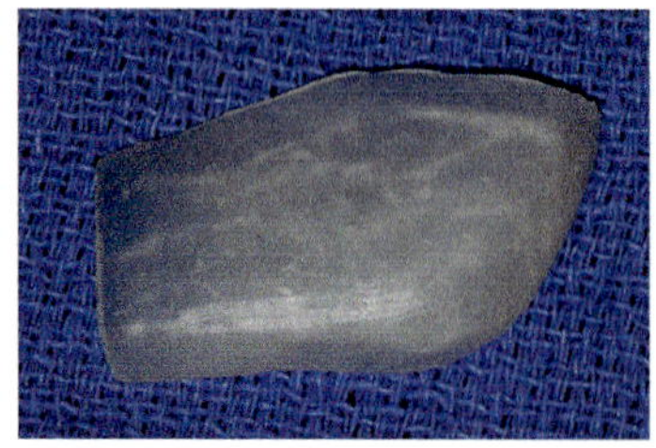

Fig. 9.150 Left mandibular custom angle implant wax prototype exterior view

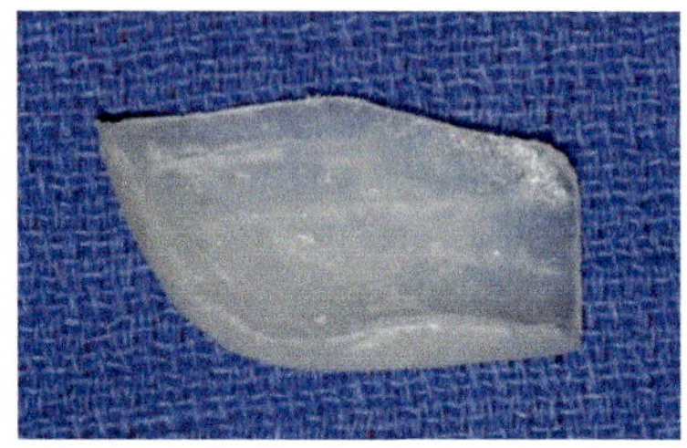

Fig. 9.151 Left mandibular custom angle implant wax prototype interior view

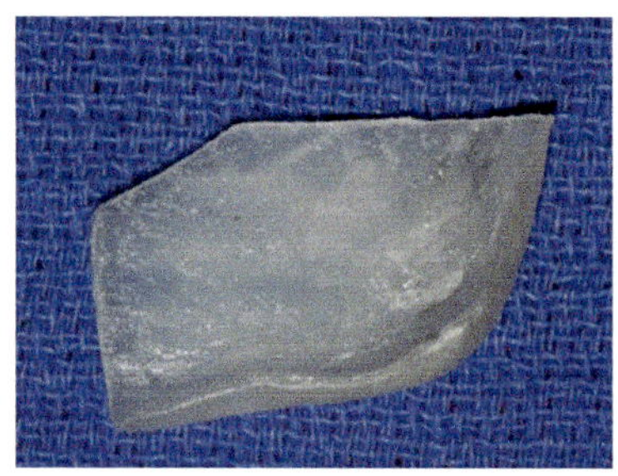

Fig. 9.152 Right mandibular custom angle implant wax prototype interior view

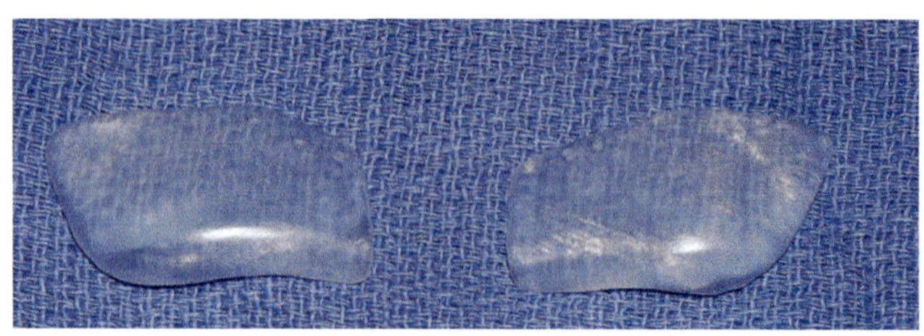

Fig. 9.153 Left and right mandibular solid silicone custom angle implants

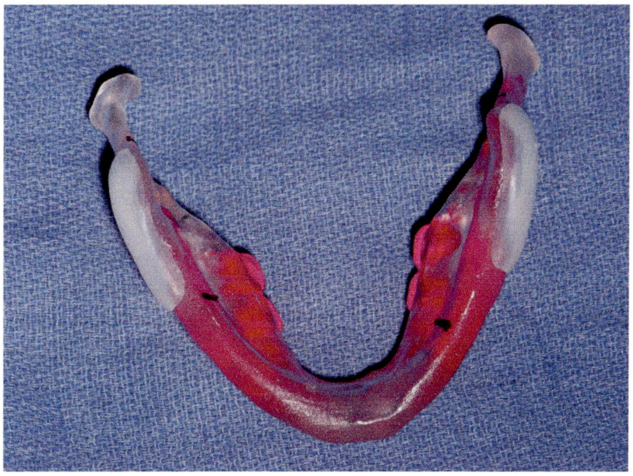

Fig. 9.154 Bilateral mandibular solid silicone custom angle implants fitted to 3-D model inferior view

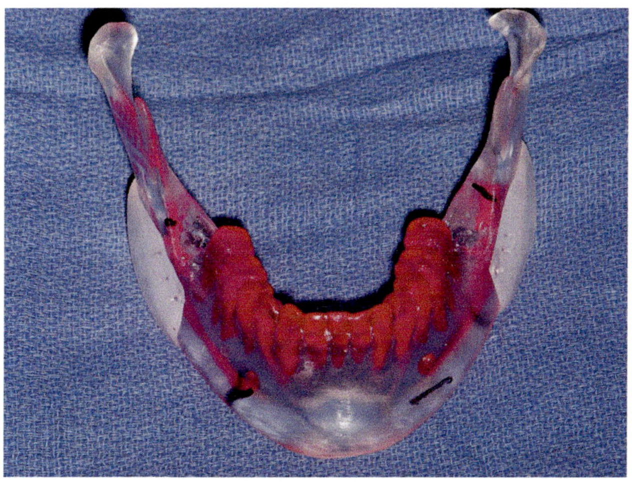

Fig. 9.155 Bilateral mandibular solid silicone custom angle implants fitted to 3-D model anterior superior view

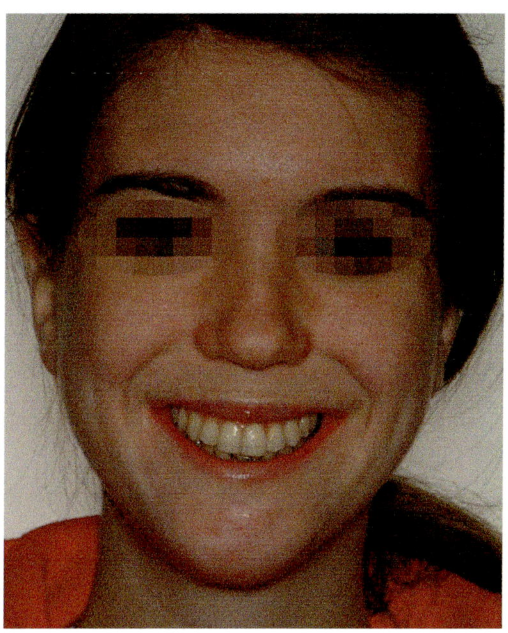

Fig. 9.156 Postoperative frontal facial view

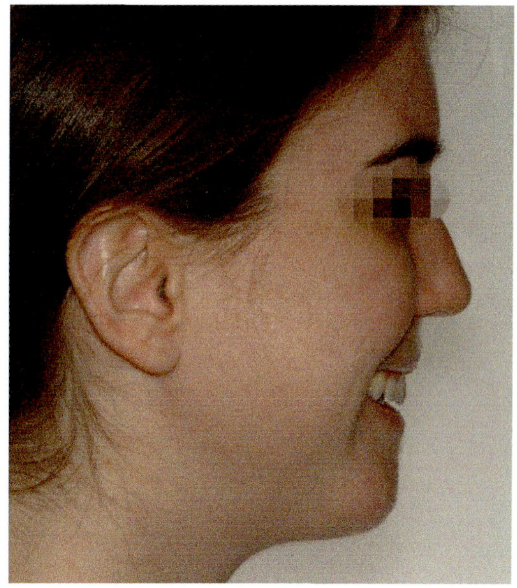

Fig. 9.157 Postoperative right lateral facial view

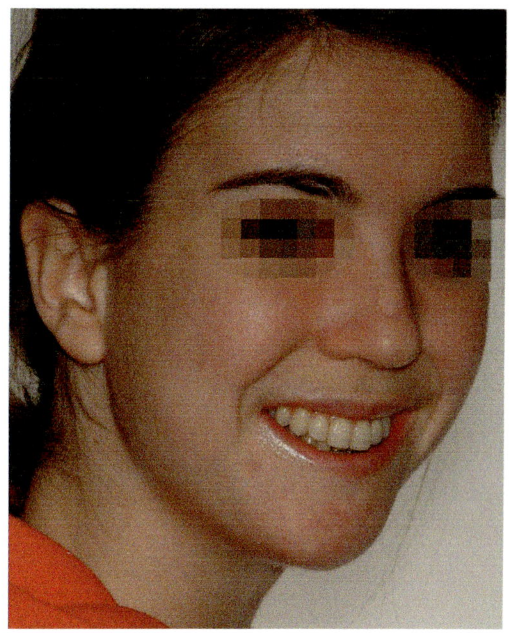

Fig. 9.158 Postoperative right 3/4 facial view

Case 6

A 19-year-old male presented with developmental asymmetry of the left mandibular ramus. A left mandibular angle custom solid silicone implant was placed (Figs. 9.159–9.170).

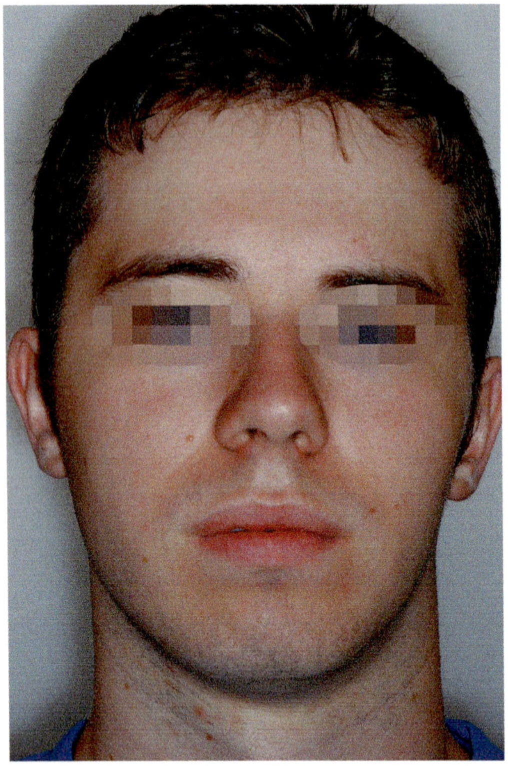

Fig. 9.159 Preoperative facial frontal view

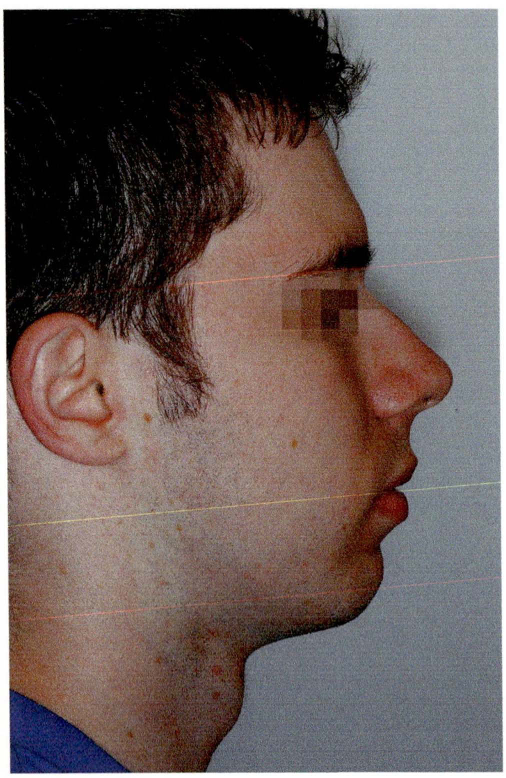

Fig. 9.160 Preoperative right lateral facial view

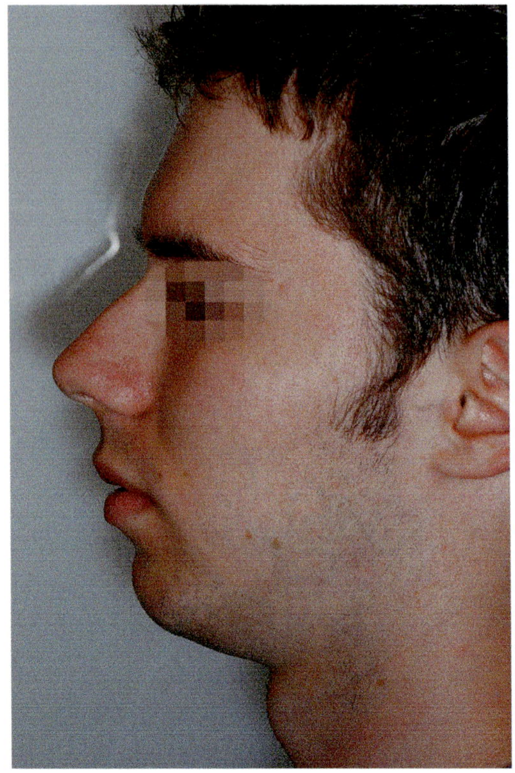

Fig. 9.161 Preoperative left lateral facial view

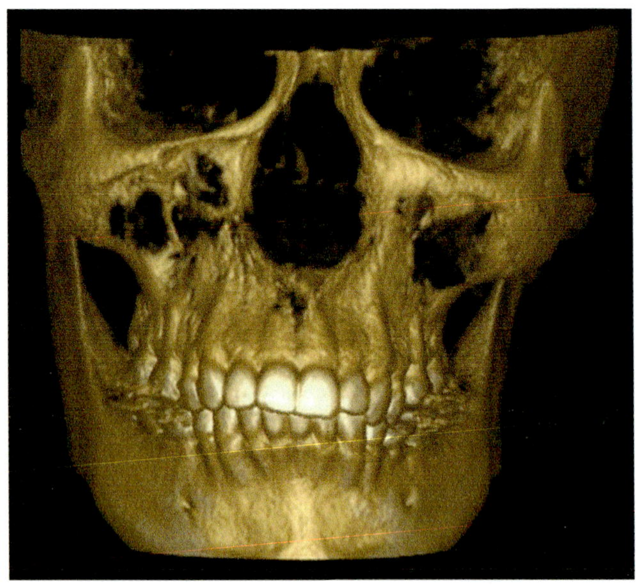

Fig. 9.162 Frontal CBCT 3-D image with left mandibular ramus hypoplasia

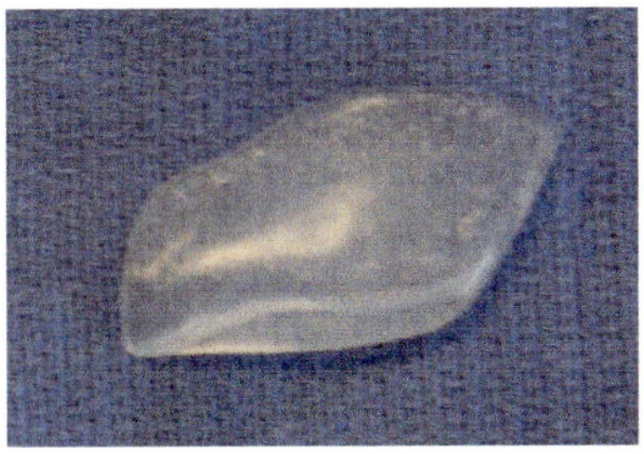

Fig. 9.163 Left mandibular custom solid silicone implant exterior view

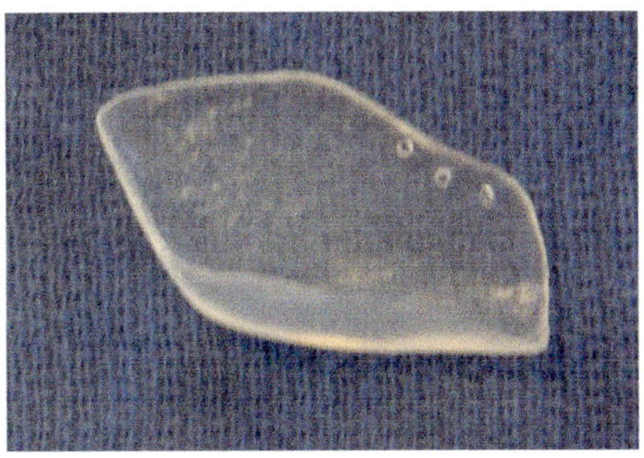

Fig. 9.164 Left mandibular custom solid silicone implant interior view. Note: 3 screw holes anterior superior border

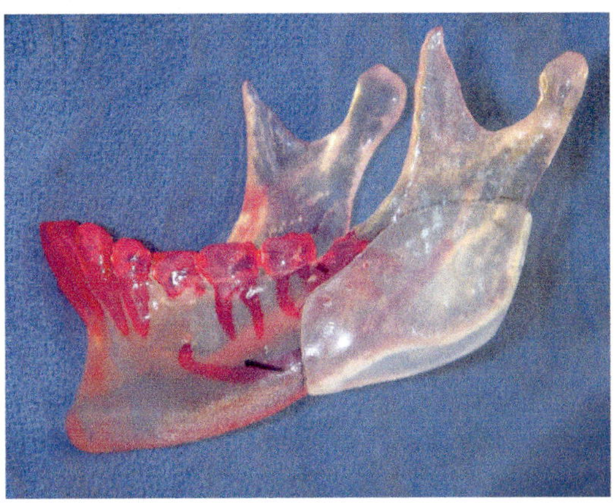

Fig. 9.165 Left mandibular solid silicone custom angle implant fitted to 3-D model lateral view

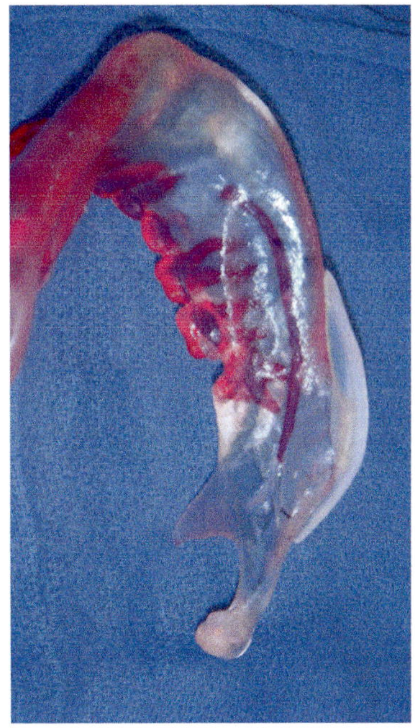

Fig. 9.166 Left mandibular solid silicone custom angle implant fitted to 3-D model inferior medial view

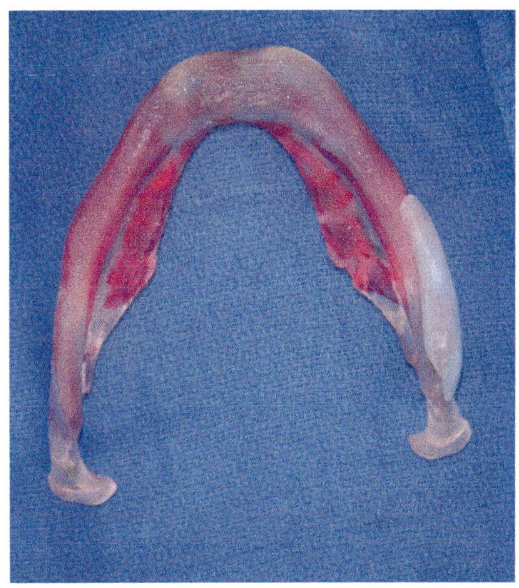

Fig. 9.67 Left mandibular solid silicone custom angle implant fitted to 3-D model inferior view

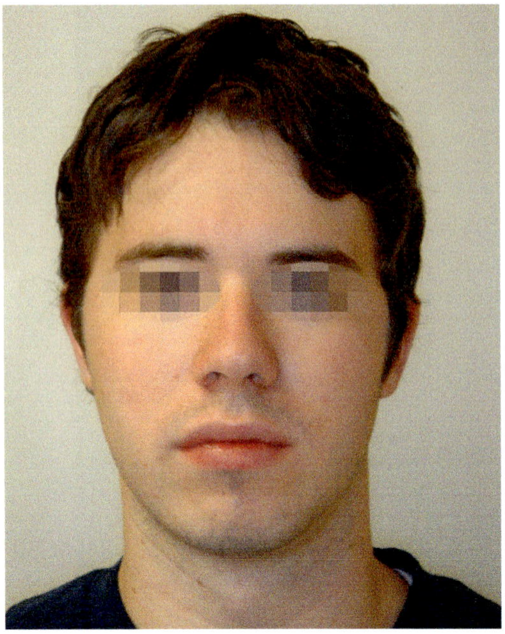

Fig. 9.168 Postoperative frontal facial view

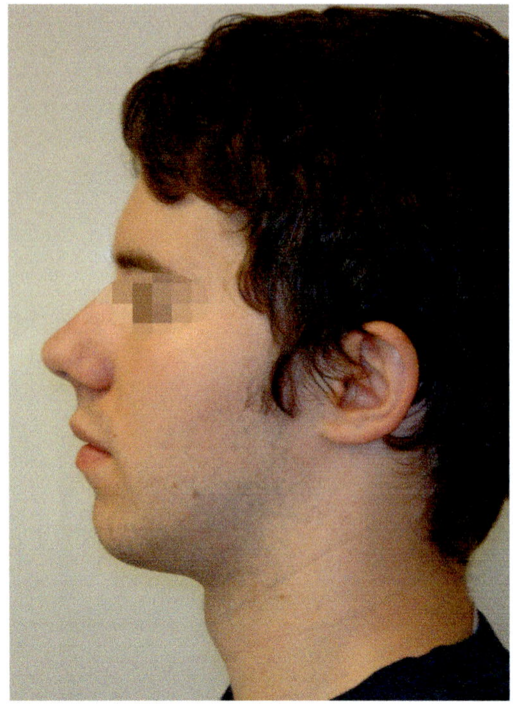

Fig. 9.170 Postoperative left lateral facial view

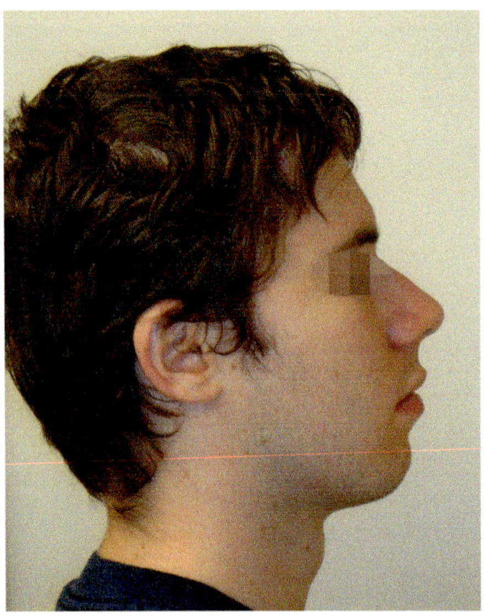

Fig. 9.169 Postoperative right lateral facial view

Combined Chin and Mandibular Angle Custom Implants: Creation of the Jawline

There are many patients for whom a combination of bilateral mandibular angle implants and chin surgery is necessary to achieve a satisfactory jaw line [41, 70]. This can be achieved using the above-described techniques, with the possibility of using either the anterior horizontal mandibular osteotomy or a chin implant depending on the mandibular bony anatomy or desired morphology of the chin. These patient types can include both nonoperated and previously operated cases. For the previously operated patient, this often includes patients who have undergone either bilateral mandibular sagittal ramus osteotomies or bilateral mandibular vertical ramus osteotomies. In some cases where the chin has been operated with an unsatisfactory result, the mandibular angles were never addressed. Soft tissue surgical procedures such as liposuction can help to provide further refinement and definition of the jawline [74, 75]. It is difficult to create an implant for intraoral placement that completely wraps around the mandible because of the presence of the bilateral mental nerves. However, custom implants have the advantage of creating feathered edges with intimate anatomic fit so as to create the appearance of a continuous smooth jaw line. Another advantage of the custom implant technique is that is possible in previously operated patients to exchange implants so that the patient does not have to be in public with a post implant removal chin deformity until soft tissue healing will allow a replacement implant to be inserted. In order to create the replacement implant, a stereolithographic model can be ordered that has the existing implant segmented and removed so that the anatomically corrected implant free mandible can be fabricated. It is then on this corrected stereolithographic implant free mandible model that the implants can be fabricated.

Case Reports

Case 7

A 59-year-old female patient had undergone previous orthognathic surgery which included a bilateral mandibular ramus sagittal split osteotomies for correction of a skeletal Class II malocclusion and placement of a PEFE implant. Postoperatively the patient was dissatisfied with loss of bilateral mandibular angle definition with the resultant step deformities from superior rotation of the proximal segments and an excessive size of the chin. Bilateral mandibular angle custom solid silicone implants were placed, and the PEFE implant was removed with a simultaneous placement of a custom solid silicone chin implant. This case demonstrates the use of 3-D modeling to allow the virtual removal of a pre-existing chin implant and creation of a 3-D model of the implant free mandible on which a custom chin solid silicone implant can be fabricated. (Figs. 9.171–9.213). (Alex M. Greenberg, DDS, Oral and Maxillofacial Surgeon, New York, NY, USA)

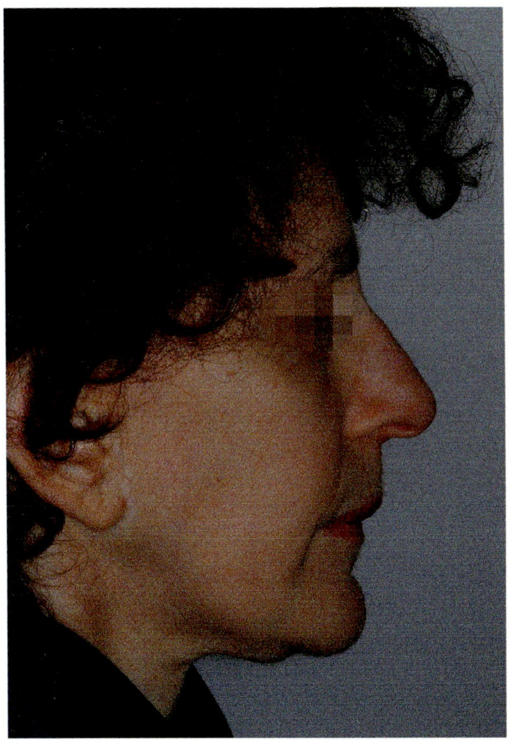

Fig. 9.171 Preoperative right lateral facial view

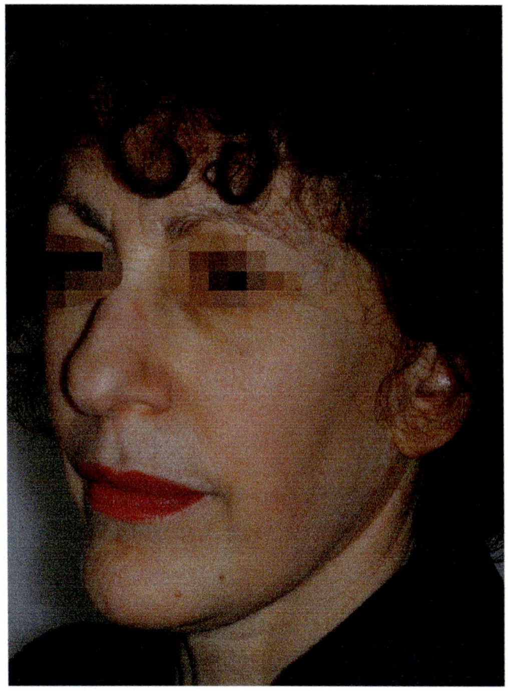

Fig. 9.172 Preoperative left 3/4 facial view

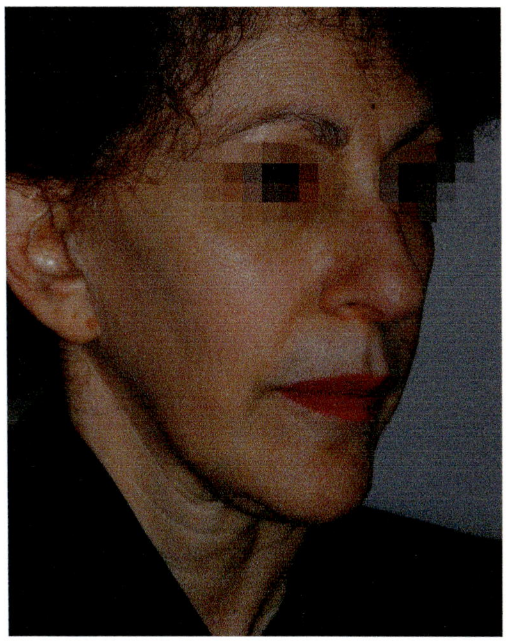

Fig. 9.173 Preoperative right 3/4 facial view

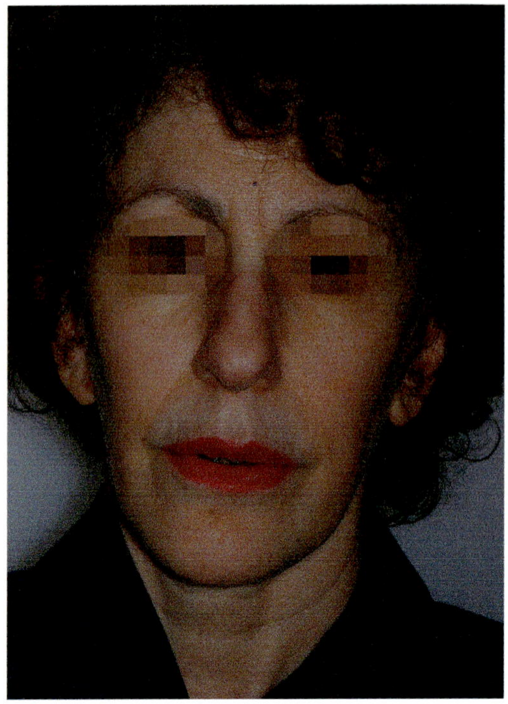

Fig. 9.174 Preoperative frontal facial view

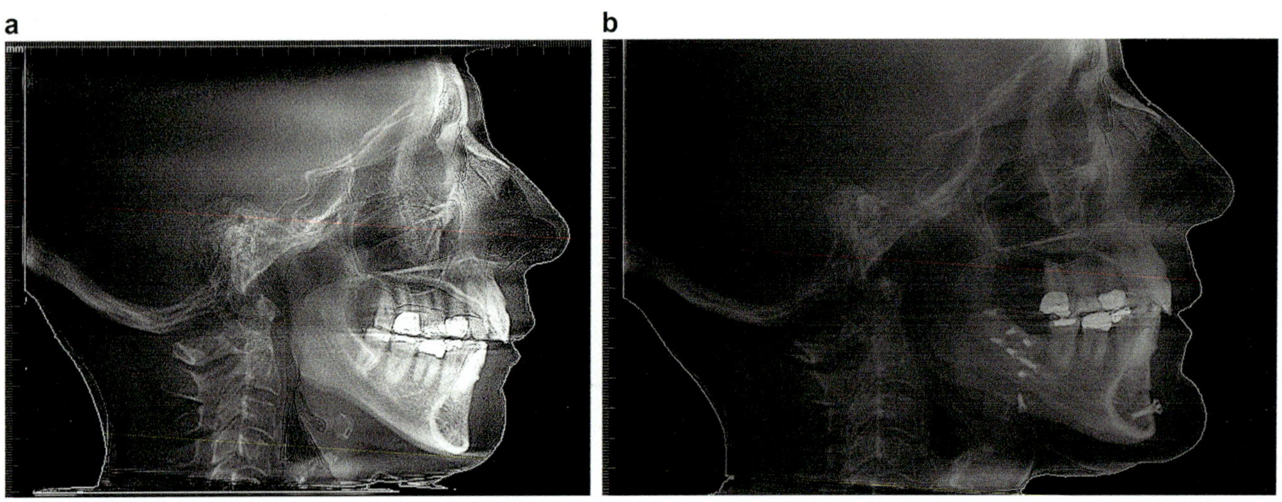

Fig. 9.175 (**a**) Preoperative preorthognathic surgery lateral cephalometric radiograph. (**b**) Postorthognathic surgery postoperative lateral cephalometric radiograph demonstrating PEFE chin implant

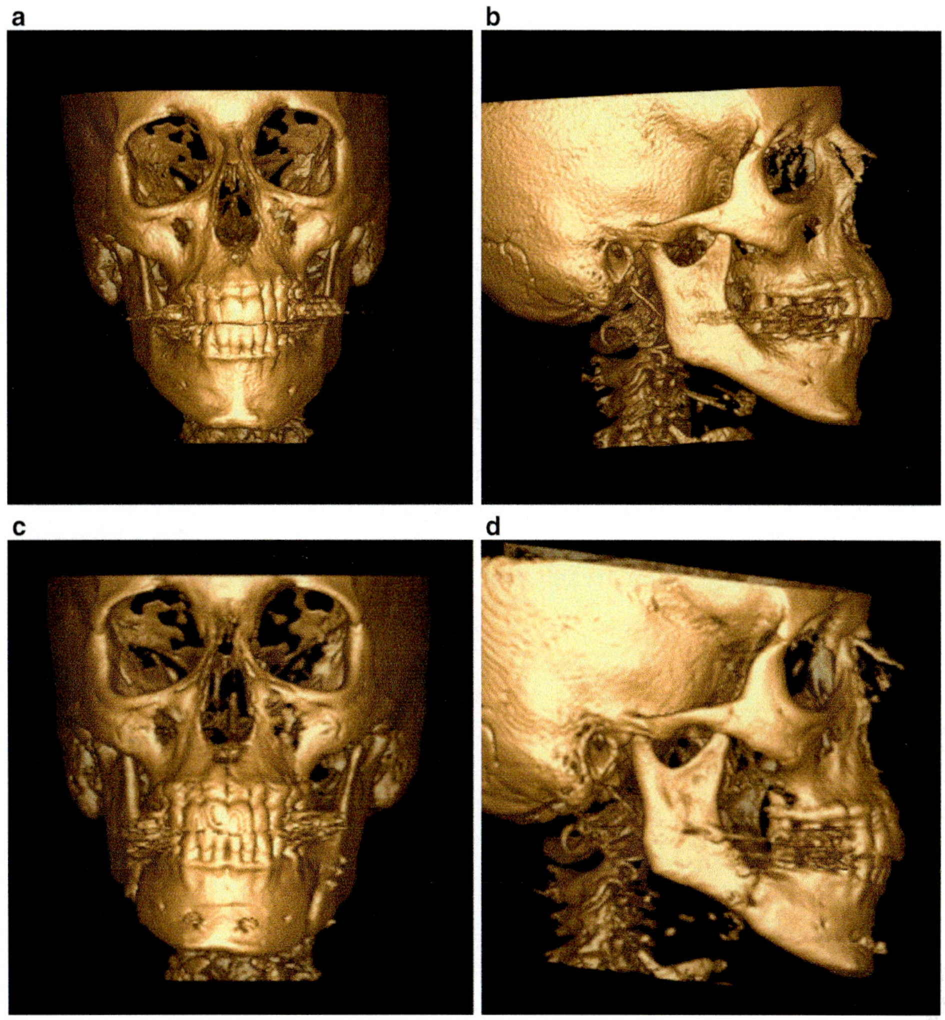

Fig. 9.176 (**a**) Preoperative preorthognathic surgery 3-D CBCT frontal view. (**b**) Preoperative preorthognathic surgery 3-D CBCT right lateral view. (**c**) Preoperative postorthognathic surgery 3-D CBCT frontal view; note narrowed mandibular angles. (**d**) Preoperative postorthognathic surgery 3-D CBCT right lateral view with right mandibular angle step defect

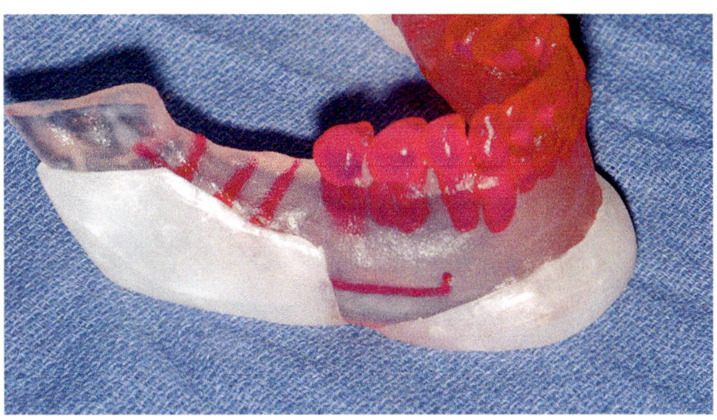

Fig. 9.177 Right mandibular custom angle and chin implant wax prototypes fitted to 3-D model right lateral view. Note: Presence of lag/positioning screws which will be left in situ

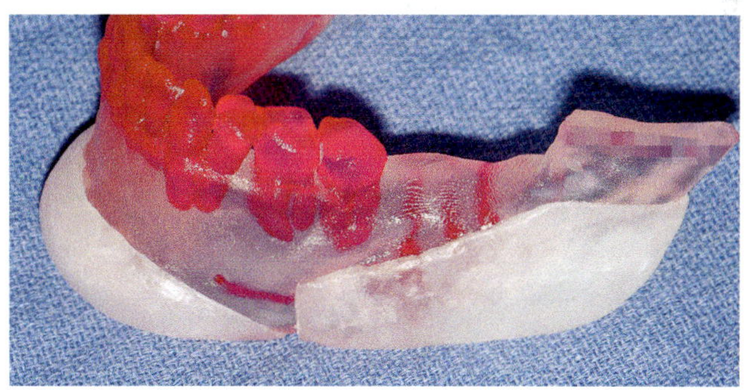

Fig. 9.178 Left mandibular custom angle and chin implant wax prototypes fitted to 3-D model left lateral view. Note: Presence of lag/positioning screws which will be left in situ

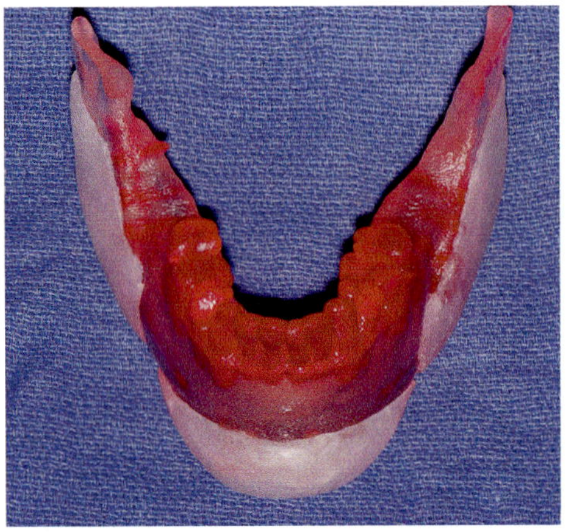

Fig. 9.179 Bilateral mandibular custom angle and chin implant wax prototypes fitted to 3-D model anterior superior view

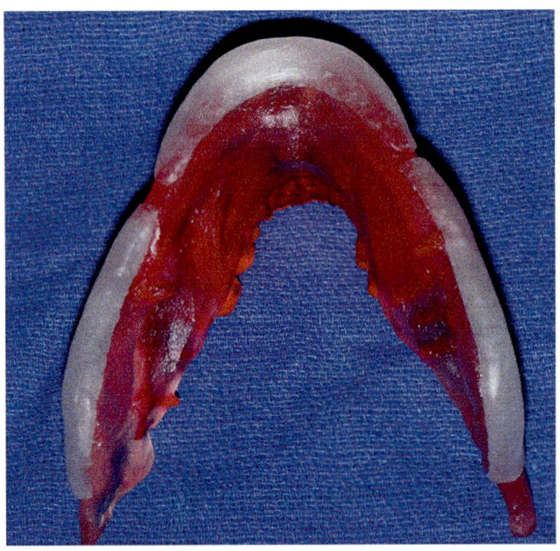

Fig. 9.180 Bilateral mandibular custom angle and chin implant wax prototypes fitted to 3-D model inferior view

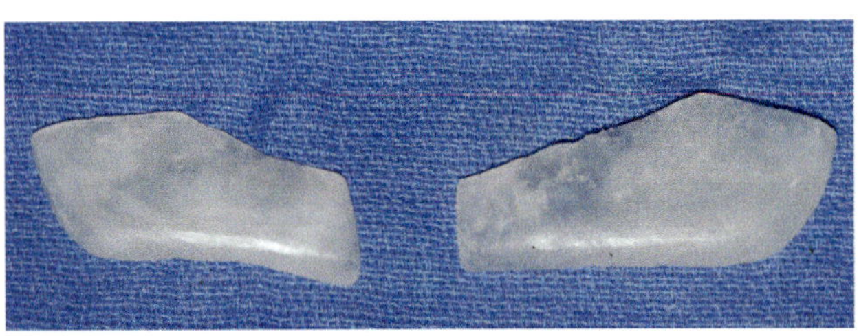

Fig. 9.181 Bilateral mandibular custom angle implants wax prototypes exterior view

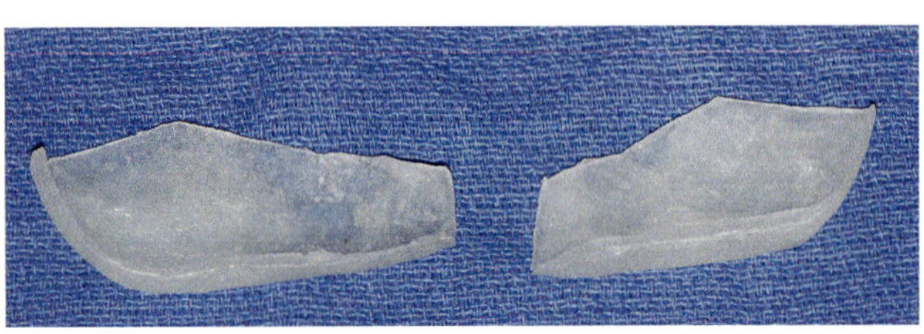

Fig. 9.182 Bilateral mandibular custom angle implants wax prototypes interior views

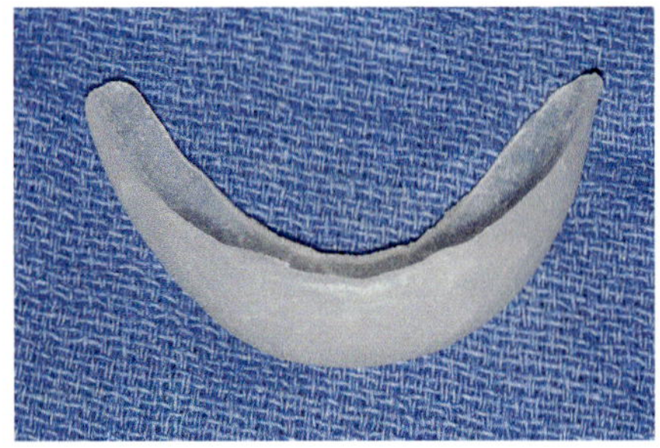

Fig. 9.183 Chin implant wax prototype anterior superior view

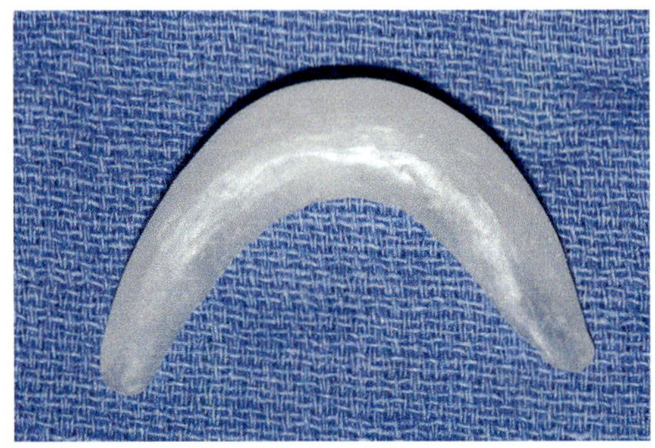

Fig. 9.184 Chin implant wax prototype inferior view

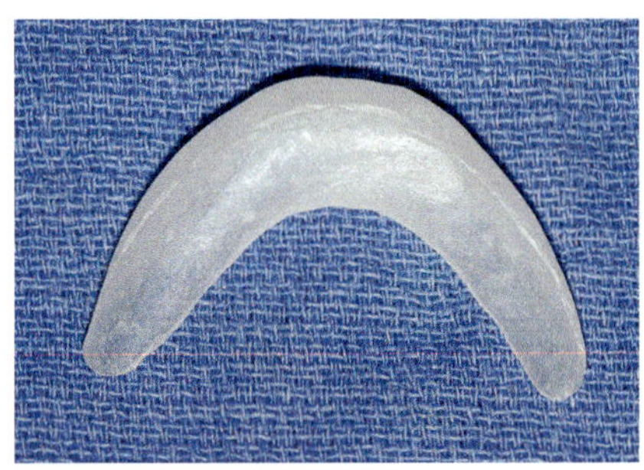

Fig. 9.185 Chin implant wax prototype superior view

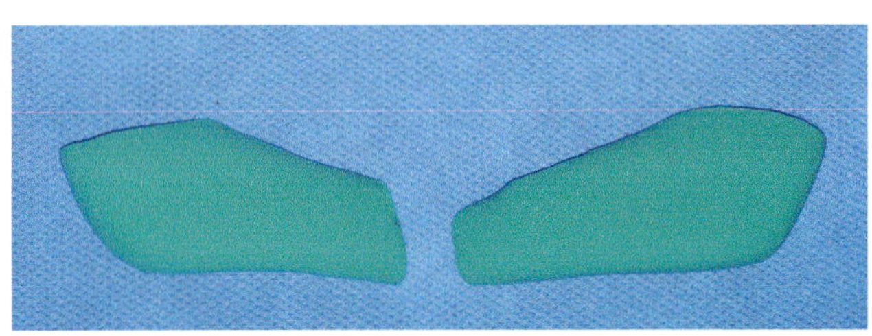

Fig. 9.186 Bilateral mandibular angle custom implant silicone prototypes exterior view

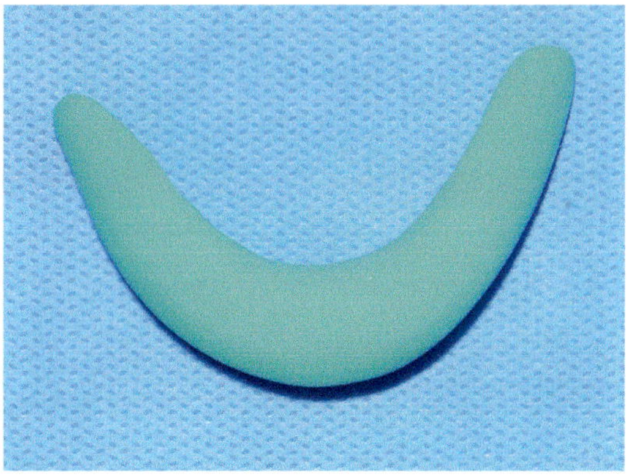

Fig. 9.187 Chin custom implant silicone prototype inferior view

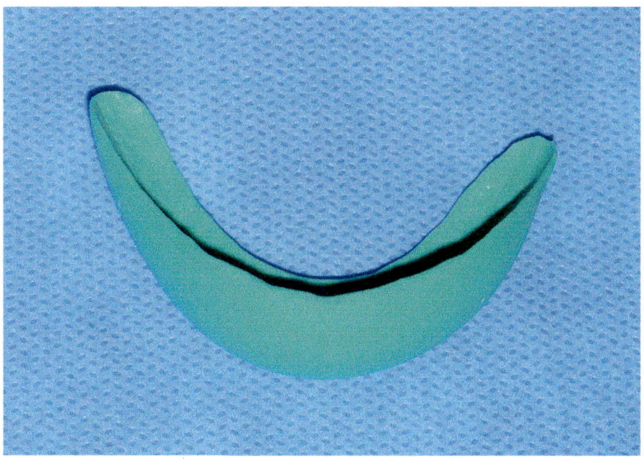

Fig. 9.188 Chin custom implant silicone prototype superior anterior interior view

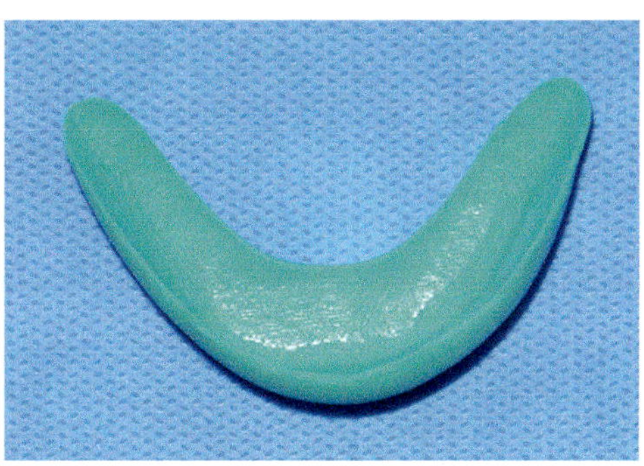

Fig. 9.189 Chin custom implant silicone prototype superior view

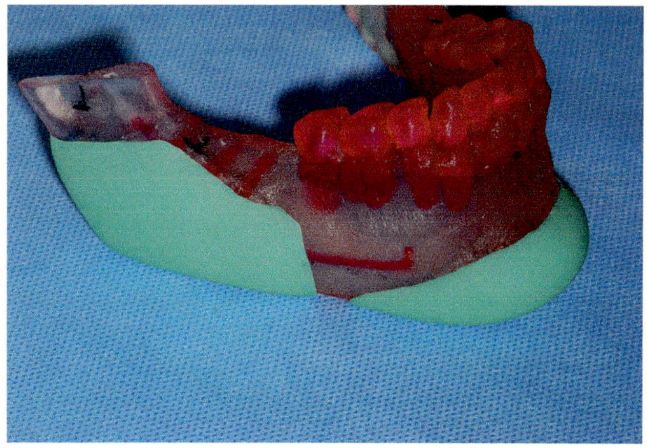

Fig. 9.190 Right mandibular custom angle and chin silicone implant prototypes fitted to 3-D model right lateral view

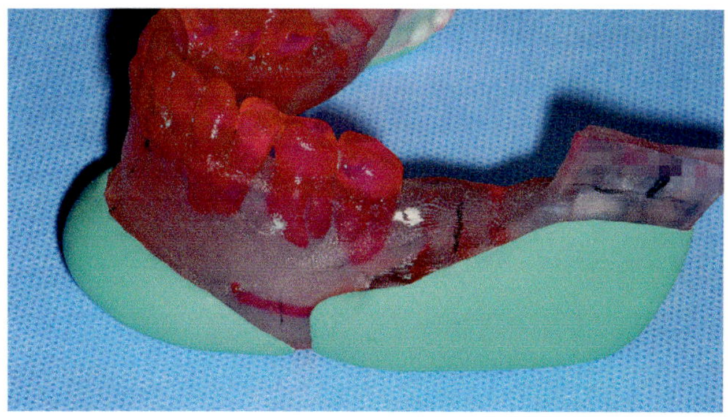

Fig. 9.191 Left mandibular custom angle and chin silicone implant prototypes fitted to 3-D model left lateral view

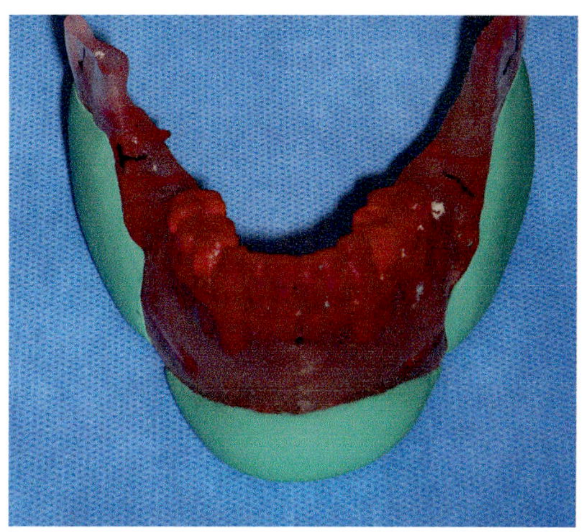

Fig. 9.192 Bilateral mandibular custom angle and chin silicone implant prototypes fitted to 3-D model anterior superior view

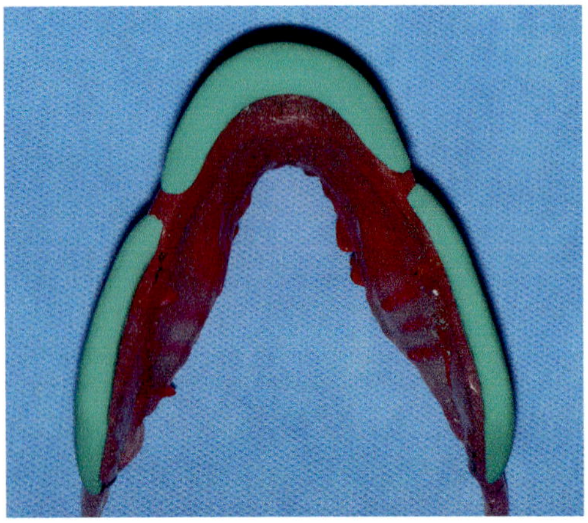

Fig. 9.193 Bilateral mandibular custom angle and chin silicone implant prototypes fitted to 3-D model inferior view

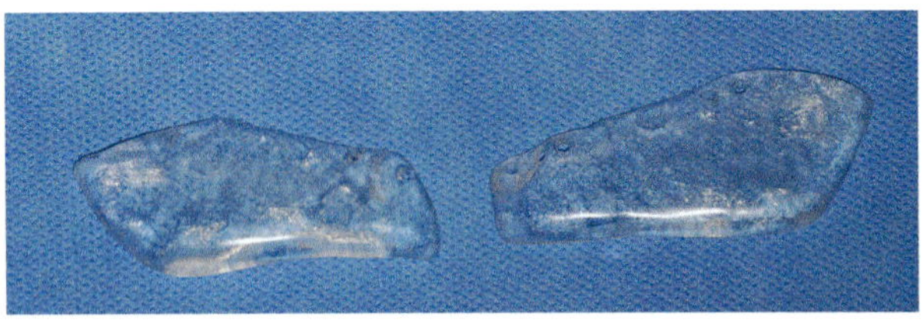

Fig. 9.194 Bilateral mandibular angle custom implant solid silicone exterior view

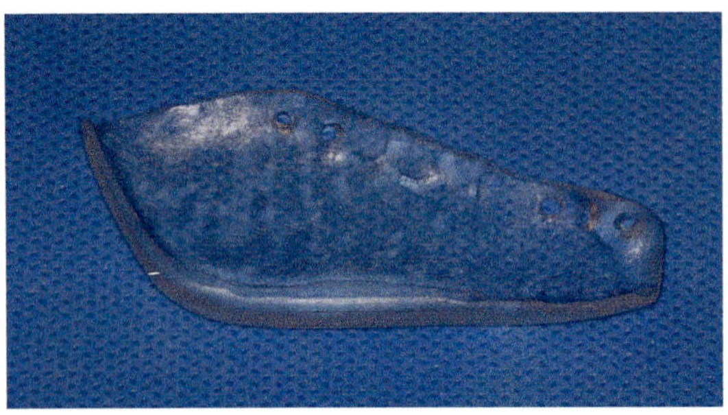

Fig. 9.195 Left mandibular custom implant solid silicone interior view. Note: screw fixation screws at anterior and posterior aspects of the superior border

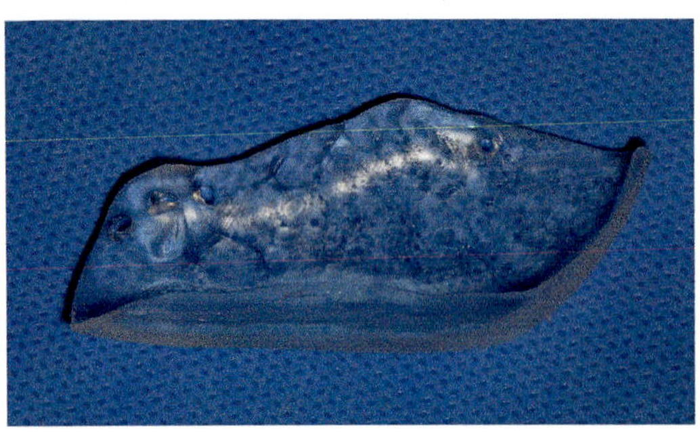

Fig. 9.196 Right mandibular custom implant solid silicone interior view. Note: screw fixation screws at anterior and posterior aspects of the superior border

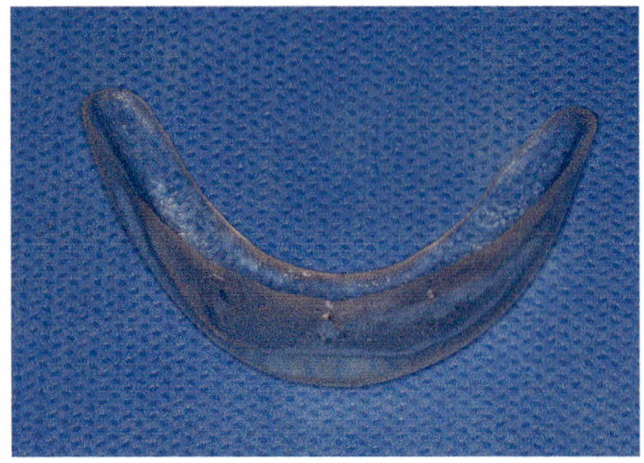

Fig. 9.197 Chin custom implant solid silicone superior anterior view. Note: 3 screw fixation holes superior border including midline

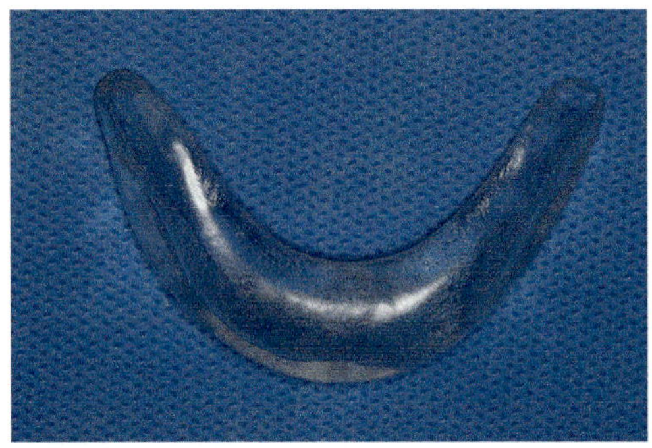

Fig. 9.198 Chin custom implant solid silicone inferior view

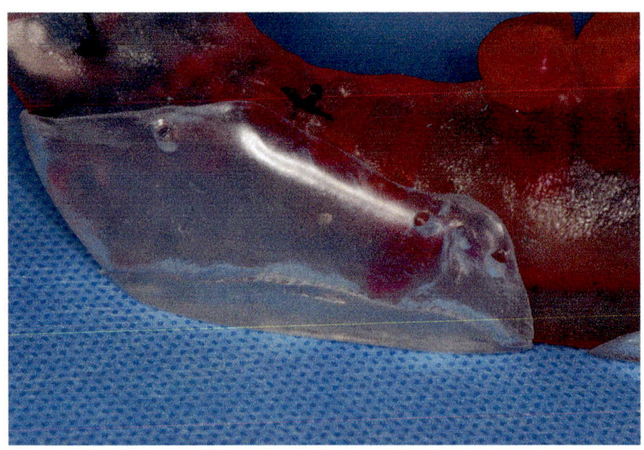

Fig. 9.199 Right mandibular angle custom solid silicone implant fitted to 3-D model. Note: screw fixation holes anterior and superior aspects of the superior border avoiding the retained lag/position screws and above the mandibular nerve

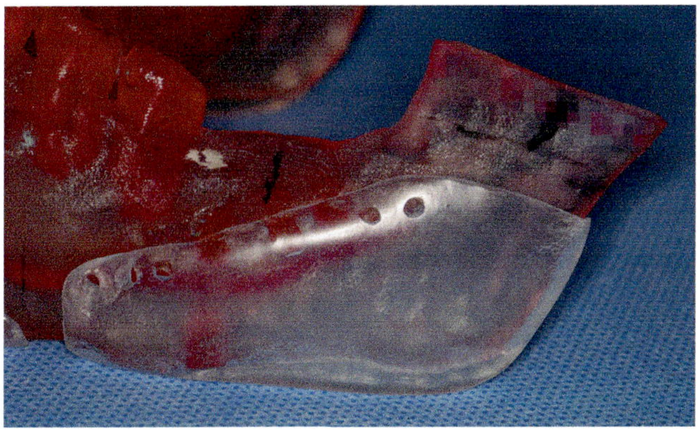

Fig. 9.200 Left mandibular angle custom solid silicone implant fitted to 3-D model. Note screw fixation holes anterior and superior aspects of the superior border avoiding the retained lag/position screws and above the mandibular nerve

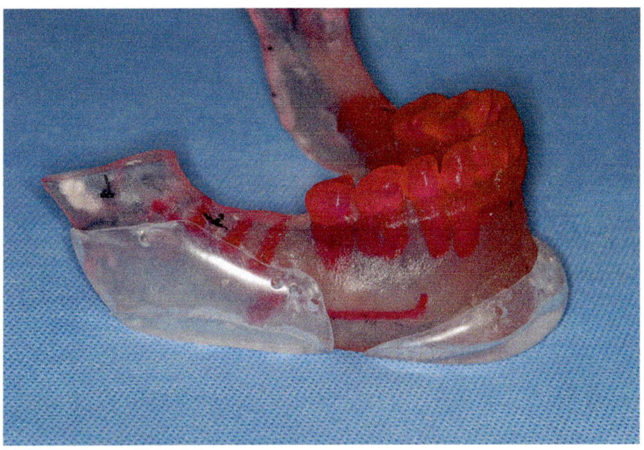

Fig. 9.201 Right mandibular angle and chin custom solid silicone implants fitted to 3-D model

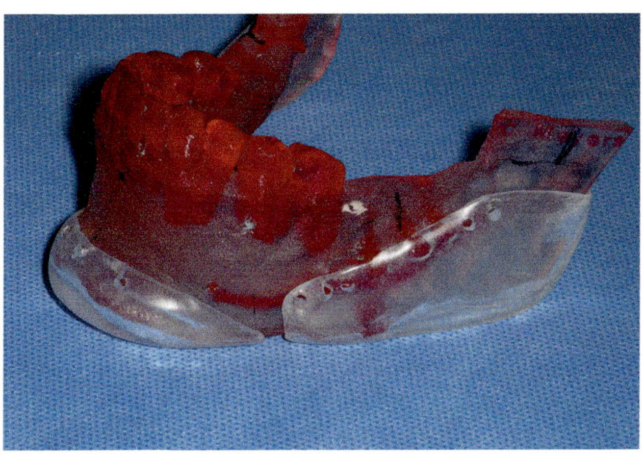

Fig. 9.202 Left mandibular angle and chin custom solid silicone implants fitted to 3-D model

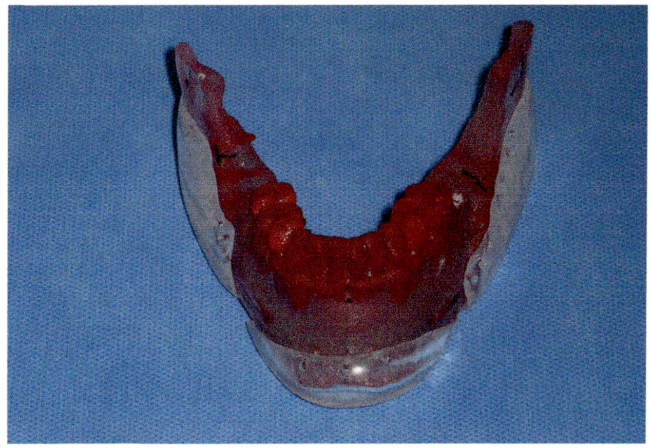

Fig. 9.203 Bilateral mandibular angle and chin custom solid silicone implants fitted to 3-D model anterior superior view

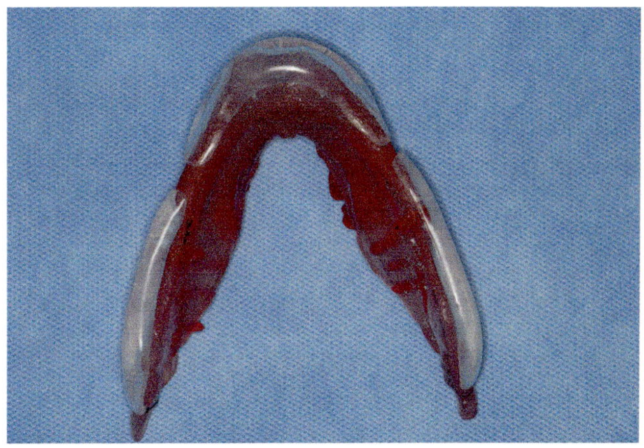

Fig. 9.204 Bilateral mandibular angle solid silicone and chin implants fitted to 3-D model inferior view

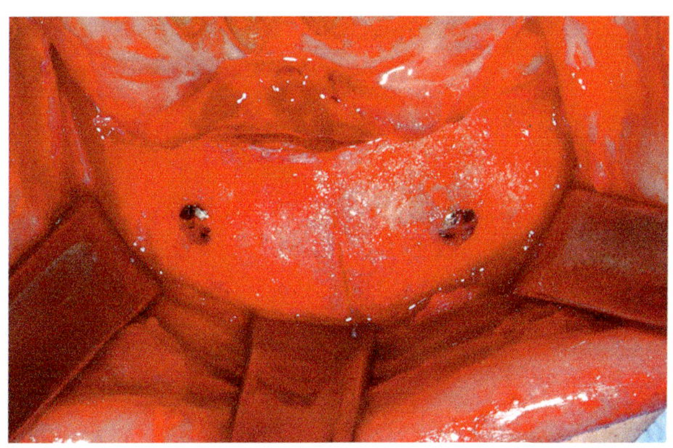

Fig. 9.205 Intraoperative view of anterior mandibular pre-existing PEFE chin implant

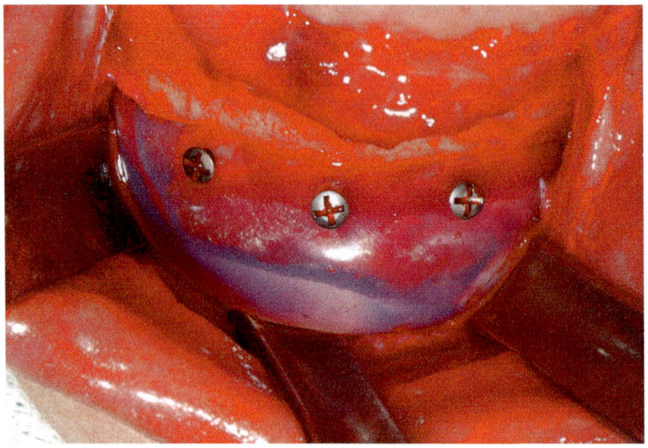

Fig. 9.206 Intraoperative view of anterior mandible following removal of pre-existing PEFE chin implant and placement of new custom solid silicone should implant with screw fixation (DuPuy Synthes Craniomaxillofacial, Paoli, PA, USA)

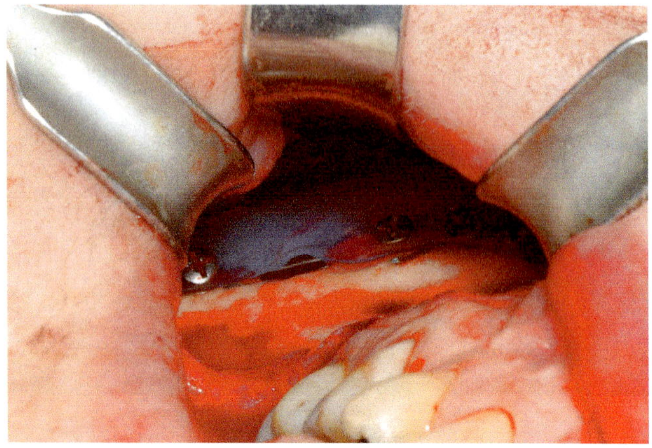

Fig. 9.208 Intraoperative view of left mandibular angle custom solid silicone implant placement with screw fixation (DuPuy Synthes Craniomaxillofacial, Paoli, PA, USA)

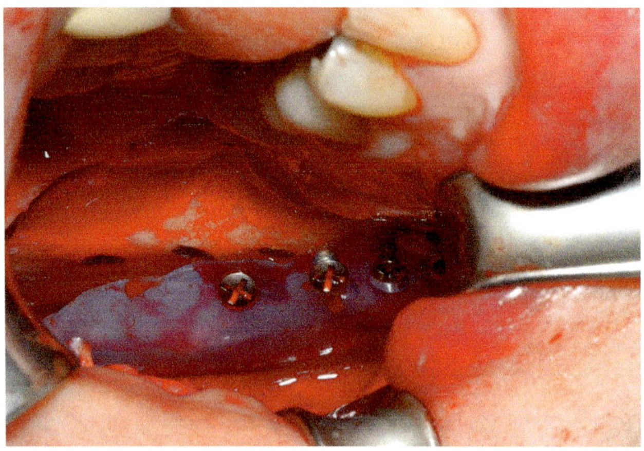

Fig. 9.207 Intraoperative view of right mandibular angle custom solid silicone implant placement with screw fixation (DuPuy Synthes Craniomaxillofacial, Paoli, PA, USA)

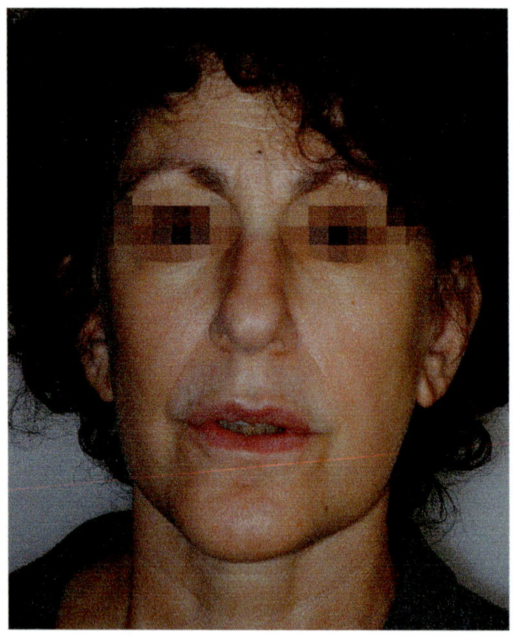

Fig. 9.209 Postoperative frontal facial view

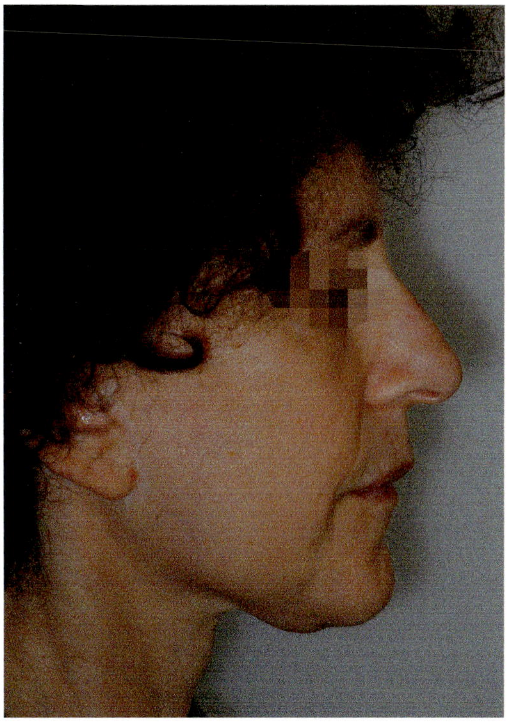

Fig. 9.210 Postoperative right lateral facial view

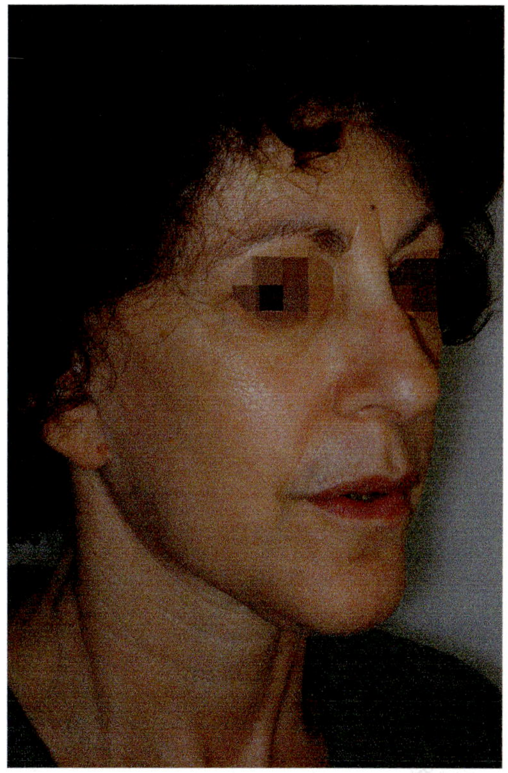

Fig. 9.212 Postoperative right 3/4 facial view

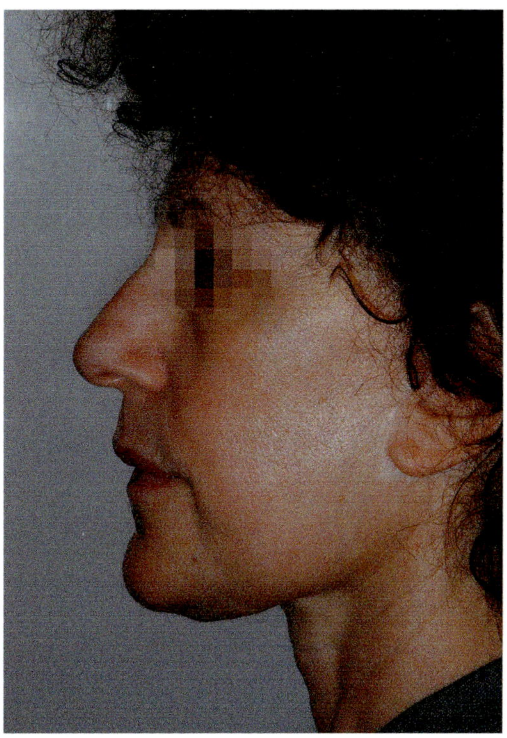

Fig. 9.211 Postoperative left lateral facial view

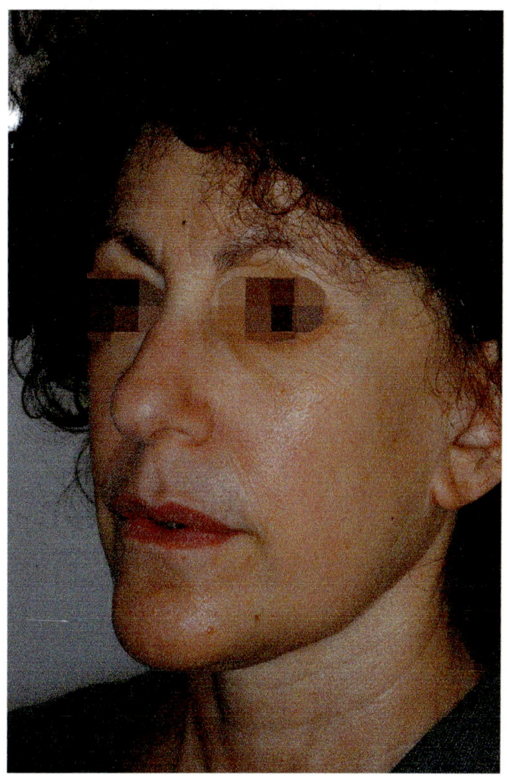

Fig. 9.213 Postoperative left 3/4 facial view

Case 8

An 18-year-old female patient presented with Class I occlusion and vertical maxillary hyperplasia and a complaint of excess display of gingiva (a "gummy smile") and lack of chin projection and jaw angle/neck definition. A LeFort I osteotomy with a wedge excision for superior repositioning, bilateral custom mandibular angle custom solid silicone implants, and chin implant were placed. This case demonstrates the use of both mandibular angle and chin implants to create a defined jaw line (Figs. 9.214–9.257). (Alex M. Greenberg, DDS, Oral and Maxillofacial Surgeon, New York, NY, USA)

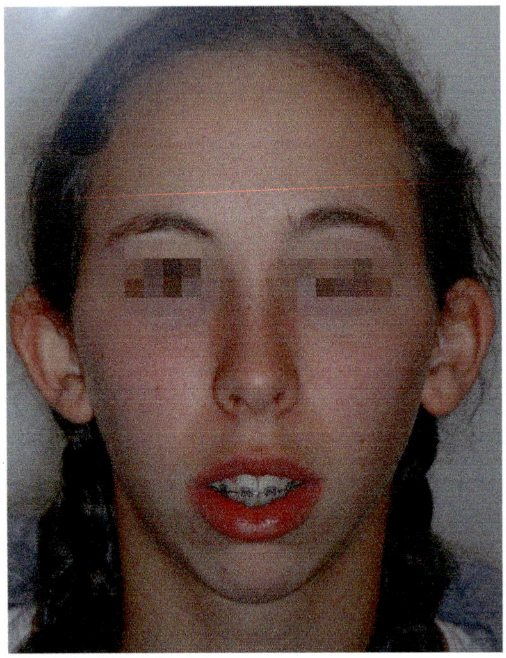

Fig. 9.214 Preoperative frontal facial view

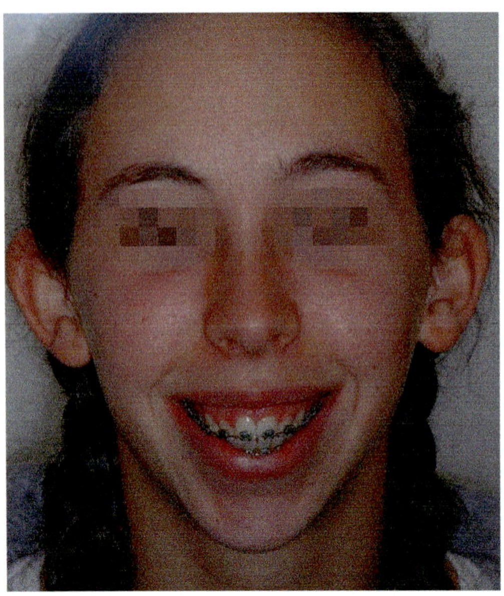

Fig. 9.215 Preoperative frontal facial view with smile

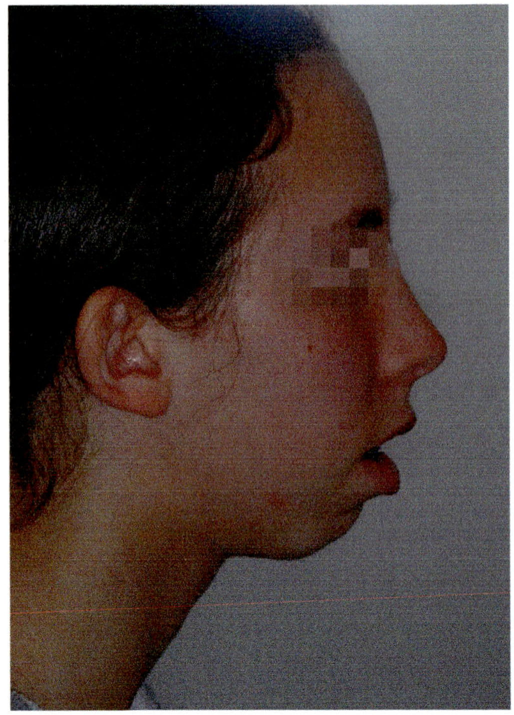

Fig. 9.216 Preoperative right lateral facial view

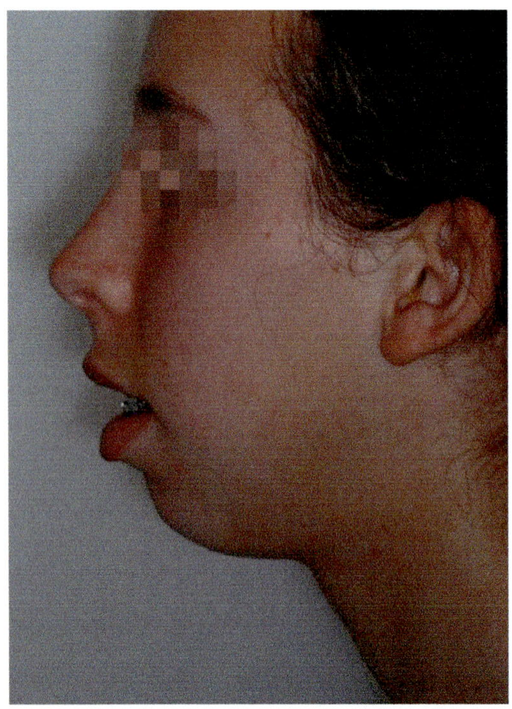

Fig. 9.217 Preoperative left lateral facial view

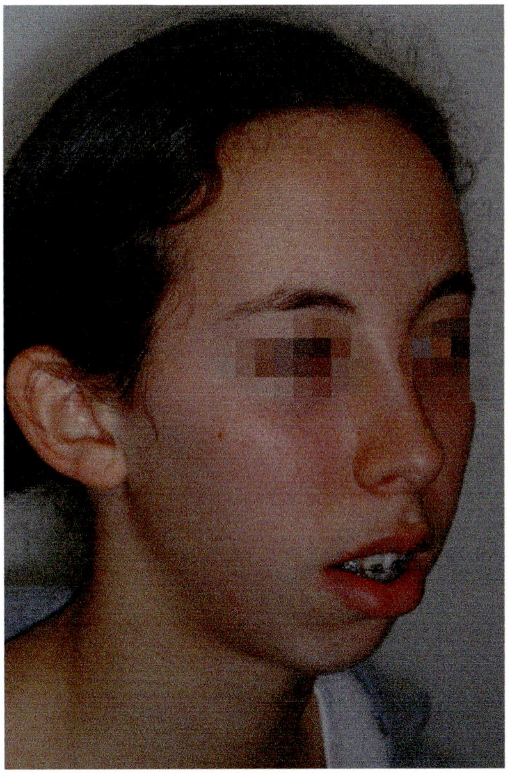

Fig. 9.218 Preoperative right 3/4 facial view

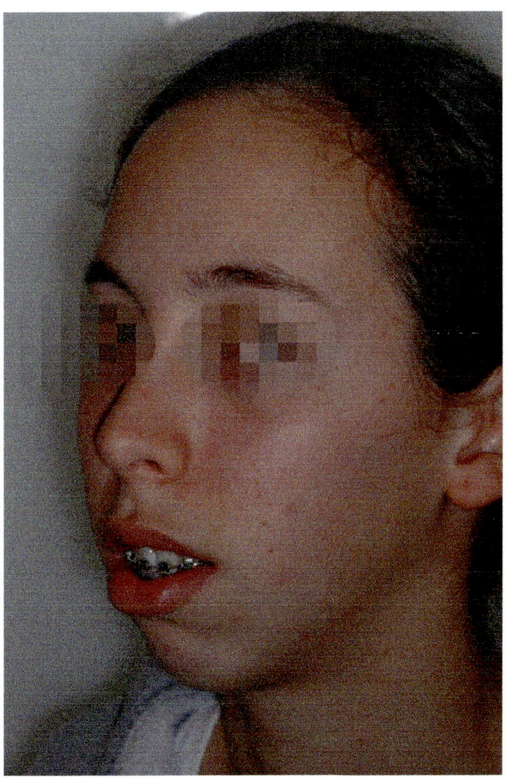

Fig. 9.219 Preoperative left 3/4 facial view

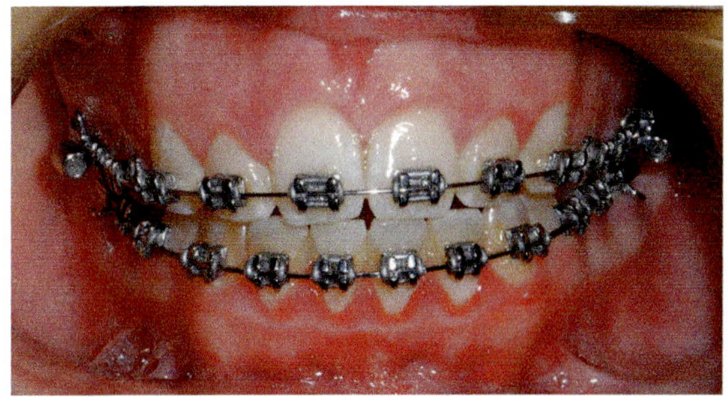

Fig. 9.220 Preoperative frontal occlusal view

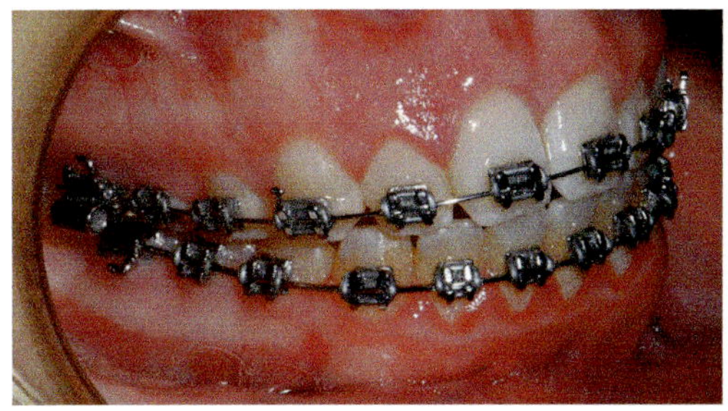

Fig. 221 Preoperative right lateral occlusal view

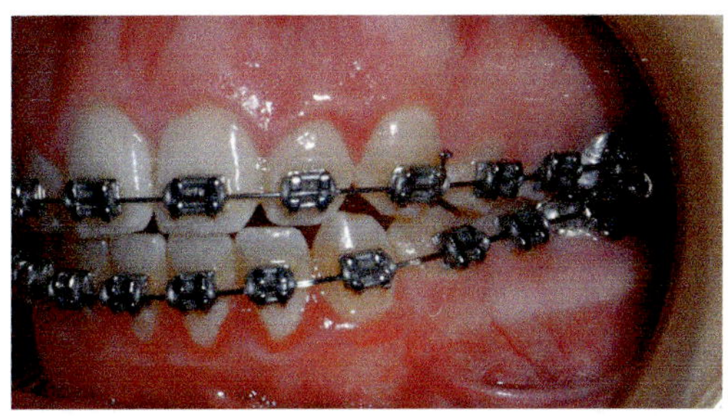

Fig. 9.222 Preoperative left lateral occlusal view

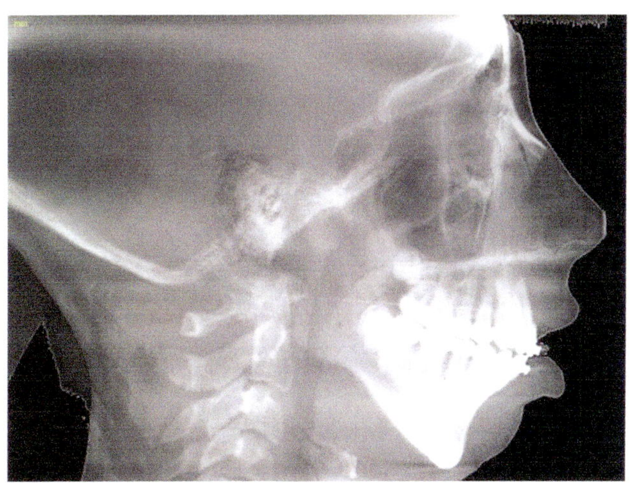

Fig. 9.223 Preoperative lateral cephalometric radiograph

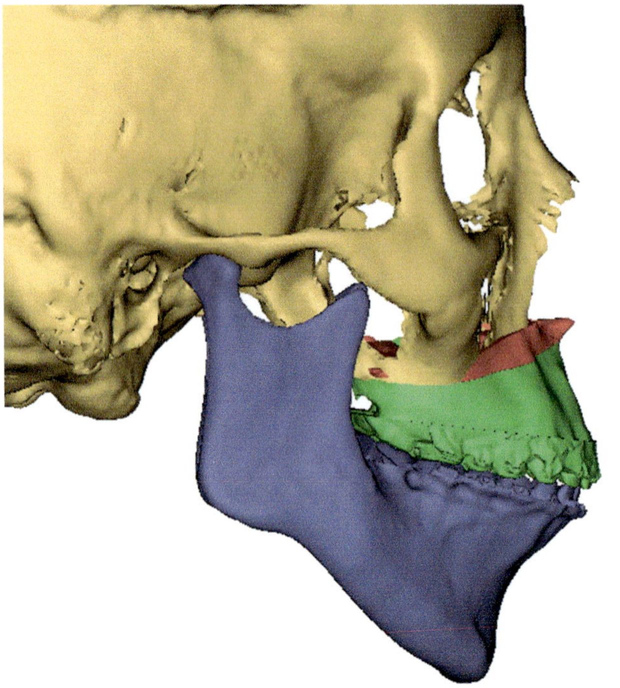

Fig. 9.224 Digital planning 3-D right lateral LeFort I osteotomy (Proplan, DuPuy Synthes Craniomaxillofacial, Paoli, PA, USA)

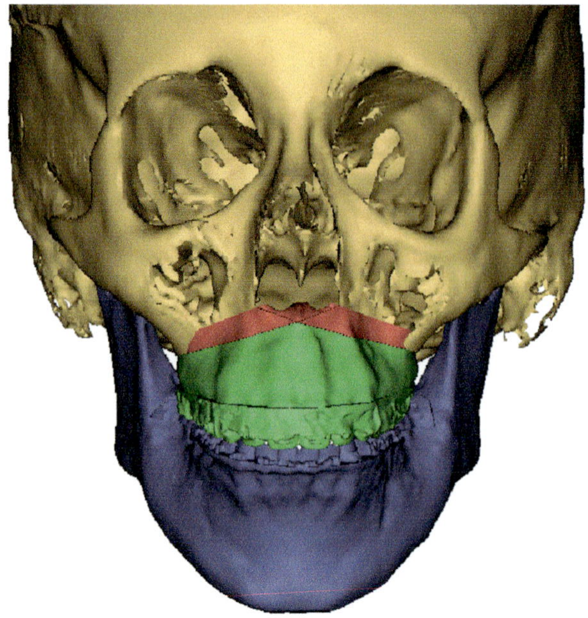

Fig. 9.226 Digital planning 3-D frontal view Lefort I osteotomy. (Proplan, DuPuy Synthes Craniomaxillofacial, Paoli, PA, USA)

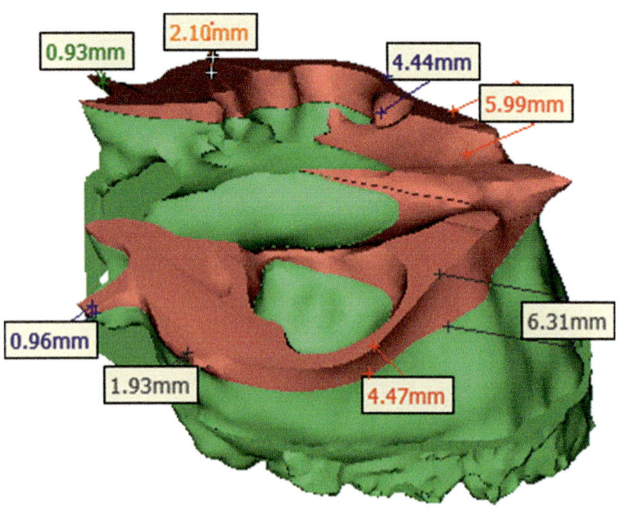

Fig. 9.225 Digital planning 3-D superior view of planned wedge excision for Lefort I osteotomy vertical impaction (Proplan, DuPuy Synthes Craniomaxillofacial, Paoli, PA, USA)

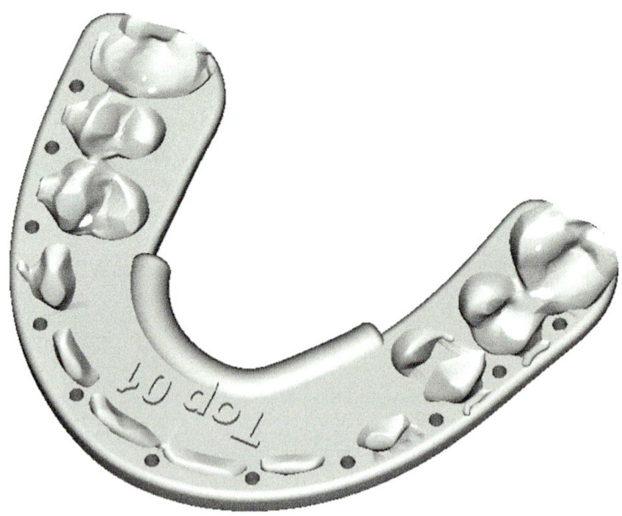

Fig. 9.227 Digital planning occlusal surgical splint (Proplan, DuPuy Synthes Craniomaxillofacial, Paoli, PA, USA)

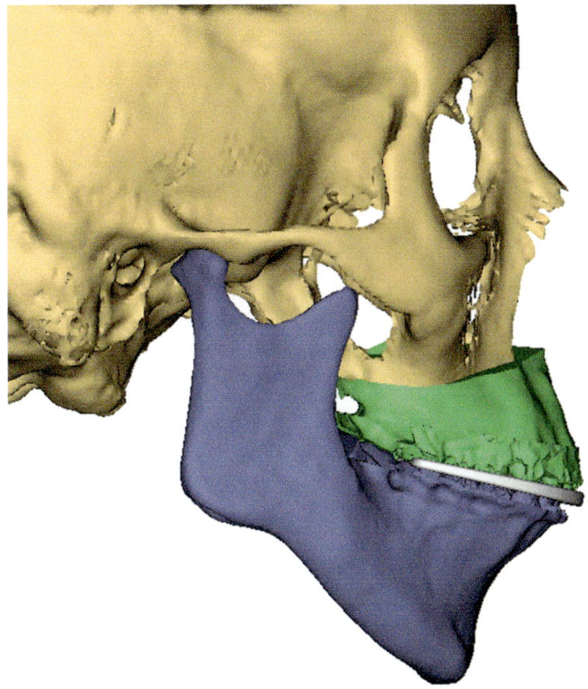

Fig. 9.228 Digital planning 3-D right side LeFort I osteotomy planned new vertical position of maxilla with final surgical splint in place (Proplan, DuPuy Synthes Craniomaxillofacial, Paoli, PA, USA)

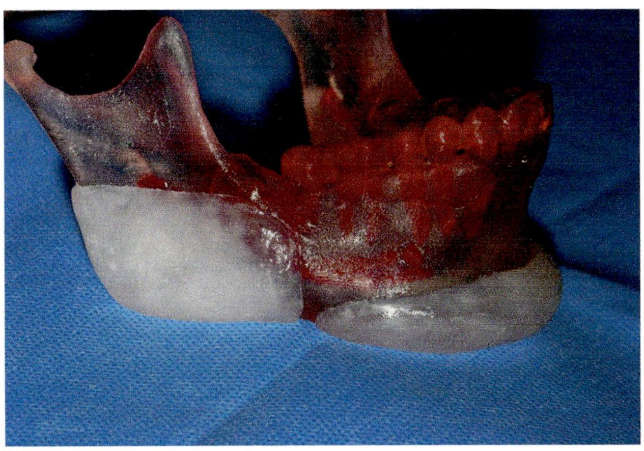

Fig. 9.229 Right mandibular angle and chin custom implant wax prototypes fitted to 3-D model

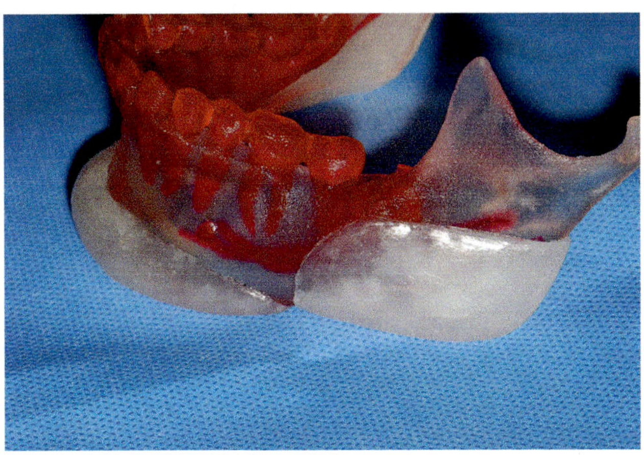

Fig. 9.230 Left mandibular angle and chin custom implant wax prototypes fitted to 3-D model

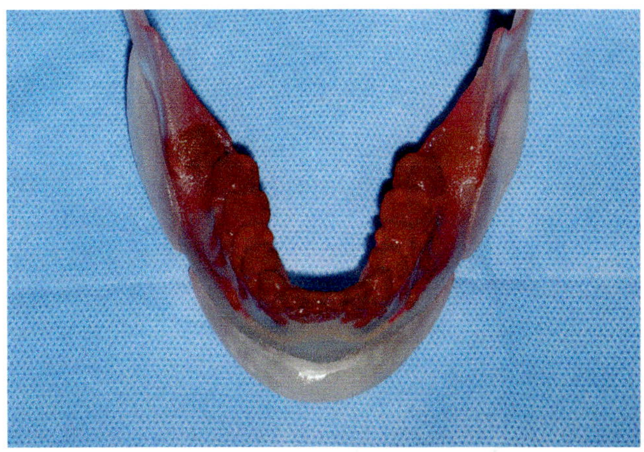

Fig. 9.231 Bilateral mandibular angle and chin custom implants wax prototypes fitted to 3-D model anterior superior view

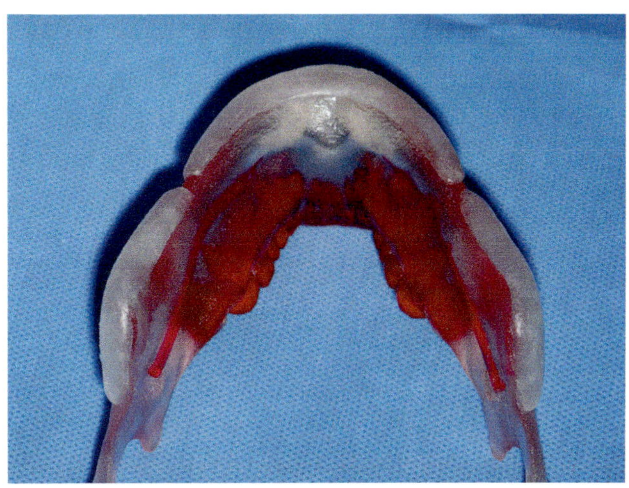

Fig. 9.232 Bilateral mandibular angle and chin custom implants wax prototypes fitted to 3-D model inferior lingual view

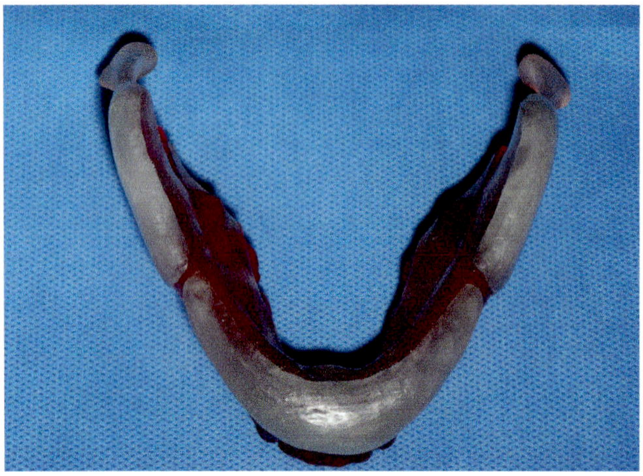

Fig. 9.233 Bilateral mandibular angle and chin custom implants wax prototypes fitted to 3-D model inferior anterior view

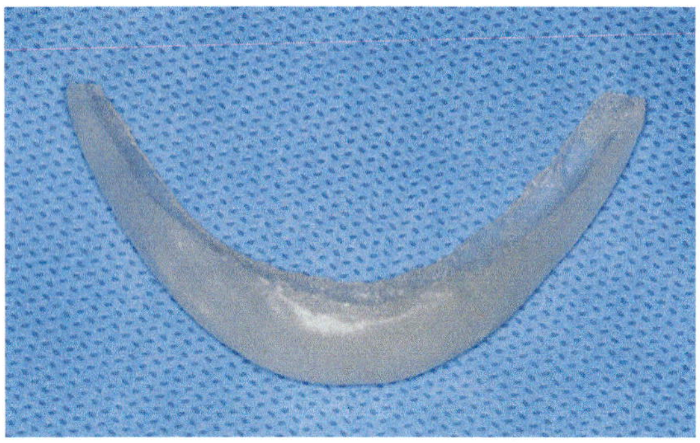

Fig. 9.234 Chin custom implant wax prototype superior anterior view

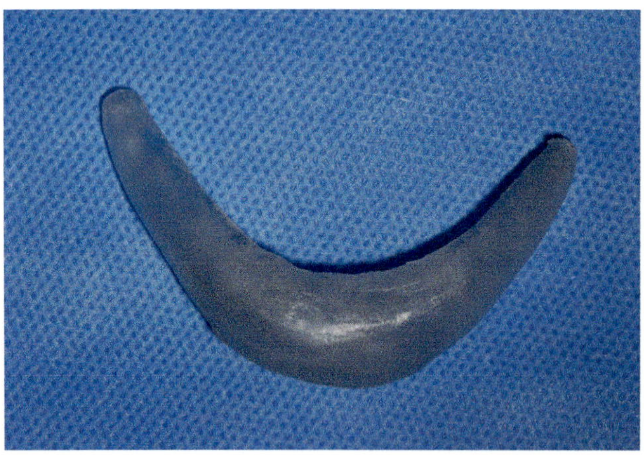

Fig. 9.235 Chin custom implant wax prototype inferior view

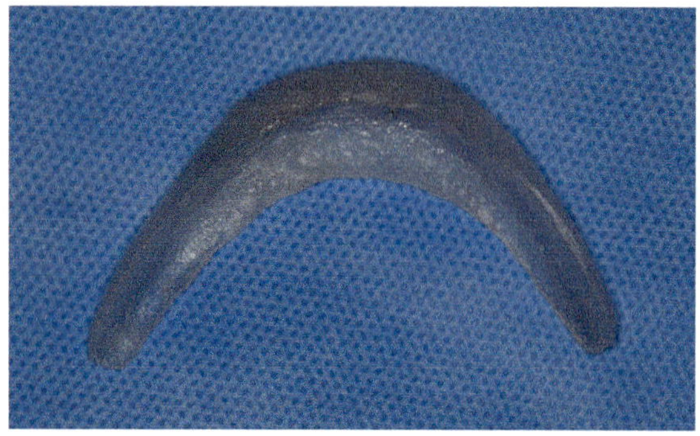

Fig. 9.236 Chin custom implant wax prototype superior interior lingual view

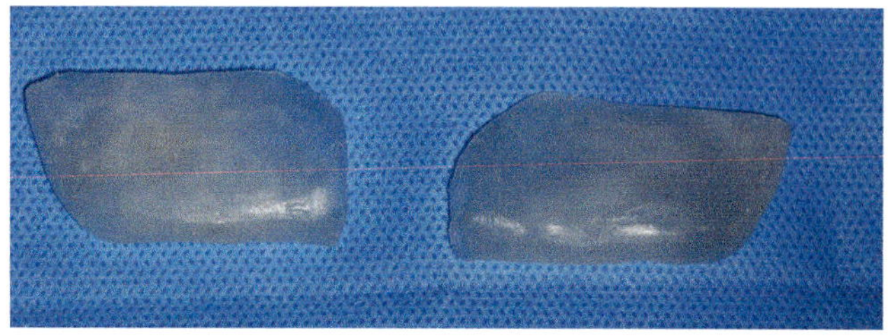

Fig. 9.237 Bilateral mandibular angle custom wax implant prototypes exterior view

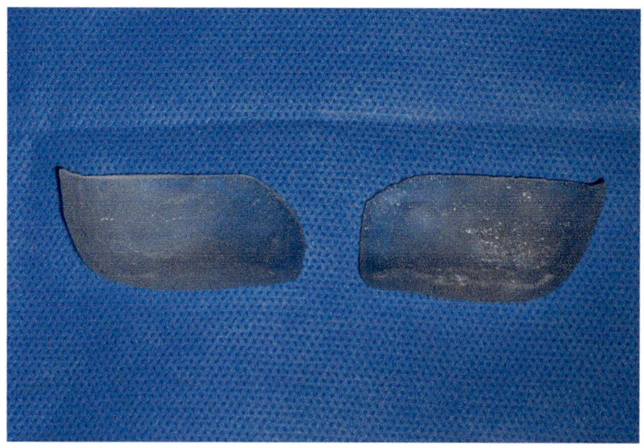

Fig. 9.238 Bilateral mandibular angle custom wax implant prototypes interior view

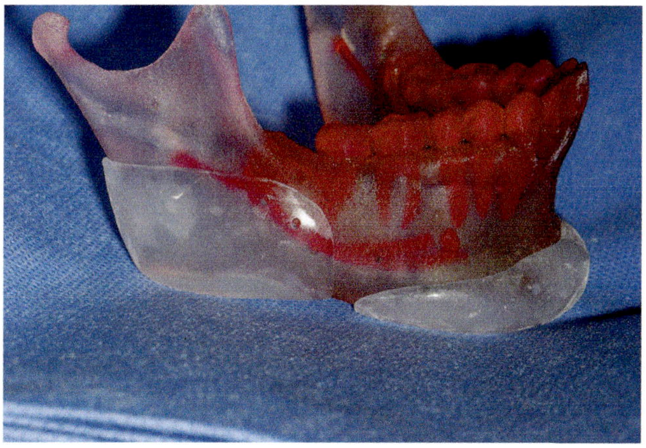

Fig. 9.239 Right mandibular angle and chin custom solid silicone implants fitted to 3-D model

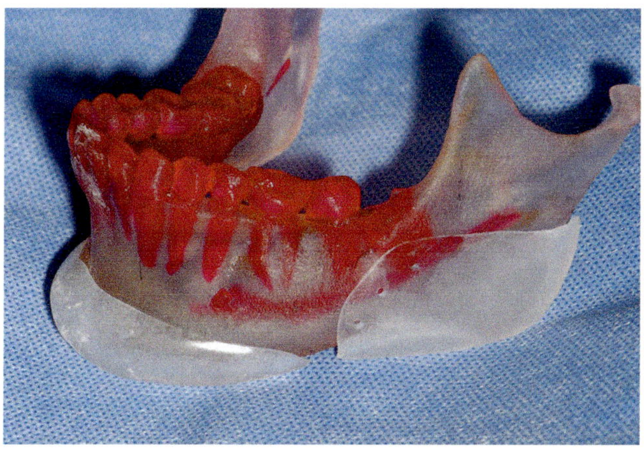

Fig. 9.240 Left mandibular angle and chin custom solid silicone implants fitted to 3-D model

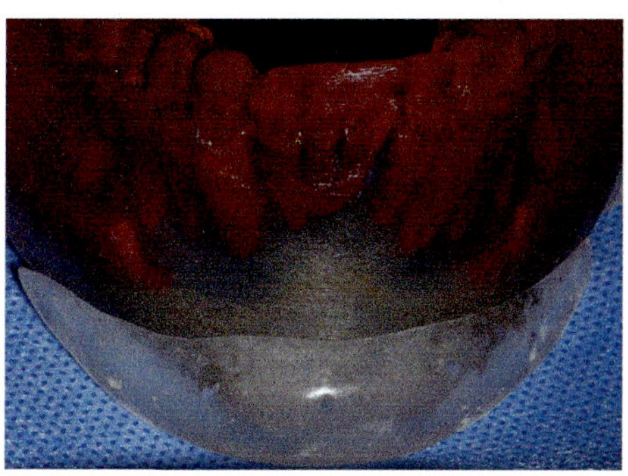

Fig. 9.241 Chin custom solid silicone implant fitted to 3-D model anterior superior view

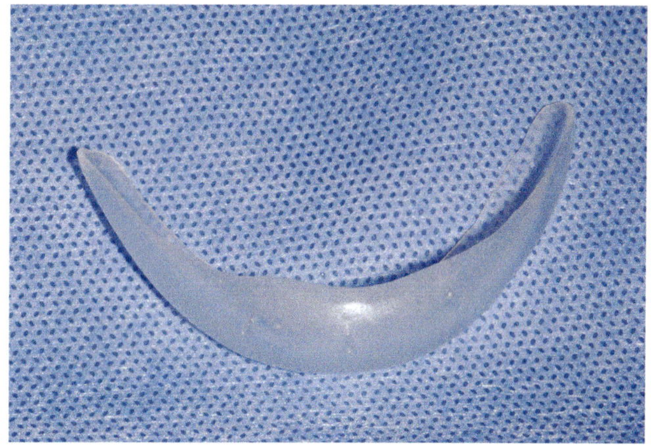

Fig. 9.242 Chin custom solid silicone implant superior anterior view

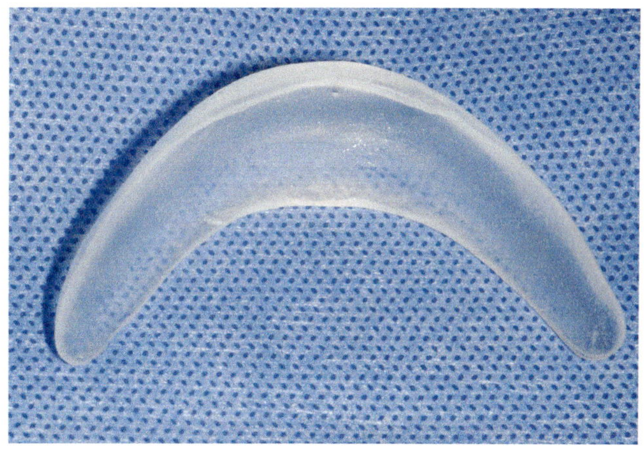

Fig. 9.243 Chin custom solid silicone implant superior lingual view

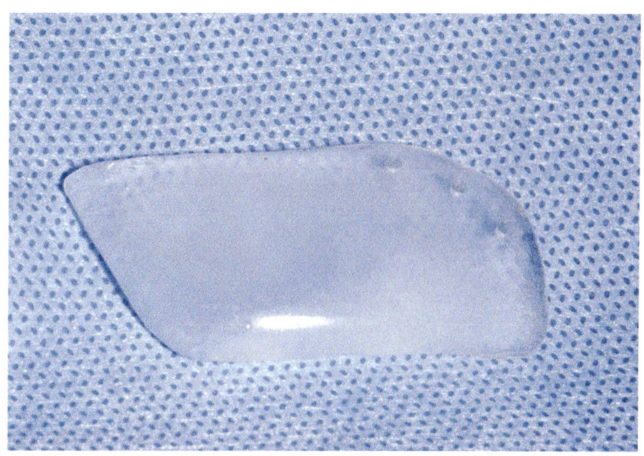

Fig. 9.244 Right mandibular angle custom solid silicone implant exterior view. Note: Anterior superior border 3 screw fixation holes

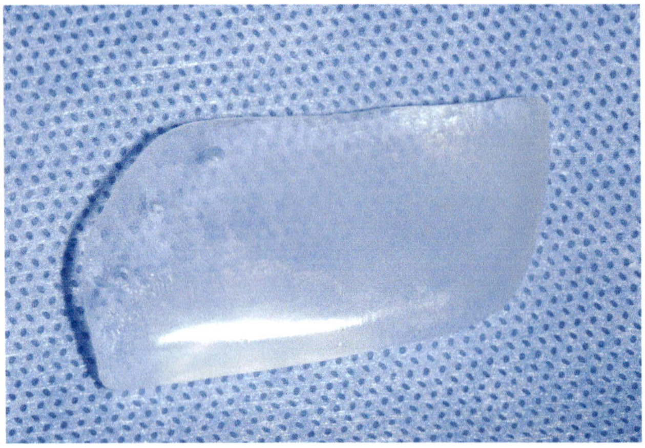

Fig. 9.245 Left mandibular angle custom solid silicone implant exterior view. Note: Anterior superior border 3 screw fixation holes

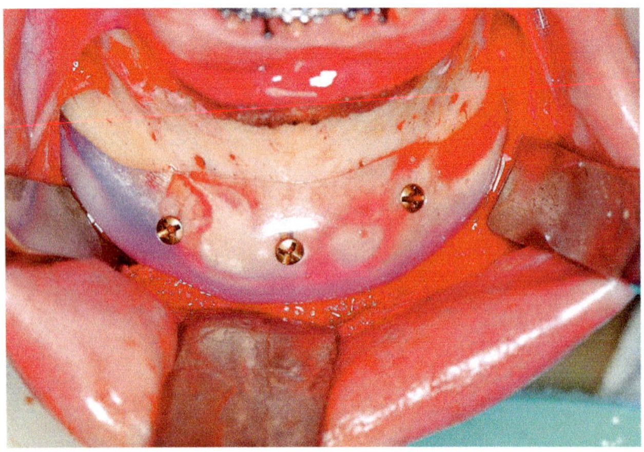

Fig. 9.246 Intraoperative view of custom solid silicone chin implant placement with screw fixation

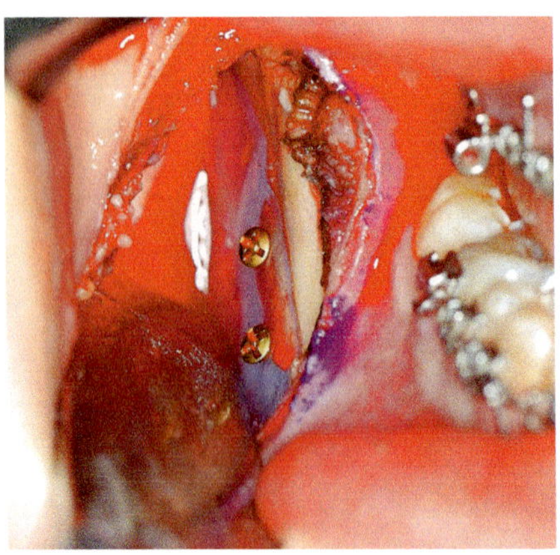

Fig. 9.247 Intraoperative view of right mandibular angle custom solid silicone implant with screw fixation

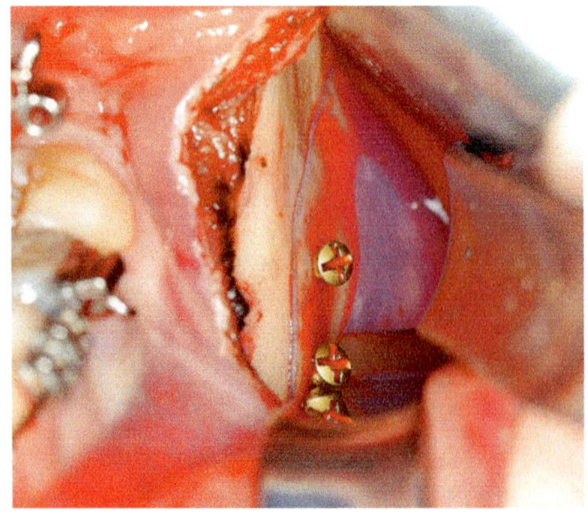

Fig. 9.248 Intraoperative view of left mandibular angle custom solid silicone implant with screw fixation

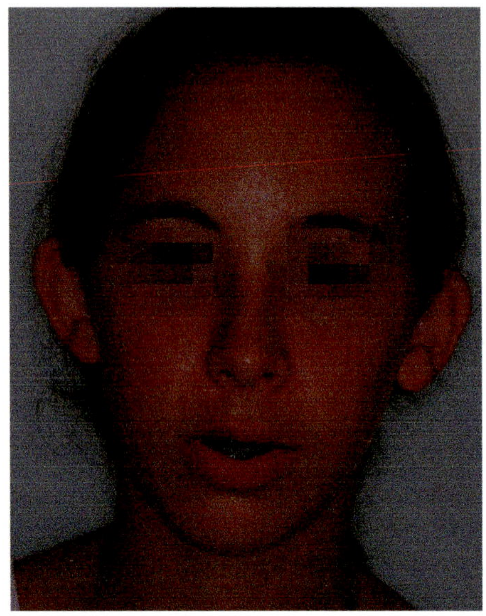

Fig. 9.249 Postoperative frontal facial view

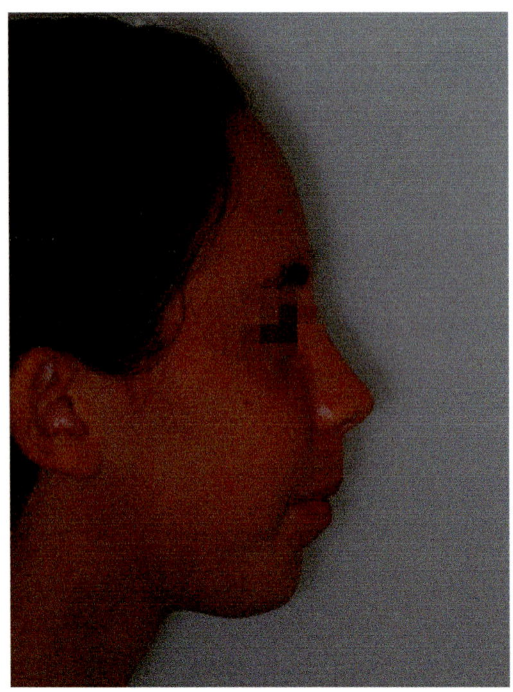

Fig. 9.250 Postoperative right lateral facial view

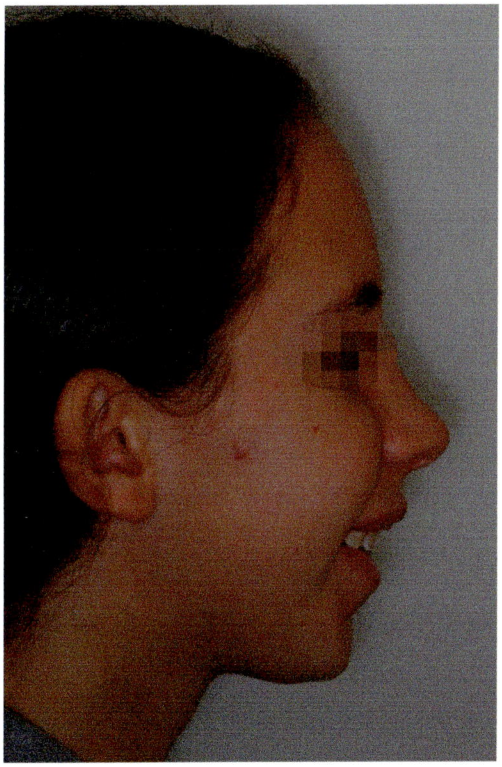

Fig. 9.251 Postoperative right lateral facial view with smile

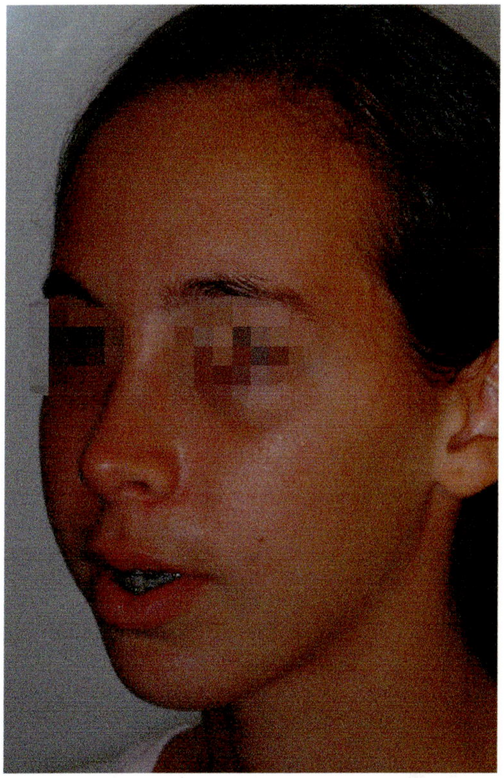

Fig. 9.253 Postoperative left 3/4 facial view

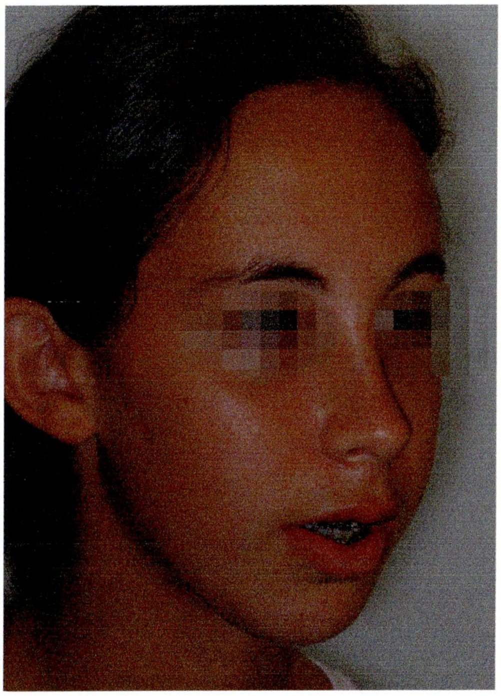

Fig. 9.252 Postoperative right 3/4 view with smile

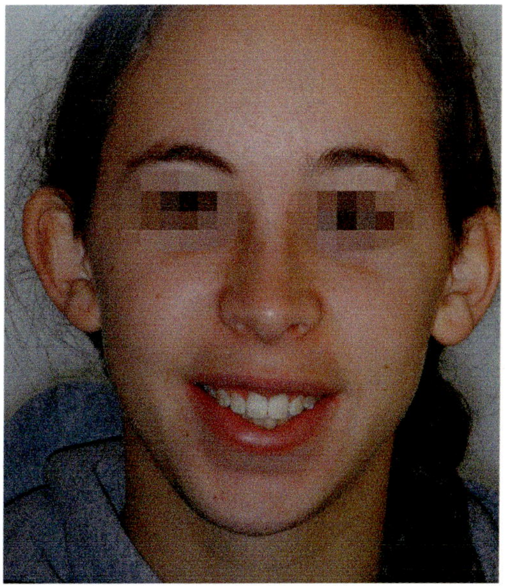

Fig. 9.254 Postoperative frontal facial view

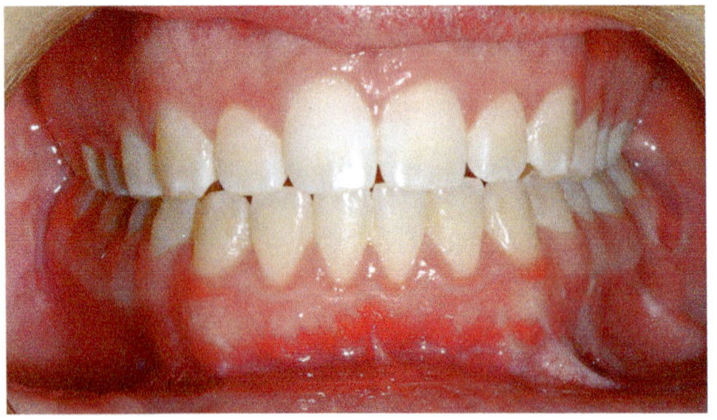

Fig. 9.255 Postoperative frontal occlusal view

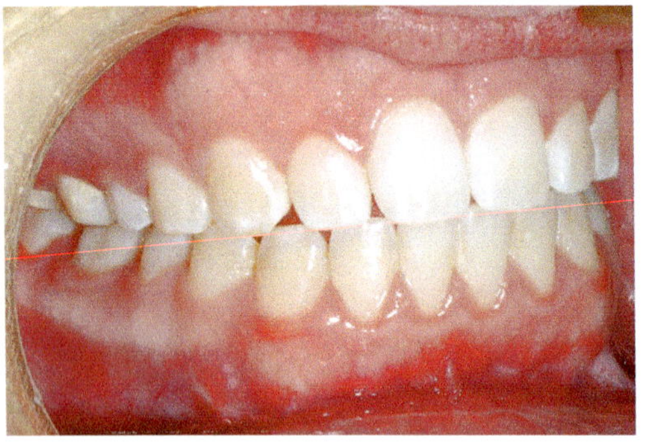

Fig. 9.256 Postoperative right lateral occlusal view

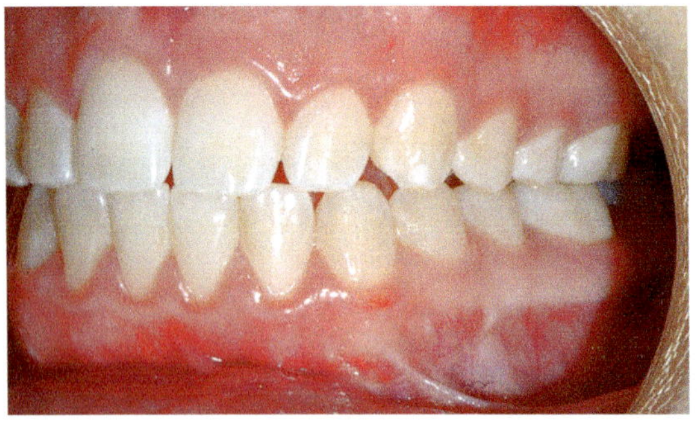

Fig. 9.257 Postoperative left lateral occlusal view

Case 9

A 37-year-old female patient presented after prior orthognathic surgery with a Lefort I osteotomy, bilateral mandibular ramus inverted L osteotomies with iliac crest bone grafts, anterior horizontal mandibular osteotomy, and ePTFE chin implant, with relapse into a Class II occlusion and dissatisfaction with the chin esthetics and loss of bilateral madibular angle definition. A Lefort I osteotomy was performed to correct the Class II malocclusion, removal of the ePTFE chin implant and bilateral custom mandibular angle custom solid silicone implants, and chin implants were performed (Figs. 9.258–9.277).

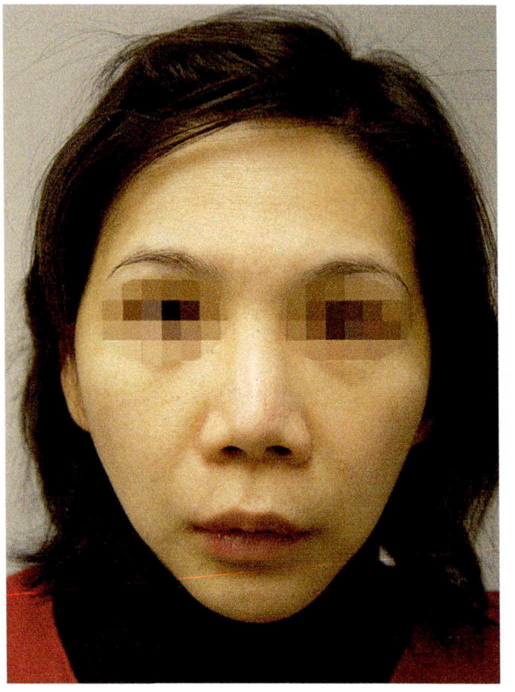

Fig. 9.258 Preoperative frontal facial view

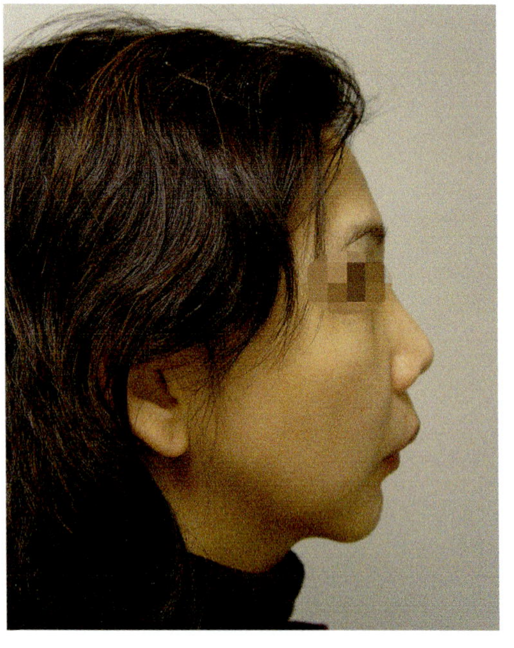

Fig. 9.259 Preoperative right lateral facial view

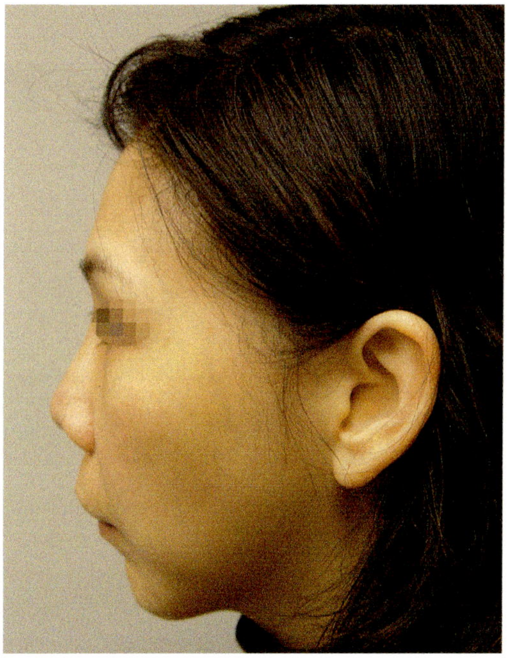

Fig. 9.260 Preoperative left lateral facial view

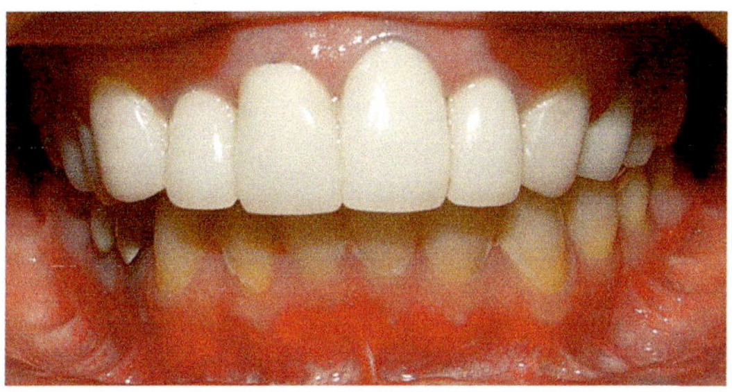

Fig. 9.261 Preoperative frontal occlusal facial view

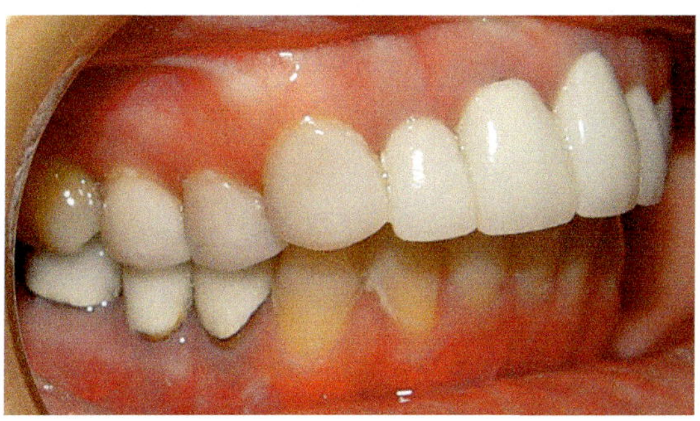

Fig. 9.262 Preoperative right lateral occlusal view

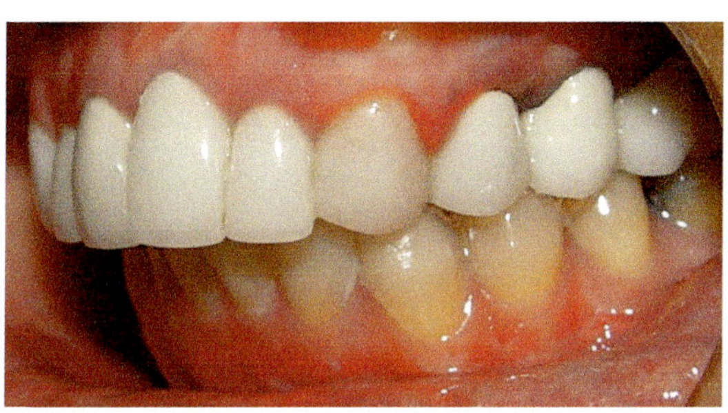

Fig. 263 Preoperative left lateral occlusal view

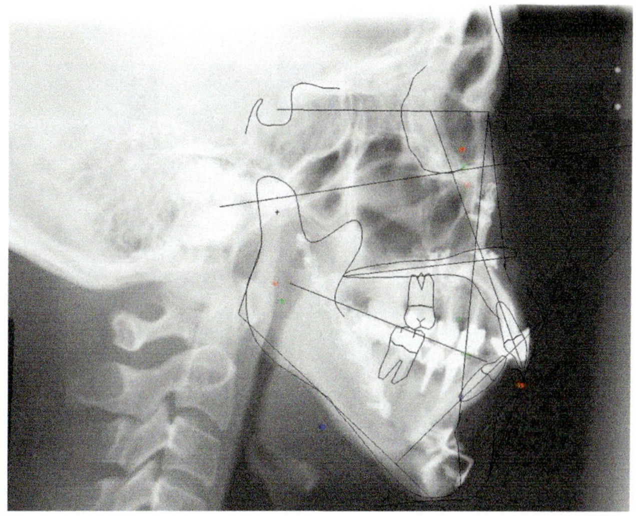

Fig. 9.264 Preoperative post orthognathic surgery cephalometric radiograph

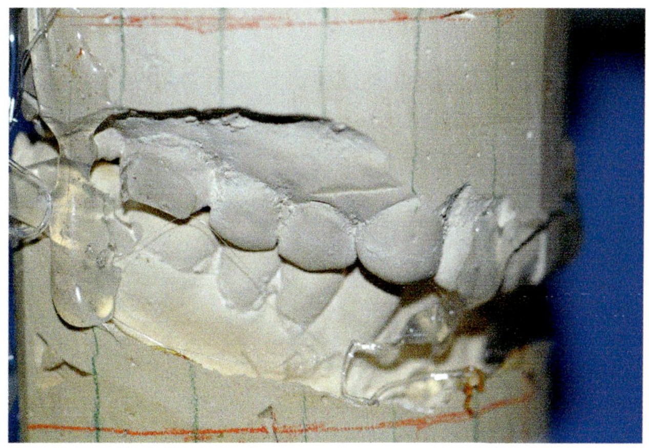

Fig. 9.265 Model surgery planning right lateral view for Lefort I osteotomy

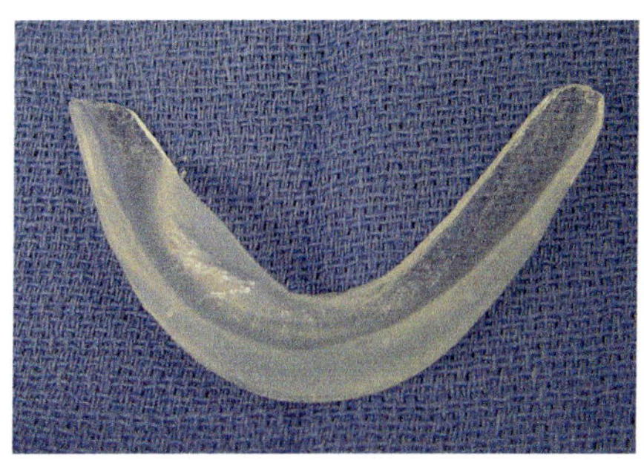

Fig. 9.266 Superior view of custom solid silicone chin implant

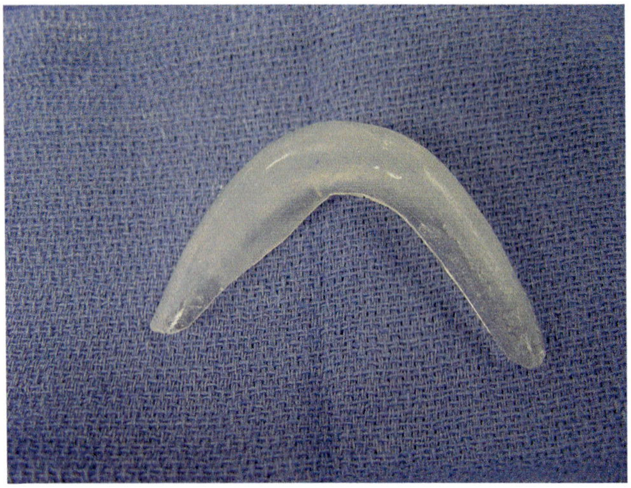

Fig. 9.267 Inferior lingual view of custom solid silicone implant

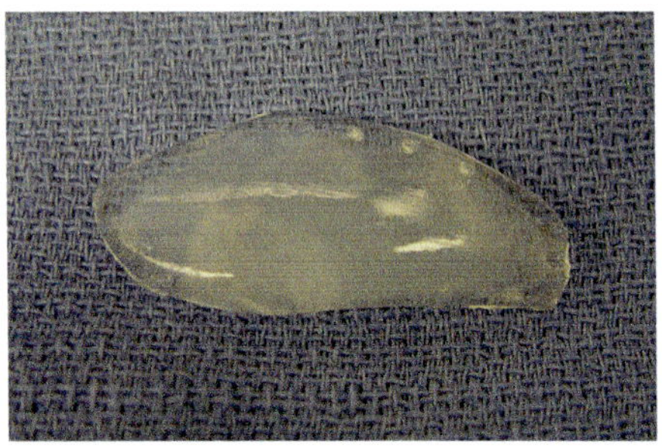

Fig. 9.268 Right mandibular angle custom solid silicone implant. Note: 3 screw holes anterior superior border

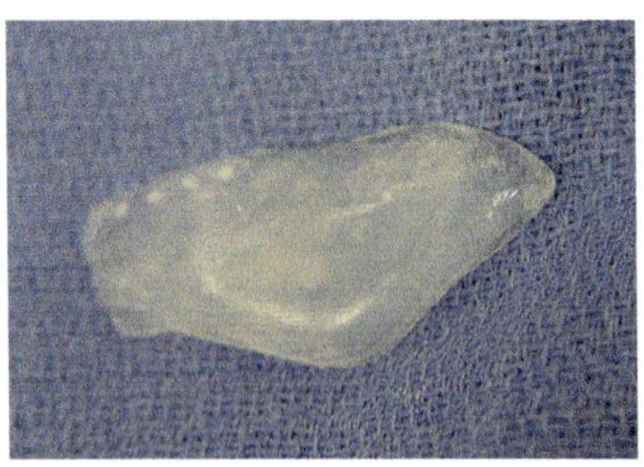

Fig. 9.269 Left mandibular angle custom solid silicone implant. Note: 3 screw holes anterior superior border

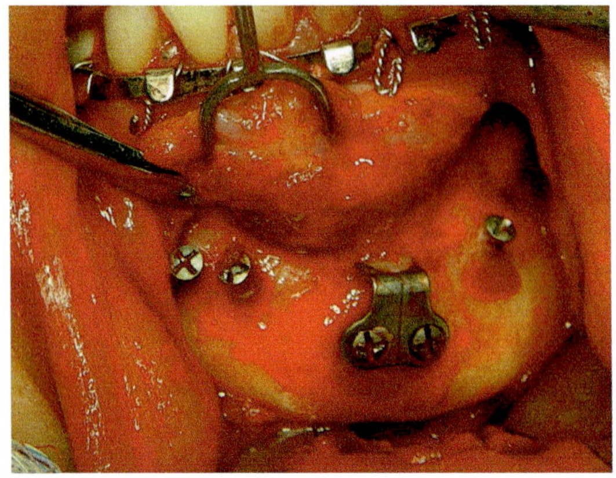

Fig. 9.270 Intraoperative view of anterior mandible with retained hardware and bony deformity

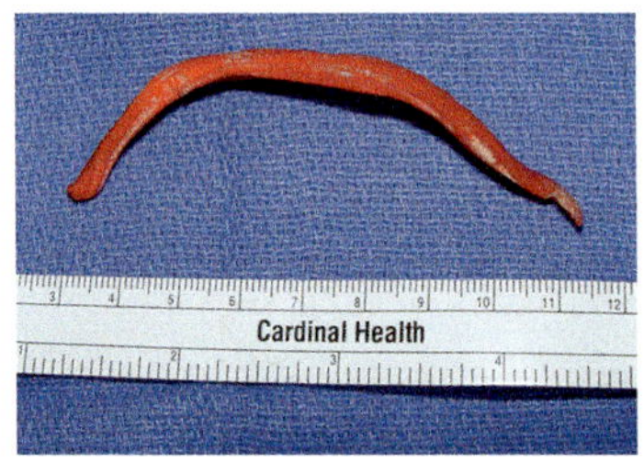

Fig. 9.271 ePTFE chin implant previously placed overlying anterior horizontal mandibular osteotomy and removed

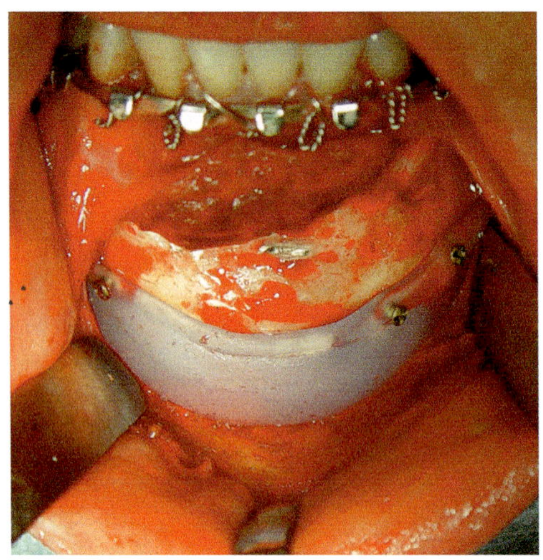

Fig. 9.272 Intraoperative view of custom solid silicone chin implant with screw fixation

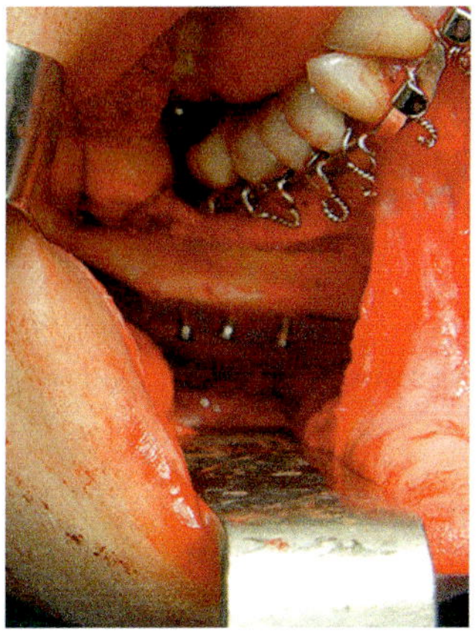

Fig. 9.73 Intraoperative view of right mandibular angle custom solid silicone implant with screw fixation

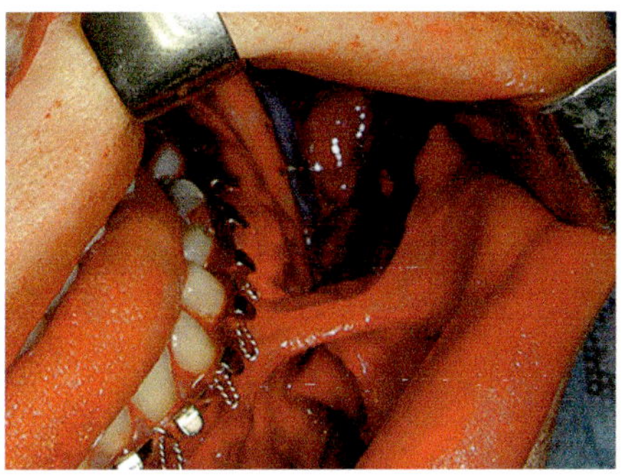

Fig. 9.274 Intraoperative view of left mandibular angle custom solid silicone implant with screw fixation. Note: Preservation of the mental nerve

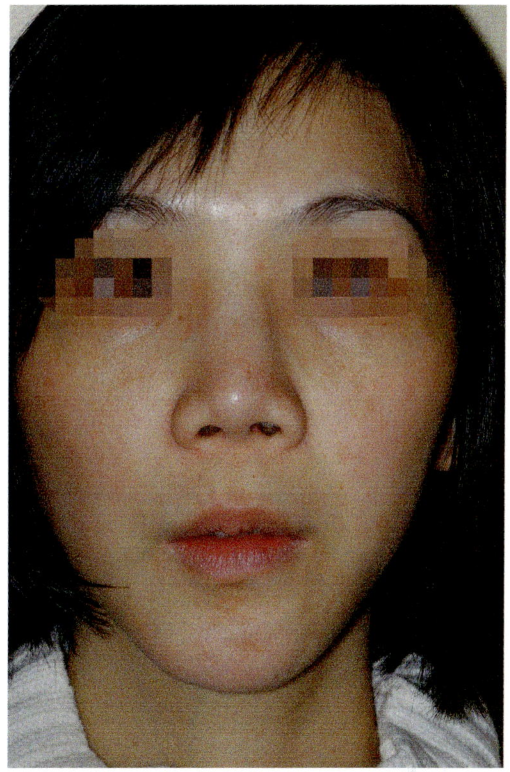

Fig. 9.275 Postoperative frontal facial view

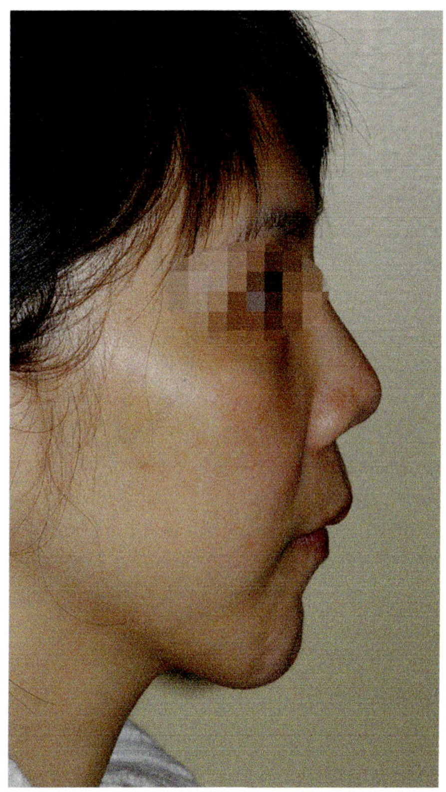

Fig. 9.276 Postoperative right lateral facial view

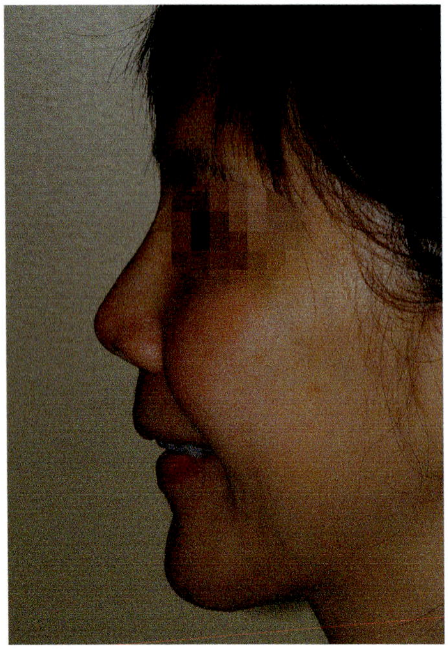

Fig. 9.277 Postoperative left lateral facial view

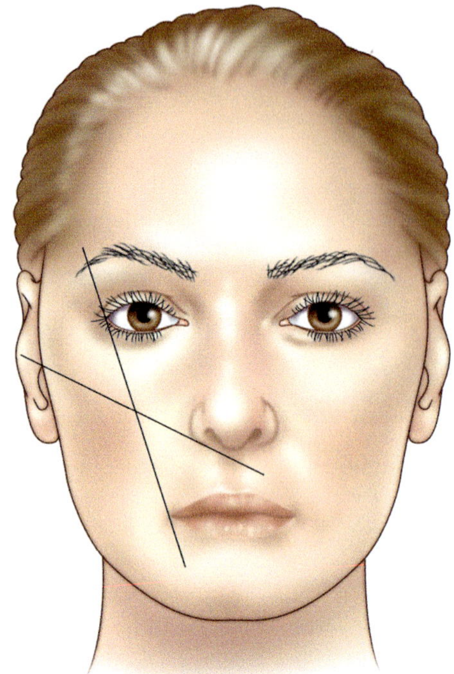

Fig. 9.278 The Hinderer method of crossed lines. Vertical line from the lateral canthus to the lip commissure. Tangential line from the tragus to the lateral ala

Zygomatic Alloplastic Augmentation

The malar region is considered to be one of the foremost aspects of facial beauty, especially in females [76, 77]. Prominent cheekbones in males can be a sign of strength, and in females, they provide an accentuation to the eyes, and the smile on animation. Individuals can present with several variations of the malar region which can be influenced by sex, ethnicity, genetics, syndromes (i.e., Treacher Collins [77]), acquired deformities (i.e., trauma, other surgeries), or unsatisfactory implants. The zygomatic regions are evaluated based on several possible analyses. Terino and Edwards [78] have described the malar region as comprising malar suborbital deficiencies and the skeletal deficiency of a combined suborbital-zygomatic region as a type 1 face. The medial extent of this deformity is the tear trough sulcus at the lid cheek junction.

Various facial analyses based on landmarks have been used to define the malar prominence for the diagnosis and placement of malar implants. Hinderer's analysis [79] for malar implants used crossed lines in which one line extends from the lateral canthus to the commissure and the other line from the ala to the tragus. The anterior medial aspect of the implant was placed within the apex of the crossed lines [79] (Fig. 9.278). The Wilkinson analysis [80] uses a vertical line drawn from the lateral canthus. The high point of the implant would be placed 1/3 of the distance from the lateral canthus to the inferior border of the mandible [80] (Fig. 9.279). Silver [81] described a malar prominence located on a triangle based on a vertical line from the lateral aspect of the limbus

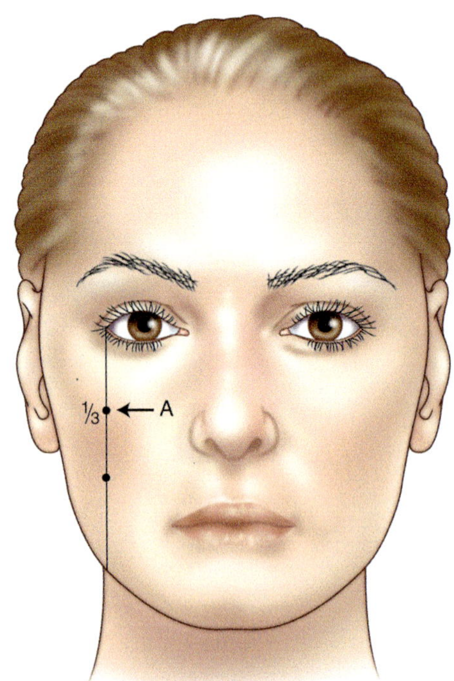

Fig. 9.79 Wilkinson's method with malar prominence 1/3 inferior on a vertical line from the right lateral canthus to the inferior border of the mandible

with the patient looking straight ahead. The vertical line creates a triangle with the apex X at horizontal line B at the midpoint between subnasale and the upper lip vermillion border. Then a line is drawn from X to the medial canthus and an equal angle line drawn from X to P lateral to the lateral canthus which will be the malar prominence [81] (Fig. 9.280). Powell's analysis [82] uses parallel lines from the lateral canthus through the lateral alar base and another from the lateral lip commissure that when crossing the Frankfort horizontal, the intersection is the malar prominence. Powell also divided the malar region into the anteromedial and posterolateral regions based on a vertical line through the lateral canthus [82] (Fig. 9.281). Prendergast and Schoenrock [83] defined the malar prominence 1/3 inferior to a line drawn from the lateral commissure through the lateral canthus (Fig. 9.282). Binder developed a set of stock implants based on three types of deformities: type 1, primary malar hypoplasia; type 2, submalar deficiency; and type 3, combined malar and submalar deficiency [84].

When evaluating the cheekbones, the patient needs to be viewed from the frontal, three-quarter, superior (bird's eye), and inferior (worm's eye) views. Differences in symmetry need to be noted. The zygoma needs to include the lateral orbital region and whether any disorders of globe position are present such as enophalmos, exophthalmos, proptosis, or soft tissue disorders of the eyelids such as lid ptosis, rhytids, and lipodystrophy. The suborbital sulcus and tear trough sulcus are also important anatomic considerations (Figs. 9.283 and 9.284). Submalar deficiency can be an aspect of aging secondary to buccal fat pad atrophy [85].

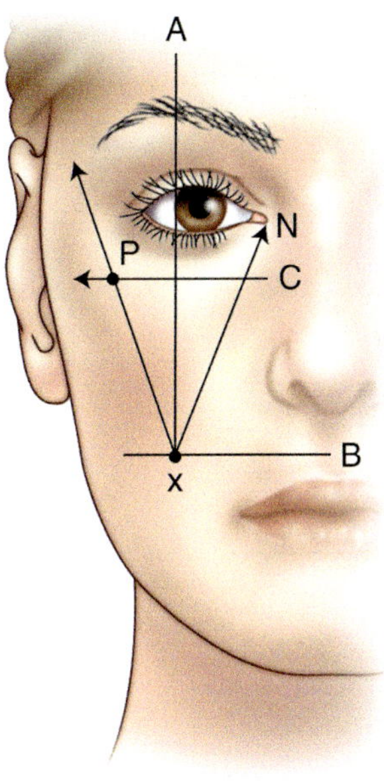

Fig. 9.280 Silver's malar prominence triangle method

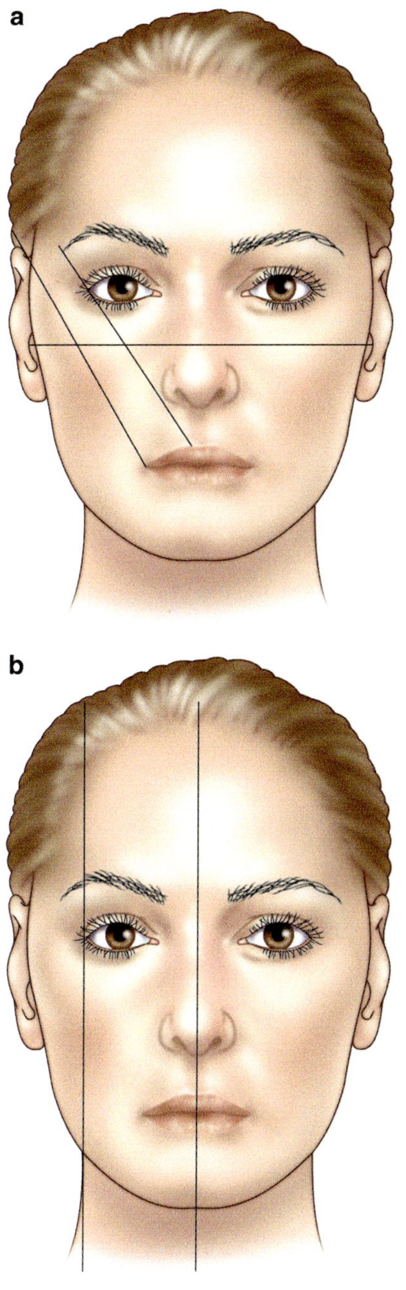

Fig. 9.281 (**a**) Powell et al.'s method. A Frankfort horizontal line is crossed by two parallel tangential lines. (**b**) Powell et al.'s method divides the malar region into posteromedial and anteromedial regions with a vertical line through the lateral canthus

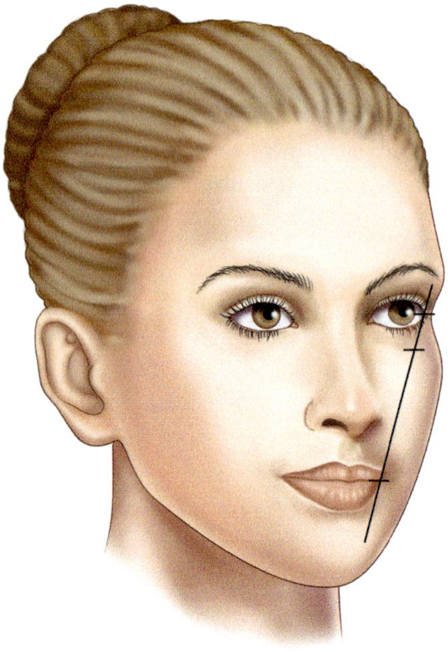

Fig. 9.282 Prendergast and Schoenrock oblique line from lateral canthus to lateral commissure with malar prominence 1/3 inferior to the lateral canthus

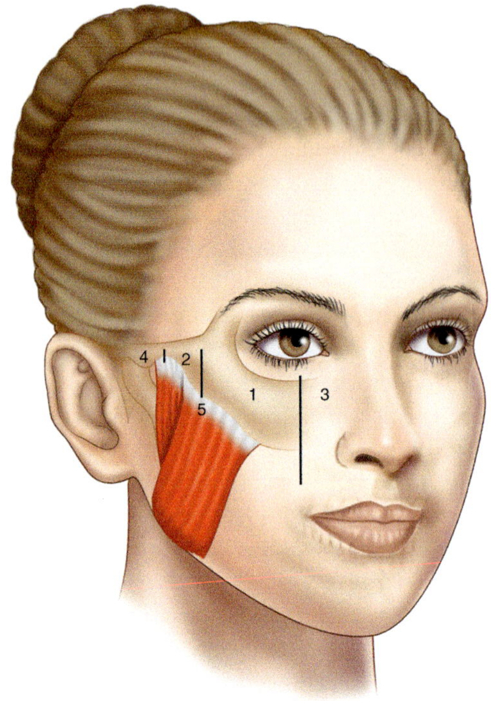

Fig. 9.283 Terino's five skeletal zones of the malar region

Fig. 9.284 Periorbital region atrophy from aging

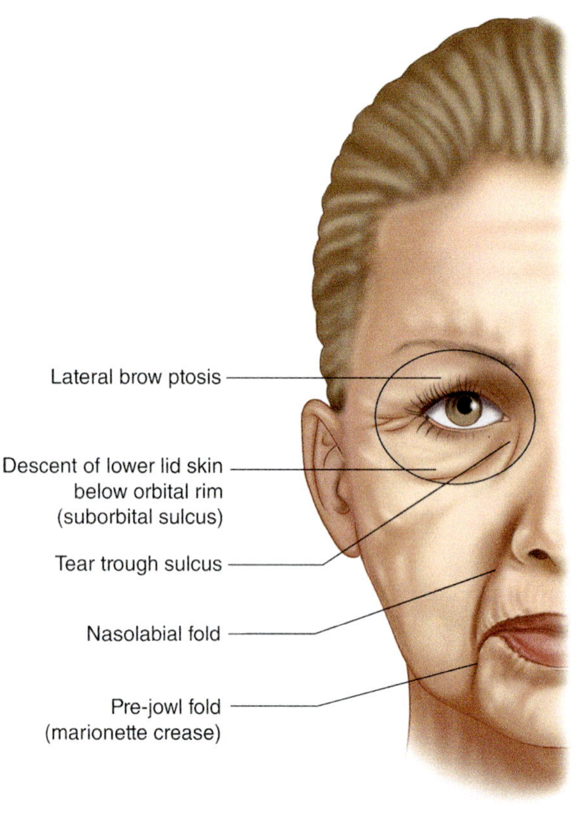

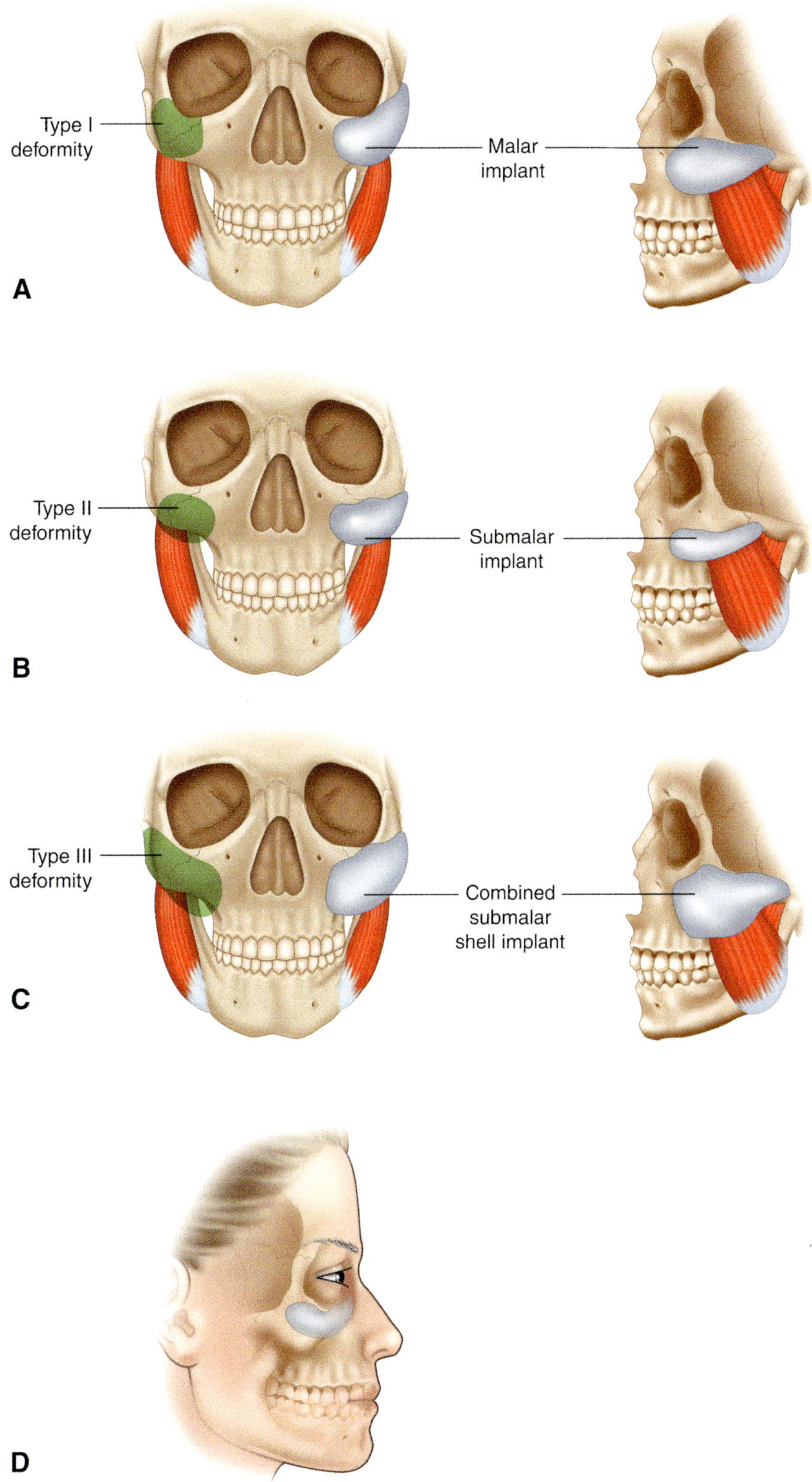

Fig. 9.285 Types of malar implants after Binder [85]. (**a**) Type I deformity malar implant. (**b**) Type II deformity submalar implant. (**c**) Type III deformity combined submalar and malar implant. (**d**) Type IV tear trough implant

Custom Malar/Zygomatic Solid Silicone Implants Using 3-D CT Models

Various methods of malar augmentation have been utilized including periorbital osteotomies of the zygoma [86, 87], reduction or augmentation with bone grafting [88], and alloplastic materials. Alloplasts have included the use of solid silicone [77, 78, 84, 85, 89], PEFE [9], HTR [11], hydroxyapatite [90], and PEEK [91]. Both the zygomatic osteotomy and alloplastic implant techniques have had limitations based on an individual's bone anatomy and morphology, as well as the commercially available preformed alloplastic implants. Stock implants include the malar, submalar, Binder, anatomic, and suborbital malar tear trough types (Figs. 9.285 and 9.1q–x). Various techniques can be employed to modify the malar region which can include osteoplasty and osteotomies for reduction or augmentation. Depending on the deformity and desired augmentation, this will help to determine the augmentation method and implant type selection, whether malar, submalar, or malar-maxillary. Numerous authors have addressed the various techniques with respect to diagnosis, treatment planning, and technique [9, 11, 76–88]. Custom malar implants carved from PEFE [9] on the operating field have been described. A recent report of custom PEEK malar implants utilizing a rapid prototyping method has been reported and may represent a future commercially available technique [91]. 3-D imaging methods can aid in the planning of the dimensions of malar implants (Fig. 9.286a, b, and c).

CT Scanning for Evaluation and Creation of a Stereolithographic Model

The patient will need to undergo CT or CBCT with the head in a natural position relative to Frankfort Horizontal. The DICOM data is then transferred to a service provider either on a disk or uploaded via a website in order to then fabricate a stereolithographic model. Stereolithographic models for malar implants must include the full orbit and zygomatic arch as well as the entire maxillary region including the dentition and should be bilateral for symmetry.

Technique for Wax Application and Carving of the Implant

The method to create a wax block outline for the malar region implant is to analyze the dimension which is desired to augment. This is often helped by the structure of the stereolithographic model and its inherent bony deficiency. This is also where the art of being able to assess the patient's esthetic features and desired contours comes into play. The review of clinical examination, facial photographs, facial moulage, and PA cephalometric and CT radiographs is essential.

The wax is utilized to form the malar implant and it is carved to the desired contours. The method for fabrication of custom solid silicone implants has been described above. Vaseline should be used to lubricate the anatomic model. The style of implant custom prepared depends on the indications for its use. These implants are placed only using an intraoral incision and in our series without a single case of wound dehiscence or loss of implant. Satisfactory capsule formation permits smooth soft tissue contours. Custom malar implants can address augmentation in the sagittal, lateral, and vertical dimensions in a predictable manner.

Care must be taken to identify the infraorbital foramen and to contour the implant around this important structure, as well as to avoid extension inside the orbital rim.

The style of implant described is a variation of the many available stock implants in which there is a rounded convex shape so as to create the anterior projection and horizontal inferior portion that blends with the borders of the zygoma and maxilla to provide a smooth malar eminence, the extent of which depends on the degree of augmentation desired. The position of the malar eminence can be determined by using the various methods of facial analysis and the facial moulage. These implants can be subtle or very large. They can extend as maxillo-malar implants if there is a combined maxillary and malar deficiency. These implants are fixed with screws to prevent their movement and to allow precise positioning. A smooth transition with feathered edges enhances the esthetic outcome and also creates a better contour. Custom implants can provide a more subtle augmentation than the available stock implants contour. Malar implants placed in the subcutaneous layer will move with the patient's facial animation as opposed to subperiosteal implants that are fixated with screws, which is a major advantage.

Choice of Implant Material Hardness

Various hardnesses of silicone are available ranging from hard, medium, soft, and extra soft. All custom implants that have been utilized to date have been medium in hardness as it provides a firm yet resilient sensation that is pleasing to the patient as it provides a more natural feeling on palpation. The medium texture implant is also easier to insert around the zygomatic body and arch due to its flexibility. The implant when received from the manufacturer should be checked on the 3-D model to ensure correct fabrication, fit, and screw hole placement. The 3-D model should be thoroughly cleaned of Vaseline prior to the fitting of the implant. The implant is then autoclave sterilized according to the manufacturer's specifications (Table 9.3).

Once placed on the operating table, the implant can be kept in a basin containing normal saline solution.

Special Circumstances

Retreatment of failed malar implants also poses similar problems as there are invariably soft tissue issues [42]. Removal of the implant without replacement can lead to unpleasant scar-

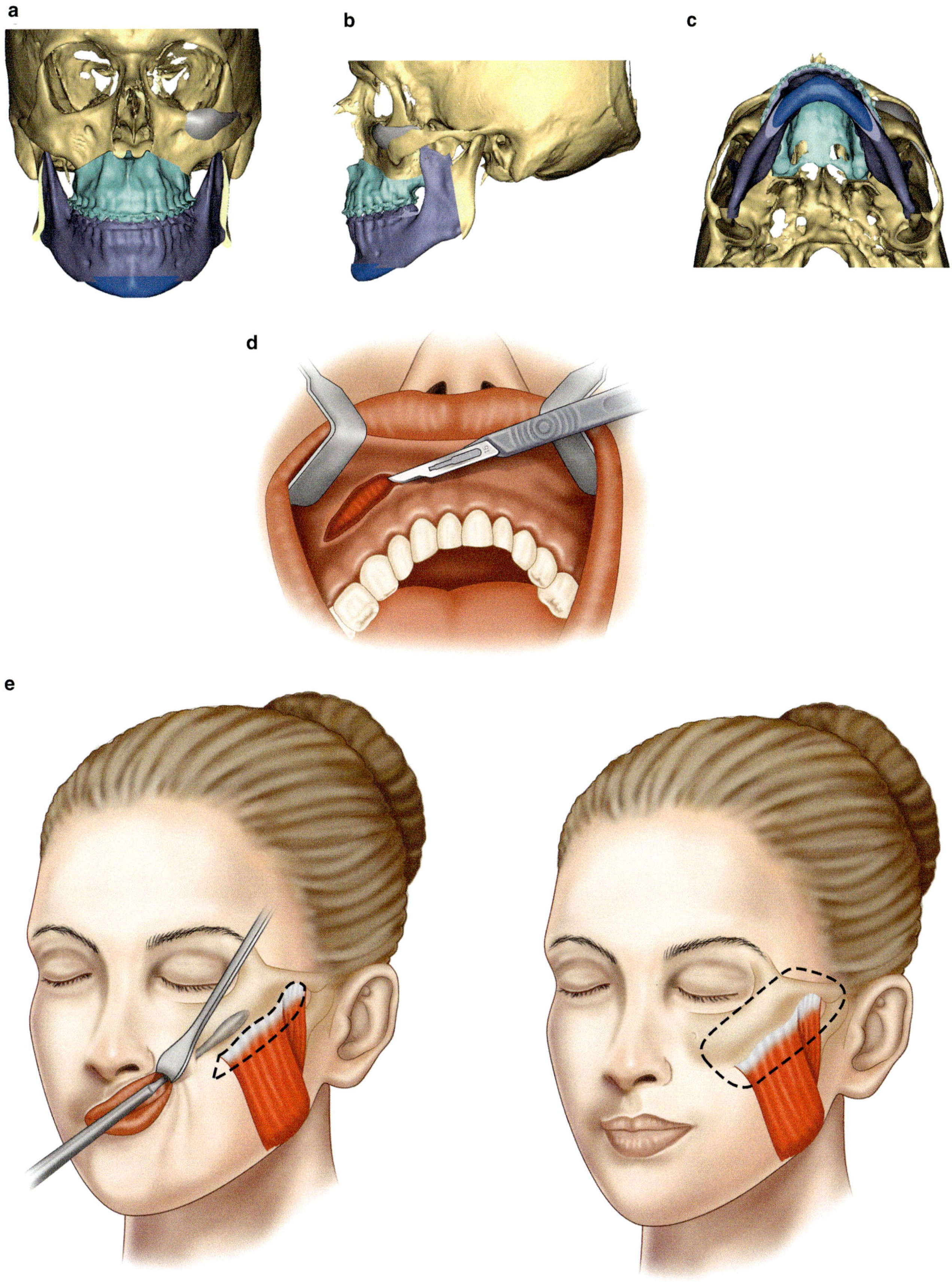

Fig. 9.286 (**a**) 3-D image of planned left malar implant frontal view. (**b**) 3-D image of planned left malar implant lateral view. (**c**) 3-D image of planned left malar implant submenton vertex view. (**d**) Malar region buccal vestibular incision. (**e**) Malar region subperiosteal dissection (Proplan, DuPuy Synthes Craniomaxillofacial, Paoli, PA, USA)

ring and wrinkling of the malar soft tissue with dimpling, atrophy, and ptosis. Custom malar implants fabricated from 3-D models can allow an immediate satisfactory reconstruction without associated soft tissue deformity of a staged approach, which can be necessary in the case of dehiscence and its associated infection. When a malar implant is present, the skull can be delineated from the implant and a model created to allow an anatomically correct custom malar implant to be fabricated. Unlike the placement of malar implant into a subcutaneous supraperiosteal "pocket" without fixation, custom solid silicone malar implants are placed on bone with screw fixation. They will not move unlike the subcutaneous supraperiosteal placed implant which moves on facial animation. Late facial atrophy from aging or HIV-related facial wasting can cause "outlining" of the implants which can require their removal and retreatment with fat transplantation or fillers.

Surgical Technique

These procedures can be performed both in the hospital and office settings under full general anesthesia or moderate sedation. The malar eminence can be marked on the skin preoperatively, but with custom implants, it is usually not necessary. Following infiltration with local anesthetic via intraoral and transcutaneous approaches, a posterior maxillary buccal incision preferably using a #15 scalpel blade created superior to the mucogingival junction is performed (Fig. 9.286d), so as to create a full-thickness mucoperiosteal flap that provides maximal coverage of the implant. The incision should be at a 90 degree angle through mucosa, submucosa, and perimandibular musculature. Utilizing a freer or #9 periosteal elevator, a full-thickness mucoperiosteal flap is reflected (Fig. 9.286e). The infraorbital nerve should be identified and preserved throughout the procedure. The implant can then be inserted and palpated externally for positioning. Because of the anatomic fit of the implant, they are usually easily positioned after which transoral screw fixation through the preplanned holes is achieved. It is preferable to place the screws into the thicker bone of the zygomatic body or zygomatic buttress.

Case Reports

Case 10

A 27-year-old female patient presented with a severe Class III skeletal malocclusion with mandibular asymmetry and prognathism and left malar hypoplasia. Following presurgical orthodontics, a LeFort I two-piece segmental osteotomy, bilateral mandibular vertical ramus osteotomies, anterior horizontal mandibular osteotomy, and placement of a left malar custom solid silicone implant were performed (Figs. 9.287–9.315).

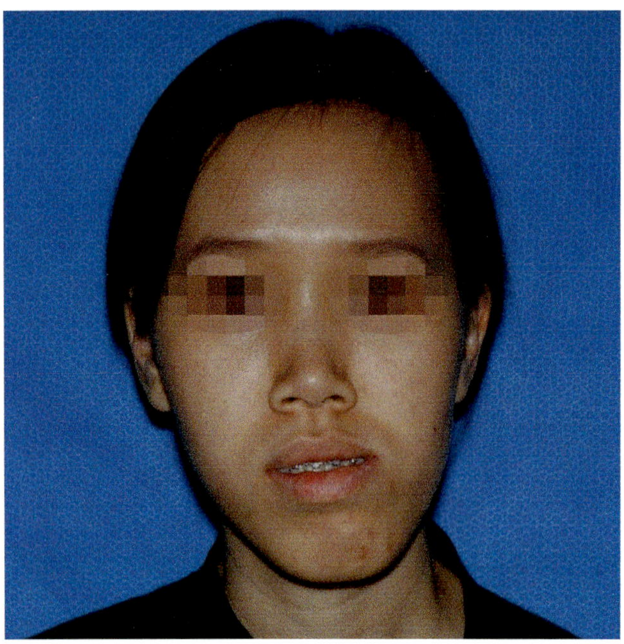

Fig. 9.287 Preoperative frontal facial view of mandibular prognathism Class III skeletal malocclusion with left malar hypoplasia and mandibular prognathism with deviation to the left

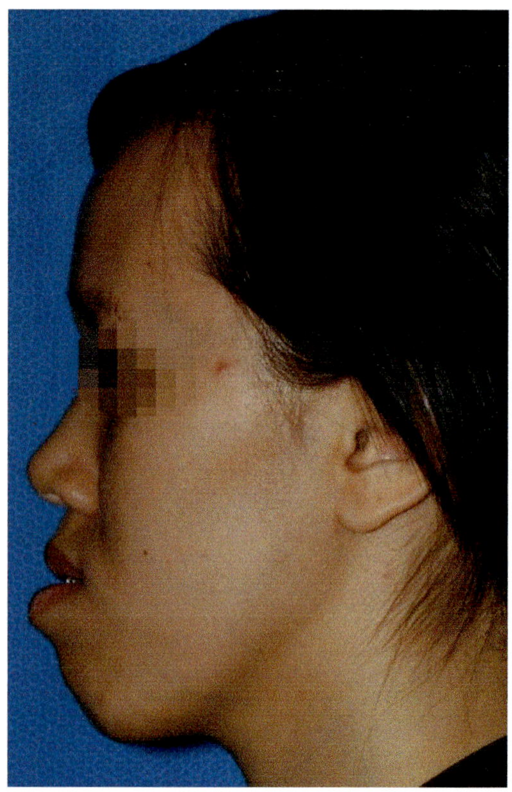

Fig. 9.288 Preoperative left lateral facial view of mandibular prognathism Class III skeletal malocclusion with left malar hypoplasia

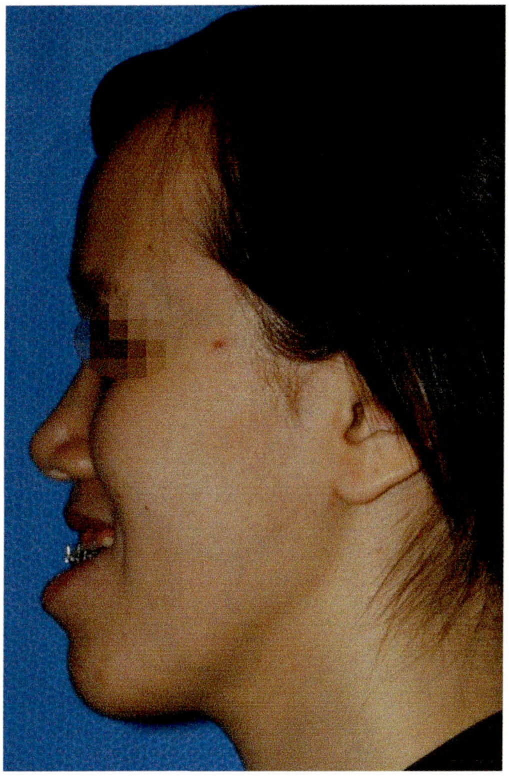

Fig. 9.289 Preoperative left lateral facial view of mandibular prognathism Class III skeletal malocclusion with left malar hypoplasia with smile

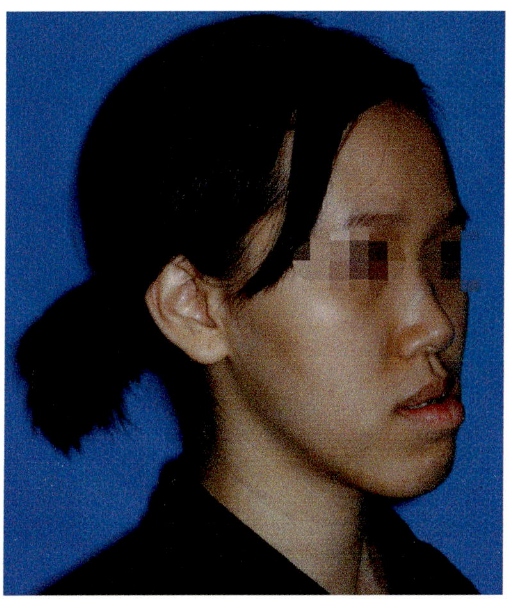

Fig. 9.290 Preoperative right 3/4 facial view of mandibular prognathism Class III skeletal malocclusion with left malar hypoplasia

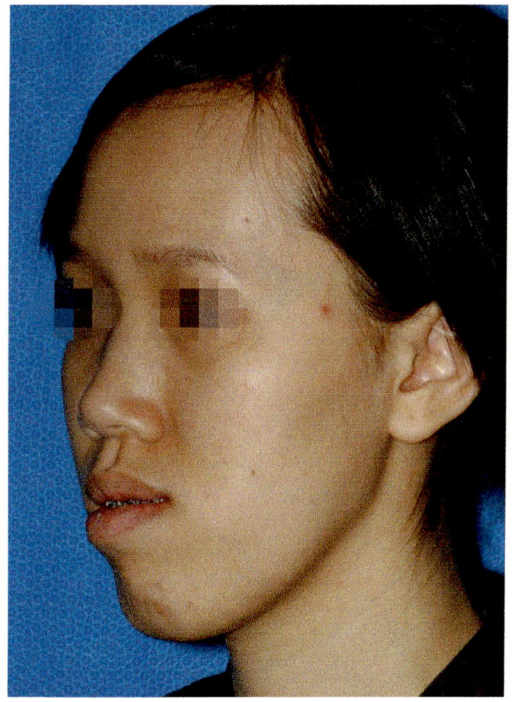

Fig. 9.291 Preoperative left 3/4 view of mandibular prognathism Class III skeletal malocclusion with left malar hypoplasia

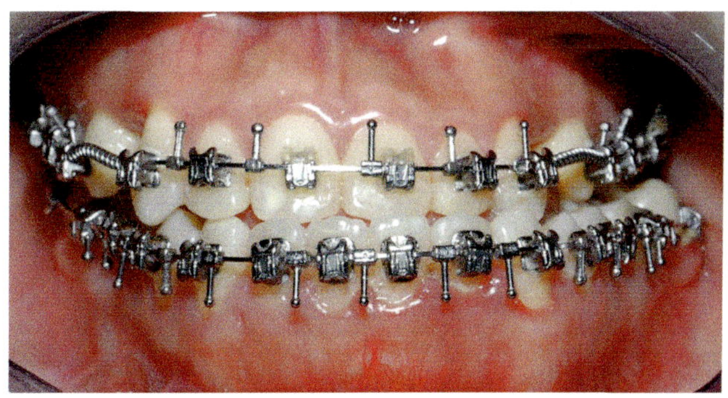

Fig. 9.292 Preoperative frontal occlusal view

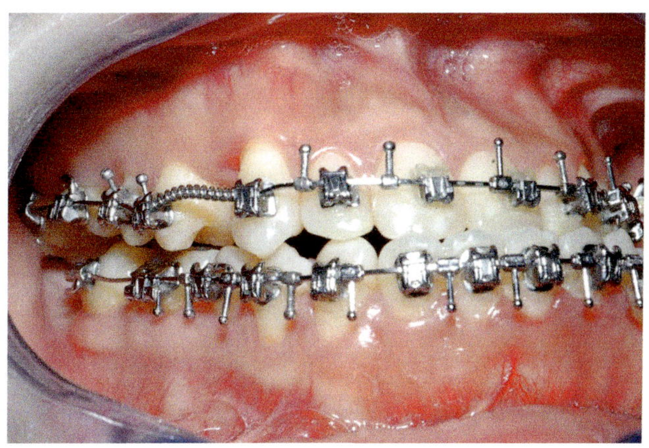

Fig. 9.293 Preoperative right lateral occlusal view

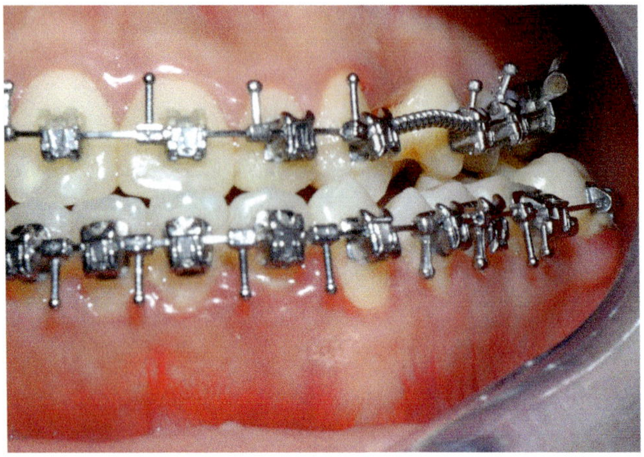

Fig. 9.294 Preoperative left lateral occlusal view

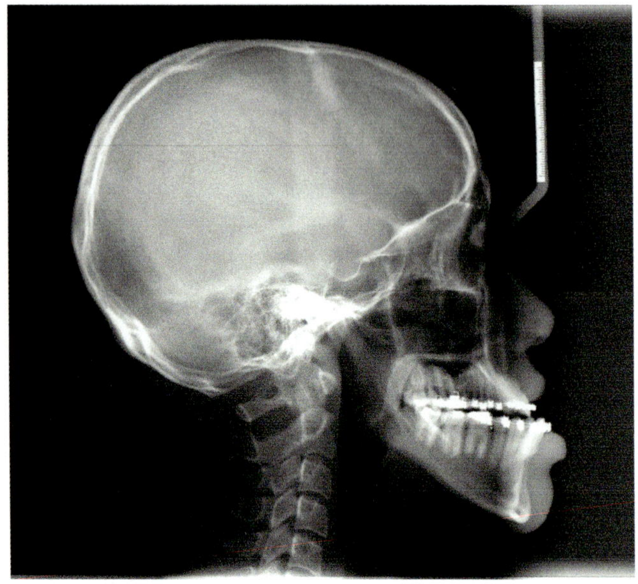

Fig. 9.295 Preoperative lateral cephalometric radiograph

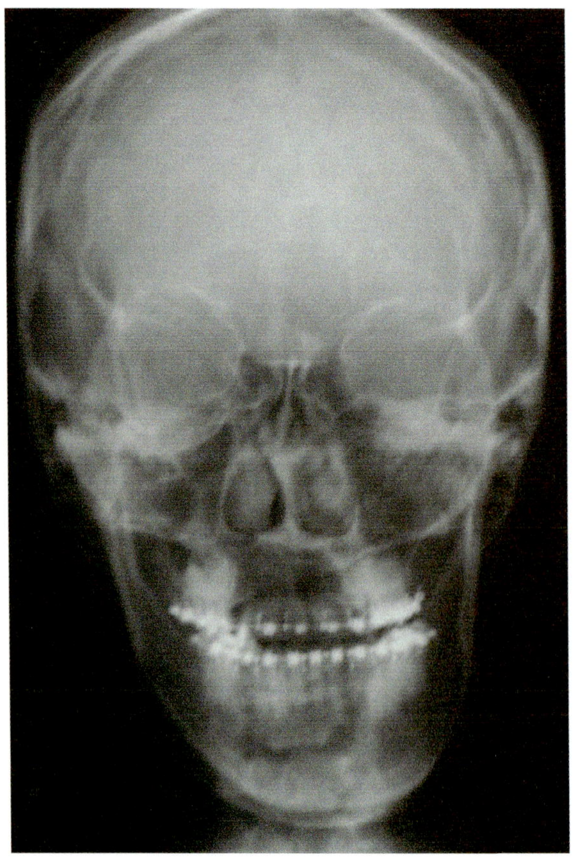

Fig. 9.296 Preoperative posterior anterior cephalometric radiograph

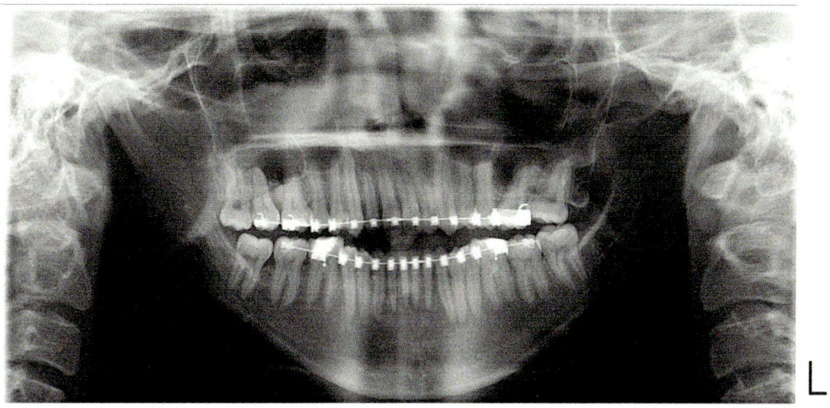

Fig. 9.297 Preoperative panoramic radiograph

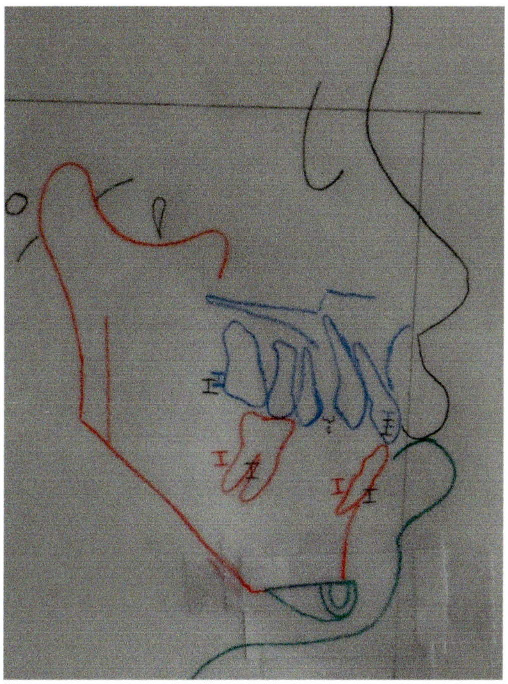

Fig. 9.298 Lateral cephalometric radiograph prediction tracing

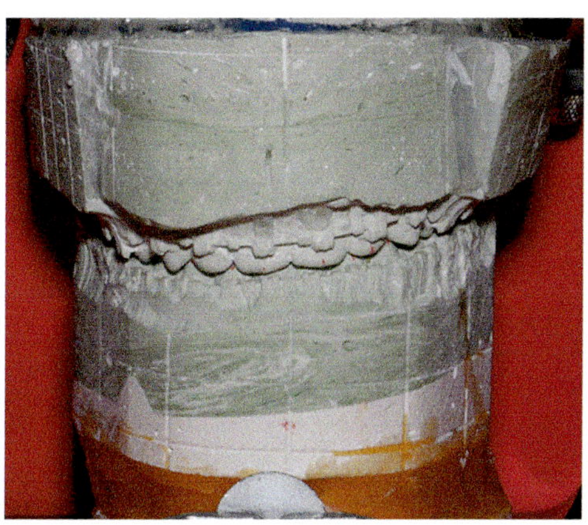

Fig. 9.299 Frontal view of model surgery

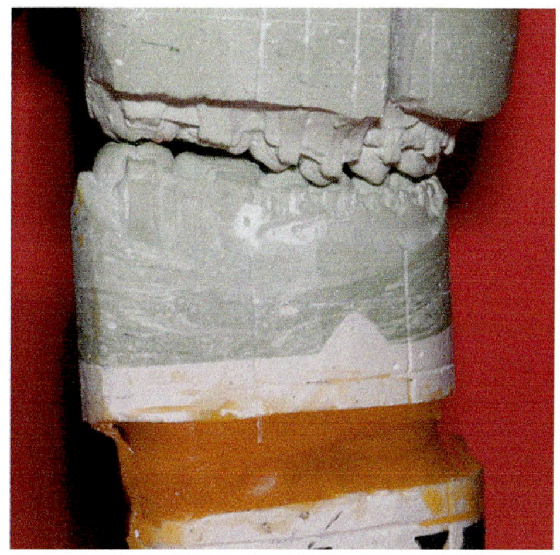

Fig. 9.300 Right lateral view of model surgery

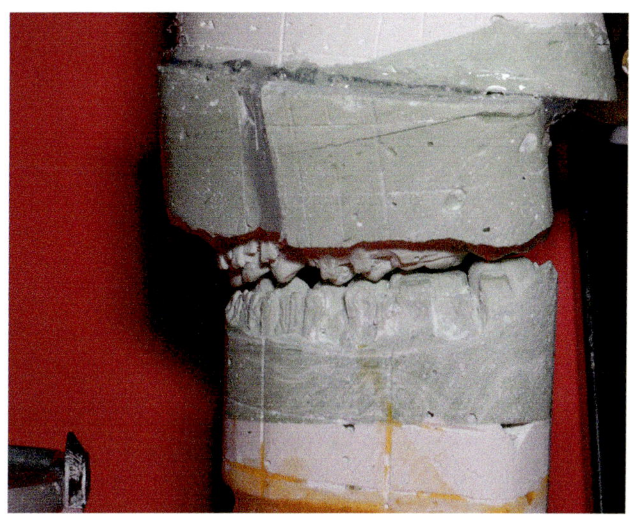

Fig. 9.301 Left lateral view of model surgery

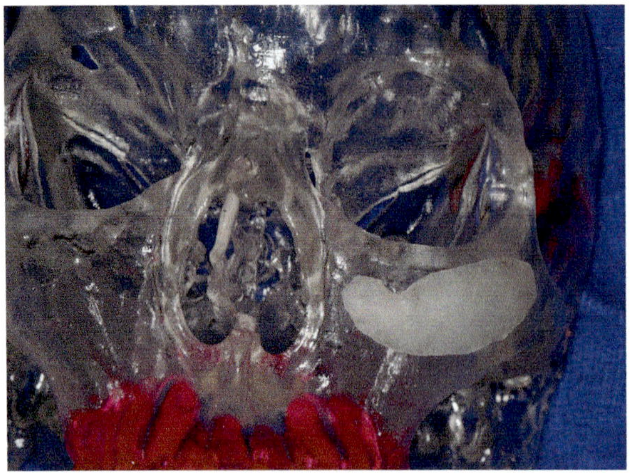

Fig. 9.302 Left malar custom implant wax prototype fitted to 3-D model frontal view. Note: Implant trimmed to avoid the infraorbital nerve

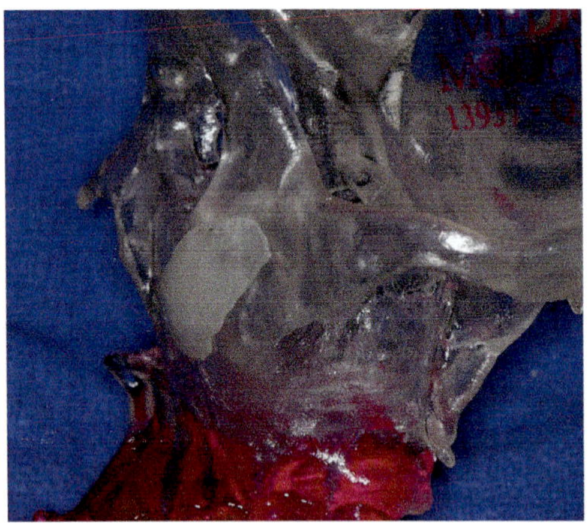

Fig. 9.303 Left malar custom implant wax prototype fitted to 3-D model left lateral view

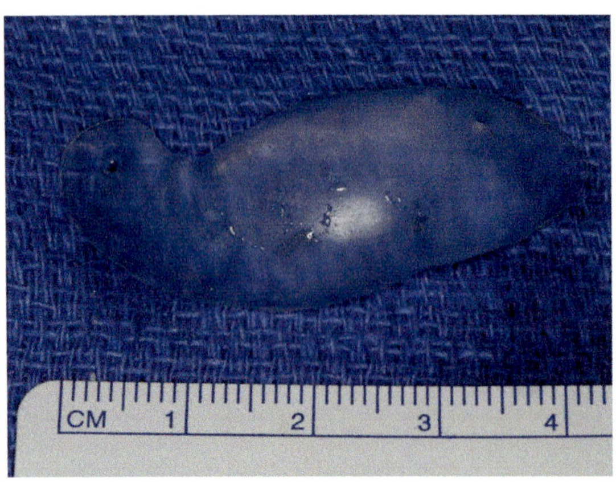

Fig. 9.304 Left malar custom solid silicone implant. Note screw holes at medial and lateral aspects

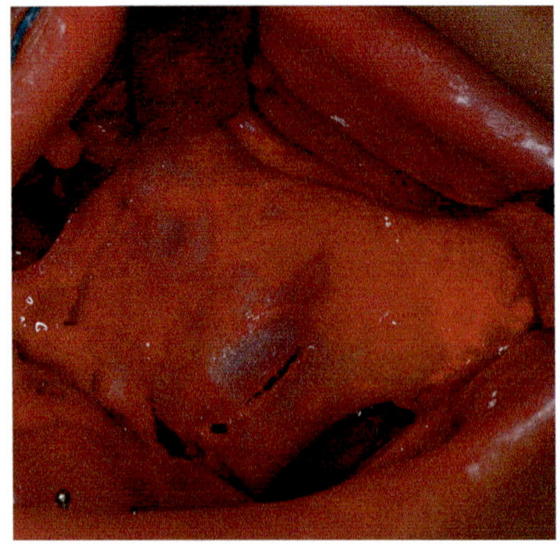

Fig. 9.305 Intraoperative view of buccal vestibular incision with exposure of the left malar region prior to LeFort I osteotomy

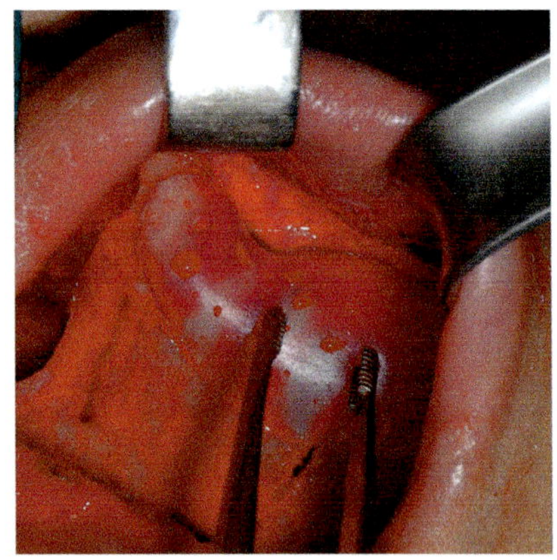

Fig. 9.306 Intraoperative view of the left malar custom solid silicone implant placement prior to LeFort I osteotomy

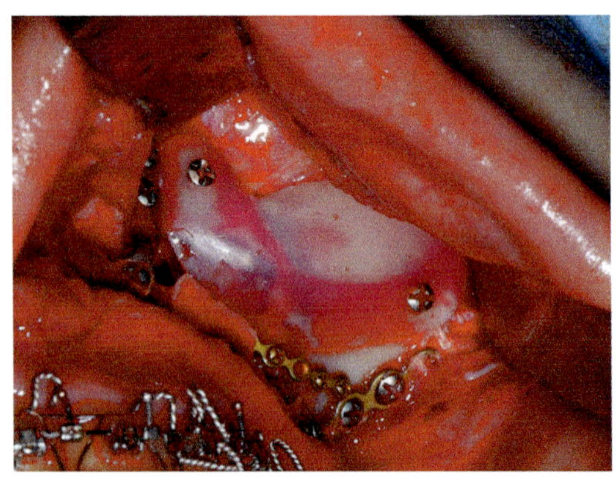

Fig. 9.307 Intraoperative view of left malar custom solid silicone implant with screw fixation following LeFort I osteotomy

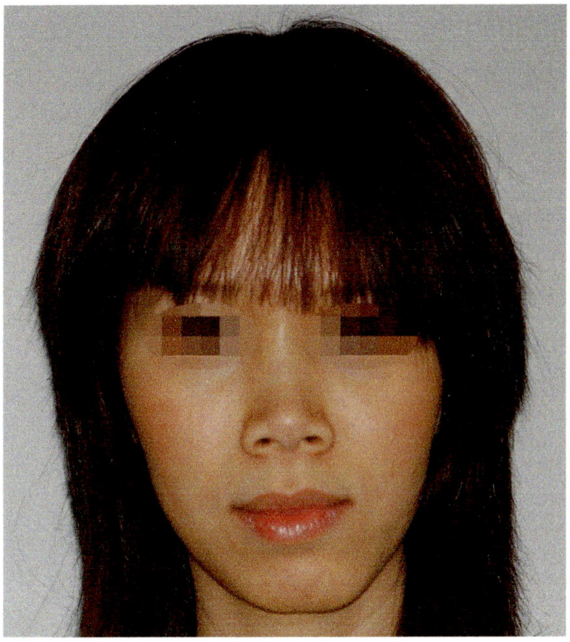

Fig. 9.308 Postoperative frontal facial view

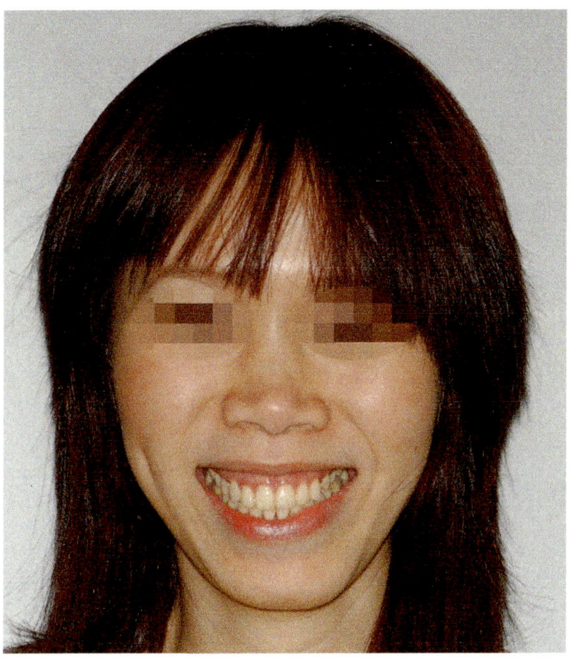

Fig. 9.309 Postoperative frontal facial view with a smile

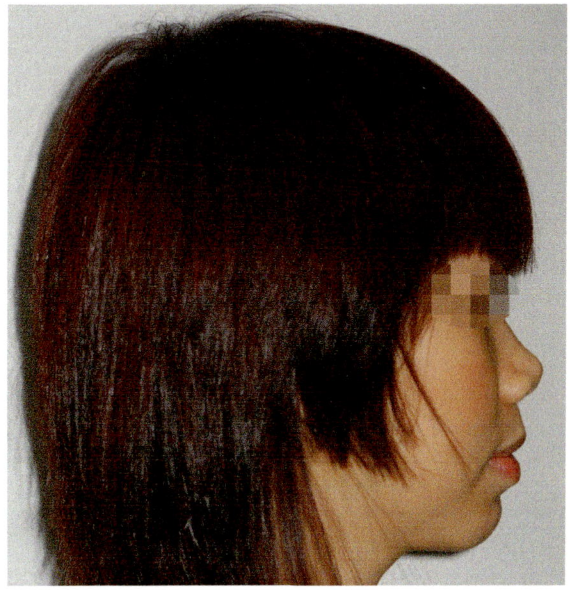

Fig. 9.310 Postoperative right lateral facial view

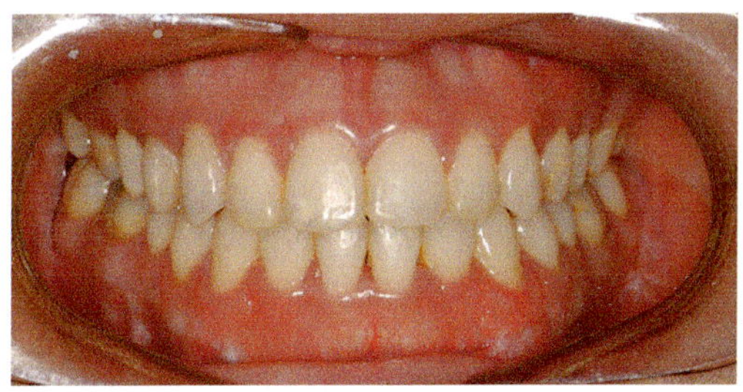

Fig. 9.311 Postoperative frontal occlusal view

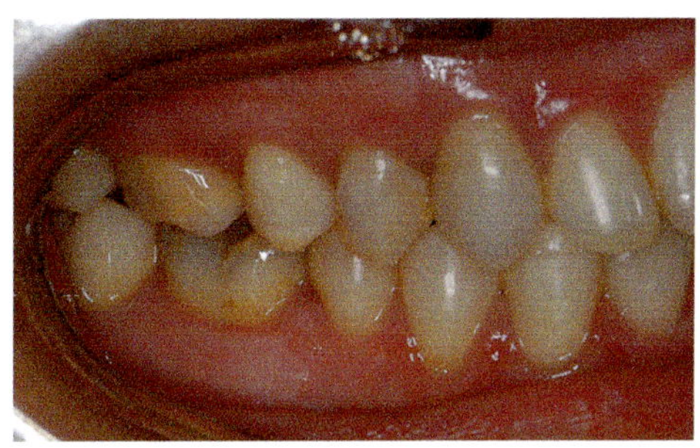

Fig. 9.312 Postoperative right lateral occlusal view

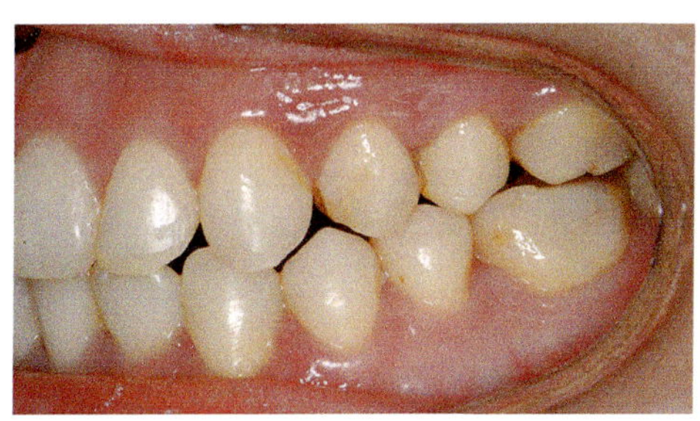

Fig. 9.313 Postoperative left lateral occlusal view

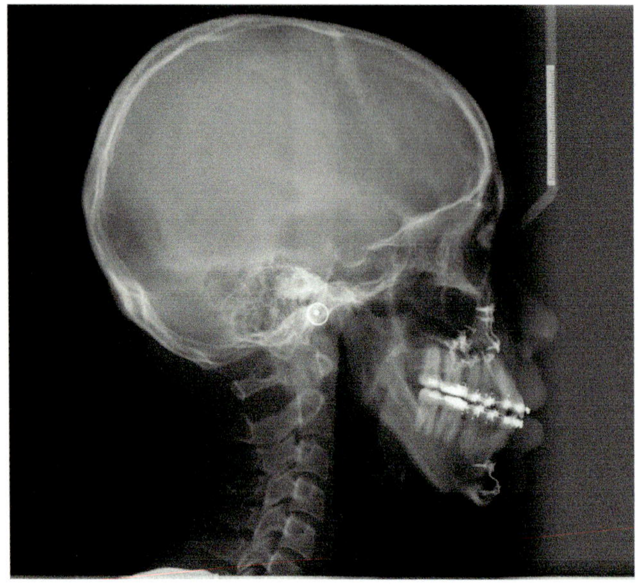

Fig. 9.314 Postoperative lateral cephalometric radiograph

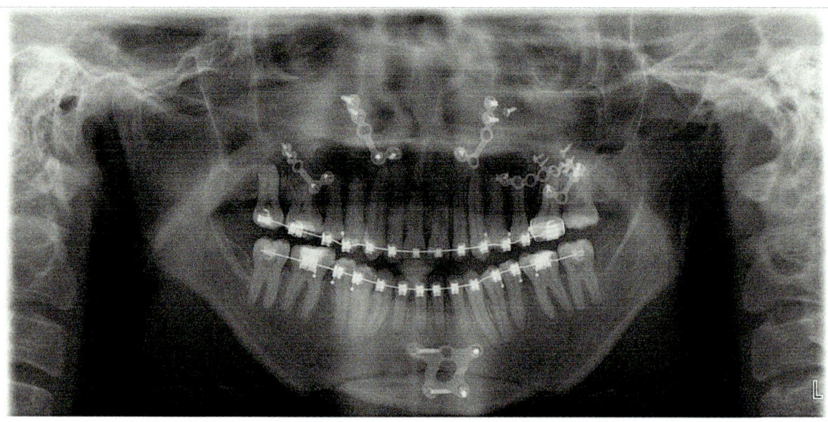

Fig. 9.315 Postoperative panoramic radiograph

Case 11

A 24-year-old female patient presented following previous right mandibular ramus sagittal split osteotomy for TMJ treatment with persistent mandibular asymmetry with deviation to the left and left malar hypoplasia. Following presurgical orthodontics, a LeFort I two-piece segmental osteotomy, bilateral mandibular vertical ramus osteotomies, anterior horizontal mandibular osteotomy, and placement of a left malar custom solid silicone implant were performed (Figs. 9.316–9.349). (Alex M. Greenberg, DDS, Oral and Maxillofacial Surgeon, New York, NY, USA).

Case 12

A 44-year-old male patient presented with a severe Class III skeletal malocclusion with mandibular asymmetry and prognathism and bilateral malar hypoplasia secondary to acromegalism. The patient had undergone trans-nasal hypophysectomy and was on hormone replacement.

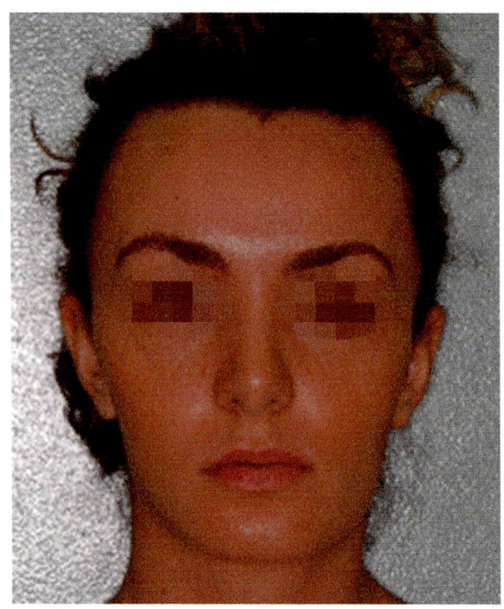

Fig. 9.316 Preoperative frontal facial view with mandibular deviation to the left and left malar hypoplasia following previous right mandibular sagittal split ramus osteotomy

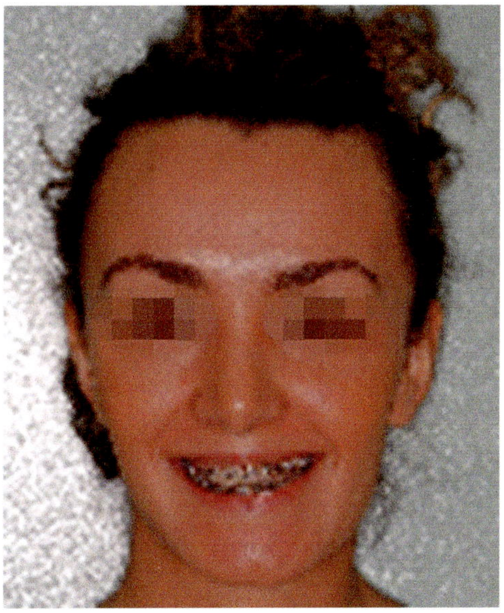

Fig. 9.317 Preoperative frontal facial view with mandibular deviation to the left and left malar hypoplasia with smile

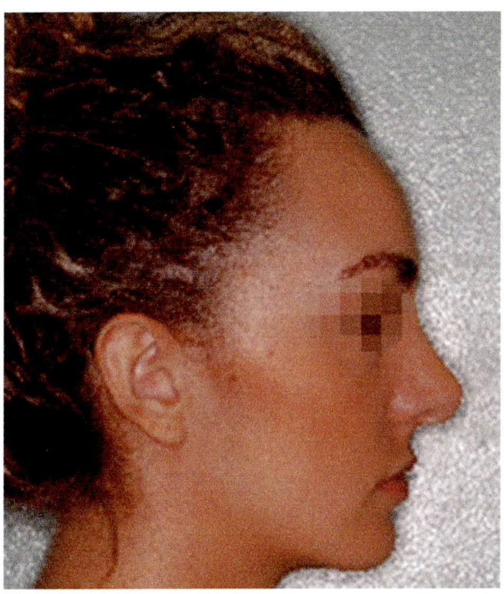

Fig. 9.318 Preoperative right lateral facial view with mandibular deviation to the left and left malar hypoplasia

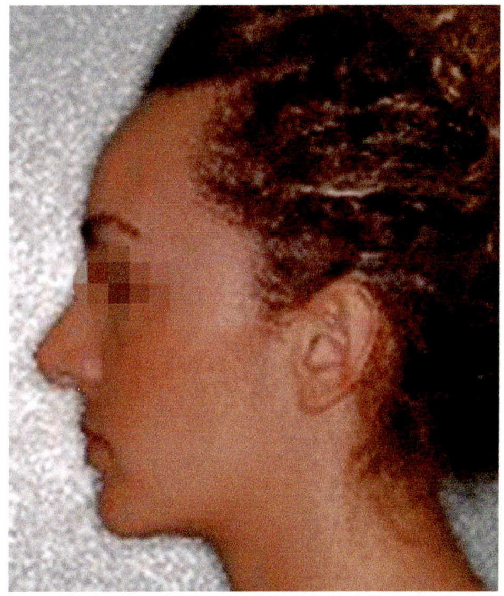

Fig. 9.319 Preoperative left lateral facial view with mandibular deviation to the left and left malar hypoplasia

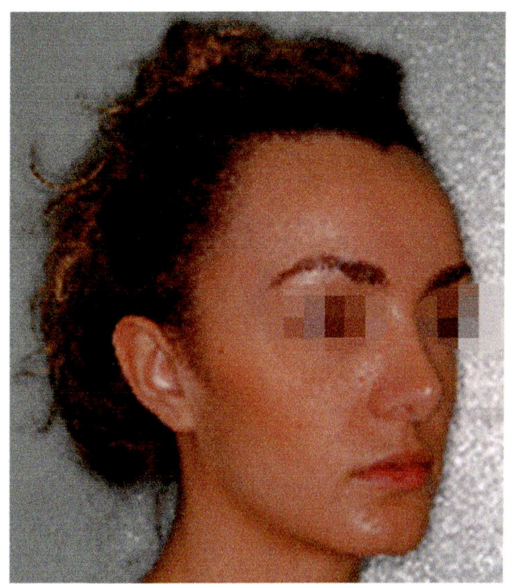

Fig. 9.320 Preoperative right 3/4 facial view with mandibular deviation to the left and left malar hypoplasia

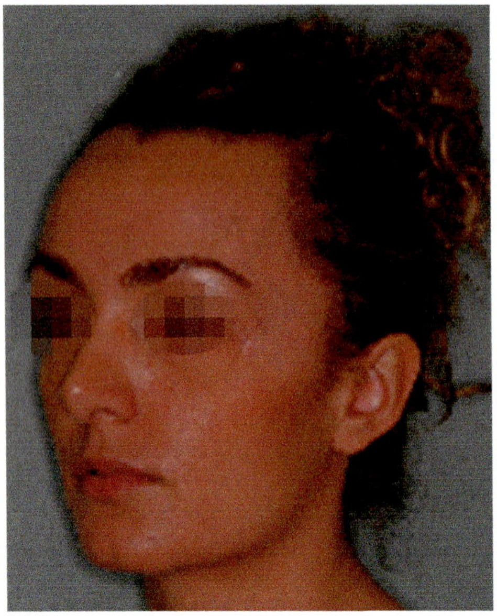

Fig. 9.321 Preoperative left 3/4 facial view with mandibular deviation to the left and left malar hypoplasia

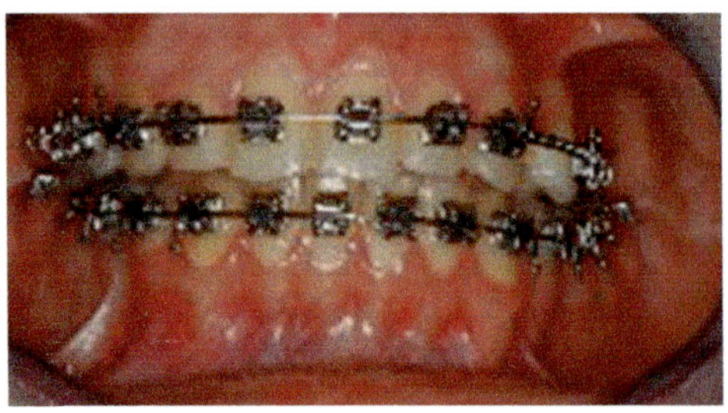

Fig. 9.322 Preoperative frontal occlusal view with Class I occlusion and mandibular deviation to the left

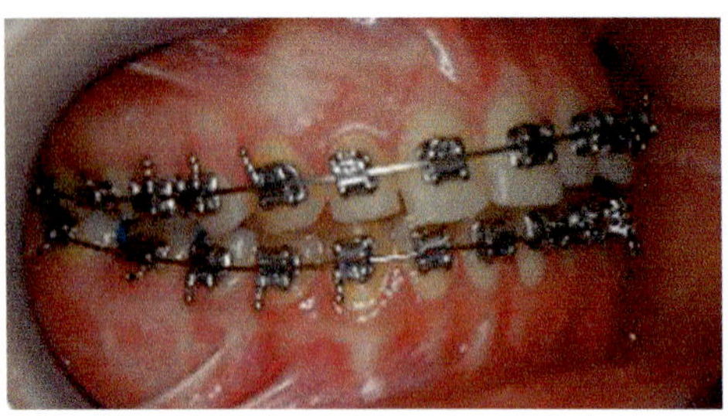

Fig. 9.323 Right lateral occlusal view with Class I occlusion and mandibular deviation to the left

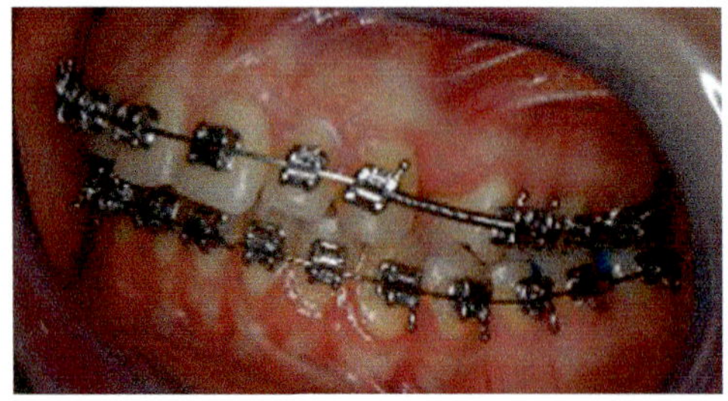

Fig. 9.324 Left lateral occlusal view with Class I occlusion and mandibular deviation to the left

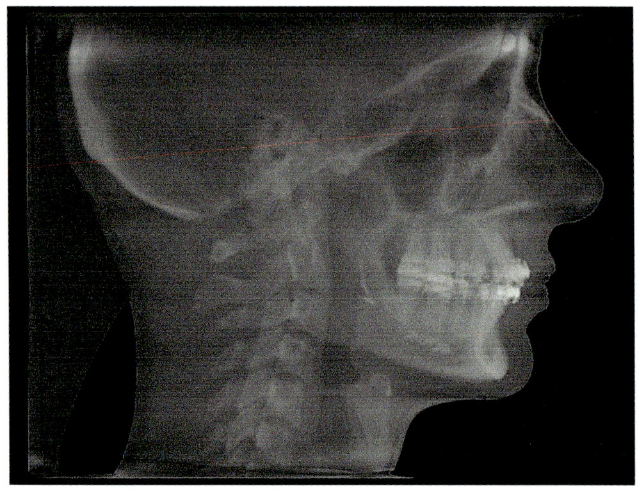

Fig. 9.325 Preoperative lateral cephalometric radiograph

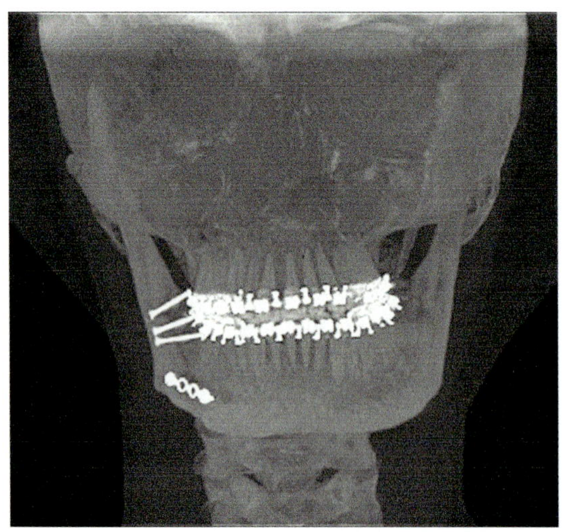

Fig. 9.326 Preoperative posterior-anterior cephalometric radiograph

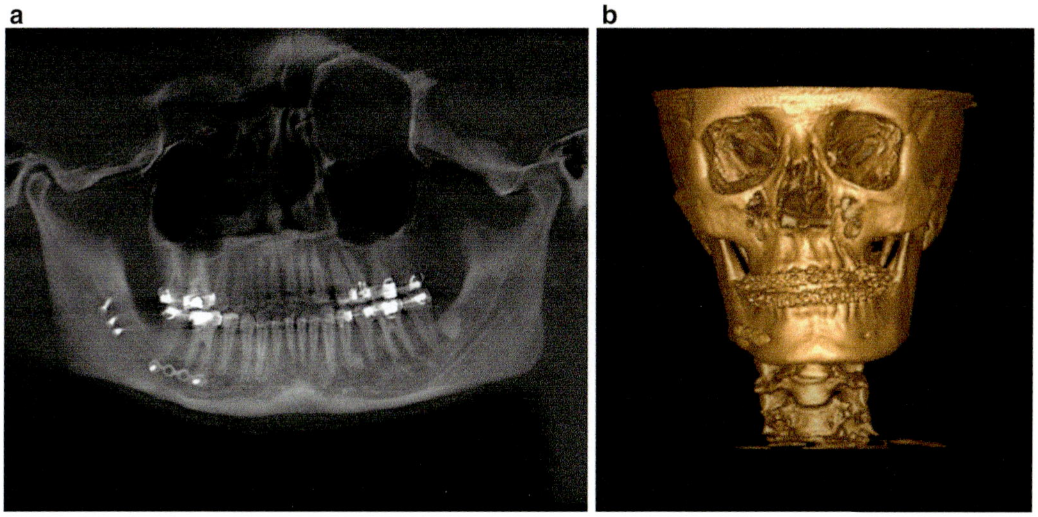

Fig. 9.327 A. Preoperative panoramic radiograph. B. Preoperative frontal 3-D CBCT image with left malar hypoplastic defect

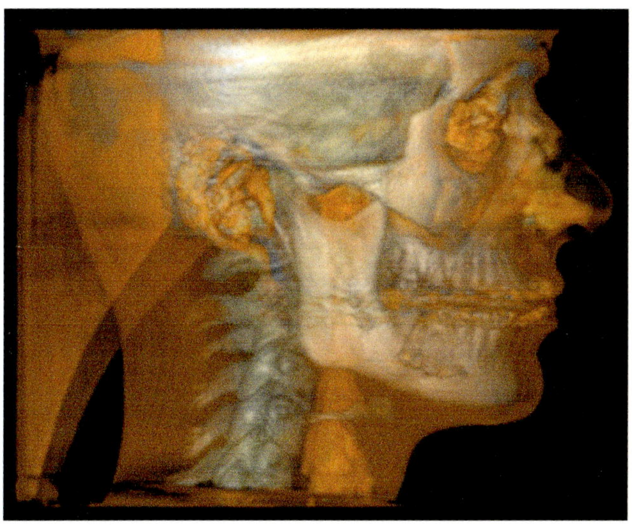

Fig. 9.328 Preoperative right lateral 3-D CBCT bone and soft tissue image

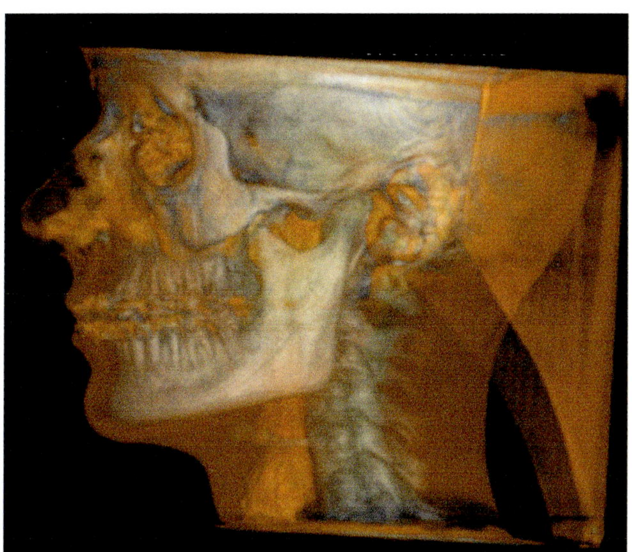

Fig. 9.329 Preoperative left lateral 3-D CBCT bone and soft tissue image with left malar hypoplastic defect

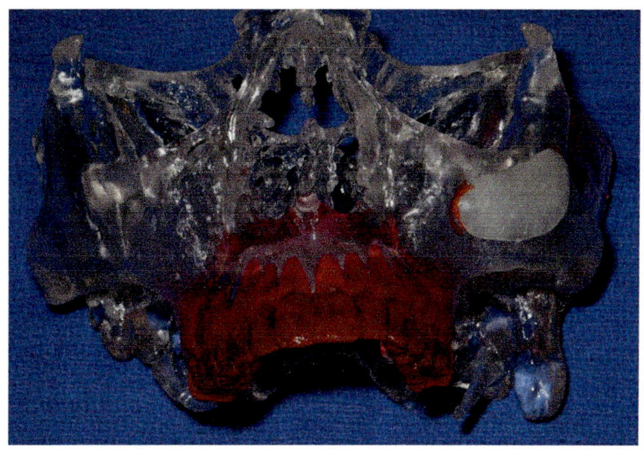

Fig. 9.330 Left malar custom implant wax prototype fitted to 3-D model frontal view

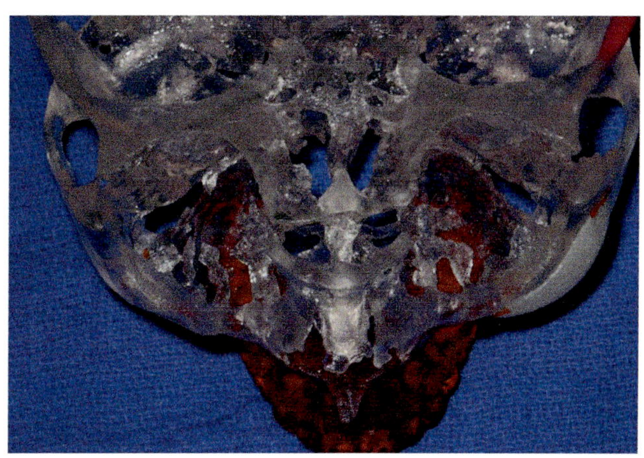

Fig. 9.331 Left malar custom implant wax prototype fitted to 3-D model superior view

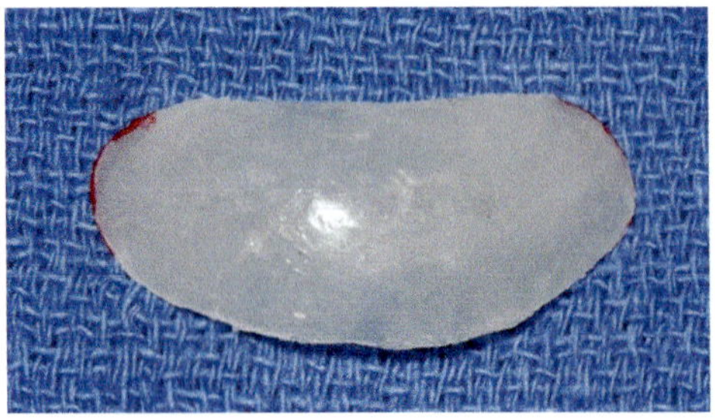

Fig. 9.332 Left malar custom implant wax prototype frontal view

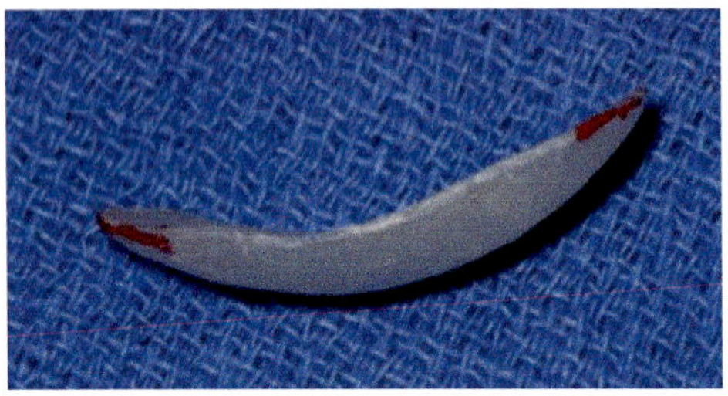

Fig. 9.333 Left malar custom implant wax prototype superior view

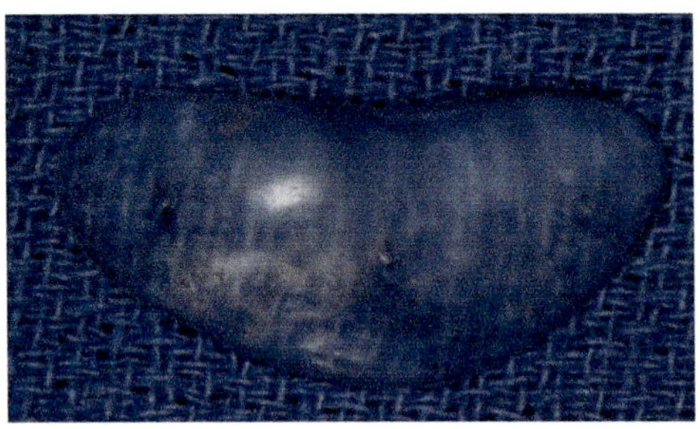

Fig. 9.334 Left malar custom solid silicone implant frontal view. Note: screw holes for fixation

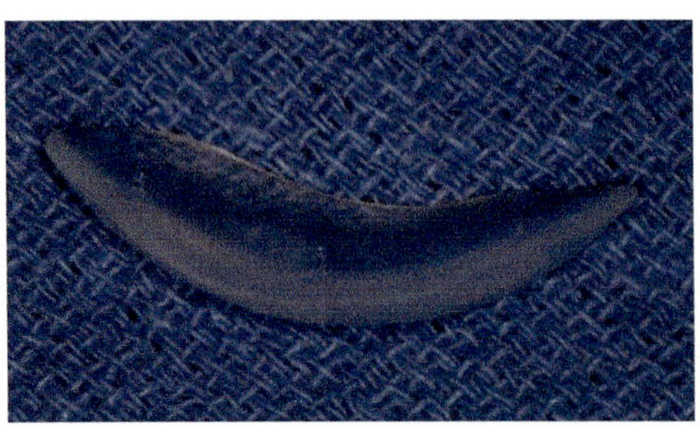

Fig. 9.335 Left malar custom solid silicone implant superior view

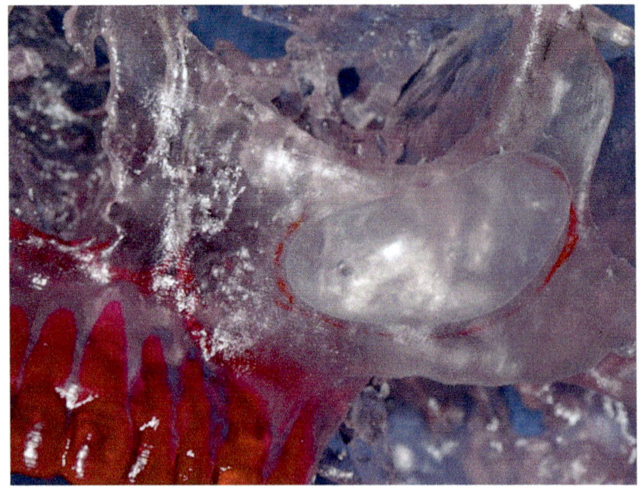

Fig. 9.336 Left malar custom solid silicone implant fitted to 3-D model frontal view

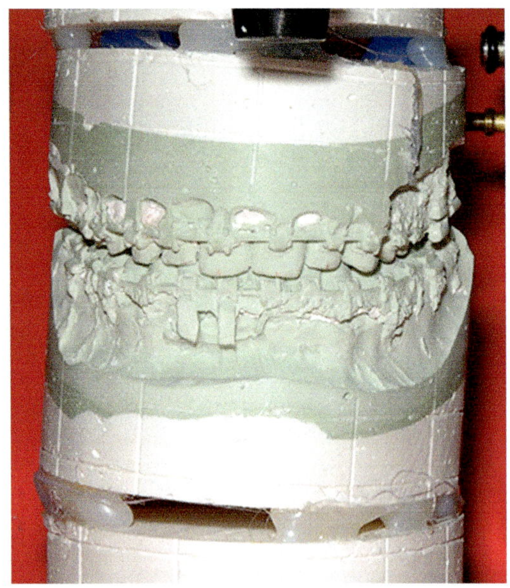

Fig. 9.337 Model surgery frontal view

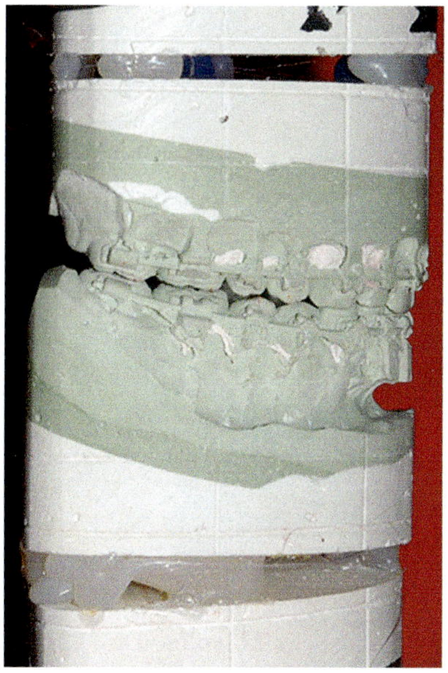

Fig. 9.338 Model surgery right lateral view

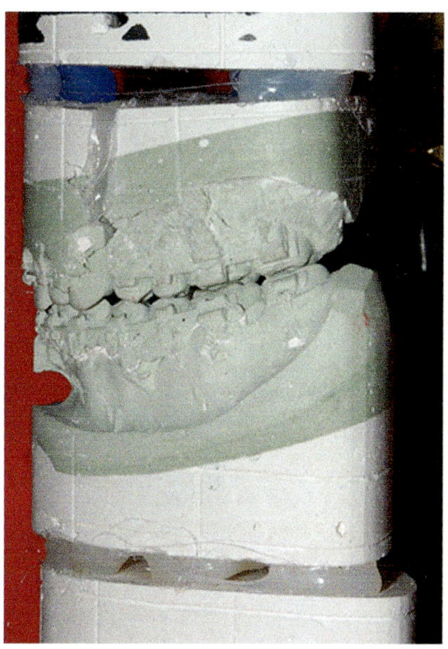

Fig. 9.339 Model surgery left lateral view

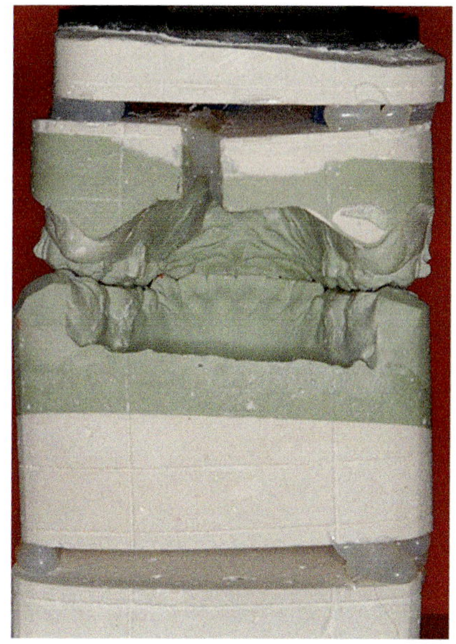

Fig. 9.340 Model surgery lingual view

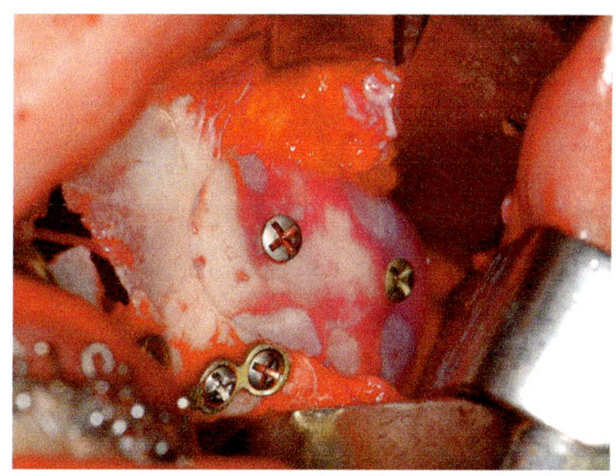

Fig. 9.341 Intraoperative view of left malar custom solid silicone implant placement with screw fixation (DuPuy Synthes Craniomaxillofacial, Paoli, PA, USA)

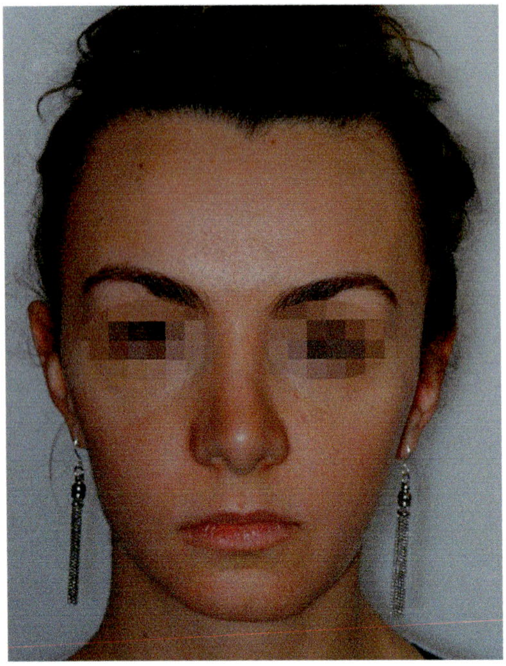

Fig. 9.342 Postoperative frontal facial view with placement of left malar custom solid silicone implant, LeFort I two-piece segmental osteotomy and bilateral mandibular vertical ramus osteotomies with bilateral symmetry and restoration of mandibular midline to facial midline

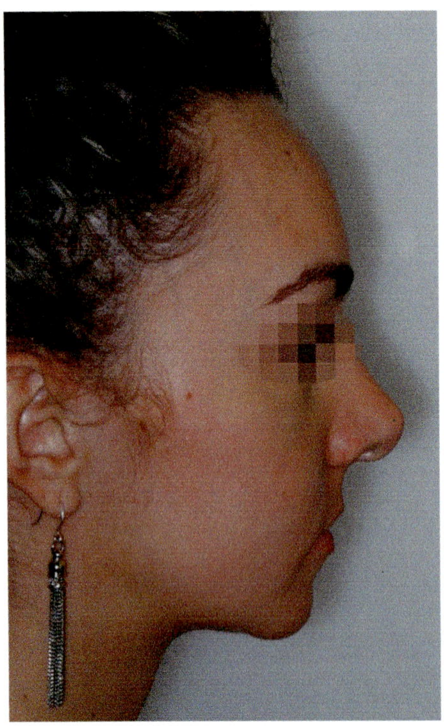

Fig. 9.343 Postoperative right lateral facial view

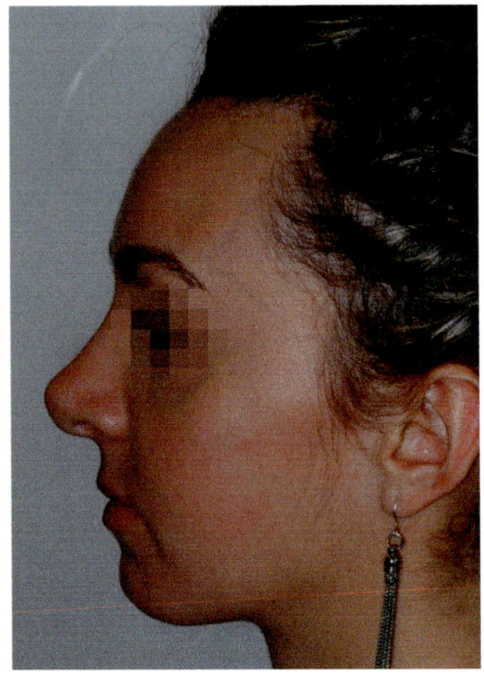

Fig. 9.344 Postoperative left lateral facial view

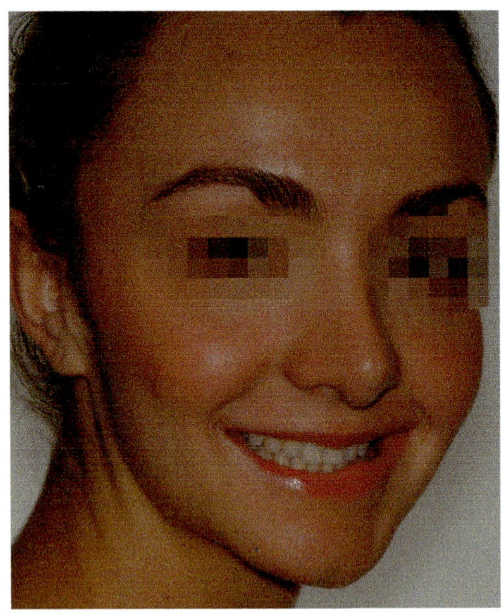

Fig. 9.345 Postoperative right 3/4 facial view

Following rapid palate expansion and presurgical orthodontics, bilateral mandibular vertical ramus osteotomies, anterior horizontal mandibular osteotomy, and placement of bilateral maxillo-malar custom solid silicone implants were performed (Figs. 9.350–9.387). (Alex M. Greenberg, DDS, Oral and Maxillofacial Surgeon, New York, NY, USA).

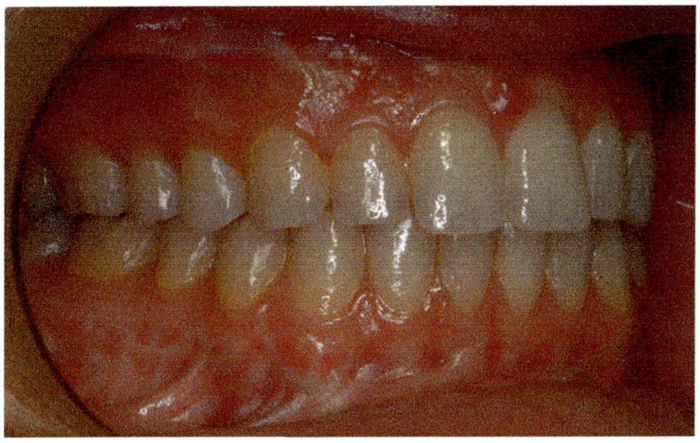

Fig. 9.346 Postoperative right lateral occlusal view

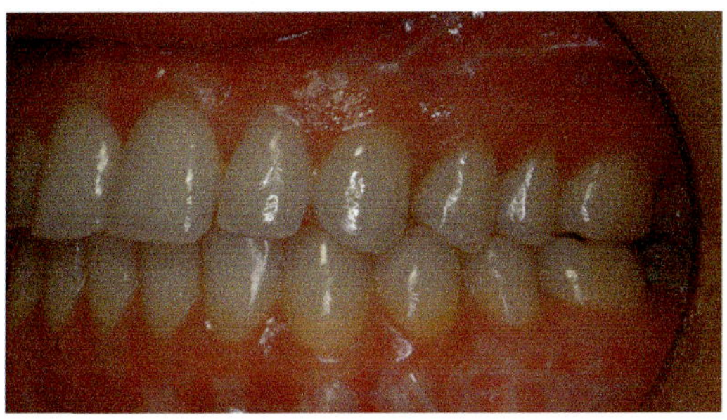

Fig. 9.347 Postoperative left lateral occlusal view

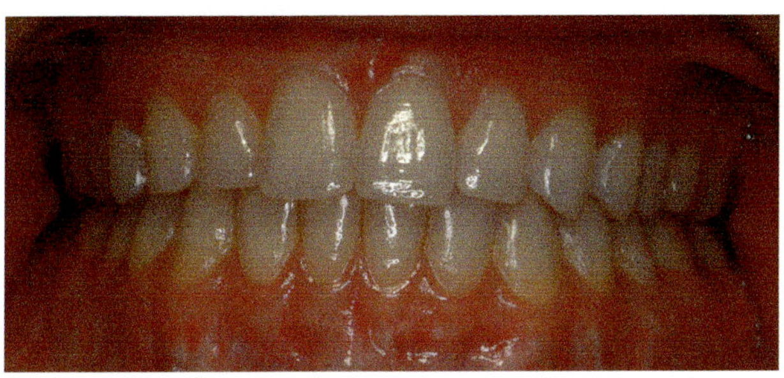

Fig. 9.348 Postoperative frontal occlusal view

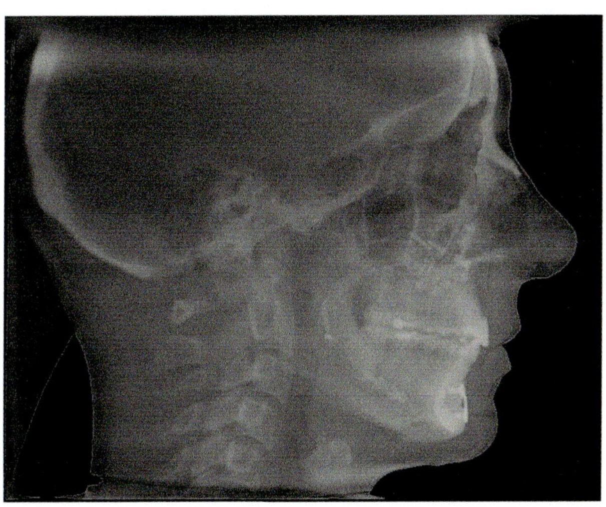

Fig. 9.349 Postoperative lateral cephalometric radiograph

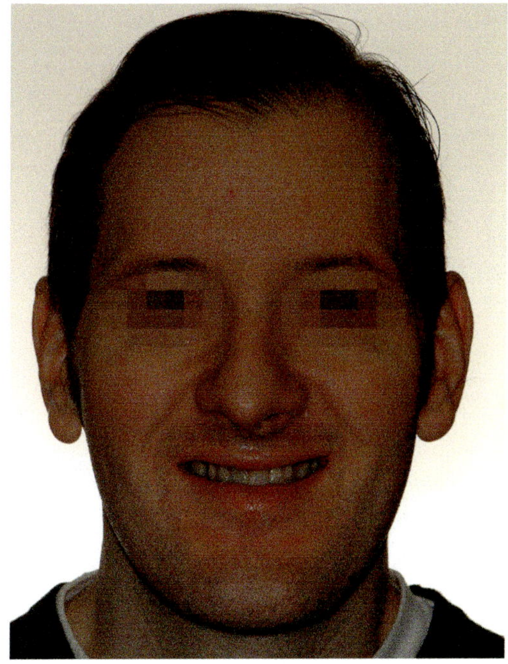

Fig. 9.350 Preoperative facial view of severe Class III skeletal malocclusion secondary to acromegalism and midfacial hypoplasia

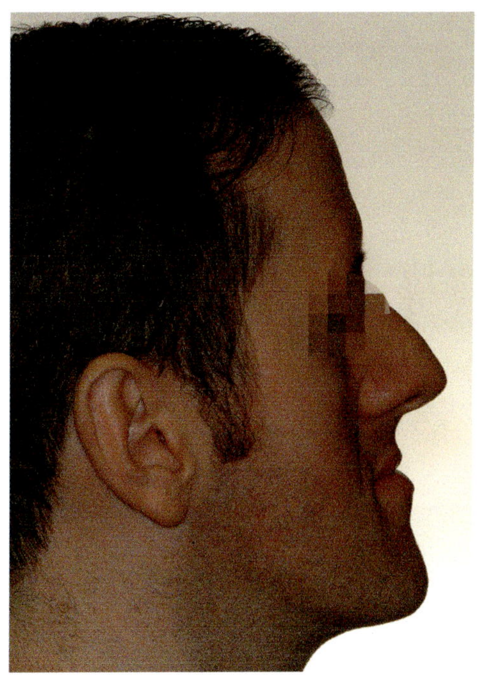

Fig. 9.351 Preoperative right lateral facial view of severe Class III skeletal malocclusion secondary to acromegalism and midfacial hypoplasia

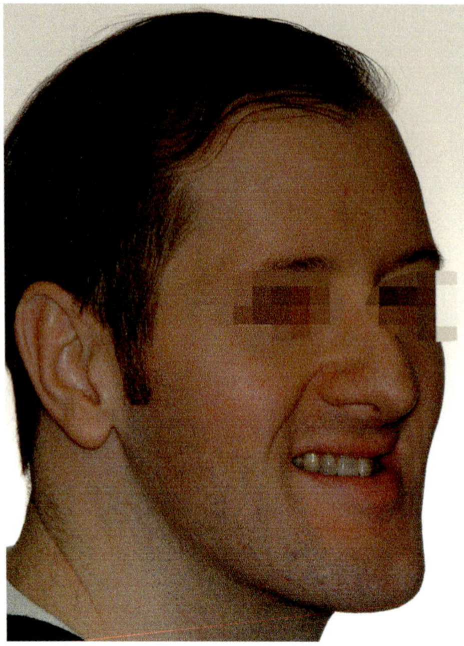

Fig. 9.352 Preoperative right 3/4 facial view of severe Class III skeletal malocclusion secondary to acromegalism and midfacial hypoplasia

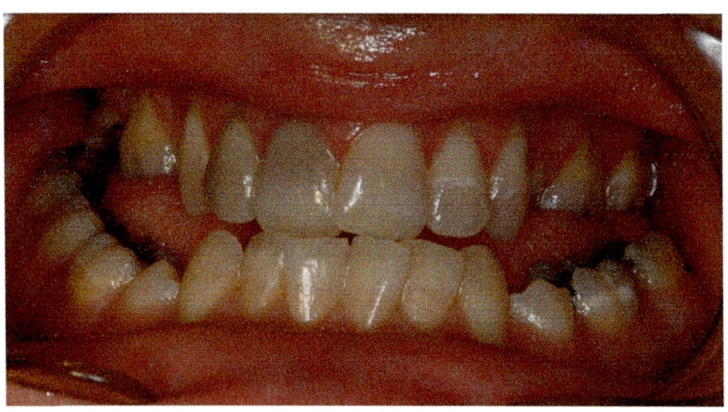

Fig. 9.353 Preoperative frontal occlusal view with Class III malocclusion and mandibular prognathism

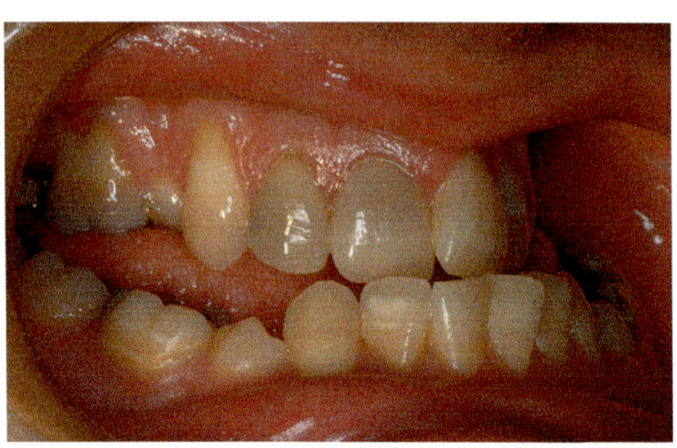

Fig. 9.354 Preoperative right lateral occlusal view with Class III malocclusion and mandibular prognathism

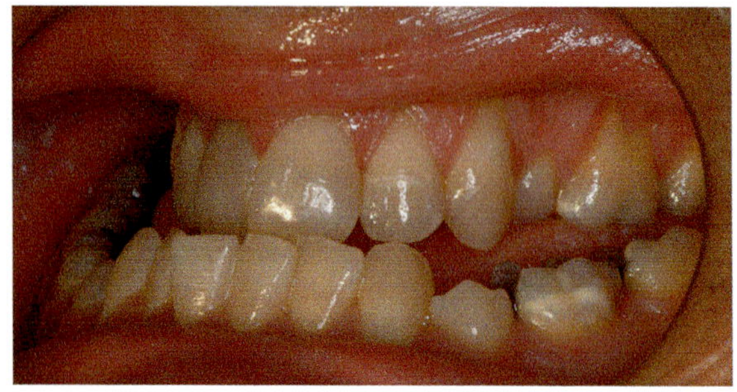

Fig. 9.355 Preoperative left lateral occlusal view with Class III malocclusion and mandibular prognathism

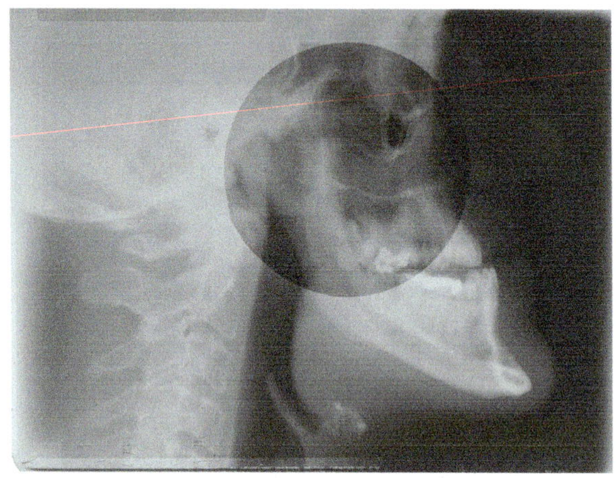

Fig. 9.356 Preoperative lateral cephalometric radiograph

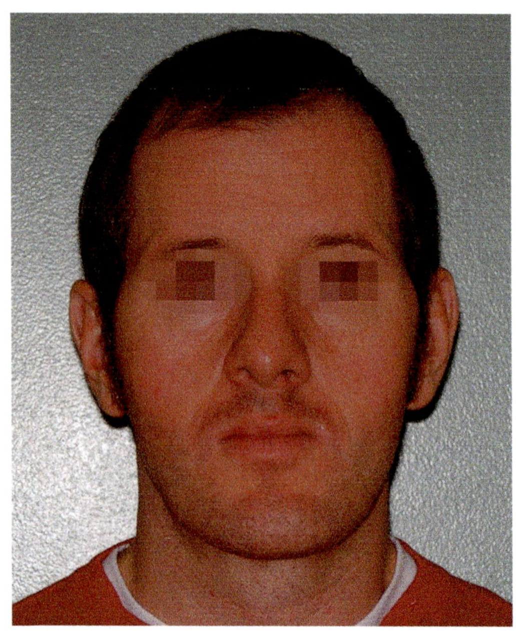

Fig. 9.357 Preoperative post orthodontic frontal facial view of severe Class III skeletal malocclusion secondary to acromegalism and midfacial hypoplasia

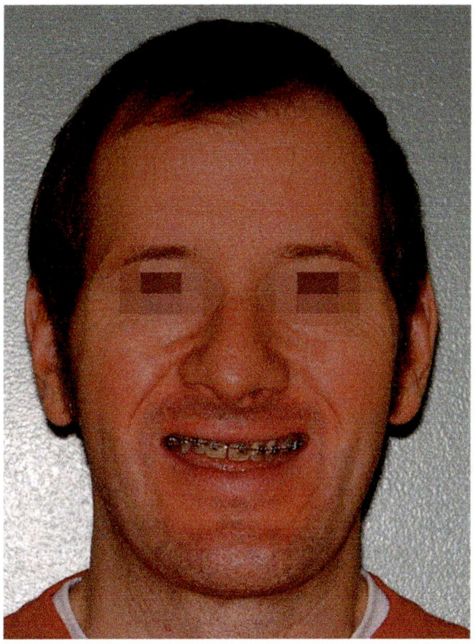

Fig. 9.358 Preoperative post orthodontic frontal facial view of severe Class III skeletal malocclusion secondary to acromegalism and midfacial hypoplasia with smile

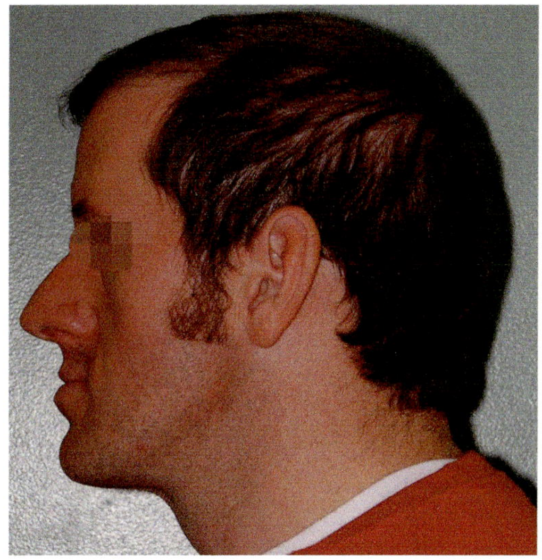

Fig. 9.360 Preoperative post orthodontic left lateral facial view of severe Class III skeletal malocclusion secondary to acromegalism and midfacial hypoplasia

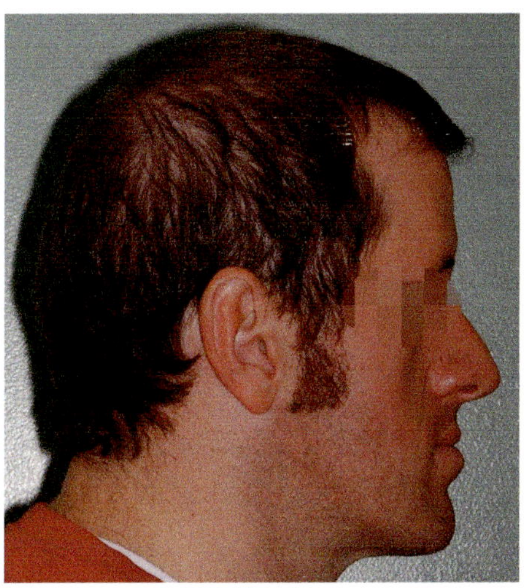

Fig. 9.359 Preoperative post orthodontic right lateral facial view of severe Class III skeletal malocclusion secondary to acromegalism and midfacial hypoplasia

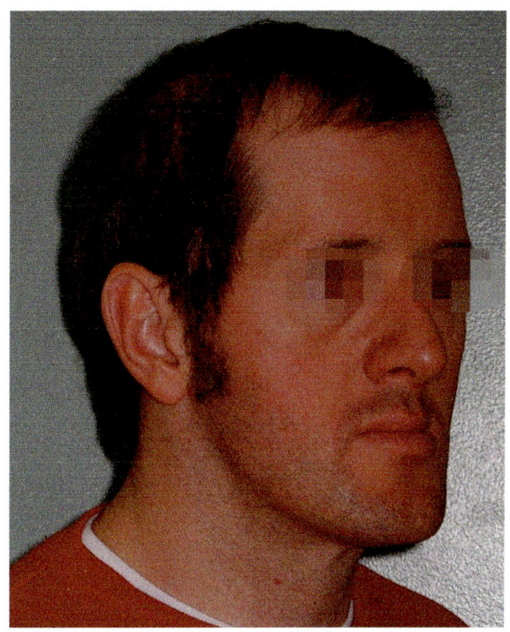

Fig. 9.361 Preoperative post orthodontic right 3/4 facial view of severe Class III skeletal malocclusion secondary to acromegalism and midfacial hypoplasia

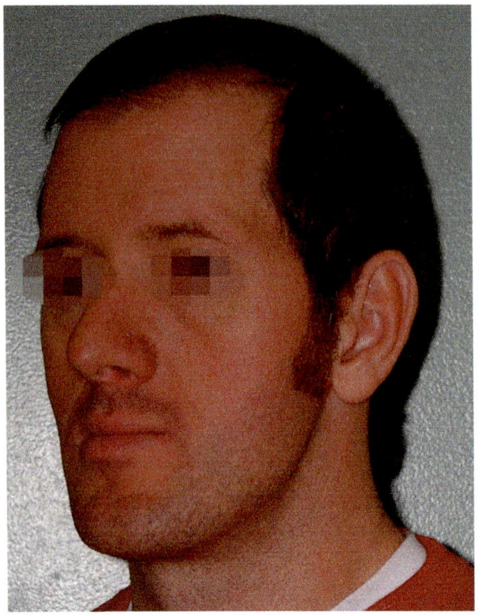

Fig. 9.362 Preoperative post orthodontic left 3/4 facial view of severe Class III skeletal malocclusion secondary to acromegalism and midfacial hypoplasia

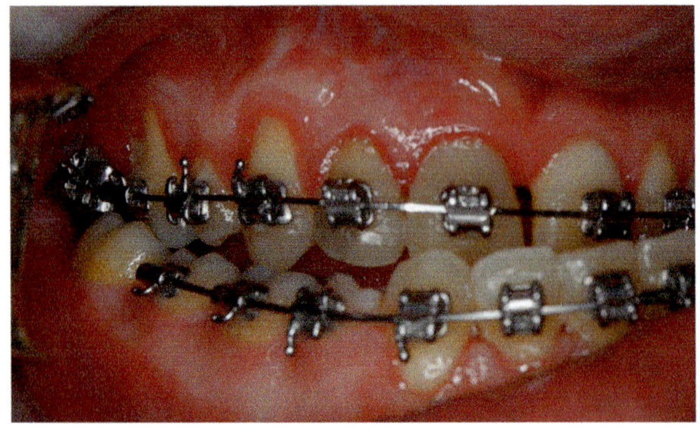

Fig. 9.364 Preoperative post orthodontic right lateral occlusal view with Class III skeletal malocclusion and mandibular prognathism

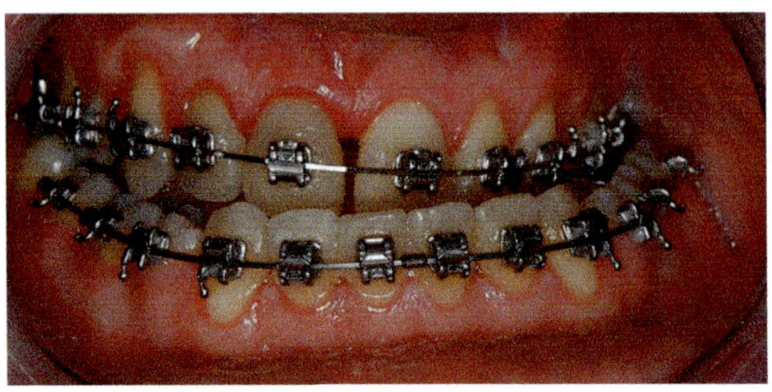

Fig. 9.363 Preoperative post orthodontic frontal occlusal view with Class III skeletal malocclusion and mandibular prognathism

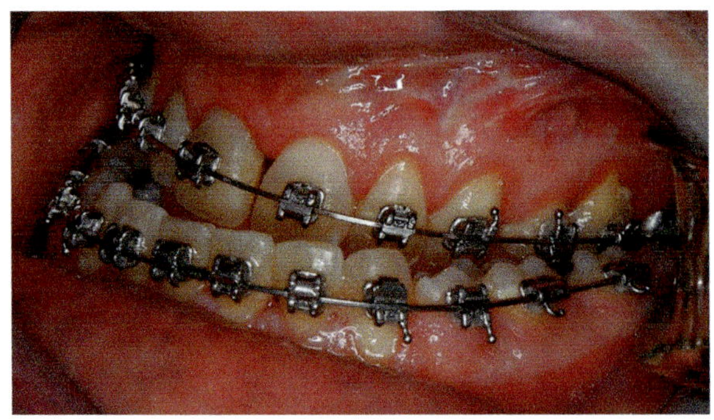

Fig. 9.365 Preoperative post orthodontic left lateral occlusal view with Class III skeletal malocclusion and mandibular prognathism

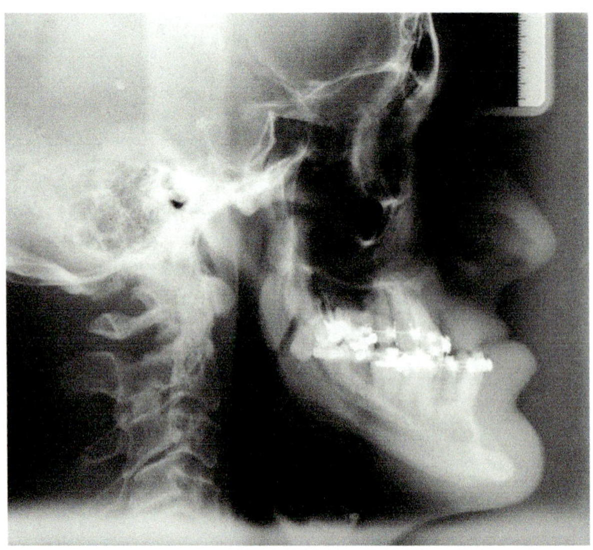

Fig. 9.366 Preoperative post orthodontic lateral cephalometric radiograph

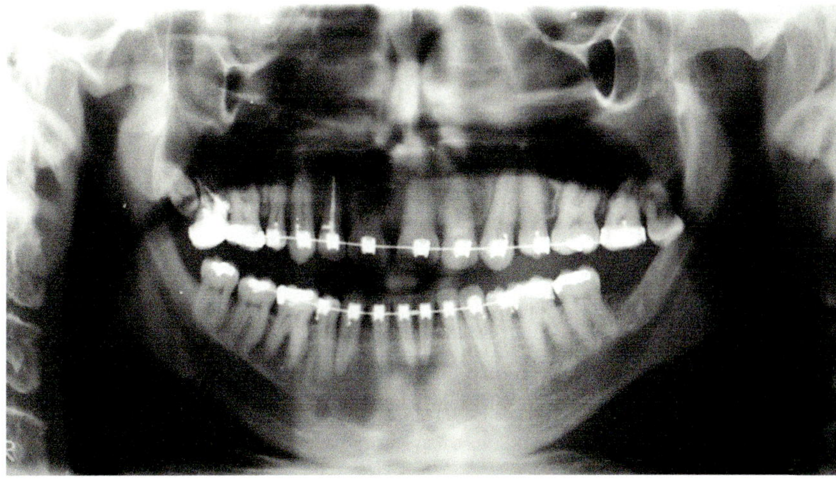

Fig. 9.367 Preoperative post orthodontic panoramic radiograph

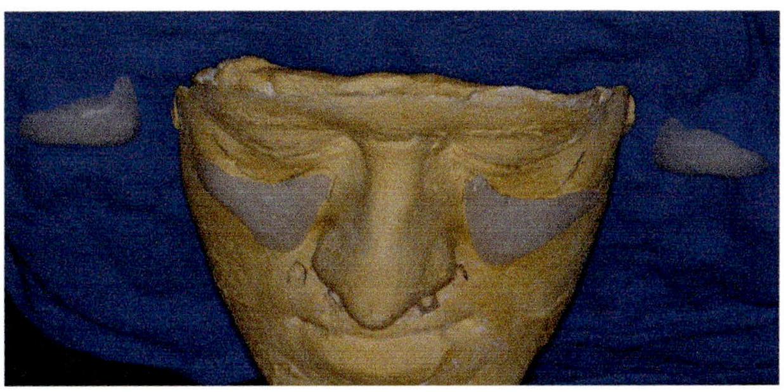

Fig. 9.368 Facial moulage with bilateral maxillo-malar wax prototypes

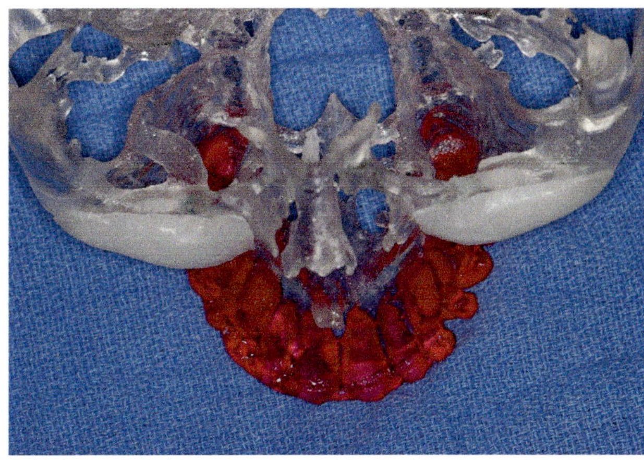

Fig. 9.370 Bilateral maxillo-malar custom implant wax prototype fitted to 3-D model superior view

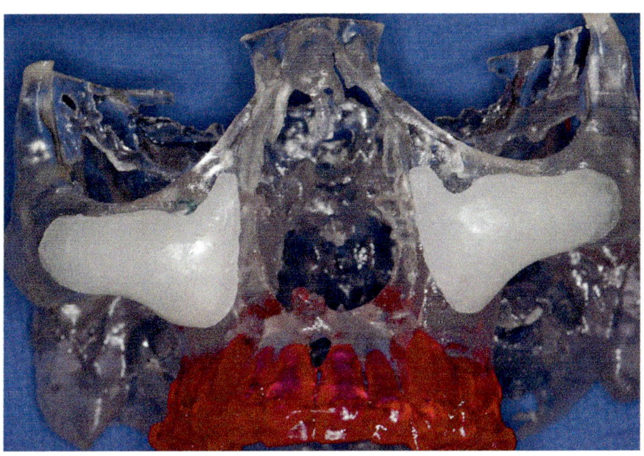

Fig. 9.369 Bilateral maxillo-malar custom implant wax prototype fitted to 3-D model frontal view

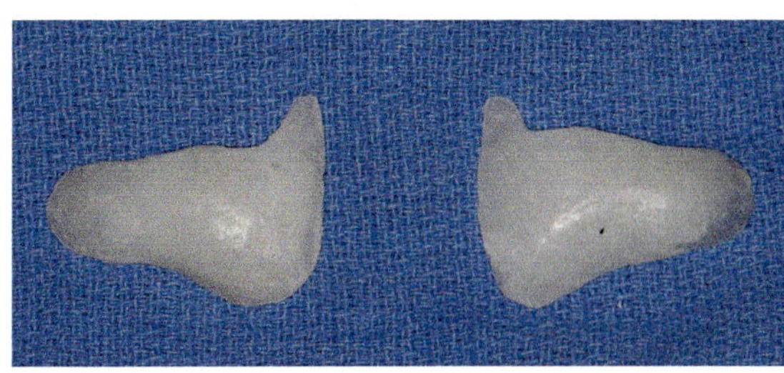

Fig. 9.371 Bilateral maxillo-malar custom implant wax prototypes, frontal views

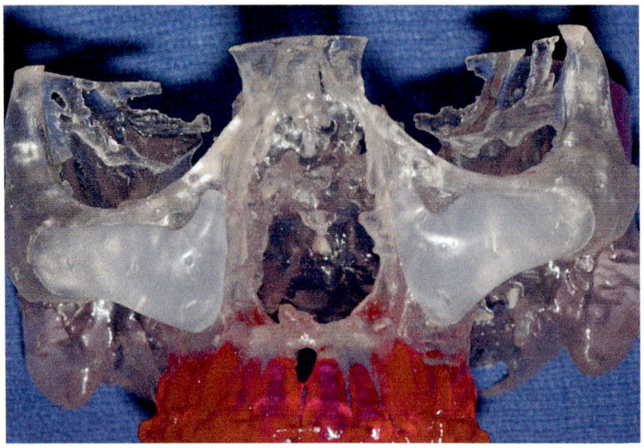

Fig. 9.372 Bilateral maxillo-malar custom solid silicone implants fitted to 3-D model frontal view. Note: Avoidance of the bilateral infraorbital foramina

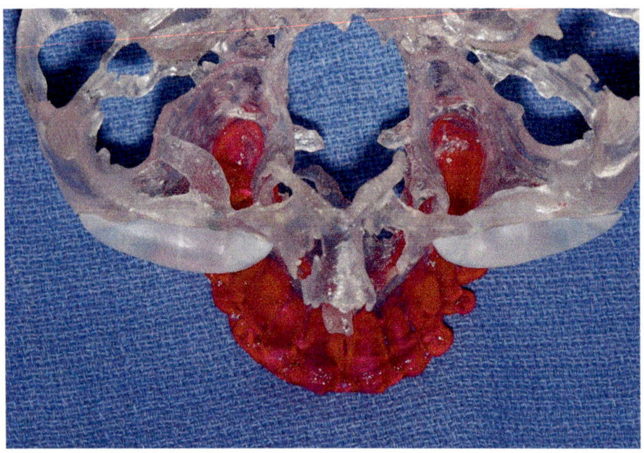

Fig. 9.373 Bilateral maxillo-malar custom solid silicone implants fitted to 3-D model superior view

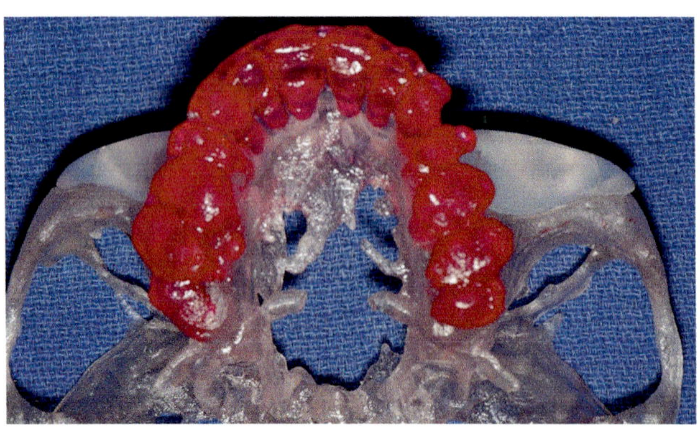

Fig. 9.374 Bilateral maxillo-malar custom solid silicone implants fitted to 3-D model inferior view

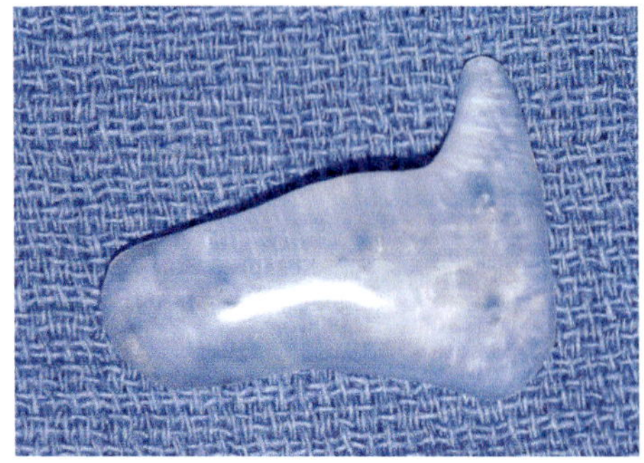

Fig. 9.375 Right maxillo-malar custom solid silicone implant frontal view. Note: Multiple screw holes

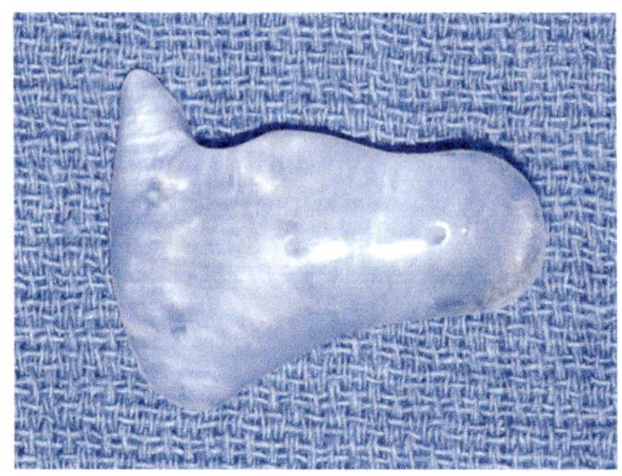

Fig. 9.376 Left maxillo-malar custom solid silicone implant frontal view. Note: Multiple screw holes

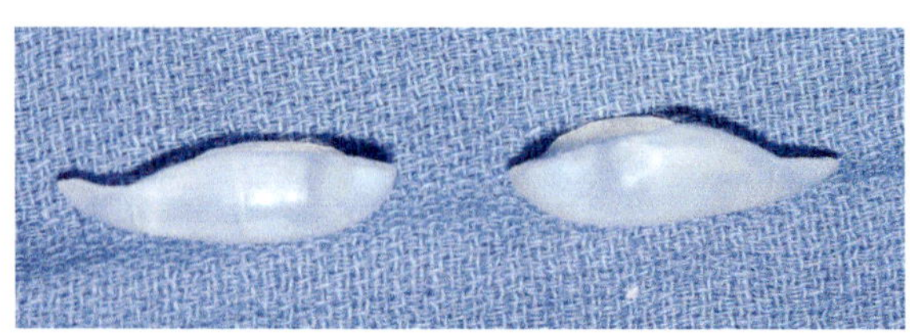

Fig. 9.377 Bilateral maxillo-malar custom solid silicone implant superior view

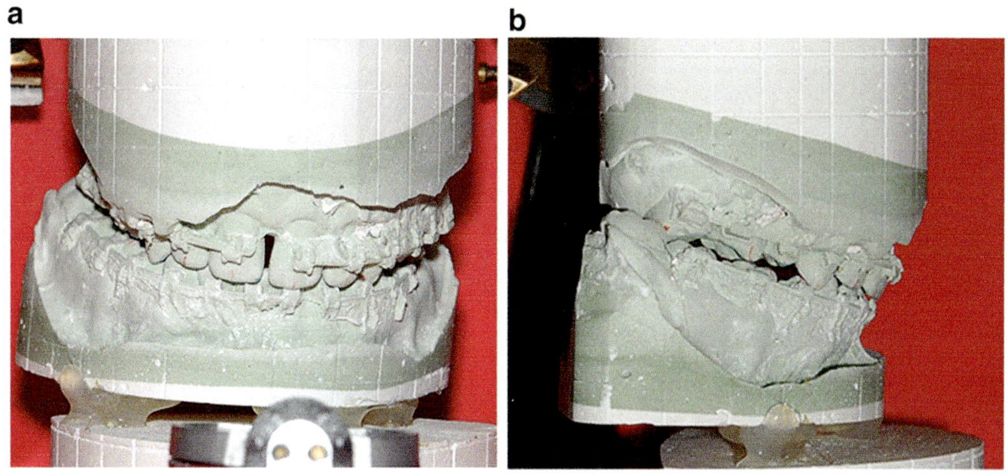

Fig. 9.378 (**a**) Model surgery frontal view. (**b**) Model surgery lateral view demonstrating large setback of the mandible

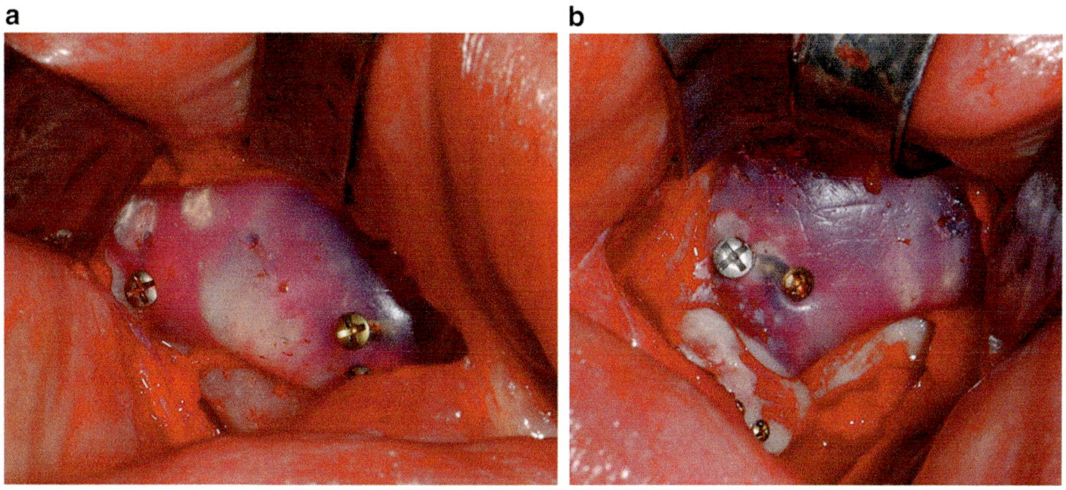

Fig. 9.379 (**a**) Intraoperative view of right maxillo-malar custom solid silicone implant placement with screw fixation. (**b**) Intraoperative view of left maxillo-malar custom solid silicone implant placement with screw fixation (DuPuy Synthes Craniomaxillofacial, Paoli, PA, USA)

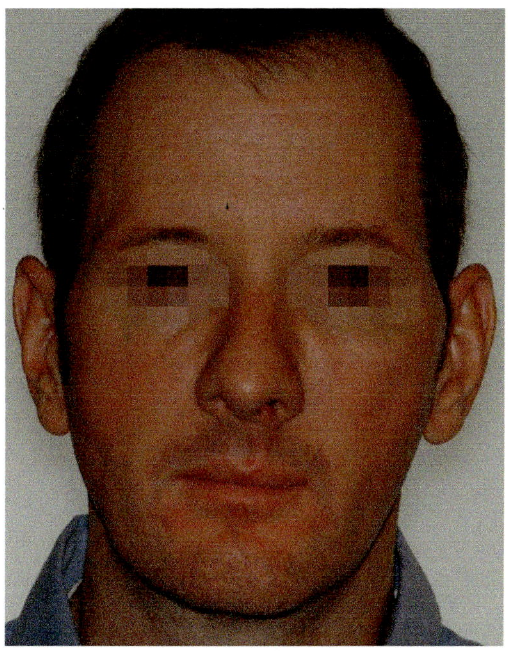

Fig. 9.380 Postoperative frontal view following placement of bilateral custom solid silicone maxillo-malar implants and bilateral mandibular vertical ramus osteotomies with anterior horizontal mandibular osteotomy

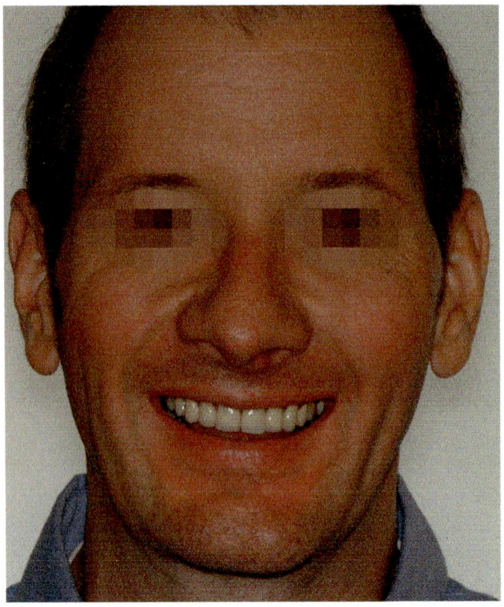

Fig. 9.381 Postoperative frontal view following placement of bilateral custom solid silicone maxillo-malar implants and bilateral mandibular vertical ramus osteotomies with anterior horizontal mandibular osteotomy with smile after dental laminate placement in the anterior maxillary dentition (Dental laminates, Dr. Joseph Haggar, New York, NY, USA)

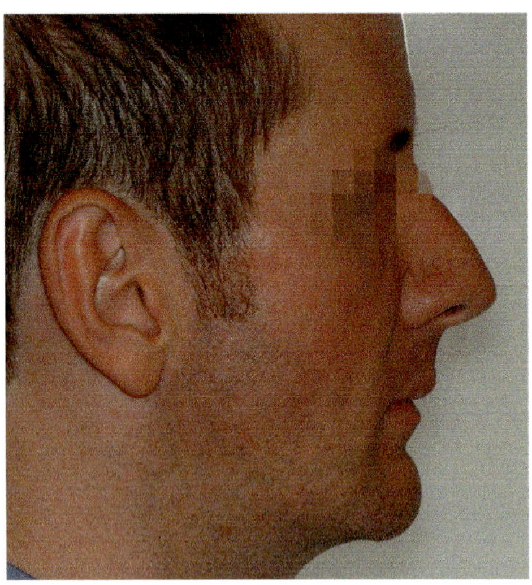

Fig. 9.382 Postoperative right lateral frontal view following placement of bilateral custom solid silicone maxillo-malar implants and bilateral mandibular vertical ramus osteotomies with anterior horizontal mandibular osteotomy after dental laminate placement in the anterior maxillary dentition (Dental laminates, Dr. Joseph Haggar, New York, NY, USA)

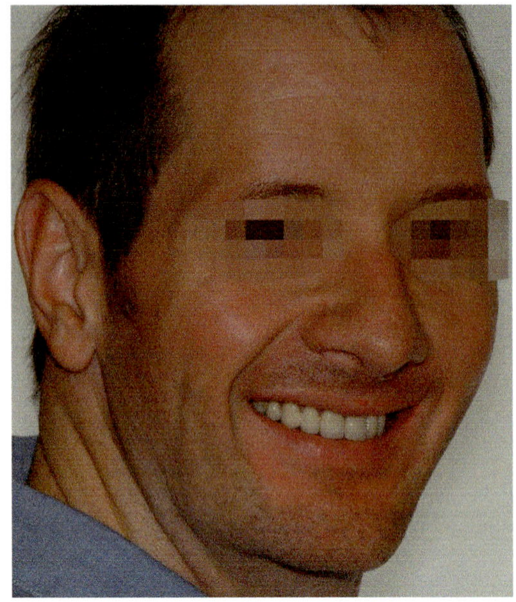

Fig. 9.383 Postoperative 3/4 view following placement of bilateral custom solid silicone maxilla-malar implants and bilateral mandibular vertical ramus osteotomies with anterior horizontal mandibular osteotomy after dental laminate placement in the anterior maxillary dentition (Dental laminates, Dr. Joseph Haggar, New York, NY, USA)

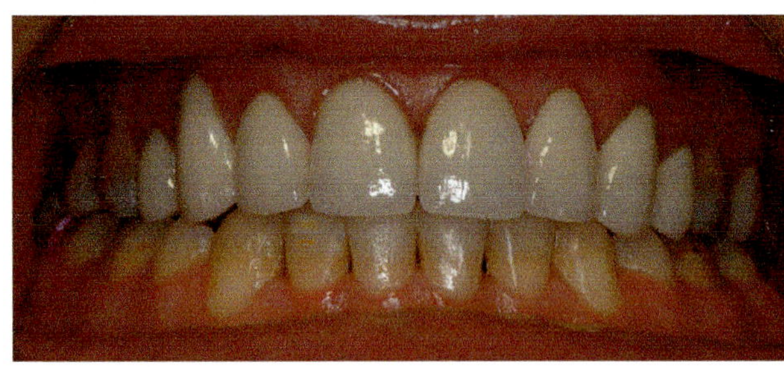

Fig. 9.384 Postoperative frontal occlusal view after dental laminate placement in the anterior maxillary dentition (Dental laminates, Dr. Joseph Haggar, New York, NY, USA)

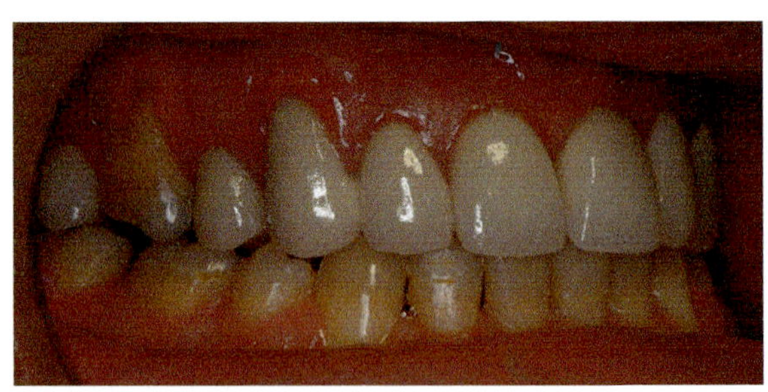

Fig. 9.385 Postoperative right lateral occlusal view after dental laminate placement in the anterior maxillary dentition (Dental laminates, Dr. Joseph Haggar, New York, NY, USA)

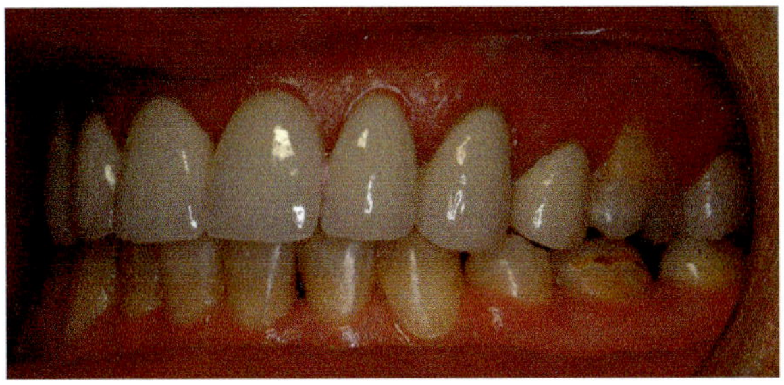

Fig. 9.386 Postoperative left lateral occlusal view (Dental laminates, Dr. Joseph Haggar, New York, NY, USA)

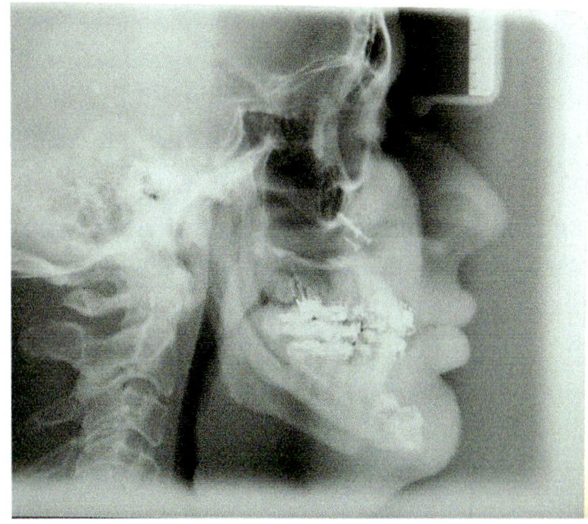

Fig. 9.387 Postoperative lateral cephalometric radiograph

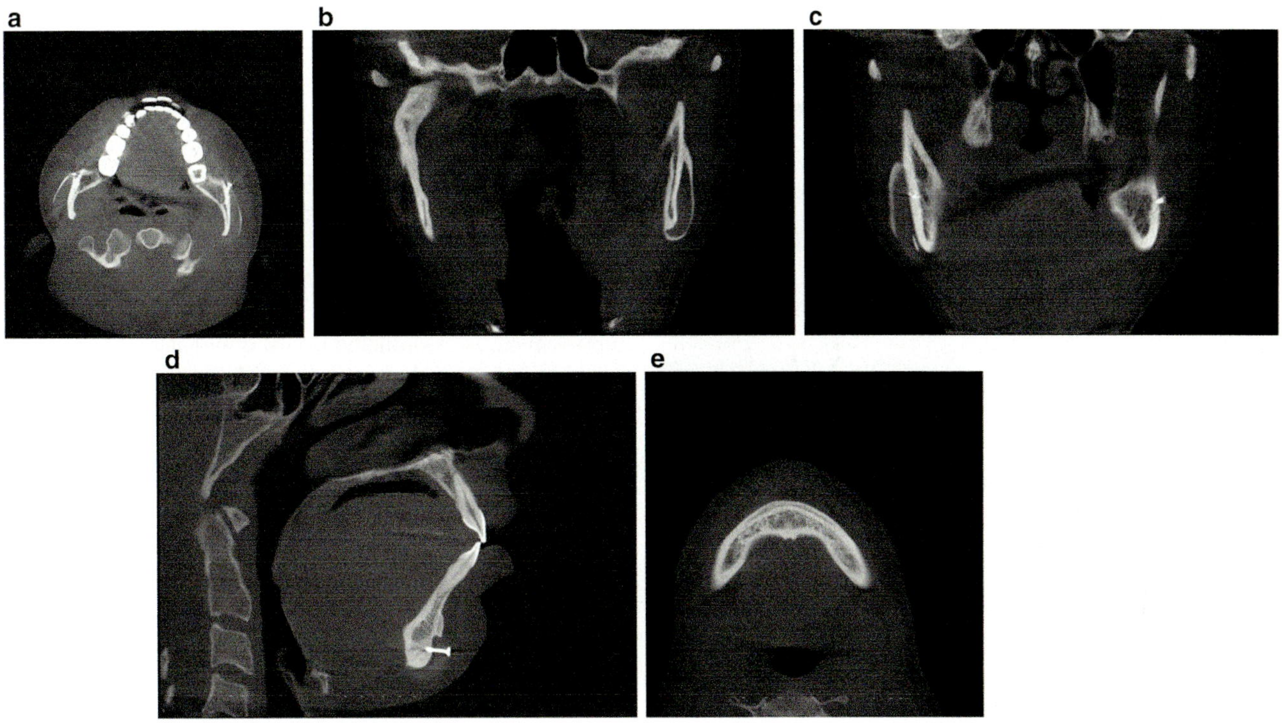

Fig. 9.388 (**a**) Bilateral mandibular angle solid silicone implants with capsule calcification axial view. (**b**) Mandibular angle solid silicone implant with capsule calcification coronal view. (**c**) Mandibular angle solid silicone implant with capsule calcification coronal view. (**d**) Solid silicone chin implant superior edge capsule calcification sagittal view. (**e**) Solid silicone chin implant superior edge capsule calcification axial view

Capsule Formation and Calcification

Solid silicone implants will develop a foreign body capsule during the initial stages of healing following placement. The thickness of the capsule is thin and does not have to be considered in planning the augmentation. However, the foreign body capsule can become calcified (Figs. 9.388a–e and 9.32a–d) which can add 1–2 mm of thickness overlying the implant and should be taken into account more for the mandibular angle than the chin or zygoma implants.

Virtual Planning and Fabrication of Patient-Specific Implants

A new process has been developed that allows the 3D virtual planning of patient-specific implants and the fabrication of prototypes that can be converted into solid silicone or ePTFE implants. The 3D Accuscan method developed by Implantech, Ventura, CA, USA, uses the patient's CT data to create either a 3D stereolithographic model with a rubber-like prototype that can be altered or a virtual model of the skull upon which a variety of custom facial implants can be planned and designed (Fig. 9.389). The contours, thickness, and shape of the implant can be planned and individualized in a 3D planning environment. The implant can then be segmented out and printed as a 3D model that can then be converted into a patient-specific implant. Whether to repair contour defects secondary to trauma or other acquired deformities or for purely cosmetic procedures, the implants can be fabricated as solid silicone. An example of a full jawline implant demonstrates this method (Figs. 9.390, 9.391, 9.392, 9.393, 9.394, 9.395, and 9.396). These implants have the advantage of providing a continuous contour along the mandible, which can be especially appealing to male patients seeking greater prominence of the jawline. The full jawline implants are inserted via a three-incision approach either as combined submental or anterior buccal and bilateral posterior buccal incisions. They can be divided in the midline for insertion with a posterior to anterior insertion to avoid injury to the mental nerves. The implant insertion is completely subperiosteal. Screw fixation can be utilized at the bilateral posterior and chin aspects of the implant for three sites of fixation, with the periosteum closed over the subperiosteal pocket. In cases where the angles are for smaller augmentation, the implant can be folded and inserted from an anterior to posterior approach. The virtual implant design technique can avoid the need for stereolithographic model fabrication, can allow web meetings between the surgeon and the laboratory technician, can obviate implant carving, and can provide patient-specific implants for the chin, angle, and malar regions.

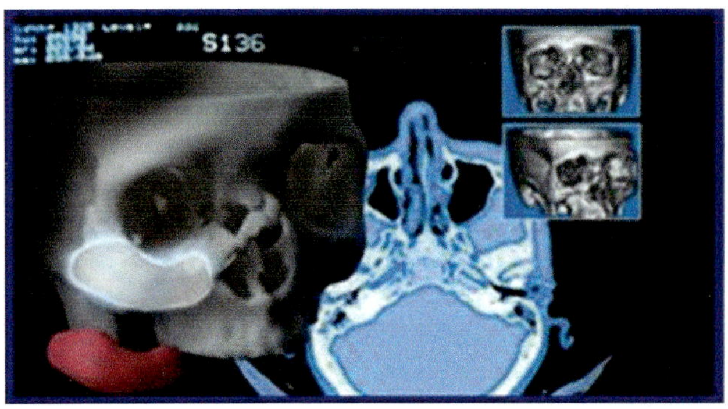

Fig. 9.389 3D Accuscan composite of the skull with malar implant prototype (3D Accuscan, Implantech, Ventura, CA, USA)

Conclusion

This chapter has reviewed facial esthetic evaluation, diagnosis, and classification of various deformities of the chin, mandibular angles, and zygomatic regions, and digital technologies available to clinicians today in order to provide custom cosmetic facial implants that are patient specific for augmentation. These implants can be for purely esthetic contour improvement, in coordination with orthognathic surgery, or for post-tumor resection or traumatic deformities. It is the clinicians choice whether to the use stock or patient-specific implants, both of which offer various advantages and disadvantages. Digital technologies have greatly increased clinician's diagnostic and treatment options and will continue to

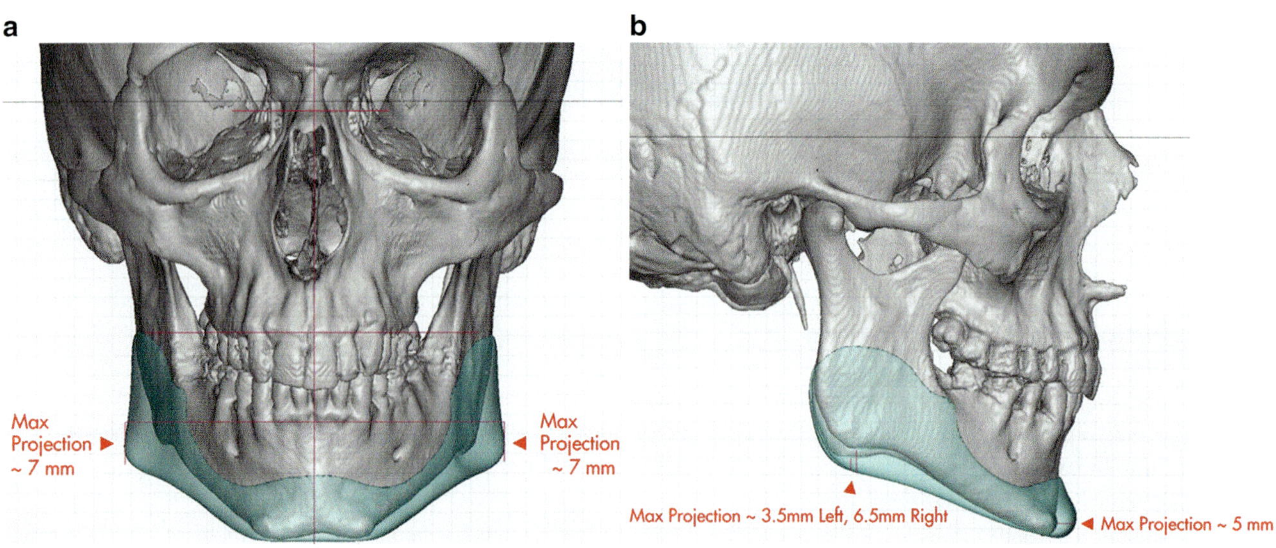

Fig. 9.390 3D Accuscan 3D skull with bilateral mandibular angle and chin (jawline) virtual transparent implant prototype with measurements for thickness: (**a**) frontal view; (**b**) right lateral view (With permission Barry Eppley, MD, DMD, Plastic Surgeon, Indianapolis, IN, USA, and Implantech, Ventura, CA, USA)

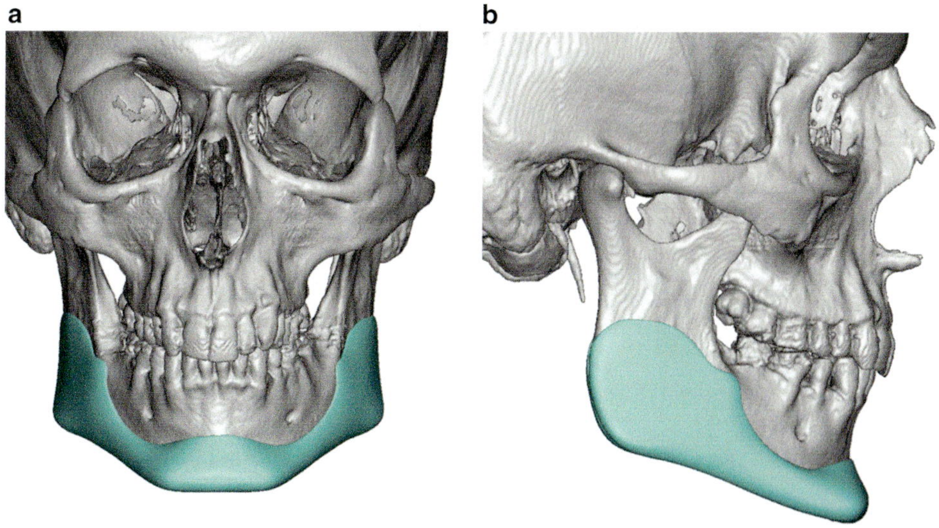

Fig. 9.391 3D Accuscan 3D skull with bilateral mandibular angle and chin (jawline) virtual nontransparent implant prototype: (**a**) frontal view; (**b**) right lateral view (With permission Barry Eppley, MD, DMD, Plastic Surgeon, Indianapolis, IN, USA, and Implantech, Ventura, CA, USA)

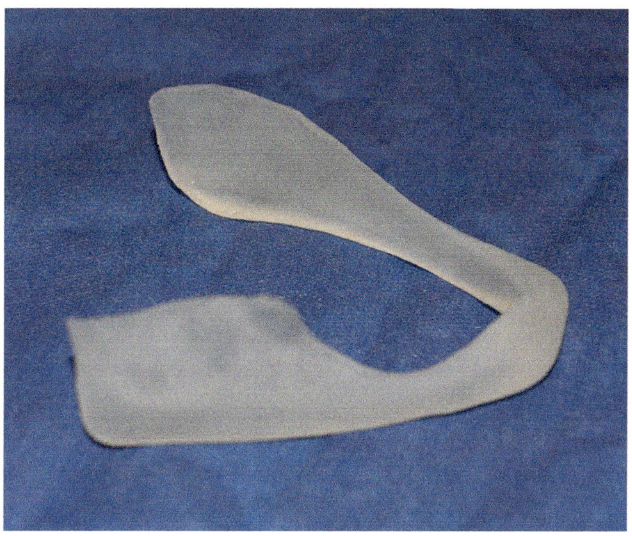

Fig. 9.392 3D Accuscan full jawline patient-specific solid silicone implant right lateral view. Note the interior detail and smooth feather edge (With permission Barry Eppley, MD, DMD, Plastic Surgeon, Indianapolis, IN, USA, 3D Accuscan, Implantech, Ventura, CA, USA)

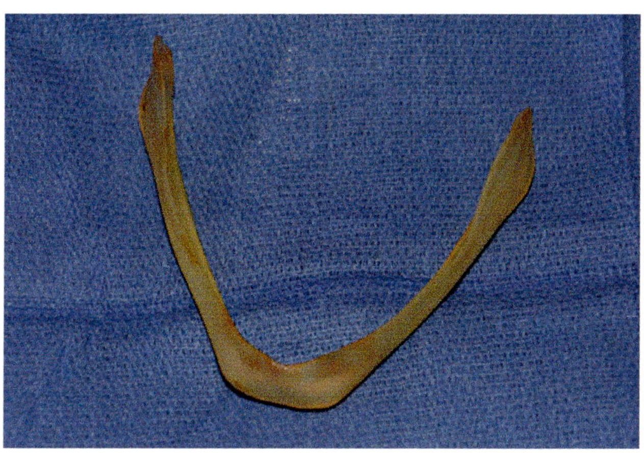

Fig. 9.393 3D Accuscan full jawline patient-specific solid silicone implant frontal lateral view. Note the betadine-soaked surface (With permission Barry Eppley, MD, DMD, Plastic Surgeon, Indianapolis, IN, USA, 3D Accuscan, Implantech, Ventura, CA, USA)

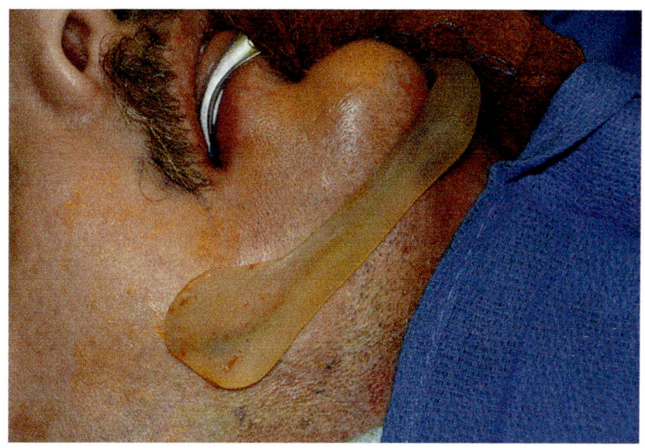

Fig. 9.394 Preoperative full jawline patient-specific solid silicone implant aligned to patient (With permission Barry Eppley, MD, DMD, Plastic Surgeon, Indianapolis, IN, USA, 3D Accuscan, Implantech, Ventura, CA, USA)

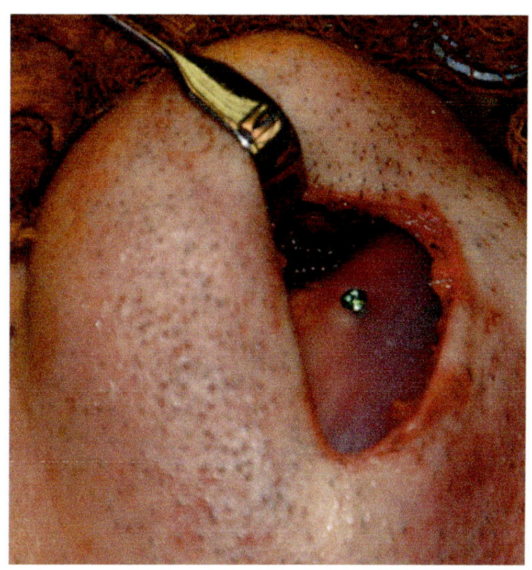

Fig. 9.395 3D Accuscan full jawline patient-specific solid silicone implant. Intraoperative view of submental incision with implant placement and single screw fixation (With permission Barry Eppley, MD, DMD, Plastic Surgeon, Indianapolis, IN, USA, 3D Accuscan, Implantech, Ventura, CA, USA)

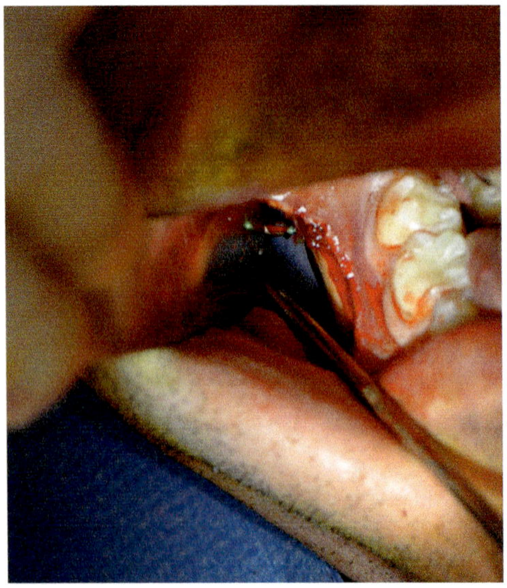

Fig. 9.396 3D Accuscan full jawline patient-specific solid silicone implant. Intraoperative view right buccal incision with implant inserted single screw fixation being placed (With permission Barry Eppley, MD, DMD, Plastic Surgeon, Indianapolis, IN, USA, 3D Accuscan, Implantech, Ventura, CA, USA)

develop and improve patient outcomes, especially in the evolving field of VSP and the virtual creation of facial alloplastic implants that can be fabricated through the use of custom-printed templates converted into various materials, and perhaps the direct fabrication of the implants themselves. Patient's final satisfaction with the cosmetic results can be a very delicate matter, especially when facial implants are performed for cosmetic improvement only. Cosmetic changes that result after the surgical correction of dentofacial deformities and tumor surgery can result in patient dissatisfaction, which can lead to alloplastic facial implant augmentation. Preoperative attention to patient's expectations and desires, and psychological aspects, plays an important role in predisposing a patient to a satisfactory outcome and can prevent patient dissatisfaction. Digital technologies will continue to evolve to provide improvements in cosmetic facial implant augmentation procedures.

References

1. O'Ryan F, Lassetter J. Optimizing facial esthetics in the orthognathic surgery patient. J Oral Maxillofac Surg. 2011;69(3):702–15
2. Holland E. Marquardt's Phi mask: pitfalls of relying on fashion models and the golden ratio to describe a beautiful face. Aesthetic Plast Surg. 2008;32(2):200–8
3. Marquardt SR. Dr. Stepehn R. Marquardt on the golden decagon and human facial beauty interview by Dr. Gottlieb. J Clin Orthod. 2002;36(6):317–8
4. Goldsmith D, Horowitz A, Orentlicher G. Facial skeletal augmentation using custom facial implants. Atlas Oral and Maxillofac Surg Clin N Am. 2012;20:119–34
5. Millard DR. Sir Harold Gillies. Ann Plast Surg. 1979;3(5):454–63.
6. Glicenstein J. Aesthetic surgery history. Ann Chir Plast Esthet. 2003;48(5):257–72.
7. Aufricht G. Combined plastic surgery of the nose and chin: resume of twenty-seven years experience. Am J Surg. 1958;95(2):231–6
8. Rubin CR, Robertson GW, Shapiro RN. Polyethylene in reconstructive surgery. Plast Reconstr Surg. 1948;3:586
9. Yaremchuk MJ. Facial skeletal reconstruction using porous polyethylene implants. Plast Reconstr Surg. 2003;111:1818–27
10. Flowers RS. Alloplastic augmentation of the anterior mandible. Clin Plast Surg. 1991;18(1):107–38.
11. Eppley BL, Sadove AM, Holmstrom H. HTR polymer facial implants: a five year clinical experience. Aesthetic Plast Surg. 1995;19:445–50
12. Farkas LG, Katic MJ, Hreczko TA, Deutsch C, Munro IR. Anthropometric proportions in the upper lip-lower lip-chin area of the lower face in young white adults. Am J Orthod. 1984;86:52–60
13. Farkas LG, Hreczko TA, Kabe MJ. Craniofacial Norms in North American Caucasians from Birth (One Year) to Adulthood. In: Farkas LG, editor. Anthropometry of the Head and Neck. 2nd ed. New York: Raven Press; 1994. Appendix A.
14. Burstone CJ. Lip posture and its significance in treatment planning. Am J Orthod. 1967;53:262
15. Burstone CJ, James RB, Legan H, Murphy GA. Norton a cephalometrics for orthognathic surgery. J Oral Surg. 1978;36(4):269–77
16. Legan HL, Burstone CJ. Soft tissue cephalometric analysis for orthognathic surgery. J Oral Surg. 1980;38:744–51
17. Ricketts RM. Esthetics, environment, and the law of lip relation. Am J Orthop. 1968;54(2):272–89
18. Steiner CC. Cephalometrics for you and me. Am J Orthod. 1953;39:729
19. Steiner CC. The use of cephalometrics as an aid to planning and assessing orthodontic treatment. Am J Orthod. 1960;46:721–35
20. Gonzalez-Ulloa M. Ptosis of the chin: the Witch's chin. Plast Reconstr Surg. 1972;50:54
21. Gonzalez-Ulloa M, Stevens SE. The role of the chin in profile plasty. Plast Reconstr Surg. 1968;41:477
22. Gonzalez-Ulloa M. Planning the integral correction of the human profile. J Int Coll Surg. 1961;36:364–73
23. Powell N, Humphreys B. Proportions of the Aesthetic Face. New York: Thieme-Stratton; 1984.
24. Romo T, Millman AL, editors. Aesthetic Facial Plastic Surgery: a Multidisciplinary Approach. New York: Thieme; 2000. p. 332–5.
25. Kiekens RM, Kvijpers-Jagtman AM, Van't Hof MA. Putatative golden proportions as predictors of facial esthetics in adolescents. Dentofacial Orthop. 2008;134(4):480–3
26. Ricketts RM. Divine proportions in facial esthetics. Clin Plast Surg. 1982;9:401
27. Shell TL, Woods MG. Facial esthetics and the divine proportion: a comparison of surgical and nonsurgical class II treatment. Aust Orthod J. 2004;20(2):51–63
28. Greenberg AM. Cone beam computed tomography scanning and diagnosis for dental implants. Oral Maxillofac Surg Clin North Am. 2015;27(2):185–202
29. Greenberg AM. Basics of cone-beam CT and CT guided dental implant surgery. Selected Readings in Oral and Maxillofacial Surgery. 2011;19(5):1–48
30. April E, Erickson A, Montano S. Clinical Anatomy. 3rd ed. Baltimore: Williams and Wilkins; 1997.
31. Filo K, Schneider T, Locher MC, Kruse AL, Lubbers HT. The inferior alveolar nerve's loop at the mental foramen and its implications for surgery. J Am Dent Assoc. 2014;145(3):260–9.s
32. Zide B, Pfeifer TM, Longaker MT. Chin surgery: I. Augmentation-the allure and the alerts. Plast Reconstr Surg. 1999;104:1843–53

33. Profitt WR, Phillips C, Turvey TA. Stability after mandibular setback: mandible only versus 2-jaw surgery. J Oral Maxillofac Surg. 2012;70(7):e408–14
34. De Lir AL, de Moura WL, Oliveira Ruellas AC, Gomez Souza MM, Nojima LI. Long term skeletal and profile stability after surgical orthodontic treatment of class II and class III malocclusion. J Craniomaxillofac Surg. 2013;41(4):296–302
35. Xu M, Chan FC, Jin X, Xu J, Lu J, Zhang C, Teng L. Hemimandibular hyperplasia: classification and treatment algorithm revisited. J Craniofac Surg. 2014;25(2):355–8
36. Reddy PS, Kashyap B, Hallur N, Sikkerimath BC. Advancement genioplasty-cephalometric analysis of osseous and soft tissue changes. J Oral Maxillofac Surg. 2011;10(4):288–95
37. Erbe C, Mulie RM, Ruf S. Advancement genioplasty in class I patients: predictability and stability of facial profile changes. Int J Oral Maxillofac Surg. 2011;40(11):1258–62
38. San Miguel Moragas J, Oth O, Buttner M, Mommaerts MY. A systemic review on soft to hard tissue ratios in orthognathic surgery part II: chin procedures. J Craniomaxillofac Surg. 2015;43(8):1530–40
39. Aston SJ, Smith DM. Taking it on the chin: recognizing and accounting for lower face asymmetry in chin augmentation and genioplasty. Plast Reconstr Surg. 2015;135(6):1591–5
40. Guyuron B, Raszewski RL. A critical comparison of osteoplastic and alloplastic augmentation genioplasty. Aesthetic Plast Surg. 1990;14:199–206
41. Terino EO, Edwards MC. Customizing jawlines: the art of alloplastic premandible contouring. Facial Plast Surg Clin N Am. 2008;16:99–122
42. Rieck KL. Taking on the chin-the art of genioplasty. Selected Readings in Oral and Maxiloofacial Surgery. 2013;21(2):1–51
43. Manji Z, Payami A, Greenberg A. Genioplasty. In: Greenberg A, Schmelzeisen R, editors. Craniomaxillofacial Reconstructive and Corrective Bone Surgery. New York: Springer Verlag; In press.
44. Frodel JL. The use of high density polyethylene implants in facial deformities. Arch Otolaryngol Head Neck Surg. 1998;124:1219–23
45. Zeph RD. Custom-designed chin augmentation. Facial Plast Surg Clin N Am. 2008;16:79–85
46. Mittelman H, Spencer JR, Chrzanowski DS. Chin region: management of grooves and mandibular hypoplasia with alloplastic implants. Facial Plast Surg Clin N Am. 2007;16:445–60
47. Romo T, Lanson BG. Chin augmentation. Facial Plast Surg Clin N Am. 2008;16:69–77
48. Simons RL. Adjunctive measures in rhinoplasty. Otolaryngol Clin North Am. 1975;8:717
49. Safian J. Progress in nasal and chin augmentation. Plast Reconstr Surg. 1966;37:446
50. Haug RH. Design and function of implants. In: Ehrenfeld M, Manson P, Prein J, editors. Principles of Internal Fixation of the Craniofacial Skeleton, Trauma, and Orthognathic surgery. New York: Thieme; 2012. p. 53–80.
51. Thomson ERE. Sagittal genioplasty: a new technique of genioplasty. Br J Plast Surg. 1985;38:70–4
52. Terino EO, Edwards MC. Customizing jawlines: the art of alloplastic premandible contouring. Facial Plast Surg Clin North Am. 2008;16(1):99–122, vi.
53. Terino EO. Implants for male aesthetic surgery. Clin Plast Surg. 1991;18(4):731–49
54. Naini FB. The origin of the zero-meridian used in facial esthetic analysis. Aesthetic Surg J. 2014;34(7):NP 72–3.
55. Avelar KL, Sa CD, Esses DF, Becker OE, Soares EC, de Oliveira RB. Unusual complication after genioplasty. J Craniofac Surg. 2014;25(2):180–2
56. Hoenig JF. Sliding osteotomy genioplasty for facial aesthetic balance: 10 years of experience. Aestehtic Plast Surg. 2007;31(4):384–91
57. Lindquist CC, Obeid G. Complications of genioplasty done alone or in combination with sagittal split-ramus osteotomy. Oral Surg Oral Med Oral Pathol. 1988;66(1):13–6
58. Zide B, MacCarthy J. The mentalis muscle: an essential component of chin and lower lip position. Plast Reconstr Surg. 1989;83(3):413–20
59. Rose EH. Autogenous fascia lata grafts: clinical applications in reanimation of the totally or partially paralyzed face. Plast Reconstr Surg. 2005;16(1):20–32. discussion 33–5
60. Zide BM. Chin disfigurement following removal of alloplastic chin implants. Plast Reconstr Surg. 1991;88:68. (Discussion)
61. Yaremchuk MJ. Improving aesthetic outcomes after alloplastic chin augmentation. Plast Reconstr Surg. 2003;112(5):1422–32. discussion 1433-4
62. Cohen SR, Mardach OL, Kawamoto HK Jr. Chin disfigurement following removal of alloplastic chin implants. Plast Reconstr Surg. 1991;88(1):62–6. discussion 67-70
63. White JB, Dufresne CR. Management and avoidance of complications in chin augmentation. Aesthet Surg J. 2011;31(6):634–42.
64. Semergidis TG, Migliore SA, Sotreanos GC. Alloplastic augmentation of the mandibular angle. J Oral Maxillofac Surg. 1996;54(12):1417–23
65. Bastidas N, Zide BM. The treachery of mandibular angle augmentation. Ann Plast Surg. 2010;64(1):4–6
66. Ousterhout DK. Mandibular angle augmentation and reduction. Clin Plast Surg. 1991;18(1):153–61
67. Roncevic R. Masseter muscle hypertrophy. Aetiology and therapy. J Maxillofac Surg. 1986;14(6):344–8
68. Ozkan BT, Tabrizi R, Cigerim L. Management of bilateral masseter muscle hypertrophy. J Craniofac Surg. 2012;23(1):e14–6
69. Lee DH, Jin SP, Cho S, Feneran A, Youn CS, Won CH, Park GH, Kim BW, An J, Chang SE, Lee MW. Rimabotulinum toxin B versus Onabotulinum toxin a in the treatment of masseter hypertrophy: a 24 week double-blind randomized split face study. Dermatology. 2013;226(3):227–32
70. Binder WJ. Custom-designed facial implants. Facial Plast Surg Clin N Am. 2008;16:133–46
71. Bell WH, Proffitt WR, White RP. Surgical Correction of Dentofacial Deformities, vol. 238. Philadelphia: WB Saunders; 1980. p. 271
72. Thomas MA. Masseter muscle reattachment after mandibular angle surgery. Aesthet Surg J. 2009;29(6):473–6
73. Epker BN. Cosmetic Maxillofacial surgery. Philadelphia: Lea and Feabiger; 1994. p. 79–94
74. Innocenti A, Andretto Amodeo C, Ciancio F. Wide undermining neck liposuction: tips and tricks for good results. Aesthetic Plast Surg. 2014;38(4):667–9
75. Adamson PA, Cormier R, Tropper GJ, McGraw BL. Cervicofacial liposuction: results and controversies. J Otolaryngol. 1990;19(4):267–73
76. Metzinger SE, McCollough EG, Campbell JP, Rousso DE. Malar augmentation: a 5-year retrospective review of the silastic midfacial malar implant. Arch Otolaryngol Head Neck Surg. 1999;125:980–7
77. Mladick RA. Alloplastic cheek augmentation. Clin Plast Surg. 1991;18(1):29–38
78. Terino EO, Edwards MC. Alloplastic contouring for suborbital, maxillary, zygomatic deficiencies Facial Plast Surg Clin North Am. 2008;16(1):33–67, v.
79. Hinderer U. Profileplasty. Int Macro J Aesthetic Plast Surg Sept. 1971;1:12
80. Wilkinson T. Complications in aesthetic malar augmentation. Plast Reconstr Surg. 1983;71:643
81. Silver WE. The use of alloplast material in contouring the face. Facial Plast Surg. 1986;3:81
82. Powell NB, Riley RW, Lamb DR. A new approach to evaluation and surgery of the malar complex. Ann Plast Surg. 1988;20:206–14

83. Prendergast M, Schoenrock LD. Malar augmentation. Arch Otolaryngol Head Neck Surg. 1989;115:964
84. Binder WJ. Submalar augmentation. Arch Otolaryngol Head Neck Surg. 1989;115:797
85. Binder WJ, Azizzadeh B. Malar and submalar augmentation. Facial Plast Surg Clin North Am. 2008;16(1):11–32. v
86. Zou C, Niu F, Yu B, Liu JF, Gui L. Zygomatic complex change after reduction malarplasty and its geometric model: a retrospective clinical study. J Oral Maxillofac Surg. 2015;73(11):2196–206
87. Layoun W, Guyot L, Richard O, Gola R. Augmentation of cheek bone contour using malar osteotomy. Aesthetic Plast Surg. 2003;27(4):269–74
88. Tessier P. The definitive plastic surgical treatment of the severe facial deformities of craniofacial dysostosis: Crouzon's and Apert's diseases. Plast Reconstr Surg. 1971;48(5):419–42
89. Quatela VC, Chow J. Synthetic Facial Implants. Facial Plast Surg Clin N Am. 2008;16:1–10
90. Waite PD, Matukas VJ. Zygomatic augmentation with hydroxyapatite: a preliminary report. J Oral Maxillofac Surg. 1986;44(5):349–52
91. Guevera-Rojas G, Figl M, Schicho K, Seeman R, Traxler H, Vacariu A, Carbon CC, Ewers R, Watzinger F. Patient-specific polyetheretherketone facial implants in a computer-aided planning workflow. J Oral Maxillofac Surg. 2014;72(9):1801–12

Navigation of Sinus and Skull Base Surgery

10

Sarah M. Kidwai, Arjun K. Parasher, Joshua B. Bederson, and Satish Govindaraj

Overview

In 1675, Molinetti described an approach to access the maxillary sinus through the anterior maxillary wall [1]. By the 1890s, Caldwell, Spicer, and Luc had fenestrated the anterior maxillary wall and created an antrostomy for drainage into the nose. This procedure, commonly known as the Caldwell-Luc procedure, became the primary choice of treatment for chronic rhinosinusitis (CRS) through the early twentieth century [1]. The first endoscopic examination of the nose was conducted with a modified cystoscope by Hirschmann in 1901 [2]. Yet, the modern era of endoscopic sinus surgery (ESS) would emerge with the development of the Hopkins rod telescope in the 1950s. Messerklinger pioneered the study of the endoscopic anatomy and pathophysiology of the paranasal sinuses, publishing his experiences in 1978 [3]. Stammberger disseminated these techniques outside of Germany and Austria, while Kennedy introduced ESS to the United States in 1985 [2]. Today, endoscopic approaches are the primary surgical modality for the treatment of CRS as well as many other sinonasal and skull base disorders.

Before the advent of endoscopy, surgery to expose intracranial lesions adjacent to the brainstem or beneath the cerebral cortex was approached via morbid external approaches. These open approaches required vigorous and often harmful degrees of retraction on the brain. With the evolution of digital navigation technologies, endoscopic skull base surgery has revolutionized the field. Current techniques allow the surgeon to approach previously inaccessible lesions, while minimizing morbidity. Navigation technology has now become a near necessity in the armamentarium of skull base surgery.

Before describing current navigation technologies in sinus and skull base surgery, the chapter begins with a review of the relevant surgical anatomy of the nose, paranasal sinuses, and skull base. This chapter will then examine the digital technologies that are used for both preoperative surgical planning and intraoperative surgical navigation with a thorough analysis of their advantages, limitations, and clinical impact. The chapter concludes with the future direction for these technologies in sinus and skull base surgery.

Part I: Anatomy of the Nose and Sinuses

An appreciation of the anatomy is crucial to successful endoscopic sinus and skull base surgery in order to limit complications and achieve optimal results for the patient. Thus, this next section will provide a thorough description of the anatomy of paranasal sinuses, skull base, and associated surgical landmarks. This section will also discuss sensory innervation, arterial supply, and common anatomical variations that are crucial components of the surgeon's knowledge base. This overview reveals the intricate and complicated anatomy of the region, which necessitates navigation technology in many surgical cases.

The Nasal Cavity

The *nose* is bound superiorly by the cribriform plate of the ethmoid bone and inferiorly by the hard palate, extending posteriorly to the choanae. The *choanae* are the anatomical openings of the nasal cavity into the nasopharynx. The perpendicular plates of the ethmoid and vomer bones, together with the quadrangular cartilage, form the *nasal septum*. The *lateral nasal wall* has three or four bony projections called the conchae, or turbinates. These turbinates increase the surface area of the nasal mucosa, provide humidification,

S.M. Kidwai (✉) • A.K. Parasher • S. Govindaraj
Department of Otolaryngology, The Mount Sinai Hospital, Icahn School of Medicine at Mount Sinai, New York, NY, USA
e-mail: sarah.kidwai@mountsinai.org; Arjun.parasher@gmail.com; satish.govindaraj@mountsinai.org

J.B. Bederson
Department of Neurosurgery, The Mount Sinai Hospital, Icahn School of Medicine at Mount Sinai, 1468 Madison Avenue, Annenberg 8-35, New York, NY 10029, USA
e-mail: Joshua.Bederson@mountsinai.org

A.M. Greenberg (ed.), *Digital Technologies in Craniomaxillofacial Surgery*, https://doi.org/10.1007/978-1-4939-1532-3_10

and create the laminar flow of air through the nose. In addition, they divide the nasal cavity into three distinct air passages. The spaces between each of the turbinates are referred to as meatuses. Each of the turbinates and meatuses is named by anatomical location: inferior, middle, or superior. Figure 10.1 shows a cadaveric view of the lateral nasal wall and the turbinates. The middle meatus contains a bulge within the lateral nasal wall, called the *bulla ethmoidalis*, which is created by the presence of the anterior ethmoidal air cells. This bulge is bound inferiorly by the *semilunar hiatus*. The mucous membrane of the nasal cavity is ciliated columnar epithelium and is specialized for olfaction within the roof of the nose and surface of the superior turbinate.

Along the floor protruding from the lateral nasal wall lays the *inferior turbinate*, which divides the pathway of the inspiratory airstream into an upper and lower pathway. The *nasolacrimal duct* opens posterior and 2 mm below the insertion of the inferior turbinate. The slit-like opening of the duct opens into the anterosuperior part of the inferior meatus, allowing tears from the lacrimal sac to be carried into the nose. At the posterior end of the inferior turbinate lies the ostium of the eustachian tube, at the same level, and sagittal plane.

Ostiomeatal Complex

The drainage pathways of these sinuses create two distinct ostiomeatal units. The *anterior and middle ethmoid cells*, the *maxillary sinus*, and the *frontal sinus* drain into the semilunar hiatus at the middle meatus. This anterior ostiomeatal unit consists of the frontal sinus ostium, frontal recess, maxillary sinus ostium, ethmoid infundibulum, and middle meatus. On the other hand, the posterior ethmoidal cells and sphenoid sinus, via the sphenoethmoidal recess, drain into the superior meatus and subsequently the nasopharynx. The posterior ostiomeatal unit consists of the sphenoid sinus ostium, sphenoethmoidal recess, and the superior meatus. ESS has gained widespread usage because of its ability to restore these normal anatomic drainage pathways.

Secretions of the sinuses are additionally carried into the nose via ciliary action. Within the *maxillary sinus*, the mucus flow originates in the antral floor and is directed centrally toward the primary ostium of the maxillary sinus, subsequently entering the middle meatus via the semilunar hiatus. In the *frontal sinus*, the mucus flow originates along the medial wall, laterally across the roof, and medially along the floor. Toward the medial floor, some mucus enters the primary ostium of the frontal sinus, while the rest is recirculated. The ostium of the frontal sinus opens into the frontal recess and subsequently into the semilunar hiatus via the ethmoid infundibulum. The ostium of the frontal sinus lies between the ethmoid bulla and agger nasi cell, a view of which is seen in Fig. 10.2. The frontal or frontoethmoid cell lies superior to the agger nasi, discussed below, and can show variable pneumatization. The frontal sinus drainage pattern varies based on the position of the *uncinate process* as illustrated in Fig. 10.3. The uncinate process extends superiorly within the lateral nasal wall. Anteriorly, the uncinate process fuses with the posterior wall of the agger nasi and the posterior wall of the nasolacrimal duct. Superiorly the uncinate process may attach to the lamina papyracea, the skull base,

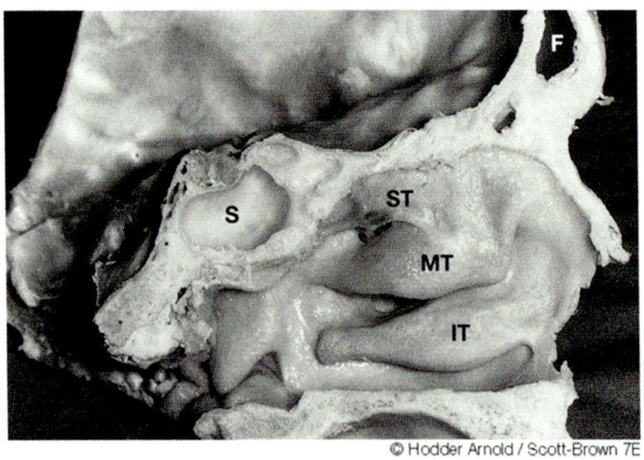

Fig. 10.1 A cadaveric image of the lateral nasal wall (*S* sphenoid sinus, *ST* superior turbinate, *MT* middle turbinate, *IT* inferior turbinate. From: Scott Brown's Otorhinolaryngology 7E (ISBN: 978-0-340-80893-1). Authors Gleeson & Clarke, Copyright (2008) Taylor & Francis Books UK. Reproduced by permission of Taylor & Francis Books UK)

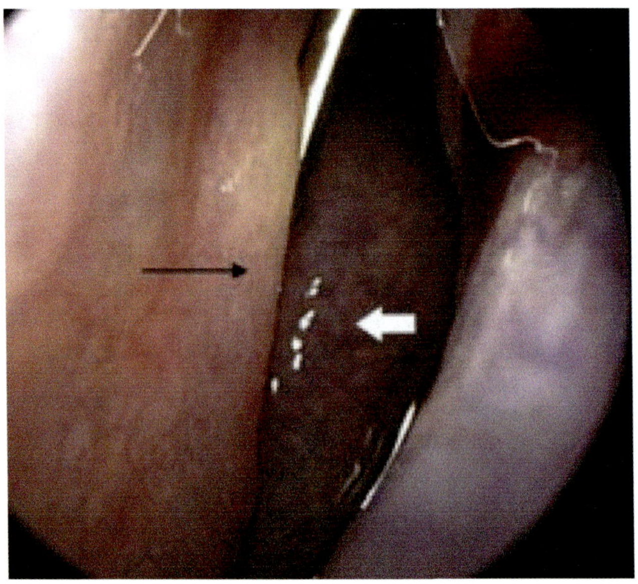

Fig. 10.2 The uncinate process (*black arrow*) and ethmoid bulla (*white arrow*) are seen (From: *Cummings Otolaryngology: Head & Neck Surgery, 5th ed.*, (ISBN: 978-0-323-05283-2). Edited by Paul W. Flint, Bruce H. Haughey, Valerie J. Lund, John K. Niparko, Mark A. Richardson, Copyright (2010) Mosby Elsevier. Reproduced by permission of Elsevier)

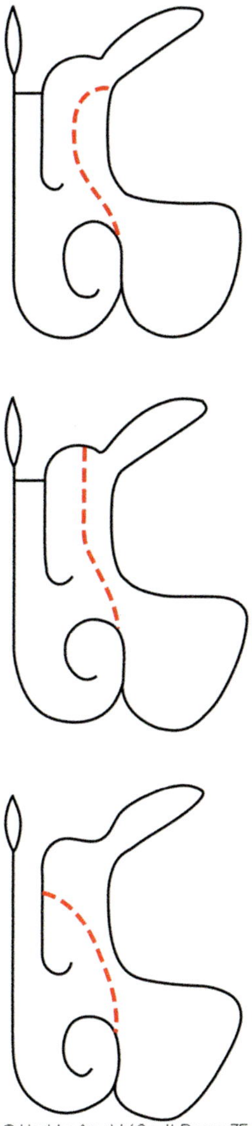

Fig. 10.3 The drainage of the frontal sinus varies based on the position of the uncinate process. The superior attachment of the uncinate process can attach to the lamina papyracea, *upper*; the roof of the ethmoid, *middle*; or the middle turbinate, *lower*. If the uncinate process attaches to the roof of the ethmoid or to the middle turbinate, the frontal sinus drains into the infundibulum. If the uncinate attaches to the lamina papyracea, the frontal sinus drains medially, next to the middle turbinate (From: Scott Browns Otorhinolaryngology 7E (ISBN: 978-0-340-80893-1). Authors Gleeson & Clarke, Copyright (2008) Taylor & Francis Books UK. Reproduced by permission of Taylor & Francis Books UK)

or the middle turbinate, all of which can cause variations in frontal sinus drainage and, thus, operative management. Preoperative identification is critical.

Maxillary Sinus

The maxilla is the second largest facial bone and forms the majority of the roof of the mouth, lateral wall, and floor of the nasal cavity and orbit. The body contains the maxillary sinus, which is relatively symmetrical with its contralateral side.

Frontal Sinus

The frontal bone forms the forehead and orbital roof. The frontal cells lie superior to the agger nasi, described below, and can show variable pneumatization. Table 10.1 describes the four pneumatization patterns, identified by Kuhn [4].

Ethmoidal Complex

Superior within the nasal vestibule is the *agger nasi*, a smooth bony swelling that lies caudal to the anterior insertion of the middle turbinate. It is an ethmoturbinal remnant present in nearly all individuals. While it may be pneumatized and thin walled, it more often has a thick bony wall and represents the most anterior ethmoid cell. Posterior to the agger nasi lies the outflow tract of the frontal sinus, the frontal recess. Because of this anatomy, the size of the agger nasi may directly influence the patency of the frontal recess. Obstruction can result in loss of ventilation and mucociliary clearance of the frontal sinus.

Posterior to the uncinate process is the *ethmoid bulla*, which is the largest of the anterior ethmoid cells. The ethmoid bulla is enclosed laterally by the lamina papyracea. The space between the ethmoid bulla and the free edge of the uncinate process defines the semilunar hiatus. Medial to this structure, the semilunar hiatus communicates with the middle meatus. Laterally and inferiorly, the semilunar hiatus also communicates with the ethmoid infundibulum, which serves as the primary drainage pathway from the maxillary sinus.

The *anterior ethmoids* are divided into infundibular cells and the ethmoid bulla. The infundibular cells include the agger nasi, the terminal cell, and the suprainfundibular cell. As mentioned above, the agger nasi lies at the attachment of the middle turbinate to the lateral nasal wall. The terminal

Table 10.1 The four types of pneumatization patterns of frontal sinus as described by Kuhn [4]

Pneumatization patterns of frontal sinus	
Type	Pattern
Type 1	A single cell superior to the agger nasi
Type 2	A tier of two or more cells above the agger nasi cell
Type 3	A single cell extending from the agger nasi cell into the frontal sinus
Type 4	An isolated cell within the frontal sinus

cell and the suprainfundibular cell are present at the superior extent of the infundibulum. The ethmoid bulla, discussed previously, is the largest cell of the ethmoid complex.

The *posterior ethmoid sinus* consists of air cells between the basal lamella and the sphenoid sinus, which vary in number, size, and shape among individuals. It lies superolateral to the sphenoid sinus. When pneumatized, the sinus extends to the lamina papyracea and anterior wall of the sphenoid. The sphenoethmoidal cell (Onodi cell) is a posterior ethmoid cell that extends superolaterally to the sphenoid sinus. The internal carotid artery and the optic nerve are within this structure.

Sphenoid Sinus

The *sphenoid sinus* is the most posterior sinus and is embedded into the clivus. It is bordered superoposteriorly by the sella turcica. The sphenoid sinus ostium is located in the anterosuperior portion of the anterior sinus wall and communicates with the sphenoethmoidal recess into the superior meatus. In order to safely enter the sinus, the surgeon must identify the location of the natural ostium, which is medial to the posterior end of the superior turbinate in 83% of cases [5]. The sphenoid sinus is surrounded by several critical structures: the internal carotid artery, the optic nerve, and the skull base.

Anterior Skull Base

The anterior skull base (ASB) is separated from the central skull base by a line running through the chiasmatic sulcus, the anterior clinoid process, along the posterior margin of the lesser sphenoid wings, and the superior rims of the greater sphenoid wings. The ASB borders the posterior wall of the frontal sinus anteriorly, the frontal bones laterally, and the planum sphenoidale or roof of the sphenoid sinus posteriorly. The components of the ASB include the orbital plates of the frontal bone, the fovea ethmoidalis, and the cribriform plate. The cribriform plate forms the medial aspect of the ASB. It is situated inferior to the ethmoid roof and is traversed by olfactory nerve fibers. It is also easily invaded by tumors. From the cribriform plate extends the fovea ethmoidalis, which forms the roof of the ethmoid sinus. The Keros classification divides the area of the olfactory fossae into three types according to the depth of the olfactory groove, described in Table 10.2.

Table 10.2 The Keros classifications of the olfactory fossa, classified by the depth of the olfactory groove within the skull base

Keros classifications	
Classification	Depth of olfactory groove
Type 1	1–3 mm
Type 2	4–7 mm
Type 3	8–16 mm

(From Keros P. on the practical value of differences in the level of the lamina cribrosa of the ethmoid. Z laryngol Rhinol Otol 1962; 41:809–13)

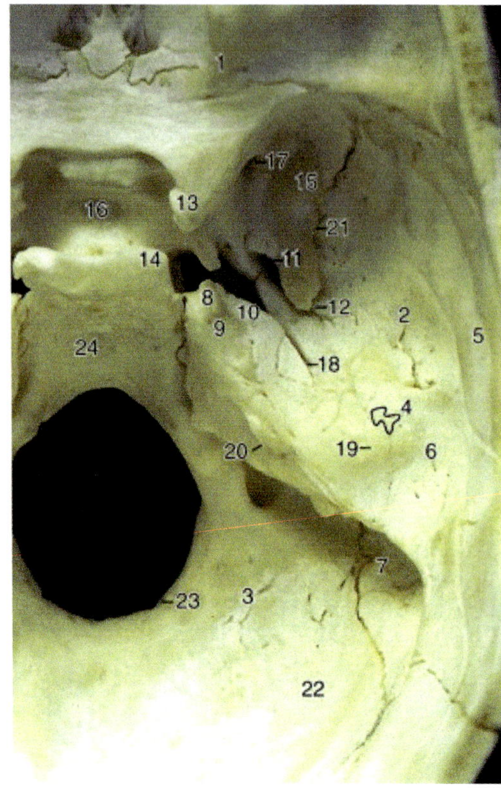

Fig. 10.4 Superior view of anterior, middle, and posterior fossae, with the projection of petrous portion of the temporal bone: *1*, anterior fossa; *2*, middle fossa; *3*, posterior fossa; *4*, petrous bone projection (*arrow*); *5*, squamous portion of the temporal bone; *6*, mastoid tegmen; *7*, sigmoid sinus impression; *8*, petrous apex; *9*, trigeminal depression (Meckel's cave); *10*, foramen lacerum region; *11*, foramen ovale; *12*, foramen spinosum; *13*, anterior clinoid process; *14*, posterior clinoid process; *15*, greater wing of sphenoid; *16*, sphenoid bone and sella; *17*, foramen rotundum; *18*, greater petrosal nerve impression; *19*, arcuate eminence; *20*, internal auditory canal region; *21*, petrosphenoidal suture; *22*, occipital bone; *23*, foramen magnum; *24*, clivus

The sella turcica and pituitary gland are part of the central skull base, while the clivus is part of the posterior skull base. These distinctions are important to make since these structures are often approached with similar surgical techniques. The ASB overlaps with the anterolateral skull base, the region between the mid-orbit, and the petrous internal carotid artery. The anterolateral skull base includes the lateral orbit, infratemporal fossa, and portions of the frontal, sphenoid, and temporal bones. This anatomical relationship is depicted in Fig. 10.4.

Sensory Innervation

The olfactory nerves (CN I) pass through the cribriform plate of the ethmoid bone into the olfactory bulb lying within the anterior cranial fossa. These fibers carry sensations of smell from the olfactory mucosa in the roof of the nasal cavity. General sensory afferent fibers to the nose are from the ophthalmic (CN V1) and maxillary (CN V2) divisions of the trigeminal nerve. The sensory innervation of the mucosa lining the anterior part of the nasal cavity is by the ethmoidal branches of the ophthalmic division of the trigeminal nerve. General sensory innervation from the lateral nasal wall and nasal septum is carried by lateral nasal branches of the maxillary division of the trigeminal nerve, and by the nasopalatine branch of the maxillary division of the trigeminal nerve, respectively. Sensory innervation to the frontal sinus is by the supraorbital branch of the CN V1 and to the sphenoid and ethmoid sinuses by the ethmoidal branches of the CN V1. Sensory innervation to the lining of the maxillary sinus is by the infraorbital branch of the maxillary division of the trigeminal nerve.

Arterial Supply

The sphenopalatine branch of the maxillary artery enters the nose from the pterygopalatine fossa, prior to splitting into the posterior lateral nasal and posterior septal branches. The sphenopalatine artery can be a persistent source for epistaxis, often requiring surgical ligation. In addition, the posterior septal branch, which passes inferior to the face of the sphenoid, serves as a key pedicle for the nasoseptal flap, a workhorse for skull base defect repairs.

The superior labial branch of the facial artery supplies the vestibule of the nose. The ophthalmic branch of the internal carotid artery supplies the roof of the nose via the anterior and posterior ethmoid arteries. Traversing posterior to the frontal recess, the anterior ethmoid artery is vulnerable to injury, resulting in significant complications including retrobulbar hemorrhage. During preoperative planning, the location of the anterior ethmoid artery – whether along the skull base or below – must be clearly identified.

Anatomical Variations

Successful surgical intervention required precise understanding of anatomical variations and appropriate preoperative planning. The *concha bullosa* is an aeration of the middle turbinate and may be unilateral or bilateral. While aeration of the inferior turbinate is uncommon, aeration of the superior turbinate can occur. If large enough, a concha bullosa in the middle turbinate may obstruct the middle meatus or the infundibulum. A *nasal septal deviation*, which may be congenital or posttraumatic, is an asymmetric bowing of the nasal septum that can impair nasal airflow, compress the middle turbinate laterally, and impair surgical instrumentation. A *paradoxical middle turbinate* occurs when the major curvature of the middle turbinate, which usually curves medially, instead projects laterally and narrows the middle meatus and infundibulum. Certain variations of the uncinate process are important to note because they may increase the risk of orbital penetration during surgery. An *atelectatic uncinate process* is a variant in which the free edge of the uncinate adheres to the orbital floor. This is often associated with a hypoplastic, opacified ipsilateral maxillary sinus. *Infraorbital cells*, a type of ethmoid air cell, extend along the medial roof of the maxillary sinus. Larger cells may cause a narrowing of the infundibulum. *Onodi cells* are lateral and posterior extensions of the posterior ethmoid cells. They result in an extension of the paranasal sinus cavity near the optic nerve, increasing its risk of injury during surgery. A *giant ethmoid bulla* can enlarge causing a narrowing or obstruction of the middle meatus and infundibulum.

Part II: Surgical Planning for Sinus and Skull Base Surgery

The previous section discussed the relevant anatomy of the sinus and skull base. This section will discuss the role of imaging in identifying anatomical landmarks and creating a surgical plan. We discuss the development of computed tomography (CT) and magnetic resonance imaging (MRI) and how these modalities have transformed the diagnosis and treatment of pathology of the sinus and skull base. Appropriate imaging is crucial for accurate diagnosis, detailed treatment planning, and optimal clinical results. This next section highlights the necessary steps for planning in sinus and skull-base surgery.

Computed Tomography

X-ray radiography has been used for years in medicine to aid in diagnosis and planning of treatment and surgery for physicians. Its use is limited, however, by the impedance of other structures that lie in the path of the X-ray beam and the two-dimensional nature of the images. X-ray radiography is also restricted by its inability to differentiate between soft tissue densities, making it difficult to recognize pathology. In 1972, the work of Allan Cormack and research by Godfrey N. Hounsfield led to the development of the first clinical CT scanner, which offered better discrimination between structures, including soft tissue, and provided a means to construct a three-dimensional image to aid in diagnosis and treatment planning.

A CT scanner works by the passage of a rotating fan beam of X-rays through a patient and the measurement of transmission of the rays at thousands of points. The obtained data is then collected by a computer, which calculates the X-ray absorption at any given spot within the patient. The data then can be either displayed on a screen or photographed. Each data point is stored in the computer memory, allowing the viewer to obtain a number of images without additional radiation. With the data, the computers can also display the data as a three-dimensional rotating image. The CT scanner offers a way to generate narrow cross-sectional images that eliminated many of the limitations of the conventional X-ray. While CT offers a reproduced local and high-contrast presentation of bony structures, patient movement and metal artifacts limit its image quality. In addition, the creation of a three-dimensional image requires additional data points, therefore requiring additional radiation exposure. These factors are compounded by the expense of CT scanners, which restricts its use in certain medical settings.

For evaluation of the paranasal sinuses and adjacent structures, CT is the modality of choice [6]. CT scan depicts fine bony anatomy of the osteomeatal channels and extent of disease. A CT scan, typically performed after medical treatment, enables a thorough evaluation of mucosal inflammation, polyp formation, anatomical variations, and bony erosion.

Magnetic Resonance Imaging

In the 1970s, Paul Lauterbar introduced the idea of applying the principles of nuclear magnetic resonance to clinical imaging. The culmination of his work became known as magnetic resonance imaging (MRI), for which he shared the Nobel Prize in Physiology or Medicine in 2003 with Peter Mansfield. MRI was first used for clinical imaging in mainstream medicine in the 1980s [7]. An MRI applies a strong magnetic field around the patient's body causing hydrogen nuclei to react to the field by aligning themselves magnetically. A radio-frequency field is then applied, and the alignment is altered, causing the nuclei to generate a rotating magnetic field detectable by a scanner, which constructs the image. Because the function of the MRI relies on hydrogen nuclei, MRI is most useful for imaging areas of the body with high concentration of hydrogen nuclei, like the brain.

Advantages of MRI are vast, including the lack of ionizing radiation making it a relatively safe procedure. As mentioned previously, MRI is also ideal for obtaining images of the central nervous system as well as stationary soft tissues [7]. Disadvantages include artifacts caused by patient motion, the high cost, length of time required for a scan, and the inability to scan patients with ferrous objects like pacemakers or cochlear implants.

For sinus imaging, magnetic resonance imaging (MRI) is particularly helpful in the evaluation of and surgical planning for the orbital and intracranial complications of inflammatory sinus disease. Furthermore, MRI has proven useful in staging neoplasms and identifying encephaloceles. To evaluate the paranasal sinuses, sagittal and axial T1-weighted images and axial and coronal T2-weighted images are ideal.

Image Fusion

There are three important tissue groups that can be appreciated within the oral and craniomaxillofacial anatomy – facial soft tissues, facial skeleton, and dentition. This triad of structures poses a challenge to optimal imaging, since no imaging technique can fully capture them completely with optimal quality. Hence, image fusion is an ideal method of imaging, which integrates different imaging techniques into one three-dimensional view. In the realm of sinus and skull base surgery, the incorporation of different imaging techniques allows for a three-dimensional view of the intricate anatomy. This modality is ideal for surgical planning.

Image Interpretation

After identification of structures on imaging, certain anatomical relationships must be noted in order to avoid complications during sinus and skull base surgery. First, the height of the ethmoid roof should be recognized, as asymmetric heights can lead to skull base defects and CSF leaks during functional endoscopic sinus surgery (FESS). Next, any dehiscence or excessive medial deviation of the lamina papyracea should be recognized. These anatomical variations can increase the risk of orbital injury during sinus surgery. Careful examination of the relationship between the sphenoid sinus and the posterior ethmoid cells with the internal carotid artery (ICA) and optic nerves is required. Expansion of the sinuses around the ICA or the optic nerve and any bony dehiscence around these structures may cause complications. The incidence of bony dehiscence around the parasellar and juxtasellar regions of the ICA is 12–22%, making its recognition crucial [8]. In order to avoid surgical complications, the relationship between the paranasal sinuses and optic nerves is also important to note. Delano characterized the relationships into four categories, described in Table 10.3 [9]. Type 2 and 3 classifications predispose the optic nerve to injury, as well as any bony dehiscence over the nerve, and

Table 10.3 Relationship between paranasal sinuses and optic nerves as described in a study by Delano [9]. The percentage of nerves studied in this study with the relationship is indicated in parentheses

Relationship between paranasal sinuses and optic nerves	
Classification	Relationship between paranasal sinuses and optic nerves
Type 1	Nerves course adjacent to the sphenoid sinus without indentation of the wall (76%)
Type 2	Nerves course adjacent to the sphenoidal sinus, causing indentation of the sinus wall (15%)
Type 3	Nerves course through the sphenoid sinus (6%)
Type 4	Nerves course immediately adjacent to the sphenoidal sinus and the posterior ethmoidal air cell (3%)

pneumatization of the anterior clinoid process. These anatomical variations should be examined with preoperative imaging in order to avoid surgical complications.

Part III: Sinus and Skull Base Surgery

Following the previous discussion of relevant anatomy and ideal imaging modalities to visualize this anatomy for optimal surgical planning, this section will review sinus surgery, specifically an external approach and its limitations, and the subsequent development of endoscopic sinus surgery. This section will conclude with the limitations of endoscopic sinus surgery, which necessitated novel approaches to the sinus and skull base.

Although the majority of sinonasal disease is now managed via endoscopic surgery, there are no absolute indications for an endoscopic approach. In fact, any sinonasal pathology may be approached endoscopically or externally. However, the development of endoscopic nasal surgery has allowed surgeons to reach disease in difficult areas of the nose, paranasal sinuses, and skull base. For certain sinonasal conditions, such as orbital or intracranial complications of acute rhinosinusitis, invasive fungal rhinosinusitis, cerebrospinal fluid (CSF) rhinorrhea, sinonasal tumors, and expansile mucoceles and polyps that cause orbital and skull base erosion, an external approach may be required. Indications for sinus surgery include:

1. Chronic rhinosinusitis
2. Recurrent acute rhinosinusitis
3. Complications of rhinosinusitis
4. Sinonasal polyposis
5. Mucoceles
6. Intractable epistaxis
7. Cerebrospinal fluid rhinorrhea and anterior meningoencephaloceles
8. Noninvasive fungal ball
9. Invasive fungal rhinosinusitis
10. Foreign body removal
11. Choanal atresia repair
12. Headaches and facial pain
13. Tumors
14. Expanded transnasal approaches to the skull base and orbit

Endoscopic Sinus and Skull Base Surgery

Initial endoscopic examination of the nose, which began in the 1970s in Europe, was ideal for magnification of the field, but did not facilitate the dexterity that was required for optimal sinus surgery. As a result, methods to visualize the nasal cavity and paranasal sinuses with angulated scopes became an area of study. Functional endoscopic sinus surgery (FESS), first introduced by Kennedy to the United States in 1985, has now become a well-established standard of care for many sinus and skull base pathologies [10]. The work of both Messerklinger and Stammberger contributed greatly to the development of FESS [11, 12]. Today, it is the standard surgical approach for the majority of sinus procedures. Prior to the advent of the endoscope, sinus surgery was primarily aimed at the frontal and maxillary sinuses, which was performed externally and with the use of a headlight transnasally. The Caldwell-Luc procedure, developed by George Caldwell in 1893 and Henry Luc in 1897, was the primary approach to the maxillary sinus [13, 14]. The procedure involved creating an opening in the canine fossa with an intranasal antrostomy. Today, the Caldwell-Luc procedure has limited indications, and FESS has instead become the preferred procedure.

FESS has the advantage of minimizing trauma to the outer skin, the oral mucosa, bony architecture of the face and the sinuses, and the respiratory and olfactory mucosa as compared to external approaches [15]. Furthermore, it provides good magnification and ideal angulations within the nasal cavity and paranasal sinuses. These advances enable improved visualization and precise instrumentation. The value of the endoscope is further appreciated by examining its portability, which permits physicians to utilize it in the office. The objective of FESS is to restore paranasal sinus function by re-creating the physiologic pattern of ventilation and mucociliary clearance. As an adjunct to medical therapy, surgery attempts to remove diseased mucosa and bone and preserve normal tissue. One aim is to widen the natural ostia of the diseased sinuses in order to allow for increased drainage and symptom relief. Toward this aim, the anterior osteomeatal complex is a primary target for the surgeon because minimal inflammation in the area can lead to disease in the maxillary, anterior ethmoid, and frontal sinuses. Bony septations should be removed, and aggressive mucosa removal should be avoided as this can cause postoperative problems with healing. Despite successful and adequate surgery, symptoms and disease may persist, requiring continuous medical therapy and, in some cases, revision surgery.

Technological advancement continually improves the endoscope to enhance the ease and safety of procedures. Increased resolution and better angular scopes are just some examples of improvements over the years. In 1959, Harold H. Hopkins developed the rod-lens system, and Karl Storz coupled this system with a fiber-optic light transmission technology in 1960. The Hopkins rod-lens telescope replaced the traditional endoscope, which caused significant scar formation, osteogenesis, and pain by denuding bone of mucosa [16]. The new rod-lens system of image transmission was much different from the traditional endoscopic. Instead of an air interspace between glass lenses, Hopkins used solid glass rods with lenses cemented between them, increasing light transmission and image definition. This new technology allowed surgeons to view quality images. These scopes provide a much wider viewing angle and smaller diameter than its predecessors, with improved resolution, contrast, and brightness. In addition to this advancement, the introduction of Tru-Cut instruments and the microdebrider allowed for clean removal of tissue without stripping of mucosa and precise surgical technique. Today, the use of high-resolution computerized tomography coupled with intraoperative techniques, such as better nasal endoscopes, has expanded the scope of endoscopic sinus surgery [17].

Limitations of Endoscopic Surgery

Despite the many advances in endoscopic sinus surgery, intraoperative complications such as bleeding, CSF leaks, orbital trauma, and, rarely, death still occur [18]. In part, these complications and surgical challenges are a manifestation of the challenges of endoscopic sinus surgery. One major disadvantage of nasal endoscopic surgery is its inherent two-dimensional view, which results from the use of a single lens within the telescopes. Given the narrow confinements of the sinonasal tract and skull base, there is little room for surgical error and an absolute requirement of technical precision. Narrow spaces coupled with anatomical variations and obscured visibility due to intraoperative bleeding make it difficult for the surgeon to locate the exact position of the surgical instrument. In order to achieve greater precision during surgery and surgical instrument localization, image-guided navigation systems were developed.

Part IV: Image-Guided Navigation Systems

This section will describe navigation technologies, also known as image-guided navigation systems that have revolutionized the field of sinus and skull base surgery. This segment will include a thorough review of the two systems used today, optical and electromagnetic systems, and reference of the commercially available systems. In concluding, this section will highlight the clinical outcomes of image-guided sinus and skull base surgery. Finally, the limitations of navigation systems and its future directions will be discussed.

In 1987, Schlondorff introduced the first navigation system for ear, nose, and throat (ENT) surgery based on preoperative CT images [19]. Anon first described computer-assisted endoscopic sinus surgery in 1994 using a frameless stereotactic system with the articulated arms of the ISG Viewing Wand (ISH Technologies Inc., Mississauga, Ontario, Canada) [20]. Since the ISG Viewing Wand, computer-assisted technology has dramatically improved with several accurate and easy-to-use tracking systems now available.

Today, these computer-assisted surgery (CAS) systems allow the surgeon to use the patient's preoperative images displayed in all three anatomic planes (coronal, axial, and sagittal) for intraoperative localization of anatomy. These systems reformat thin-cut CT and/or MRI scans to create three-dimensional views, allowing the surgeon to more accurately target pathology and steer away from areas of danger. In addition to anatomical localization, these systems help to identify surgical instruments within a surgical field, calculate the precise location of the instrument tip in relation to the patient, and project the instrument location onto previously obtained imaging studies. The surgeon can navigate through downloaded CT and MR image or a combination of the two data sets fused together or superimposed [21]. Such fusion data sets are useful in complex cases of noninflammatory disease that may involve the skull base.

Since their initial use, these image-guided systems have now become a near necessity in complex skull base procedures. These navigation systems are best applied when additional information beyond the endoscopic or surgical view is beneficial to the operative procedure and surgical outcome. The use of these systems, however, should always depend upon disease-specific and surgeon-related factors, including clinical experience and familiarity to the technology, on a case-by-case basis. These systems are often used in the resection of extensive disease or revision surgery, in which pathology, extensive scarring, adhesions, and prior instrumentation may destroy traditional anatomic landmarks [16]. Navigation aids in identifying these distorted landmarks and distinguishing pathological regions from normal areas [22, 23]. In certain malignancy cases, navigation systems can reveal the complete extent of tumor invasion, which may not be apparent through the endoscope, thus allowing for complete tumor resection [24]. The American Academy of Otolaryngology – Head and Neck Surgery supports the use of CAS in special situations such as:

1. Revision sinus surgery
2. Distorted sinus anatomy of development, postoperative, or traumatic origin
3. Extensive sinonasal polyposis
4. Pathology involving the frontal, posterior, ethmoid, and sphenoid sinuses
5. Disease abutting the skull base, orbit, optic nerve, or carotid artery
6. CSF rhinorrhea or conditions where there is a skull base defect
7. Benign and malignant sinonasal neoplasms

Image Registration

An image-guidance system requires a system of image registration in order to use preoperative images of the patient's anatomy for intraoperative use. The accuracy of surgical navigation depends on the quality of image registration. In the registration process, the navigation system maps points from the patient's head while on the operating table to corresponding points on the CT scan using a transformation matrix. From these matched points, the navigation system correlates the scan with real-time operative positioning. Thus, any errors in the image registration process could result in inaccurate mapping between the patient's true position and the CT scan.

There are two primary methods of image registration, optical and electromagnetic. Both systems offer an accuracy of within 2 mm [25]. Each of these systems accounts for intraoperative head movement by securing a headset onto the patient. Some commercially available navigation systems are listed in Table 10.4 with details about the type of tracking system and reported accuracies. Figure 10.5 depicts the process of registration by the surgeon using the BrainLAB system by VectorVision.

Electromagnetic Navigation Systems

Electromagnetic systems use a radio-frequency transmitter within the headset and a receiver positioned within the instrument. The headset and instrument are attached via wires to the system hardware. These systems are at risk for interference from metal instruments within the field or metal operating room table. For this reason, the use of electromagnetic navigation systems must be avoided in patients with electronic devices within the brain or nervous system. In such patients, optical tracking systems can be used as an alternative. Use of electromagnetic navigation systems is no longer contraindicated in patients with cardiac pacemakers.

Table 10.4 Reported accuracies of commercially available navigation systems

Commercially available navigation systems			
System (vendor)	Tracking system	Registration type	Reported accuracy
InstaTrack, (GE Navigation & Visualization, Lawrence, MA)	Electromagnetic	Automatic PPR CBR	2.28 mm 1.97 mm 1.50 mm
LandmarX, (Medtronic Xomed, Jacksonville, Fl)	Optical	Automatic PPR CBR	N/A 1.69 mm No report
Stryker Navigation System, (Stryker Leibinger, Kalamazoo, MI)	Optical	Automatic PPR CBR	N/A 1.6 mm No report
VectorVision, (BrainLAB, Heimstetten, Germany)	Optical	Automatic PPR CBR	No report 1.57 mm 2.4 mm

Adapted from Ref. [26], with permission from Elsevier, NY, NY

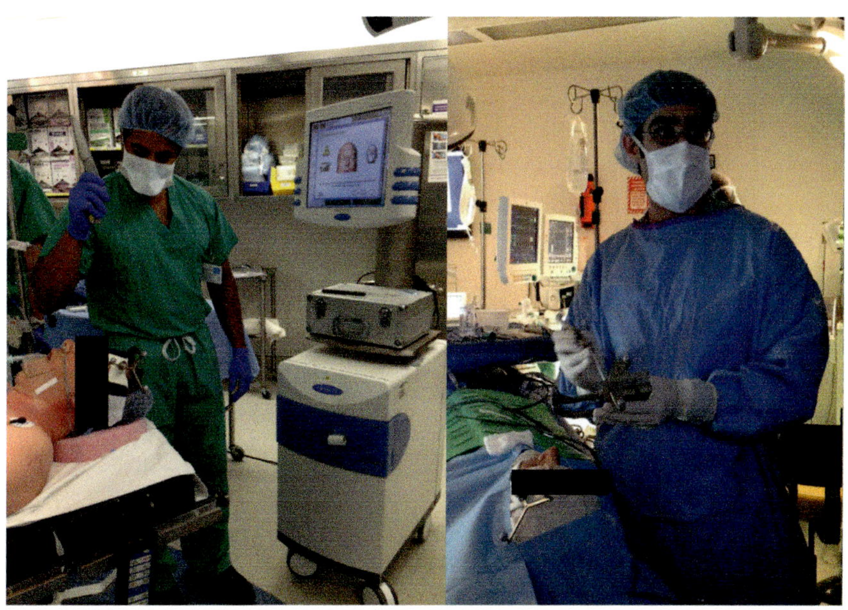

Fig. 10.5 Picture showing surgeons during process of registration for BrainLAB by VectorVision. *Left*, the surgeon registers the patient's preoperative CT images to the headset; *right*, the surgeon registers the suction instrument to the preoperative CT images

The Fiagon Electromagnetic Navigation System, a system widely used in Germany, consists of a navigation screen, navigation module, and tracking pointer. Other systems have similar interfaces and components. Within the 18″ navigation screen, there are four windows. Three windows display raw CT and/or MRI data in the axial, coronal, and sagittal planes, and the fourth window displays the video image of the surgical field as viewed by the endoscope. The navigation module contains a DVD or CD drive, USB port, plug points for navigation sensor, patient localizer, and pointer system, which consists of a connecting plug, sensor cable, and pointer [27].

To begin the process of image registration and image guidance, preoperative CT and/or MRI data is saved in a DICOM 3.0 format on a CD and loaded onto the workstation. A secured headset is strapped to the patient and moves along with the patient's head in order to maintain registration throughout the surgical procedure. After appropriate registration, a tracking probe is used to show position with respect to the orthogonal CT images of the patient, and a cursor moves across the CT image in accordance with the movement of the probe. See Fig. 10.6 for schematic depicting the steps necessary for image registration and usage of the image-guidance system.

For optimal image registration, three bony prominences are selected that are located directly beneath the skin in order to create a triangular electromagnetic field. Two reference points are the lateral canthi of the right and left eyes and the third reference point in the base of the philtrum. These reference points are then touched with the tip of a reference pointer. For the Fiagon navigation system, a surface registration is used, while for the Instatrak 3500 Plus, an automatic registration system is used. During automatic registration, the patient wears the same headset during preoperative CT scan and the surgical procedure. The headset enables a process of correlating the patient's medical images to the patient's actual anatomy automatically. The electromagnetic sensors, which are attached to the instrument and headset, register to show the position of the instrument tip with respect to the CT images of the patient. This registration method varies from system to system [22].

Optical Navigation Systems

Optical navigation or tracking systems, on the other hand, use infrared light and a camera positioned above the patient's head to track the headset and instruments, which are affixed with reflective spheres. A source emits infrared light that reflects off the spheres back to the camera. While this is a wireless system, it requires a clear pathway between the tracking device and instruments. If the pathway between the tracking device and instruments is disturbed at any point during surgery, the images on the navigation screen are distorted. Metson compared the two systems and found no significant differences in blood loss or complications [25]. For image registration, either point merge protocol or surface merge protocol is used. In a point merge protocol, anatomical fiducial points are used for marking, whereas in the surface merge protocol, contour mapping is used for marking. Figure 10.7 shows intraoperative use of the BrainLAB image-guidance system by VectorVision during a repair of a cerebrospinal fluid (CSF) leak. Table 10.5 highlights the key differences between electromagnetic and optical tracking navigation systems.

Data Integration

The computer workstation integrates this data set with continuous information from the tracking system and projects the location of the tracked instrument onto all three CT views on the workstation [28]. The CT images are taken preoperatively and do not change during surgery. Any movement of the instrument tip is shown superimposed onto the preoperative CT images in real time. Data from digital angiography, ultrasound, and PET scans can be fused for further aid in navigation. Advanced features of the software also allow for three-dimensional reconstruction, addition and subtraction tools, and cutout view reconstruction of CT images for intricate preoperative planning. Today's technology also allows any rigid surgical instrument to be tracked, including angled suctions, curettes, drills, and microdebriders. The tracking of curved and powered instruments allows for localization in difficult-to-access areas.

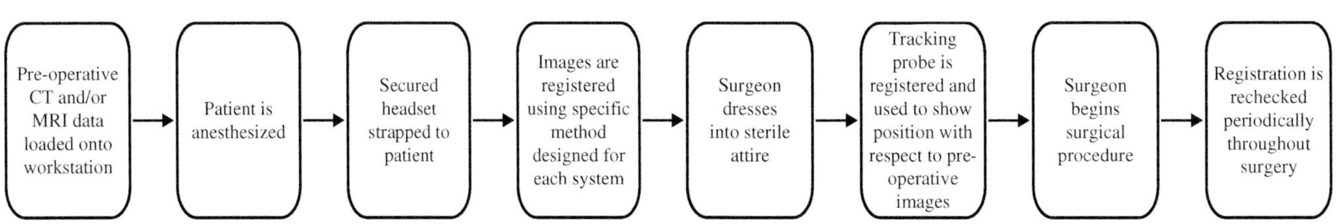

Fig. 10.6 Schematic drawing of the steps necessary for optimal image registration and use of the image-guided systems

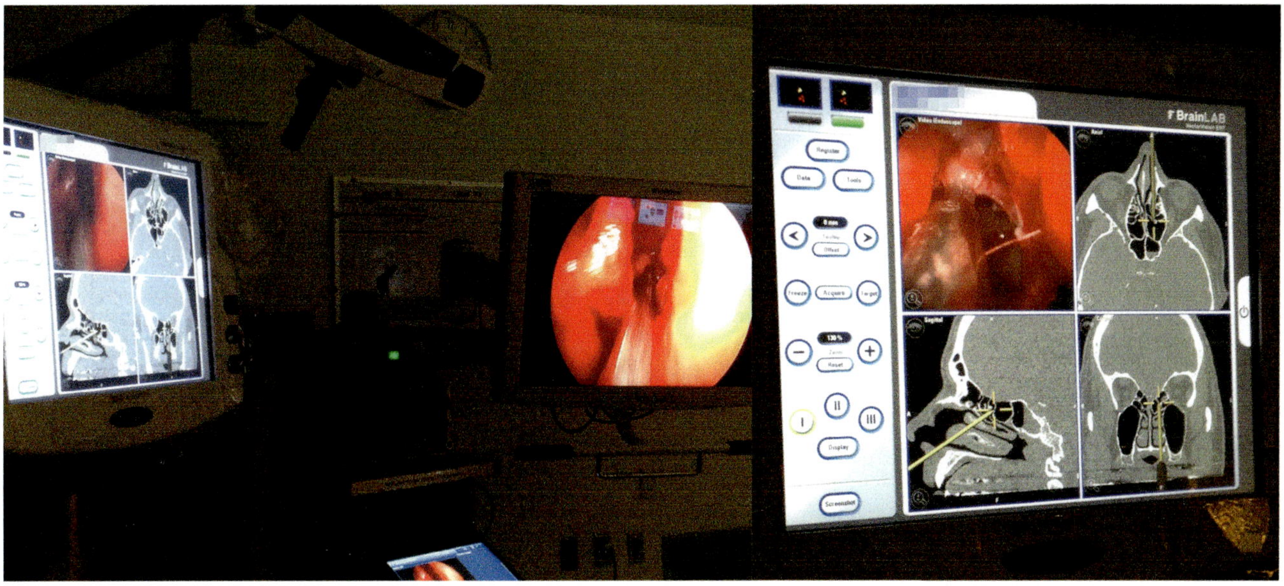

Fig. 10.7 Intraoperative use of the BrainLAB system by VectorVision. (**a**) The BrainLAB monitor on the *left* and the endoscopic camera view on the *right*. (**b**) A close-up of the preoperative CT scans with instrument tracking shown as *yellow* markings on the CT scan

Table 10.5 Comparison between optical and electromagnetic tracking systems

Optical and electromagnetic tracking systems		
	Electromagnetic tracking system	Optical tracking system
Registering probe	Electromagnetic sensor that is integrated within the headset	Four infrared light-emitting diodes with exact positions of the diodes measured by an infrared 3-D-based localizer
Headset	Headset with navigation sensor is placed on patient's head	Headset that allows attachment of reference frame with light-emitting diodes is placed on patient's head
Registration	Surface registration is used in the Fiagon system; automatic registration is used in the Instatrak 3500 Plus and fusion systems	Point merge protocol or surface merge protocol
Registration verification	Registration is verified by localizing bony landmarks on the face	Registration is verified by localizing bony landmarks on the skull and nasal cavity
Instrument localization	The surgical instrument can be localized within a triangular electromagnetic field at any point during surgery to verify exact anatomical location	The surgical instrument can be localized at any time unless there is an interruption in the line of sight between the overhead digitizer, surgical instrument, or the surgeon's operating hand

Reproduced from Ref. [27], with permission

Clinical Outcomes

While image-guided systems have been in use for years, no clear benefit of image guidance has been demonstrated. Tabaee et al. evaluated incidences of intraoperative complications, major postoperative complications, revision procedures, and postoperative SNOT-20 symptom scores and found no significant difference in patients who underwent image-guided versus non-image-guided ESS [29]. However, a higher incidence of CSF leak was noted in the group that received ESS without image guidance.

Another study found no significant reduction in complications with the use of image guidance [30]. In this study, optical and electromagnetic-based image-guidance systems were used during endoscopic surgery on patients with disease of the paranasal sinuses, orbit, skull base, and temporal bone. This intervention group was compared to controls who underwent similar surgery without image guidance. The study found a complication rate of 2.7% in the image-guidance group and a complication rate of 4.7% in the control group, but a statistically significant difference was not noted between these two groups.

One study, by Fried et al., does confirm a lower major complication rate for sinus surgery using navigation technology [31]. In this study, major complications were defined as inadvertent entry into any area beyond the nasal cavity and paranasal sinuses, a postoperative bleed requiring return to the operative room, and having to abort an operation for any reason. The study concluded that navigation technology may reduce some of the adverse intraoperative events associated with ESS and allow for a more thorough procedure due to increased ease of access to the sinuses. This study did, however, find a greater operative time and blood loss in the cohort that received sinus surgery using navigation technology.

Other studies have shown, however, that more complicated sinus procedures, such as frontal sinus surgeries that require localization of complex frontal sinus outflow anatomy, have a significantly reduced rate of complications when using image guidance [32, 33]. In addition, approaches to the sellar, parasellar, and orbital areas have been significantly safer and can now be explored with greater precision and accuracy since the use of navigation systems [24]. For example, a study by Sadoughi has shown the sphenoid sinus often has altered anatomy that can be approached with greater surgical precision with the aid of navigation systems [34].

Limitations of Image Guidance

One major limitation of image guidance is the increased costs associated with the use of systems. These costs, which can be attributed to many different sources, are likely to decrease as the learning curve associated with the technology improves. Metson et al. showed an average increase in operative time of 17.4 min/case, but this is likely to decrease with improved efficiency of the surgeon, leading to overall decreased operative time [25]. Even with the increase in operative time, the possibility of a decreased complication rate for more advanced procedures may represent a cost benefit.

Another source of increased cost is the initial purchase of the system by the institution and subsequent increased billing expenditures each time the system is used. At Massachusetts Eye and Ear Infirmary, the use of an image-guidance system is based on a hospital charge of $182 and anesthesia charge of $66 for each 15-minute interval of operating room time. According to Metson, hospital charges increased by approximately $496 per case [25].

Another major limitation of image guidance is the potential for technical errors intraoperatively. This may be related to headsets, which are placed intraoperatively, moving after registration and thereby contributing to inaccuracy of anatomy localization. This issue can be avoided by frequent corroboration with clinical landmarks and evaluation of the headset for any movement during the procedures. Additionally, preoperative CT scans may not accurately reflect the intraoperative disease process. To address such issues, attempts have been made to overcome this drawback by acquiring intraoperative CT scans. Brown et al. reported that near-real-time image-guided surgery using intraoperative fluoroscopic CT scans was possible [35]. This system allows for reconstruction of CT-like images from a series of intraoperative fluoroscopic scans that can be integrated into an image-guided system. In another study by Jackman et al., 20 subjects undergoing ESS received intraoperative CT scans which were obtained in less than 40 seconds and could be loaded to an image-guidance system [36]. They report that information gained from these intraoperative scans led to additional surgery in 30% of patients, which may have otherwise required a revision surgery without the intraoperative information.

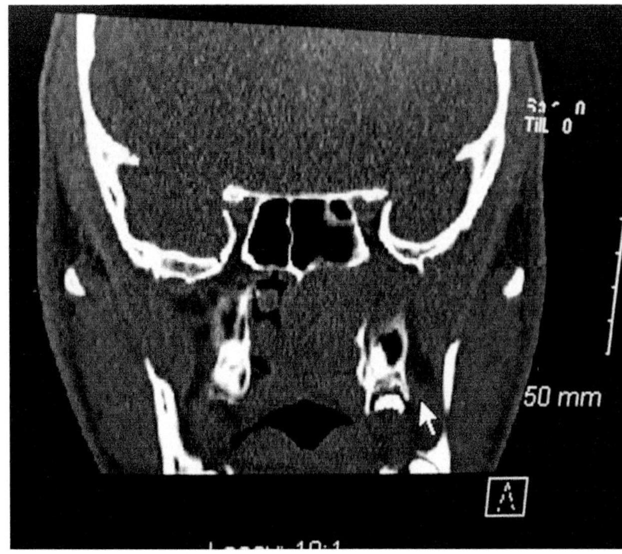

Fig. 10.8 Coronal-cut CT scan in bone window through the posterior nasopharynx showing the extension of the lesion into the sphenopalatine fossa

Clinical Case Report

An 18-year-old male presented with nasal congestion and history of frequent bilateral epistaxis for several months. The bleeding was heavy, often with large clots. CT scan of the sinuses revealed a large left sphenopalatine fossa hypervascular mass, 4.3 × 3.1 cm in size, with heterogenous enhancement with extension into the posterior nasopharynx. This is shown in Fig. 10.8. These findings were most consistent with a juvenile nasopharyngeal angiofibroma. The patient underwent endoscopic removal of the lesion after preoperative embolization. Image-guided surgery was used to guide the resection. The Fusion ENT Navigation System (Medtronic, Minneapolis, MN, USA) was used and is shown in Fig. 10.9. With the help of the image guidance, endoscopic transnasal removal of the tumor from the difficult-to-access sphenopalatine fossa was possible. The patient did well postoperatively.

Future Directions

Research and development efforts to improve navigation systems in sinus and skull base surgery are ongoing and widespread. One particular area of focus is integration of MRI and CT images to provide both enhanced visualization of intracranial soft tissues and enhanced delineation of bony

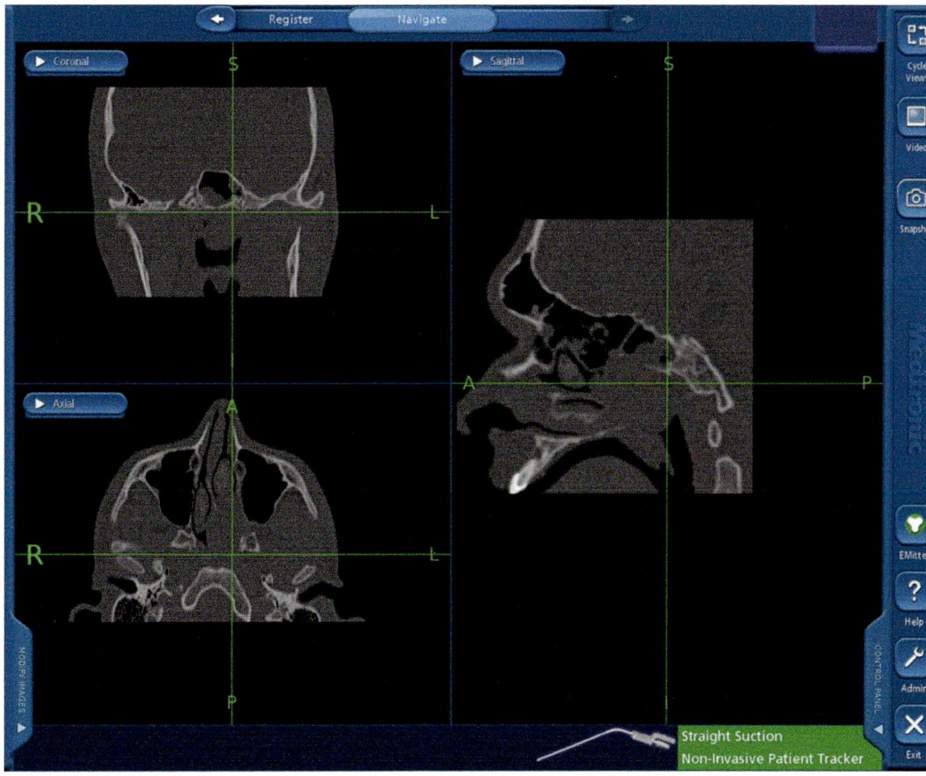

Fig. 10.9 Image of Fusion ENT Navigation System screen while being used intraoperatively (Medtronic, Minneapolis, MN, USA)

structures. Particularly in joint cases between neurosurgeons and otolaryngologists, this area of navigation technology may represent a significant opportunity to optimize surgical outcomes.

Further advances strive to make the process of registration and usage of the navigator less time-consuming and more user-friendly. New areas of investigation include the integration of robotic surgery with navigation systems to develop advanced surgical techniques. In these robot-assisted surgeries, there are four articulated arm ports. While two of the arm ports carry right and left surgical arms, one carries a dual-channel endoscope coupled with a camera for 3-D visualization of the surgical field, and the fourth is used as a spare arm. These robotic surgeries allow for two-handed tremor-free procedures and eliminated the need for manual stabilization [37]. The integration of navigation systems to robot-assisted sinus and skull base surgery is a scope of further development.

Conclusion

This chapter has discussed sinus and skull base anatomy relevant for sinus surgery, the developments in sinus and skull base surgery, and the need for novel techniques like navigation. The contribution of these technologies to craniomaxillofacial surgery has been significant, and the introduction of navigation systems to sinus and skull base surgeries has revolutionized the field. Previously difficult surgeries have been facilitated by the ability to localize the surgical instruments, and their trajectory on a continuous basis. While the systems may pose an increased initial expense, navigation systems have provided a significant advantage, allowing increased and precise access to the sinus and skull base. Improved delineation of anatomical landmarks with this technology has enabled the expansion of endoscopic sinus and skull base surgery. With continued development and research within the field of image-guided surgery, new discoveries will continue to advance the field in order to further facilitate surgery, eliminate costs, and decrease complication rates.

References

1. Lund V. The evolution of surgery on the maxillary sinus for chronic rhinosinusitis. Laryngoscope. 2002;112:415–9.
2. Vining EM, Kennedy DW. The transmigration of endoscopic sinus surgery from Europe to the United States. ENT J. 1994;73:456–60.
3. Stammberger H. The evolution of functional endoscopic sinus surgery. ENT J. 1994;73:451–5.
4. Kuhn FA. Chronic frontal sinusitis: the endoscopic frontal recess approach. Operat Tech Otolaryngol Head Neck Surg. 1996;7:222–9.
5. Kim HU, Kim SS, Kang SS, Chung IH, Lee JG, Yoon JH. Surgical anatomy of the natural ostium of the sphenoid sinus. Laryngoscope. 2001;111:1599–602.

6. Zinreich SJ, Benson ML, Oliverio PS. Sinonasal cavities: CT normal anatomy, imaging of the osteomeatal complex, and functional endoscopic surgery. In: Som P, Curtin H, editors. Head and Neck Imaging. 3rd ed. St. Louis: Mosby; 1996.
7. Mettler FA. Chapter 1: Introduction. In: Mettler FA, editor. Essentials of Radiology. Third ed. Philadelphia: Saunders by Elsevier; 2014.
8. Johnson DW, Hopkins RJ, Hanafee WN, Fisk JD. The unprotected parasphenoidal carotid artery studied by high-resolution computed tomography. Radiology. 1985;155:137.
9. Delano M, Fun FY, Zinreich SJ. Optic nerve relationship to the posterior paranasal sinuses: a CT anatomic study. AJNR Am J Neuroradiol. 1996;17:669.
10. Kennedy DW. Functional endoscopic sinus surgery: technique. Arch Otolaryngol. 1985;111:643–9.
11. Messerklinger W. Endoscopy of the Nose. Baltimore: Urban & Schwarzenberg; 1978.
12. Stammberger H. Endoscopic endonasal surgery – concepts in treatment of recurring rhinosinusitis. Part I. Anatomic and pathophysiologic considerations. Otolaryngol Head Neck Surg. 1986;94:143–7.
13. Caldwell GW. The accessory sinus of the nose, and an improved method of treatment for suppuration of the maxillary antrum. N Y Med J. 1893;58:526–8.
14. Tange RA. Some historical aspects of the surgical treatment of the infected maxillary sinus. Rhinology. 1991;29:155–62.
15. Hosemann W, Gode U, Wagner W. Epidemiology, pathophysiology of nasal polyposis, and spectrum of endonasal sinus surgery. Am J Otolaryngol. 1994;15:85–98.
16. Palmer O, Moche JA, Matthews S. Endoscopic surgery of the nose and paranasal sinus. Oral Maxillofac Surg Clin N Am. 2012;24:275–83.
17. Al-Swiahb JN, Al Dousary SH. Computer-aided endoscopic sinus surgery: a retrospective comparative study. Ann Saudi Med. 2010;30:149–52.
18. Sindwani R. Image-guided surgery of the paranasal sinuses and skull base. Mo Med. 2008;105:257–61.
19. Schlöndorff G, Mosges R, Meyer-Ebrecht D, Krybus W, Adams L. CAS (computer assisted surgery). A new procedure in head and neck surgery. HNO. 1989;37:187–90.
20. Anon JB, Rontal M, Zinreich SJ. Computer-assisted endoscopic sinus surgery-current experience and future developments. Op Tech Otolaryngol Head Neck Surg. 1995;6:163–70.
21. Sindwani R, Bucholz R. The next generation of navigational technology. Otolaryngol Clin N Am. 2005;38:551–62.
22. Javer AR, Genoway KA. Patient quality of life improvements with and without computer assistance in sinus surgery: outcomes study. J Otolaryngol. 2006;35:373–9.
23. Ceylan S, Koc K, Anik I. Extended endoscopic approaches for midline skull-base lesions. Neurosurg Rev. 2009;32:309–19.
24. Ahn JY, Jung JY, Kim J, Lee KS, Kim SH. How to overcome the limitations to determine the resection margin of pituitary tumours with low-field intra-operative MRI during trans-sphenoidal surgery: usefulness of gadolinium-soaked cotton Pledgets. Acta Neurochir. 2008;150:763–71.
25. Metson R, Gliklich RE, Cosenza M. A comparison of image guidance systems for sinus surgery. Laryngoscope. 1998;108:1164–70.
26. Knott PD, Batra PS, Citardi MJ. Computer aided surgery: concepts and applications in rhinology. Otolaryngol Clin North Am. 2006;39:503–22.
27. Irugu DVK, Stammberger HR. A note on the technical aspects and evaluation of the role of navigation system in endoscopic endonasal surgeries. Indian J Otolaryngol Head Neck Surg. 2014;66:S307–13.
28. Reardon EJ. The impact of image-guidance systems on sinus surgery. Otolaryngol Clin N Am. 2005;38:515–25.
29. Tabaee A, Hsu AK, Shrime MG, Rickert S, Close LG. Quality of life and complications following image-guided endoscopic sinus surgery. Otolaryngol Head Neck Surg. 2006;135:76–80.
30. Metson R, Cosenza M, Gliklich RE, Montgomery WW. The role of image-guidance systems for head and neck surgery. Arch Otolaryngol Head Neck Surg. 1999;125:1100–4.
31. Fried MP, Moharir VM, Shin J, Taylor-Becker M, Morrison P. Comparison of endoscopic sinus surgery with and without image guidance. Am J Rhinol. 2002;16:193–7.
32. Sindwani R, Metson R. Impact of image-guidance on complications during osteoplastic frontal sinus surgery. Otolaryngol Head Neck Surg. 2004;131:150–5.
33. Sindwani R, Metson R. Image-guided frontal sinus surgery. Otolaryngol Clin N Am. 2005;38:461–71.
34. Sadoughi B, Brown SM, Nachlas NE, Fried MP Image-guided surgery. http://emedicine.medscape.com/article/875524 (2010). Accessed 7 Apr 2014.
35. Brown SM, Sadoughi B, Cuellar H, von Jako R, Fried MP. Feasibility of near real-time image-guided sinus surgery using intraoperative fluoroscopic computed axial tomography. Otolaryngol Head Neck Surg. 2007;136:268–73.
36. Jackman AM, Palmer IN, Hiv AG, Kennedy DW. Use of intraoperative CT scanning in endoscopic sinus surgery: a preliminary report. AM J Rhinol. 2008 Mar–Apr;22(2):170–4.
37. O'Malley BW Jr, Weinstein GS. Robotic skull base surgery. Arch Otolaryngol Head Neck Surg. 2007;133:1215–9.

Cranioplasty: Development and Clinical Use in Neurosurgery

11

Kyle J. Riley, Anthony B. Costa, Joshua B. Bederson, and Raj Shrivastava

The Role of Cranial Implants

Purpose

Cranioplasty is the repair of a cranial defect or deformation through the use of a cranial implant. Its basic goals are straightforward: to provide the functionality and structure of the missing cranial bone and to support the soft tissues [1]. Cranioplasty is undertaken to protect the brain from damage that could occur from the defect, cosmetic enhancement, and psychosocial considerations. It has been shown to improve electroencephalographic abnormalities, cerebral blood flow, cerebrospinal fluid dynamics, and cerebral metabolism [2, 3]. See Fig. 11.1a–c for images that illustrate a patient specific digitally fabricated cranial implant.

Ideal Implant Material

The characteristics identified that embody the ideal implant include: (1) malleable to allow for precise fit and complete closure, (2) strong but not heavy, (3) infection resistant, (4) non-thermally conductive, (5) implant ease, (6) biocompatible and chemically inert, (7) readily available, (8) low cost, and (9) radiolucent [3]. Implant materials each have their own advantages and disadvantages. There is no one material considered ideal for all circumstances.

K.J. Riley (✉)
Icahn School of Medicine at Mount Sinai,
1468 Madison Avenue, Annenberg 8-35, New York, NY 10029, USA
e-mail: kyle.riley@icahn.mssm.edu

A.B. Costa • J.B. Bederson • R. Shrivastava
Department of Neurosurgery, The Mount Sinai Hospital, Icahn School of Medicine at Mount Sinai, 1468 Madison Avenue, Annenberg 8-35, New York, NY 10029, USA
e-mail: anthony.costa@mssm.edu; joshua.bederson@mountsinai.org; raj.shrivastava@mountsinai.org

Historical Development and Perspective

The evolution of cranioplasty has been driven by warfare, new technologies, and surgical experience.

Archeological evidence supports the practice of cranial reconstruction dating back to at least 3000 BC in many ancient civilizations such as the Incans, the Britons, and the North Africans [4, 5]. These findings reveal that the Incans used precious metals and natural materials to repair head trephinations [4–6]. The material used was predicated on the person's socioeconomic status: gold and silver for the nobility and shells and gourds for the common man [3, 4]. Although the precise reasons for trephinations are unknown, archeological evidence suggests that warfare played a large role [7]. It is estimated that traumatic injuries, primarily from battle, account for 28–46% of the trephinations [7]. Historical findings of trepanation are more abundant than cranial repair [4, 6]. One theory suggests that the precious metals used were removed before burial which would cause the rate of cranial reconstructions to be underreported [4, 6].

Further evidence of cranioplasty practice and advancement was limited until 1505 AD when Ibrahim Bin Abdullah, an Ottoman military surgeon, wrote, in his surgery textbook *Alâim-i Cerrâhin* (*Wonders of Surgeons*), the first known documented description of cranioplasty. This described the use of goat and canine xenografts for cranial repair [5, 7]. In Europe, Fallopius and Petronius recommended a gold plate to repair a skull defect in the late sixteenth century [3–7]. Before the rediscovery of Ibrahim's book, Job Janszoon van Meekeren, a Dutch surgeon, provided the first report of a successful bone graft cranioplasty in 1668. Bone from a dead dog's cranium was used to repair the cranial defect a man received from a sword wound [3–5]. The bone grafts from many different animals were tested including dog, ape, rabbit, and calf. In 1901, Marchand found that animal horns worked well. Additional procedures by other surgeons using ivory, ox, and buffalo horn reported similar results [3–5].

A.M. Greenberg (ed.), *Digital Technologies in Craniomaxillofacial Surgery*, https://doi.org/10.1007/978-1-4939-1532-3_11

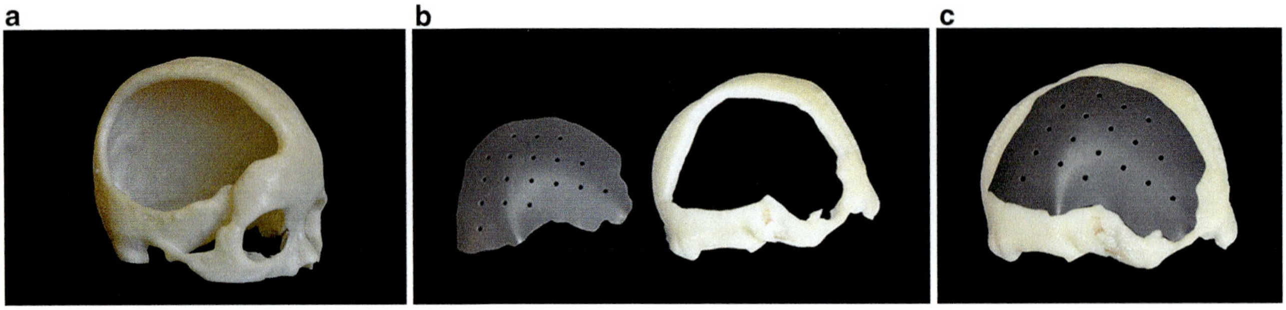

Fig. 11.1 (**a**) Skull model for designing a patient specific digitally fabricated cranial implant, (**b**) implant with skull model, (**c**) implant simulation in skull

Ultimately, the use of xenografts was replaced by more successful techniques.

Cranioplasty was also practiced using allografts. In 1915, Morestin experimented with cadaver cartilage. World War I was underway, and this became a popular technique. However, its popularity decreased because of its lack of strength and calcification problems. In 1917, Sicard and Dambrin tried cadaveric skull, but it failed due to high infection rate and bone resorption issues [3–5].

The first documented human autologous bone graft is credited to Walther in 1821 who, after a trephination, replaced the bone plug and observed partial healing [3–5]. By his successful reimplantation of calvarial bone fragments in 1878, William Macewen, a Scottish physician, may be considered the father of modern autologous bone grafting [4, 5]. From 1890 to 1917, autologous graft sources for cranioplasty included temporalis muscle and fascia, whole ribs, scapula, ilium and split ribs [5], and split-thickness calvarial grafts [4]. As currently practiced, the use of autologous split rib grafts for large cranial defects was pioneered by Longacre and DeStefano in 1957 [5].

During the Crimean War (1853–1856) and the US Civil War (1861–1865), the availability of general anesthesia and military field hospitals improved medical care for injured soldiers, yet the mortality rate for those with head wounds (73.7% and 71.1% respectively) remained high [7]. Despite the heavy use of grenades, improved antiseptic and sterile techniques combined with new surgical practices (surgical debridement and primary closure of open wounds) helped to reduce the head wound mortality rate in WWI to 35%. With antibiotics, improved techniques, and better implant materials, the rate dropped to 14% during WWII [7].

Cranioplasty materials continued to evolve. Gold and silver were two of the materials used for cranial repair in antiquity and throughout World War I but were discontinued by the mid-1900s [6]. Platinum, lead, and aluminum were tested through the early twentieth century [6]. During the mid-twentieth century, the alloys tantalum, vitallium, and steel were used. Tantalum was extensively utilized during and after World War II [6]. In 1965, titanium use began. Because of various issues with other metals that titanium does not exhibit, like the softness with gold and silver [6], seizures with aluminum [3], thermal conductivity that caused temperature-dependent headaches with tantalum [3, 6], and toxicity with lead [6], titanium is the lone metal still in use for cranial reconstruction [6].

Various nonmetals including celluloid, gum cork, plaster of Paris, sheet mica, and hard rubber have been tried and rejected for cranioplasty due to product issues or undesirable side effects [4].

Commonly known by the trade name Plexiglas, methyl methacrylate (MMA) was first used as a cranial implant material in the 1940s [3, 5]. With its malleability, the lack of thermal conduction, radiolucency, and low cost, MMA was useful in treating the large number of cranial defects soldiers sustained during World War II [6]. With the aforementioned advantages and with shorter operating times and without the issues of donor site pain and morbidity associated with autologous bone implants, the popularity of MMA increased rapidly [5]. It is still an extensively used non-bone graft implant material [8, 9].

Current Cranial Implant Materials and Technology

This section describes some of the common cranial materials and technology being used in cranioplasty procedures.

Autologous Bone

Autologous bone is often called the "gold standard" because of its many positive properties, including cost, biocompatibility, and regeneration potential [5]. As early as the late nineteenth century, it was recognized that most transplanted bone cells die but are slowly replaced by living cells [4]. This process, called osteoconduction, is how autologous bone grafts heal, and it requires a good blood supply and rigid fixation of the implant for osteoblast migration [1, 9]. As regenerative capacity decreases with age, this osteogenic healing activity may not complete when a large cranial defect is repaired with a large bone flap [9]. Additionally, if revascularization is incomplete or fails, then necrosis, resorption, and/or infection are common complications [9]. Reported bone flap resorption rates have been as high as 50% [5]. Additional drawbacks include limited malleability, and if the original bone flap is not usable, potential donor site issues can include limited material availability, pain, and morbidity [5, 9].

Metal

Titanium is used for fixation devices like microplates and screws, can be used to secure other implant materials, and also as the implant itself either as a plate, mesh, or mesh substrate for other materials [9]. Advantages of titanium include its malleability, biocompatibility, low infection rates, and strength [3, 6]. If a primary autologous bone implant has failed, titanium is often used as the secondary repair mechanism [6]. The disadvantages of titanium include its cost and image artifact on imaging [3].

Acrylics

MMA or PMMA (polymethyl methacrylate) continues to be widely used [5, 6]. PMMA comes as a powder and is mixed with a monomer to form a malleable putty that can be intraoperatively formed to the desired shape. It hardens in 4–6 minutes in an exothermic reaction that requires irrigation to prevent damage to the surrounding tissue. While PMMA has good strength and biocompatibility properties, it is brittle and lacks osteointegration. Reported complication rates range from 5% to 40% [3, 5].

Ceramic

Calcium phosphate (CaP), a ceramic, which as a paste hydrolyzes into hydroxyapatite (HA), may be used over a titanium mesh. The titanium mesh is needed to provide support as HA is extremely brittle. Advantages of HA are its biocompatibility – chemically, it's the closest synthetic material to bone, it is contourable, and it may support osteoconduction and osteoinduction [1, 5, 6, 9].

Plastics

Porous polyethylene and polyether ether ketone (PEEK) are plastic hydrocarbon polymers that are nondegradable, durable, and inert. These plastics are prefabricated and can be custom shaped to handle large defects [1, 5]. The advantage of porous polyethylene is that it may support vascularization and bony ingrowth [1, 5, 6], although this has been brought into doubt [1, 5]. Advantages of PEEK are its small rate of reported complications, strength, and it is easily removed [1, 5, 6].

Additive Manufacturing

Additive manufacturing (AM), commonly called three-dimensional (3D) printing, is a current technology supporting the development of better materials. First introduced in the late 1980s, it is now a booming industry as lower costs and advancements in computer technologies have driven usage in manufacturing and consumer markets [10]. Its use in the medical field is also growing rapidly in a number of diverse applications. 3D printing supports cranioplasty graft design and has improved the fit of premade cranial grafts that were previously done manually [9]. Computer-aided design (CAD) and AM have been used to create highly accurate skull phantoms and molds from which prefabricated patient-specific cranial implants have been cast [11, 12]. It has been demonstrated that even relatively low-cost 3D printers (US $2000) can be used for this purpose [11].

CAD, AM, and other computer-aided fabrication techniques are also being used to create patient-specific implants (PSIs) that have been successfully implanted with low resultant rates of complications [13, 14]. Lethaus et al. conducted a retrospective study comparing 17 patients who had cranioplasty operations using PSIs to 16 patients whose operations used stored bone grafts. Of the PSIs, nine were milled titanium implants, one was a 3D selective laser sintering (SLS) printed titanium implant, and seven were computer numerical control (CNC) milled PEEK implants. Of the stored bone, six had been stored in the abdominal wall, and ten had been stored by cryopreservation. Analysis of the post-operational complications revealed that the PSI group had a statistically significant lower rate of complications (5.9%), compared to the stored bone group (43.8%) [14].

In the area of surgical practice and teaching, 3D printing of patient-specific anatomy offers neurosurgeons the opportunity to develop skills (e.g., tumor excisions, before operating on a patient [15, 16]), perform pre- and intraoperative surgical planning, and improve communication with patients. Here, 3D models can be used during consultation enabling significantly improved knowledge transfer about the procedure and concerns of the patient with a realistic model of the surgery [17]. Examples of these types of models are given in Figs. 11.2 and 11.3. In both cases these models were printed on ProJet Series 660 3D printer (3D Systems, Rock Hill, SC, USA) by curing gypsum powder with superglue layer-by-layer, adding color in an ink-jet-like fashion. These

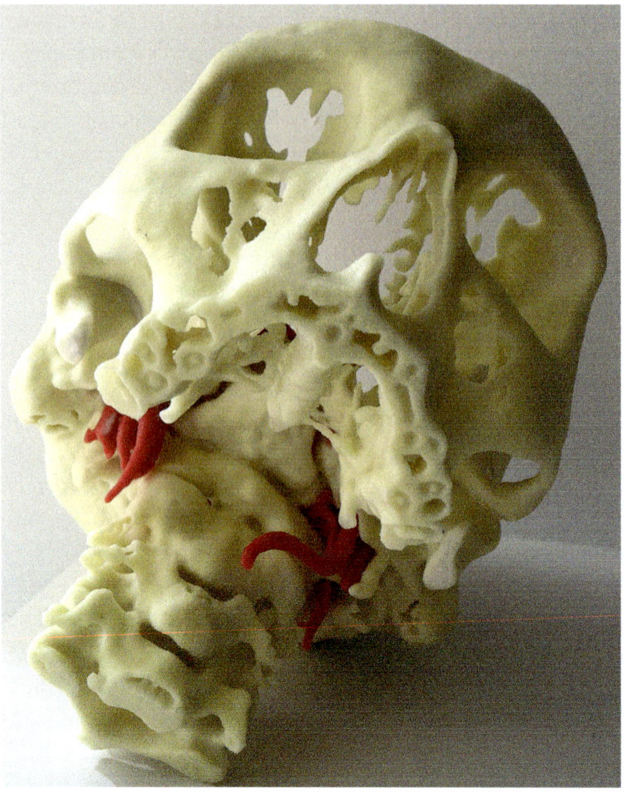

Fig. 11.2 A preoperative model for the planning of odontoidectomy for a patient with type 1 Chiari malformation through transnasal endoscopic approach, noting the abnormally medial left carotid artery

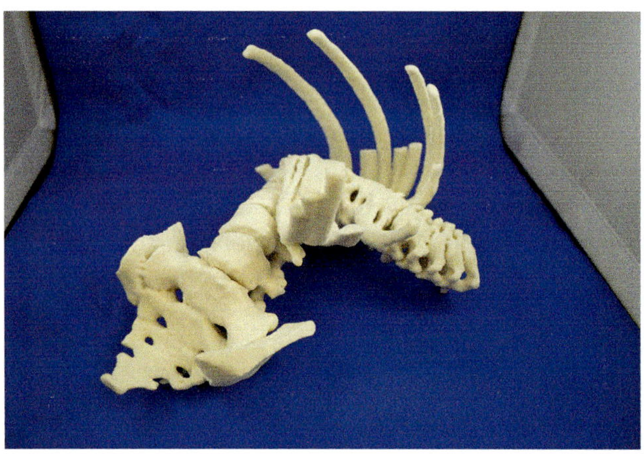

Fig. 11.3 A pre- and intraoperative planning model for the case of complex juvenile scoliosis

types of printers are popular for medical modeling purposes, especially because they create structures with an arbitrary number of colors with hard, bone-like durable materials which accurately reflect large-scale features.

Preprocessing techniques, where radiological scan sequences are interpreted numerically to generate patient-specific models, are similar in the case of preoperative modeling and implant design. The process of segmentation, or the process of partitioning a radiologic scan sequence into regions corresponding to physiological structures of interest (e.g., bone/skull, soft tissue, nerves, blood vessels, tumors), is the most significant of the tools used to generate patient-specific models, implants, and implant molds. These tools are established and undergoing active research, though methods used for segmenting bone are comparatively simple to those used for soft tissue analysis, and are therefore available in a variety of open-source and commercial software packages. Industry-leading examples of these packages include *3D Slicer* [18], a powerful open-source publically supported package; *Seg3D2* (University of Utah, Center for Integrative Biomedical Computing, Salt Lake City, UT, USA), another open-source package implementing a variety of image-analysis primitives which, when combined, can develop very complex models; and *Mimics* (Materialize, Plymouth, MI, USA), a well-known commercial package for medical image analysis and modeling which provides powerful, high-end automated processing of radiological scan data. Most of these types of software packages ultimately rely on a back-end of generic image-processing software libraries, such as the Insight Toolkit (ITK, Kitware, Clifton Park, NY, USA) or OpenCV [19], which implement the fundamental algorithms used by the user-end packages, but are not typically used directly except by software developers.

Each of these tools provides functionality used directly for the generation of patient-specific cranioplasty models and molds. Bone is easily segmented from helical CT data because it contrasts extremely well relative to all other structures in a given scan sequence and immediately proximate to the bone itself. Techniques such as *thresholding* (where image voxels are labeled as bone if they fall within a certain brightness in the image), *restricted thresholding* (the same as thresholding but with a user-driven region selection in the image), *neighborhood connected* (initial seeds within the bone are "grown" algorithmically by considering the relationship of each labeled voxel with its surroundings; if the "connected," or surrounding, voxels are sufficiently similar to the initial seed point, those voxels are included in the model), and *Otsu thresholding* and *canny edge detection* (where the borders between contrasting structures, like bone and tissue in helical CT, are easily demarcated) are commonly used and typically sufficient for the purposes of skull modeling. More powerful tools are occasionally implemented when structures are not easily differentiated in the image. However, as the tools become more complex, they also become more manual and expert driven, significantly increasing the time to model. Therefore, high-quality radiological sequences are a fundamental prerequisite to medical modeling in all its forms.

Postprocessing techniques, those that prepare the final model for printing, typically come in the form of cleanup (extraneous structure removal, model smoothing) and growth modeling (where the surface of the model is "grown" to create a mold). In the case of cleanup, image granularity in the raw radiological volume leads to "steps" in the resulting model which are not representative of the anatomy, but naïve smoothing removes material and therefore does not faithfully recreate the modeled structure. Surface-preserving smoothing tools are numerous, and implementations like Laplacian-based or Taubin smoothing are used instead and are commonly implemented in 3D printing postprocessing tools such as MeshLab [20] and ITK. Equivalently, cleanup methods which remove extraneous structures (especially those that are not connected to the model itself, if they exist) like connected component and growth methods which expand the initial structure smoothly along the model's surface normals for mold generation are available in MeshLab, 3D Slicer, Seg3D2, Mimics, and indeed a host of other similar applications. A smoothed and adequately postprocessed model is at this point ready for slicing and printing with the appropriate 3D printer software.

Clinical Applications: Trauma and Tumor Surgery

Causes

Trauma, neurosurgical procedures, and infections are common causes of skull defects. Across all age groups, brain tumor surgery and decompressive craniectomies are the reasons for most cranial defects [3, 8]. A cranioplasty is often performed after a craniectomy for diagnoses including benign tumor, malignant tumor, trauma, infection, intracranial ischemia, intracerebral hemorrhage, extradural hematoma, and subdural hematoma [21, 22]. It may also be performed to alleviate complications like subdural effusion, seizures, and herniation of the cortex through the bone defect that have arisen after the craniectomy [22]. For children under three, congenital anomalies and growing skull fractures are also causes for cranioplasty [8].

Demand

In recent years, decompressive craniectomies have increased considerably due to advances in medical care, particularly intensive care [23]. Likewise, today's soldiers are surviving traumatic brain injuries sustained during combat at an exponentially higher rate due to improvements in body armor and a rise in early decompressive craniectomies [1, 5, 7]. This lower patient mortality rate coupled with the increase in craniectomy procedures has increased the need and number of cranioplasties [23].

Complication Rate

Compared to other non-emergent neurosurgical procedures, the complication rate for a cranioplasty is much higher [2]. Complication rates are approximately 12% to 50% [24], and there is as high as a 25% reoperation rate [5]. These risks are demonstrated in a retrospective study by Broughton et al. [25] that assessed the outcomes of 87 cranioplasties, performed over a 7-year period in a regional neurosurgical center: 30% of the patients experienced complications, 20% were major, and 10% were minor. Most complications took place in the first few weeks to months after the procedure. Sixteen patients incurred 18 major complications: 9 infections (10.3%), 5 extradural hemorrhages, 2 symptomatic pneumocephalus, 1 persistent subgaleal collection needing a shunt, and 1 survived a postoperative cardiac arrest. Two patients died (2.3% mortality rate).

Infections

Infections are the most frequent complication after a cranioplasty [26]. Postoperative infections rates can be high as these studies illustrate: Broughton et al. 10.3% [25], Pittulainen et al. 15.48% [22], and Zanaty et al. 26.43% [27]. Native skin flora, like *Staphylococcus* and *Propionibacterium*, are the most common sources of an infection [26].

Surgical-Specific Factors

Surgical-specific factors such as timing and cranial implant material and their impact on complication and infection rates are being assessed.

Timing

The ideal time frame between a craniectomy and a cranioplasty to limit complications has not been established and remains controversial [2]. There are studies that report higher rates of complications and infections with early versus later cranioplasty, studies that report lower rates, and some that found no relationship [2]. What is recognized is that the time delay can be significant and is situation specific. In Ng et al. [21], a retrospective review of 12 patients who underwent PEEK implant cranioplasty performed by one surgeon, the cranioplasty followed their decompressive craniectomy by an average of 10 months, with a range of 3–40 months. Piitulainen et al. [22], in a retrospective review of 100 cranioplasties on 84 different patients with 4 different implant materials (20 autograft, 20 bioactive fiber-reinforced composite, 31 hydroxyapatite, and 29 other synthetic materials), found the time between craniectomy and cranioplasty ranged from 0 to 3815 days, with a mean of 390.4 days.

Materials

Although autologous bone implants have been identified as the gold standard, it has been found that for large cranial defects these implants have increased resorption rates that may, especially for older adults, indicates the use of an alloplastic graft implant [1, 23]. Iaccarino et al. [28] performed a 6-year prospective study of 96 patients (14 and older) that included 31 autologous bone implant patients to 65 alloplastic implant patients – 50 hydroxyapatite (HA), 13 polymethyl methacrylate (PMMA), and 2 polyether ether ketone (PEEK). A statistical analysis showed a higher complication rate with the autologous bone group compared to the alloplastic group.

Yadla et al. [29] performed a systematic review of the literature which pooled data from 18 retrospective studies totaling 2254 procedures. Their analysis found no statistically significant differences in the rates of infection: between autogenous grafts and allografts, between subcutaneous and extracorporeal preservation (freezing) of autogenous graft, or between early and later cranioplasty. Subsequent retrospective studies [26, 27] also found no statistical difference among the same surgery-specific factors with respect to rates of infections.

Patient-Specific Factors

Some studies indicate that patient-specific factors may be more important than surgery-specific factors with regard to the risk of post-cranioplasty complications [27, 30]. A retrospective study of 348 patients by Zanaty et al. [27] looked at the variables: age, sex, race, hypertension, diabetes, smoking status, reason for craniotomy, urgency status, and cranioplasty location. Analysis showed a postoperative complication rate of 31.32% including infection (overall 26.43%, deep 11.49%), seizures (14.37%), hydrocephalus (13.51%), reoperation for hematoma evacuation (6.9%), and death (3.16%). The study identified the following predictors: complication predictors were hypertension, increasing age, and hemorrhagic stroke; infection predictors were older age, hemorrhagic stroke, post-cranioplasty hydrocephalus, and bilateral convexity cranioplasty; and mortality predictors were diabetes, seizures, bifrontal cranioplasty, and repeated surgery for hematoma evacuation.

A retrospective study of 195 procedures on 180 patients [30] found: the strongest predictor of any postoperative complication was preoperative radiation; no predictive factor for postoperative infection; the presence of preoperative infection increased the odds of cranioplasty material exposure; and patients whose cranial defect was frontally located or who had preoperative radiation were more likely to undergo a secondary cranioplasty.

Pediatric Cranioplasty Considerations

Cranioplasties in adults and older children are performed using a wide variety of materials from autologous bone grafts to synthetic materials. For young children the continued growth of their cranium and the resulting bone contour changes put limits on what can be successfully used. Studies have found autologous bone to be the best material as the bone flap will reintegrate as the child matures [3, 5]. However, there are concerns with its supply given the inadequate calvarial thickness in young children and the limited bone that may effectively be available from other sites [5]. High bone resorption rate is also a concern with pediatric cranioplasties using autologous bone graft. A retrospective study of 61 pediatric patients (under 18 years of age) by Piedra et al. [24] demonstrated this issue. The young patients were divided into two groups by timing of cranioplasty: 28 patients in Group 1 (<6 weeks) and 33 patients in Group 2 (≥6 weeks). The bone resorption rate was high and ranged from 14% for Group 1 to 42% for Group 2, indicating that for pediatric cases, early cranioplasty (<6 weeks) may be more appropriate.

Cranial Implant Research Directions

Research to find better implant materials and techniques continues. One area of active cranial implant research involves tissue engineering which investigates the use of resorbable scaffolds, growth factors, and various types of cells [1, 3, 5, 9].

In a study to develop an osteoconductive scaffold for capillary and osteoprogenitor cell ingrowth, Tseng et al. [31] used gamma rays to cross-link two biodegradable polymers, acrylic acid and N-isopropylacrylamide, to make a powder which was then mixed with platelet-rich plasma (PRP) treated with thrombin to release osteoinductive agents. This PRP-treated scaffold, which, when implanted in New Zealand White rabbits after a 15 mm diameter cranial bone defect was created, showed significant new bone growth compared to the control groups.

Smith et al. [32] used a commercially available acellular collagen sponge as their scaffold to compare five modes of treatment: no repair (control 1), untreated scaffold (control 2), adipose-derived stem cell-infused scaffold, low-dose bone morphogenetic protein BMP-2 osteoinduced adipose-derived stem cell-infused scaffold, and high-dose BMP-2-infused scaffold. A 15 by 15 mm craniectomy defect was created in New Zealand White rabbits and repaired with one of the 5 types of prepared scaffolds. The results showed that after 6 weeks, only the high-dose BMP-2-infused scaffold had a significantly greater level of defect ossification 96.9% over the controls which were 32.8% and 34.4%, respectively.

Animal model studies have found bone morphogenetic protein BMP-2 to have a defect ossification level of over 95% compared to controls which were under 35% [32, 33], but, using a modified punch-out compression test, the BMP-2-generated bone did not have as robust biomechanical properties as native bone [33]. As BMP-2 is a potent morphogen, there are concerns in administrating the high doses needed to induce ossification [34]. Inkjet-based bioprinting technologies that allow for precisely customized low-dose protein patterns have been used with BMP-2 in mice. Acellular dermal matrix (ADM) discs that had been printed with BMP-2 bio-ink were implanted with their printed surface directly on the dura mater, which acted as the source of osteoprogenitors. It was found that bone was generated to cover an average of 66.5% of the defect's surface area [34].

Other studies have investigated stem cells including using induced human pluripotent stem cells (iPSCs), a stem cell that can be generated from adult cells, which have been shown to produce calcium mineralization in in vitro [35] and human true bone in vivo (mouse model) [35, 36].

Inadequate native bone sources and issues with limited ossification with respect to alloplastic implants have propelled osseous reconstruction of the craniofacial skeleton to become a subject of tissue engineering efforts. There have been some promising results with in vitro and in vivo in animal model studies, but much more research is still needed.

Summary

Ongoing advances in technology, materials, and surgical practices have enabled neurosurgeons to repair increasingly complex cranial defects. Yet, complications and infections are common. Cranioplasty protocols tend to be surgeon or institution specific with observational data and personal preference playing a large role [29]. Neurosurgeons and researchers continue to study a variety of factors to help define the optimal materials and approaches for particular clinical scenarios. However, varying and inconsistent study results have made a consensus difficult.

References

1. Goldstein JA, Paliga JT, Bartlett SP. Cranioplasty: indications and advances. Curr Opin Otolaryngol Head Neck Surg. 2013;21(4):400–9.
2. Paredes I, Castano-Leon AM, Munarriz PM, Martinez-Perez R, Cepeda S, Sanz R, et al. Cranioplasty after decompressive craniectomy. A prospective series analyzing complications and clinical improvement. Neurocirugia (Astur). 2015;26(3):115–25.
3. Shah AM, Jung H, Skirboll S. Materials used in cranioplasty: a history and analysis. Neurosurg Focus. 2014;36(4):E19.
4. Sanan A, Haines SJ. Repairing holes in the head: a history of cranioplasty. Neurosurgery. 1997;40(3):588–603.
5. Feroze AH, Walmsley GG, Choudhri O, Lorenz HP, Grant GA, Edwards MS. Evolution of cranioplasty techniques in neurosurgery: historical review, pediatric considerations, and current trends. J Neurosurg. 2015;123(4):1098–107.
6. Harris DA, Fong AJ, Buchanan EP, Monson L, Khechoyan D, Lam S. History of synthetic materials in alloplastic cranioplasty. Neurosurg Focus. 2014;36(4):E20.
7. Bonfield CM, Kumar AR, Gerszten PC. The history of military cranioplasty. Neurosurg Focus. 2014;36(4):E18.
8. Aydin S, Kucukyuruk B, Abuzayed B, Aydin S, Sanus GZ. Cranioplasty: review of materials and techniques. J Neurosci Rural Pract. 2011;2(2):162–7.
9. Bonda DJ, Manjila S, Selman WR, Dean D. The recent revolution in the design and manufacture of cranial implants: modern advancements and future directions. Neurosurgery. 2015;77(5):814–24. discussion 24
10. Klein GT, Lu Y, Wang MY. 3D printing and neurosurgery – ready for prime time? World Neurosurg. 2013;80(3–4):233–5.
11. Tan ET, Ling JM, Dinesh SK. The feasibility of producing patient-specific acrylic cranioplasty implants with a low-cost 3D printer. J Neurosurg. 2015;124(5):1531–7.
12. Kim BJ, Hong KS, Park KJ, Park DH, Chung YG, Kang SH. Customized cranioplasty implants using three-dimensional printers and polymethyl-methacrylate casting. J Korean Neurosurg Soc. 2012;52(6):541–6.
13. Gilardino MS, Karunanayake M, Al-Humsi T, Izadpanah A, Al-Ajmi H, Marcoux J, et al. A comparison and cost analysis of cranioplasty techniques: autologous bone versus custom computer-generated implants. J Craniofac Surg. 2015;26(1):113–7.
14. Lethaus B, Bloebaum M, Essers B, ter Laak MP, Steiner T, Kessler P. Patient-specific implants compared with stored bone grafts for patients with interval cranioplasty. J Craniofac Surg. 2014;25(1):206–9.
15. Waran V, Narayanan V, Karuppiah R, Owen SL, Aziz T. Utility of multimaterial 3D printers in creating models with pathological entities to enhance the training experience of neurosurgeons. J Neurosurg. 2014;120(2):489–92.
16. Rehder R, Abd-El-Barr M, Hooten K, Weinstock P, Madsen JR, Cohen AR. The role of simulation in neurosurgery. Childs Nerv Syst. 2016;32(1):43–54.
17. Liew Y, Beveridge E, Demetriades AK, Hughes MA. 3D printing of patient-specific anatomy: a tool to improve patient consent and enhance imaging interpretation by trainees. Br J Neurosurg. 2015;29(5):712–4.
18. Fedorov A, Beichel R, Kalpathy-Cramer J, Finet J, Fillion-Robin JC, Pujol S, et al. 3D slicer as an image computing platform for the quantitative imaging network. Magn Reson Imaging. 2012;30(9):1323–41.
19. Bradski G. The OpenCV library. Dr Dobb's Journal of Software Tools. 2000;25(11):120, 2–5.
20. Taubin G, editor. Curve and surface smoothing without shrinkage. Fifth International Conference on Computer Vision (ICCV '95); Conference was June 20–23, 1995 Massachusetts Institue of Technology, Cambridge, Massachusetts.
21. Ng ZY, Nawaz I. Computer-designed PEEK implants: a peek into the future of cranioplasty? J Craniofac Surg. 2014;25(1):e55–8.
22. Piitulainen JM, Kauko T, Aitasalo KM, Vuorinen V, Vallittu PK, Posti JP. Outcomes of cranioplasty with synthetic materials and autologous bone grafts. World Neurosurg. 2015;83(5):708–14.
23. Schoekler B, Trummer M. Prediction parameters of bone flap resorption following cranioplasty with autologous bone. Clin Neurol Neurosurg. 2014;120:64–7.
24. Piedra MP, Thompson EM, Selden NR, Ragel BT, Guillaume DJ. Optimal timing of autologous cranioplasty after decompressive craniectomy in children. J Neurosurg Pediatr. 2012;10(4):268–72.
25. Broughton E, Pobereskin L, Whitfield PC. Seven years of cranioplasty in a regional neurosurgical centre. Br J Neurosurg. 2014;28(1):34–9.
26. Morton RP, Abecassis IJ, Hanson JF, Barber J, Nerva JD, Emerson SN, et al. Predictors of infection after 754 cranioplasty operations

and the value of intraoperative cultures for cryopreserved bone flaps. J Neurosurg. 2016;125(3):766–70.
27. Zanaty M, Chalouhi N, Starke RM, Clark SW, Bovenzi CD, Saigh M, et al. Complications following cranioplasty: incidence and predictors in 348 cases. J Neurosurg. 2015;123(1):182–8.
28. Iaccarino C, Viaroli E, Fricia M, Serchi E, Poli T, Servadei F. Preliminary results of a prospective study on methods of cranial reconstruction. J Oral Maxillofac Surg. 2015;73(12):2375–8.
29. Yadla S, Campbell PG, Chitale R, Maltenfort MG, Jabbour P, Sharan AD. Effect of early surgery, material, and method of flap preservation on cranioplasty infections: a systematic review. Neurosurgery. 2011;68(4):1124–9. Discussion 30
30. Reddy S, Khalifian S, Flores JM, Bellamy J, Manson PN, Rodriguez ED, et al. Clinical outcomes in cranioplasty: risk factors and choice of reconstructive material. Plast Reconstr Surg. 2014;133(4):864–73.
31. Tseng CL, Chang GW, Ou KL, Chou WT, Wu TH, Fang HW, et al. Cranioplasty using a novel osteoconductive scaffold and platelet gel. Ann Plast Surg. 2016;76(Suppl 1):S125–9.
32. Smith DM, Cooper GM, Afifi AM, Mooney MP, Cray J, Rubin JP, et al. Regenerative surgery in cranioplasty revisited: the role of adipose-derived stem cells and BMP-2. Plast Reconstr Surg. 2011;128(5):1053–60.
33. Cray J Jr, Henderson SE, Smith DM, Kinsella CR Jr, Bykowski M, Cooper GM, et al. BMP-2-regenerated calvarial bone: a biomechanical appraisal in a large animal model. Ann Plast Surg. 2014;73(5):591–7.
34. Smith DM, Cray JJ Jr, Weiss LE, Dai Fei EK, Shakir S, Rottgers SA, et al. Precise control of osteogenesis for craniofacial defect repair: the role of direct osteoprogenitor contact in BMP-2-based bioprinting. Ann Plast Surg. 2012;69(4):485–8.
35. Phillips MD, Kuznetsov SA, Cherman N, Park K, Chen KG, McClendon BN, et al. Directed differentiation of human induced pluripotent stem cells toward bone and cartilage: in vitro versus in vivo assays. Stem Cells Transl Med. 2014;3(7):867–78.
36. Levi B, Hyun JS, Montoro DT, Lo DD, Chan CK, Hu S, et al. In vivo directed differentiation of pluripotent stem cells for skeletal regeneration. Proc Natl Acad Sci U S A. 2012;109(50):20379–84.

Digital Planning in Pediatric Craniofacial Surgery

12

Samer Elia Haber, Anup Patel, and Derek M. Steinbacher

Abbreviations

2D:	Two-dimensional
3D:	Three-dimensional
CAD:	Computer-aided design
CAM:	Computer-aided manufacturing
CT:	Computed Tomography
DICOM:	Digital imaging and communications in medicine
HFM:	Hemifacial microsomia
VSP:	Virtual Surgical Planning

Introduction

Pediatric craniofacial surgery involves comprehensive restitution of form and function while treating dysmorphology, disease, and defects. Both soft tissue and osseous reconstructions are performed, often in concert. The anatomy is complex and *the paucity of the blood reserve* requires efficient and precise intervention. The *topographic relations* and compartments between anatomic structures are critically important to the reconstruction. Planning such intricate surgery preoperatively is of utmost importance ensuring that geometric and quantitative factors, particularly relating to the craniofacial skeleton are completely evaluated and correctly operated.

In the past two decades, progress in virtual three-dimensional simulation has opened the door to multiple techniques for surgical planning. Nevertheless, before we develop these techniques, it must be stressed that they are neither meant to nor will replace a surgeon's clinical judgment or technical skill. Three-dimensional reconstruction of computed tomography (CT) scan images has made it possible to (1) visualize bony and soft tissue craniofacial structures, (2) examine the effects of different possibilities for surgical intervention to assist in decision-making, (3) preoperatively "rehearse" the task at hand in a virtual environment, (4) fabricate stereolithographic models and tools to be used peroperatively, and (5) assist in intraoperative positioning of surgical equipment using real-time face detection coupled with reconstruction of preoperative CT images [1].

The purpose of this chapter is to provide an overview of the current applications of virtual imaging in planning and performing craniofacial surgery in the pediatric setting.

Principles

The fields of computer prototyping and simulation have witnessed major progress during the past two decades thanks to the rapid evolution of a complex infrastructure: (1) computer processing speed, (2) informatics and software engineering, (3) sensing technologies, and (4) computer communication (internet, WiFi, Bluetooth, cellular phones, etc.) [2].

Advanced imaging techniques such as computed tomography (CT) are used to create two-dimensional images in the digital imaging and communications in medicine (DICOM) format. These files are processed to create three-dimensional reconstructions using one of the various programs available on the market, thus improving the understanding of anatomical relationships [3].

Interactive 3D models can be viewed from different perspectives and a surgical plan devised using simulation. This is commonly known as computer-aided design (CAD), and it has been used to create digital atlases of normal craniofacial anatomy, craniofacial pathology, and craniofacial procedures which are currently published online [4, 5].

As to the application of these techniques in patient care, bone cutting and bone realignment as well as secondary soft

S.E. Haber
Plastic and Maxillofacial Surgery Department, Hôtel Dieu de France Hospital, Beirut, Lebanon

A. Patel
Yale Plastic Surgery, New Haven, CT, USA

D.M. Steinbacher (✉)
Craniomaxillofacial Surgery, Yale University School of Medicine, New Haven, CT, USA
e-mail: derek.steinbacher@yale.edu

A.M. Greenberg (ed.), *Digital Technologies in Craniomaxillofacial Surgery*, https://doi.org/10.1007/978-1-4939-1532-3_12

tissue deformation can be simulated in order to preoperatively give a preview of what the patient will look like postoperatively. This is done using a 3D photo (laser surface scanner) in addition to the traditional CT scan while taking into consideration gravity, skin turgor, and the elastomechanical properties of the multiple layers of soft tissue [6].

In addition to better visualization, rapid prototyping allows the materialization of detailed 3D models using a 3D printer. This is known as computer-aided manufacturing (CAM). CAD/CAM technology has made it possible to preoperatively evaluate surgical outcomes for different treatment options. It yields superior precision with less operative time, risks, and costs.

In addition to individualized anatomical models, CAD/CAM technology enables the surgical team to generate patient-specific implants (PSIs), as well as individualized surgical tools such as cutting jigs and molding plates to be used intraoperatively as a guide [7].

Another application for DICOM images at the operative site is intraoperative navigation. A preoperatively acquired 3D reconstruction of CT images is constantly projected during the operation. A localizer tracks the patient's head position using fiducial markers placed on stable and reliable anatomical points. A surgical probe can then be used alone or mounted on the surgical instruments, which will be directly visualized in relation to the patient's anatomy [8, 9].

The applications of 3D technology in surgical planning can hence be summarized as follows:

(a) Diagnosis: 3D visualization helps to better demonstrate the bony anomaly.
(b) Quantitative measurement and analysis: can be compared to the norms or the ideal.
(c) Reconstructive goals: derived from the comparison between the existing deformity and the norm/ideal we intend to attain.
(d) Virtual surgical simulation: this step offers the advantage of an unlimited number of trial-error possibilities. Unexpected anatomic problems are identified and solved. Once the desired surgical goals are visualized, new quantitative measurements are taken with the structures in their projected position.
(e) Manufacture of surgical cutting guides and jigs: osteotomy sites and movement of the anatomic constituents are translated with great precision through computer-aided manufacture (CAM).
(f) Postoperative comparison of actual and planned results.

Applications

Craniosynostosis

When open repair for craniosynostosis correction is indicated, 3D planning has potential use and benefit. The main goals of digital operative planning are to reduce operative time and to increase the predictability of the results. Early reports and suggestions of 3D analysis of craniofacial conditions have been in the literature for decades now [10–14].

Computer-aided design (CAD) was first used for craniosynostosis repair in 1996 [15].

It consisted of a mere 3D interactive mathematical model of the patient's skull that allowed preoperative procedural planning.

In 2001, Mommaerts et al. took it a little further when they used the computer-generated 3D model to determine the dimensions of 2D templates that were preoperatively manually cut out of thick aluminum foil, autoclaved, and transferred to the cranium to guide the osteotomies [16].

Computer-aided manufacturing (CAM) was introduced in 2011 when Burge et al. utilized a previously generated "Super Skull" model [17] – based on the study of 103 CT scans of normocephalic children aged 8–12 months – to generate customized stainless steel templates of the fronto-orbital region that most closely reproduce a normal head shape. They then use these templates to help aid the fabrication of the supraorbital bandeau intraoperatively [18].

In 2013, Mardini et al. and Seruya et al. combined the techniques described by Mommaerts et al. and Burge et al. while applying them to the entire skull. Using 3D planning software, a patient's skull can be compared to its age and size-matched "Super Skull" counterpart, and it generates templates (CAM) for intraoperative osteotomy and remodeling of the calvarium as well as positioning guides for accurate skull vault shaping [19, 20].

Using CAD/CAM for guidance via templates and jigs appears to improve operative time as well as accuracy and reproducibility of the surgical outcome [21–28].

The limited downside of requiring a preoperative planning session is outweighed by the decreased intraoperative stress – as the surgery has already been performed once virtually, enabling multiple vantage points not present intraoperatively – and the ability for early recognition of obstacles and interferences.

Posterior Calvarial Distraction Osteogenesis

Posterior calvarial expansion is indicated for intracranial decompression as the first phase of treatment for patients with multisuture syndromic craniosynostosis. It provides a more profound enlargement of intracranial volume compared with the anterior cranial vault advancement while leaving the fronto-orbital bandeau intact, hence allowing enhanced control of the surgical correction of the facial deformity at a later stage [29–32].

The technique involves a posterior craniotomy creating a posterior bone flap that is left attached to the dura. At least two distraction devices are then applied with one footplate affixed to the more anterior stable bone and activation arms let out anteriorly (Fig. 12.1).

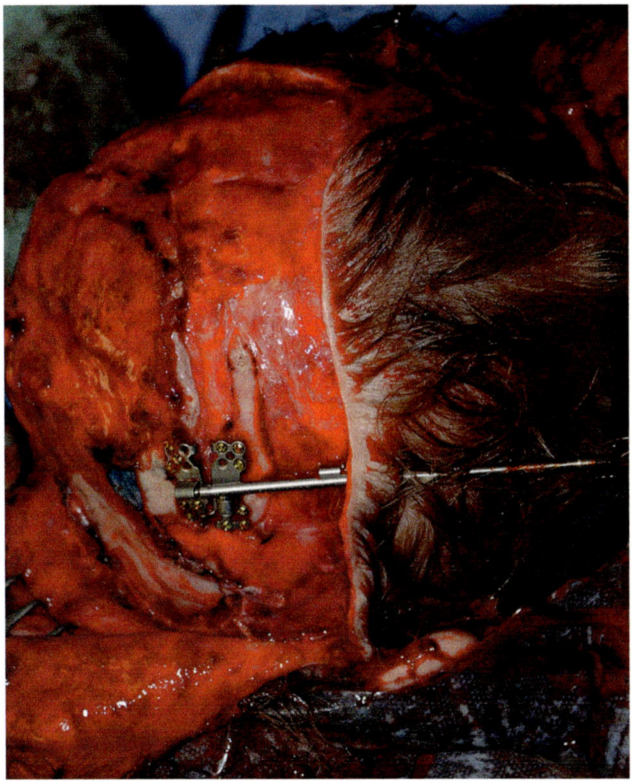

Fig. 12.1 Intraoperative placement of a posterior cranial vault distraction device (DuPuy Synthes Craniomaxillofacial, Paoli, PA, USA)

The scalp is closed and, following latency, the device activated. Installation of the devices is subject to parallax errors, and it should follow the appropriate vector – typically this is posterior and slightly inferior. Planning helps to guide the placement of the craniotomy and of the devices to achieve the appropriate vector [29, 33–39].

LeFort III and Frontofacial Monobloc Advancement

Multiple syndromes (Crouzon, Apert, Pfeiffer, Saethre-Chotzen) are characterized by craniofacial dysmorphology that involves fronto-orbital and/or midface retrusion. This retrusion is measured relative to the apex corneae (acor) – the most anteriorly projecting point of the ocular cornea – which constitutes the most reliable landmark in the correction of these conditions. The sagittal orbital-globe relationship corresponds to the projection of four specific bony points and their respective soft tissue counterparts on an anteroposterior axis with *acor* as the reference point [40, 41]. These four points are:

- Os (resp. os for soft tissue): Orbitale superius at the mid-superior orbit
- Oi (resp. oi for soft tissue): Orbitale inferius at the midinferior orbital rim (*Oi* corresponds to *Orbitale – Or* in the traditional cephalometric studies)
- Ol (resp. ol for soft tissue): the deepest convexity of the lateral orbital rim
- N (resp. n for soft tissue): nasion

Corrective surgery (LeFort III procedure and frontofacial monobloc advancement) aims to redefine these relations to match previously established normative measures for bony and soft tissue landmarks [40]. *Os* has been shown to advance in a soft tissue: skeletal movement ratio of 0.9:1 following the surgical advancement of *Os* [41].

Digital planning has been employed in these types of procedures with distractor placement in syndromic craniosynostosis. It simulates the osteotomy and advancement as well as the gain in intraorbital volume [42].

Another method is direct intraoperative visualization of otherwise hidden osteotomy sites (pterygoid and periorbital) using the StealthStation intraoperative navigation system (Medtronic Sofamor Danek, Memphis, TN, USA) [43].

Cranial Defects

Pediatric cranial defects originate from trauma, congenital anomaly, and surgery (craniosynostosis repair, tumor excision). Dural osteoinductive potential is lost or markedly reduced between 9 and 11 months of age, thus significantly impairing the ability to close large cranial defects after that age limit [44].

This means that for children older than 1 year of age who have a cranial defect, a proper reconstructive technique must be performed in order to provide a solid protection for the nervous system underneath and for aesthetic reasons as well. Autologous bone grafting provides the most suitable technique thanks to the biocompatibility, resistance to infection, strength characteristics, and the remodeling capacity in the growing child. However, for large defects and in the absence of sufficient autologous bone, alloplastic materials or bone substitutes ought to be employed. Computer-aided design (CAD) of prefabricated cranial plates provides better-fitting implants with less operative time without the need of peroperative modeling of the implants [45].

Initially, computer-aided manufacturing (CAM) was used in indirect methods where the computer generates a mold for the fabrication of the prosthesis or for shaping of autologous bone grafts. In this regard, stereolithographic models can reproduce complex 3D shapes through the use of laser beam polymerization of liquid ultraviolet light-sensitive resin. These models have been used to mold titanium plates for cranial reconstruction [46], carbon fiber-reinforced polymer [47], and hydroxyapatite implants for very large cranial defects [48].

CAM has more recently been used in the direct fabrication of implants using solid free-form fabrication technology without the need for a model or a mold, which yields even more precision (0.1%) [49], predictability, and less operative time.

Computer-aided manufacturing (CAM) of custom-made implants have been made from titanium, methyl metacrylate, hydroxyapatite, porous polyethylene, polymethyl methacrylate-polyhydroxyethyl-calcium hydroxide coated, and polyetherketone (PEEK) [50].

Nonetheless, these non-resorbable alloplastic materials are not very well adapted in the pediatric setting with a 3.7% infection rate and a 23% long-term failure rate [51]. The optimal material to be used in pediatric calvarial reconstruction is the one that protects the nervous system, does not interfere with cranial growth, and has osteoconductive and osteoinductive properties [52, 53].

Tissue engineering of cranial defect implants is accomplished by producing a bioresorbable scaffold which is seeded with autologous cells (osteoblasts, bone marrow-derived stem cells, or adipose-derived stem cells).

Tissue-engineered implants are non-immunogenic. The ideal material used should retain its physical properties for at least 6 months with a resorption rate that matches tissue infiltration and osteointegration (12–18 months) [54].

Polycaprolactone currently seems like a good fit for the ideal implant, and it has been applied for delayed large calvarial reconstructions in a two-stage approach in humans [55].

Orbital Translocation

As delineated by Mulliken in 1996, digital planning using CT scan images is the most accurate method to control the sagittal orbital-globe relationship in orbital translocation surgery [40].

As opposed to the traditional exophthalmometers, this technique is free from parallax errors even in the most asymmetric facial deformity, because it does not involve optical measurements. The same principles of CAD/CAM technology are applied here through translation of the measured movements into appropriate surgical guides and cutting jigs in order to restore normal anatomic relations.

Micrognathia

Distraction osteogenesis is indicated for neonatal micrognathia airway obstruction that is refractory to conservative measures. Through visualization of the bone structure, bony relationships, and the oropharyngeal lumen, three-dimensional CT scan reconstructions allow careful examination of the jaw disharmony (ANB angle, Wits appraisal, mandibular length, etc.), the tightness of the airway space, choanal atresia, and the tongue position (useful to plan floor of mouth releases). It is valuable in determining anatomic pitfalls to avoid during surgery such as nerves and tooth buds, and in accurately planning the vector of distraction using a "reverse engineering" strategy where the desired final position is applied to the digital model and the required advancement deduced from it. Three-dimensional planning has thus been of invaluable importance in establishing a treatment plan in Pierre Robin sequence [56].

Three-dimensional CT scan reconstruction is also applied in the generation of individualized surgical equipment that is specific to each case. In this regard, D'Hauthuille et al. compared two different approaches to mandibular distraction osteogenesis using computer-assisted techniques [57].

The Rapid Prototyping Technique

An individualized stereolithographic template or guide is designed in a way to specifically fit the predefined area of osteotomy and screw fixation, using three different spatial planes of contact with the bone. This resin template has four drilling cylinders and a split hole that correspond to the exact location of screw fixation and sagittal osteotomy, respectively. This allows for rapid and precise intraoperative positioning of the mandibular distractor according to the predefined vector of distraction.

Computer-Assisted Surgery

This technique employs real-time peroperative surgical navigation using infrared camera tracking of the head's position, along with the previously taken two-dimensional CT scan images that are matched with the head's position. Maxillomandibular fixation is necessary both at the time of the CT scan preoperatively and during the operation to ensure the solidarity of the mandibular complex with the position of the upper face. The surgical instruments, including the drill, are also calibrated for intraoperative computer visualization. The vector axis is defined preoperatively, and the drill holes are thus positioned accordingly under direct peroperative control.

Both techniques yield comparable accuracy, but the rapid prototyping technique has greater surgeon satisfaction and less operative time despite longer preoperative planning.

Older tracheostomy-dependent children with micrognathia can also beneficiate from distraction osteogenesis, and virtual planning constitutes a powerful surgical tool in this regard [58].

Hemifacial Microsomia (HFM)

The most prominent feature of hemifacial microsomia is the mandibular deformity, and it provides the basis for the Pruzansky classification which is the most commonly used for this disease. Since McCarthy et al. described the use of distraction osteogenesis in the mandible in 1992 [59], this technique has been widely employed in children with HFM with superb results on the short term. However, more recent publications with lengthier follow-up report a high rate of relapse on the long run (up to 100% relapse rate) requiring orthognathic surgery after skeletal maturation both for distraction osteogenesis and bone grafting [60–63].

Despite failure of this treatment on the long term, the child's social and psychological development and the quality of life are significantly improved after surgical correction in the early school years [64]. Digital planning has been utilized for mandibular distraction osteogenesis in HFM children [65].

It helps to guide the osteotomy and the position of the distractor and to determine the amount of distraction needed.

The desired effect is translation and rotation of the mandible, with the contralateral unaffected condylion as the center of rotation [66].

The main caveat noted was discordance between the planned position of the mandible and the actual postoperative position, and this was attributed to the forces generated by the lateral pterygoid muscle and the remaining soft tissue [67].

Mandibular Defects: Reconstruction Using Free Fibula Flap

In the pediatric population, extensive mandibular defects are caused by oncologic and traumatic etiologies [68]. 3D reconstruction of CT images is useful in the diagnosis of the mandibular defect, and it assists in the indication for surgery. It is helpful in assessing the anatomy of the mandibular complex, especially in the determination of the temporomandibular joint status and whether or not it needs reconstruction.

The application of virtual planning to mandibular reconstruction via free fibular flap transfer [69, 70] – and onlay fibular graft [71] – allows precise osteotomies of the fibular bone. Its utility lies in the ability to accurately estimate the dimensions of the required flap. The size of the missing bone and the angle of the mandible can all be derived from the contralateral side of the mandible by judiciously rotating the 3D image around the contralateral condyle (center of rotation) until the lower interincisal line intersects with the midline and/or proper dental occlusion is achieved in centric relation; the required flap shape can hence be conceptualized by subtracting the intact hemimandible from the mirror image of the contralateral side of the mandible. A 3D image of the donor site can then be used to elaborate the technical steps needed for shaping the fibular bone. Osteotomy sites and drill hole locations are determined and then translated into cutting jigs, repositioning guides, and pre-bent *custom* plates to be used peroperatively. The location and length of the pedicle is also studied on the 3D images and the recipient vessels identified.

In a case study concerning an adult patient with a large mandibular defect, digital planning allowed precise fibular bone shaping with concomitant placement of dental implants and prosthesis in one single surgical procedure. This was done using a preoperatively fabricated cutting guide that contained drilling cylinders for accurate implant placement. A neogingiva was created through split-thickness skin grafting of the flap [72]. Nevertheless, evidence of the applicability of such an endeavor in the pediatric setting is still missing.

Orthognathic Surgery

Virtual planning has provided the means for a veritable paradigm shift in orthognathic surgery. It is more accurate and less time-consuming than the classic model surgery, and it renders the lengthy laboratory work for splint fabrication somewhat preposterous. A 3D image of the patient's facial bone structure allows accurate cephalometric measurements, evaluation of the occlusal cant, and diagnosis of the jaw disharmony. In cleft patients, it allows visualization of the cleft gap. Simulation of the desired movements is then carried out to achieve centric relation and centric occlusion. This requires identification of the osteotomy lines while avoiding the anatomic pitfalls (infraorbital nerve, inferior alveolar nerve, tooth roots, tooth buds, etc.) and studying the location and amount of bony contact after correction. Once the simulation is achieved, quantitative measurements are drawn from the 3D virtual model in order to translate the movements to the operating field. The decision is made as to which jaw will be moved first, and 3D-printed splints are devised that concretize the measurements for intraoperative usage: an *intermediate splint* serves to correctly position one jaw based on the location of the second jaw. After the first jaw is safely secured using plates and screws, the second jaw is mobilized and correctly positioned to the first jaw using another splint – the *final splint*. Thus, the preplanned new jaw position is acquired. A genioplasty can also be planned using the same technology, using a genioplasty splint or guide to translate the computer-based virtual osteotomy and movement [73–76].

Intraoperative navigation has also been used for intermediate splint fabrication [77].

Clinical Cases

Case 1

A 6-month-old child with metopic synostosis, trigonocephaly (Fig. 12.2), confirmed on CT scan, narrow endocranial

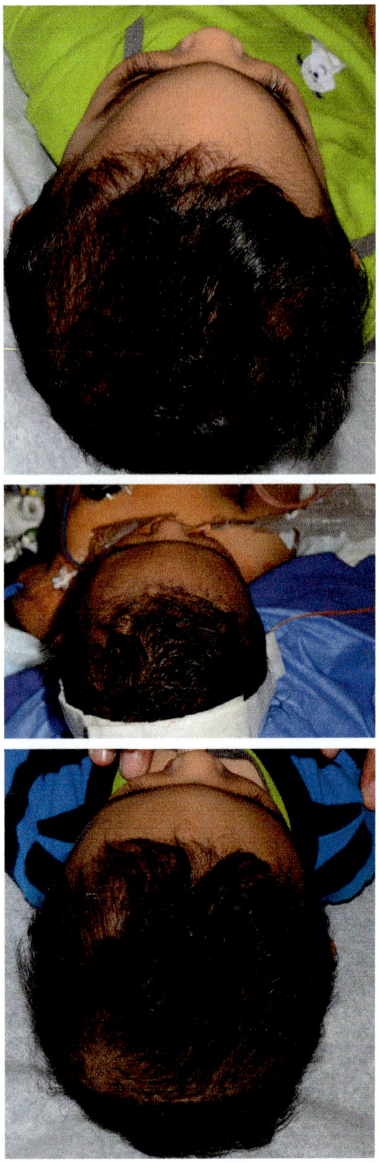

Fig. 12.2 A 6-month-old child with trigonocephaly. (*Upper*) preoperative picture; (*middle*) immediate postoperative picture showing correction of cranial shape; (*lower*) 3-year follow-up showing persistence of good results

bifrontal angle 123°. 3D planning was used to widen this angle to a more normal 151° using a positioning template (Figs. 12.3 and 12.4).

Case 2

This case is about an older child with Crouzon syndrome. She has undergone LeFort III osteotomy and advancement (Fig. 12.5). 3D planning allows one to see the orbital-globe relationship, occlusion, facial height, and set these dimensions as metrics to plan and execute the surgery.

Case 3

This case is about a younger child with Apert syndrome. Frontofacial monobloc advancement with distractor placement (Fig. 12.6) was performed and 3D planning assisted in determining the osteotomy line and burr hole positions, as well as ensuring the proper vector and avoiding anatomical pitfalls such as skull defects.

Case 4

This is a child with retrusion and hypoplasia of the midface who has undergone LeFort III osteotomy and advancement. 3D reconstruction of CT scan images assisted in the diagnosis and treatment planning through simulation of the osteotomy lines and of the mobilization required (Fig. 12.7).

Case 5

This case is an example of digital planning in orthognathic surgery. The patient has a maxillary retrusion that requires surgical correction. Digital planning was used to simulate the consecutive steps of the surgical procedure: mandibular repositioning was undergone first via bilateral sagittal split osteotomy using an intermediate splint. Then, the maxillary advancement was carried out using the final splint fixated on the repositioned mandible. Both of these splints had previously been generated through computer-assisted manufacturing. Finally, a sliding genioplasty was performed as visualized on the digital plan to refine facial aesthetics (Fig. 12.8).

Case 6

A 15-year-old Apert patient with frontal defects and retrusion along with microretrognathism. After completion of craniofacial growth, a cranial titanium mesh was custom made to correct both retrusion and the defect. A simultaneous LeFort I osteotomy with a 23.5 mm advancement, 5 mm lengthening, and 10° downward rotation was performed (Fig. 12.9).

Case 7

A child with left-sided orbital dystopia (5mm downward) undergoes a four-wall box orbital translocation. Virtual surgical planning allows accurate measurements, precise surgical steps, and the translation of this plan into precision custom-made surgical cutting jigs and repositioning guides

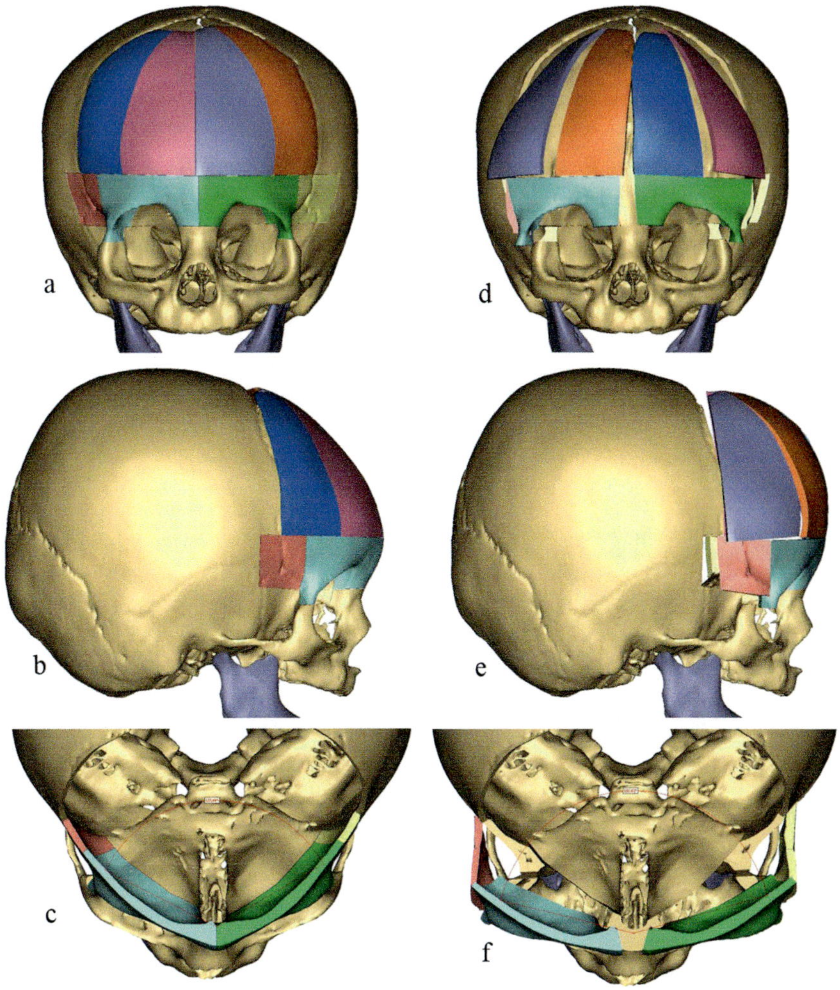

Fig. 12.3 Surgical planning for the patient shown in Fig. 12.2. (**a–c**) Preoperative: narrow endocranial bifrontal angle (123°); (**d–f**) projected postoperative state: endocranial bifrontal angle 151° (Proplan, DuPuy Synthes Craniomaxillofacial, Paoli, PA, USA)

(Figs. 12.10 and 12.11). Two guides were manufactured for this operation: the first one serves to guide the osteotomy and to specify the locations of the drill holes. It mimics and complements the shape of the left superior orbital rim. Once the osteotomies and the drill holes are made, the second guide serves to reposition the entire orbit in its new position relative to the contralateral orbit. Hence, the second surgical guide spans the entire fronto-orbital bandeau in its new postoperative shape. This patient had a 5mm translocation upward of the left orbit.

Case 8

This is an example of the application of digital planning in neonatal micrognathia in a tracheostomy-dependent child (Figs. 12.12 and 12.13). It determines the osteotomy sites and distractor type and locations along with the amount and vector of distraction as well as the projected final result. It also simulates the relief of airway obstruction after mandibular distraction.

Case 9

This is a patient with right-sided hemifacial microsomia showing an occlusal cant of more than 6° (Figs. 12.14 and 12.15). 3D planning helped determine:

- The vector for mandibular distraction: vertical and slightly anterior.
- The type and size of device needed: straight distractor.
- The amount of distraction required: appropriate length.
- Determine and guide the osteotomy and device position while bearing in mind the topographic relations to close-by structures (in this case, the inferior alveolar nerve): a surgical guide was manufactured and used to place the corticotomy and screw holes.

Case 10

Digital planning was undergone for bilateral mandibular distraction in an older tracheostomy-dependent child with neo-

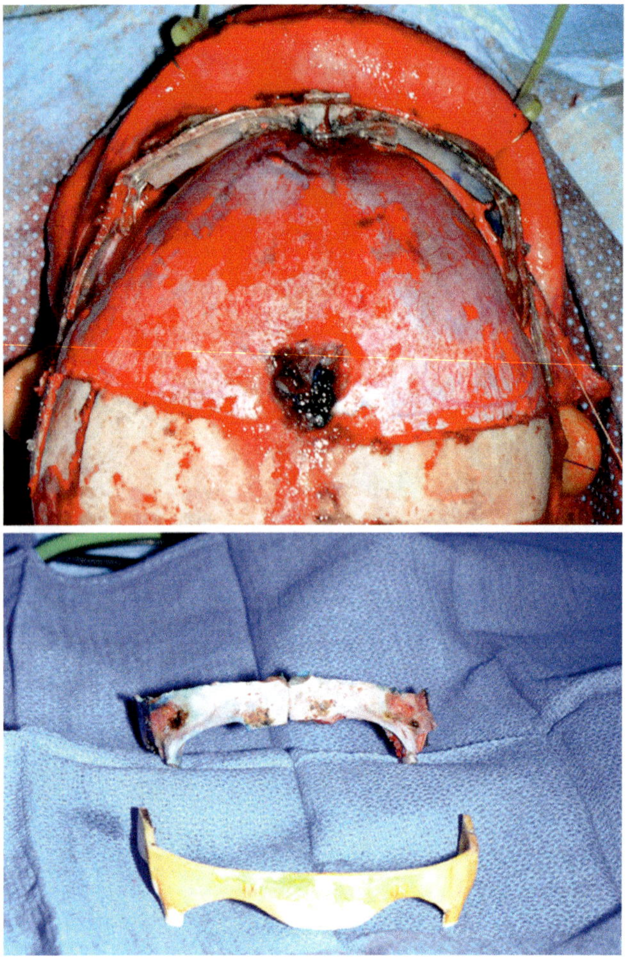

Fig. 12.4 Intraoperative photos of the fronto-orbital bandeau with the surgical guide (*lower*) and in situ (*upper*)

natal micrognathia (Figs. 12.16 and 12.17). The same objectives cited in case 8 were also attained here for the relief of airway obstruction.

Case 11

A patient has a jaw disharmony with right-sided deviation of the maxillary and mandibular bones. Pre- and postoperative pictures show the correction of jaw position and cant after maxillary LeFort I osteotomy and bilateral sagittal split mandibular osteotomies with genioplasty (Fig. 12.18). 3D planning of the surgical procedure helped to precisely determine and execute the location of the osteotomies and the direction and amount of the bone mobilization (Figs. 12.19, 12.20, and 12.21).

Case 12

This child suffers from severe neonatal micrognathia causing airway obstruction as shown by the chronic tracheostomy placement (Fig. 12.22).

Digital planning assisted in the strategic elaboration of every step of the mandibular reconstruction using a free vascularized fibular bone flap including harvesting, shaping, pedicle length, and inset of the flap (Fig. 12.23).

Conclusion

The implementation of computer-based surgical planning in pediatric craniofacial surgery has revolutionized patient care in this subpopulation. It allows outcome prediction with accuracy, and it provides individualized precision tools to assist the surgeon during the intervention. The increased costs of these various techniques should be weighed against the decrease in operative time, operative risk (bleeding, anesthesia exposure in the growing child), and improved results as well as the major decrease in the learning curve for apprentice surgeons or surgeons in training performing complex operations. This review delineates the spectrum of the various applications of 3D planning in pediatric craniofacial surgery: craniosynostosis, cranial defects or dysmorphology, orbital repositioning or translocation, mandibular reconstruction using free fibula flap, mandibular distraction for micrognathia with airway obstruction (neonatal and in older children), and orthognathic surgery. In all of these conditions, 3D planning assists in the cephalometric study, diagnosis, treatment simulation, surgical guide manufacture, and evaluation of the simulated surgical steps. However, a surgeon must be ready to act outside the given plan should these techniques fail, or expose the patient to unnecessary risks or becomes located at an institution that does not have this expensive equipment. We underline the fact that these digital software and 3D printing based techniques, despite their great accuracy and precision, are not meant to replace a surgeon's technical abilities or sense of clinical judgment.

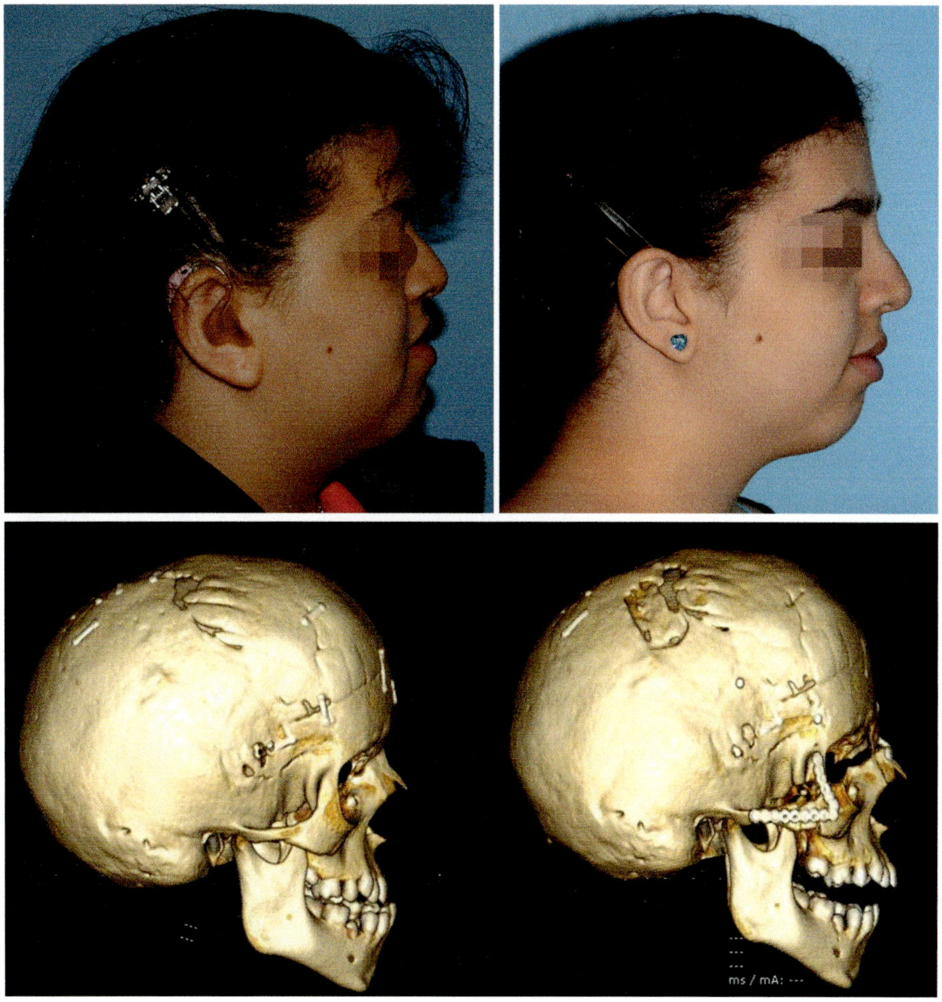

Fig. 12.5 Older child with Crouzon syndrome. Pictures and 3D reconstruction of CT images before and after LeFort III osteotomy

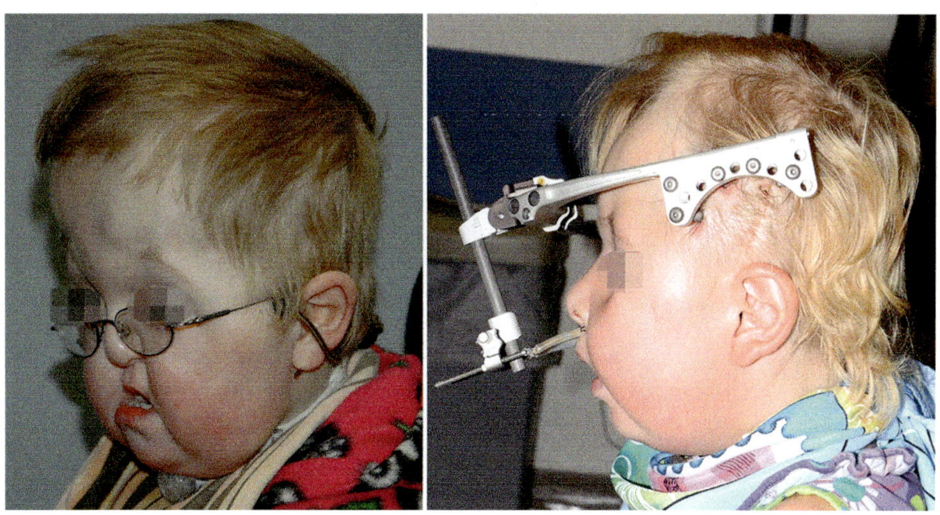

Fig. 12.6 (*left*) Child with Apert syndrome showing turribrachycephaly and maxillary hypoplasia. (*right*) Same patient after frontofacial monobloc distraction

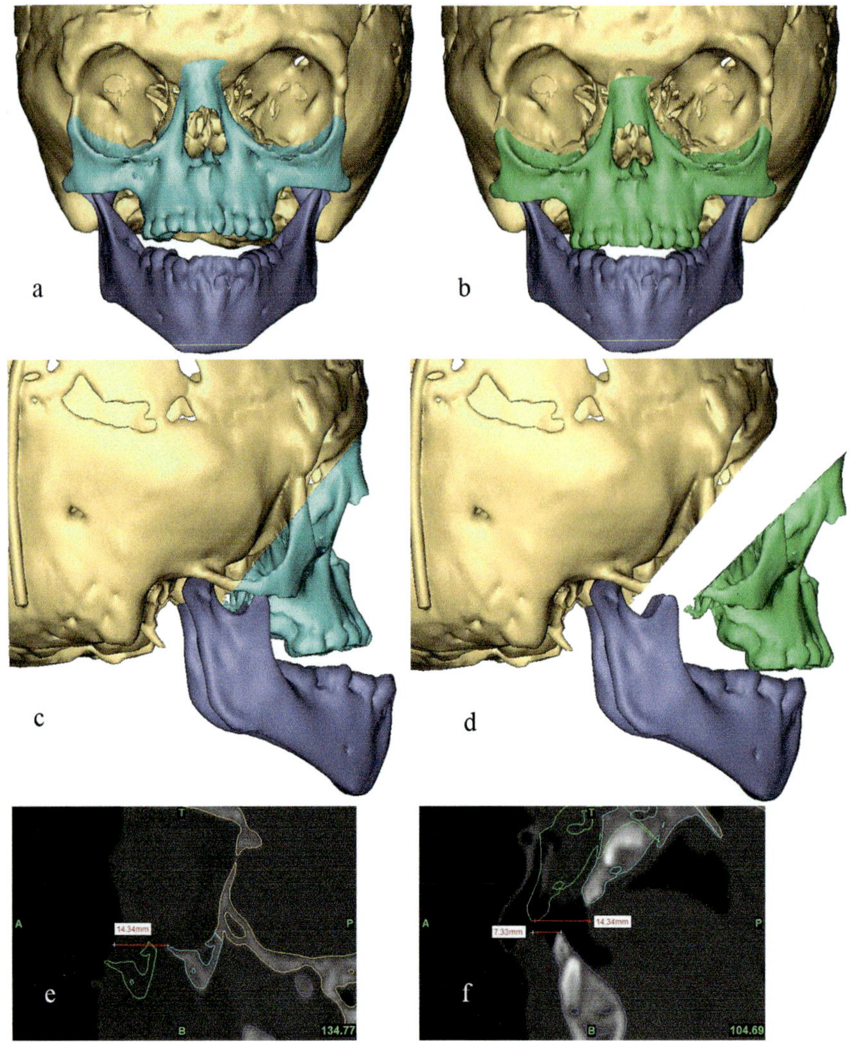

Fig. 12.7 Surgical planning for a LeFort III advancement procedure in a child with midface retrusion (case 4): (**a**, **c**) preoperative; (**b**, **d**) projected postoperative position; (**e**, **f**) 14.34 mm advancement, 7.33 mm downward movement (Proplan, DuPuy Synthes Craniomaxillofacial, Paoli, PA, USA)

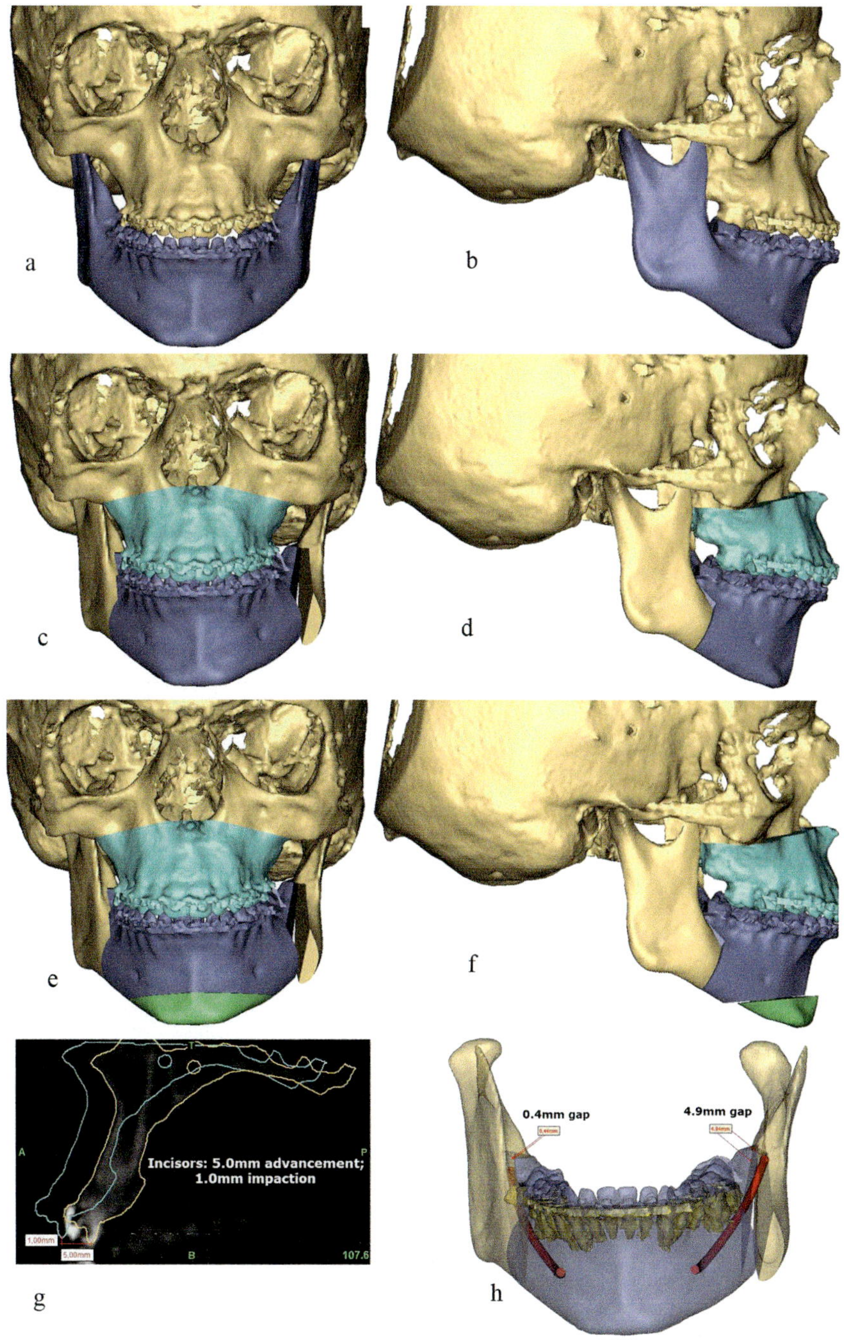

Fig. 12.8 Surgical planning for a patient with maxillary retrusion (Case 5). The mandible was mobilized first via bilateral sagittal split osteotomy and was positioned using an intermediate splint. Then the maxilla underwent a LeFort I osteotomy, and a 5 mm advancement with 1 mm impaction was applied using a final splint (**a**–**d**, **g**, **h**). A sliding genioplasty was performed with 5 mm advancement (**e**, **f**) (Proplan, DuPuy Synthes Craniomaxillofacial, Paoli, PA, USA)

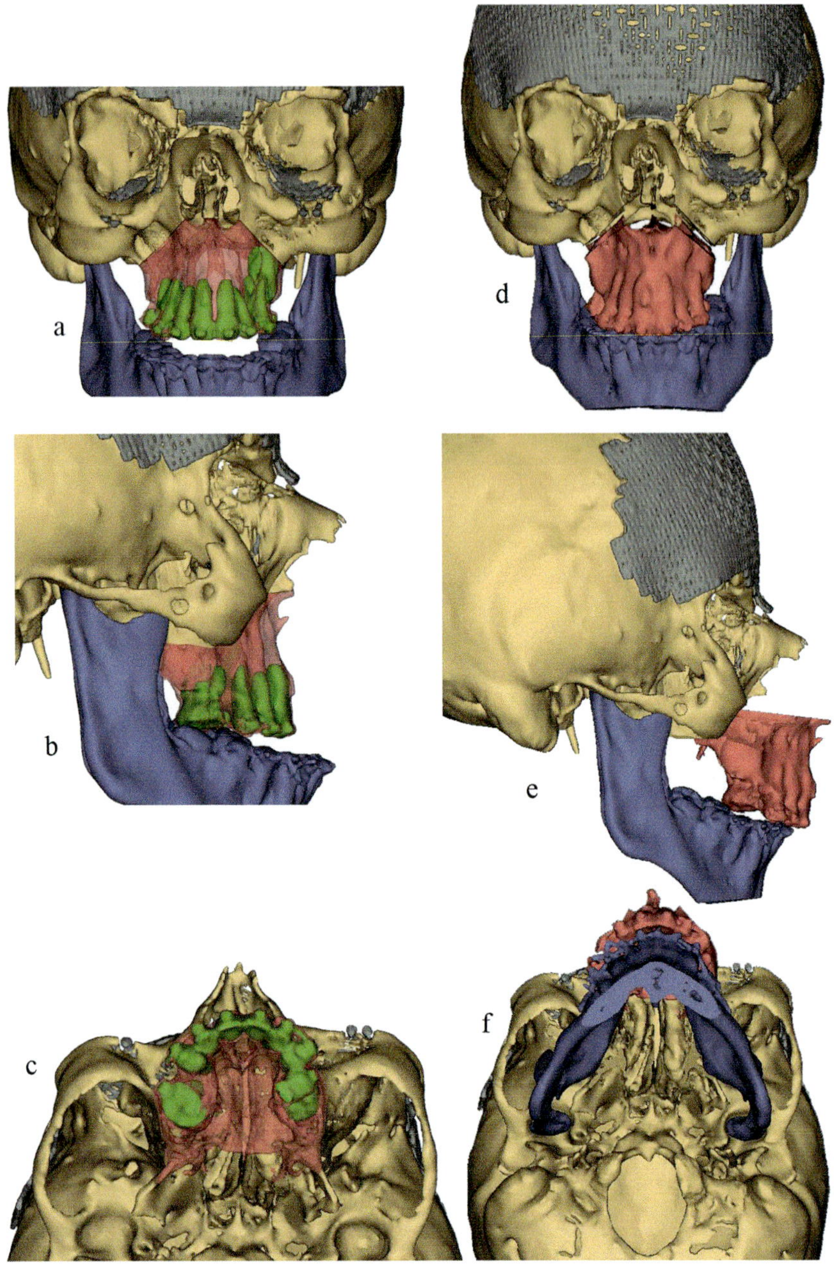

Fig. 12.9 Digital planning of the patient in Case 6. Preoperative 3D reconstruction (**a**–**c**) shows frontal defects and retrusion with major maxillary hypoplasia and retrusion and Angle Class III malocclusion. Simulated surgery shows LeFort I osteotomy and advancement along with a titanium mesh that was custom made for this patient based on this digital reconstruction. These 3D planning images (**d**–**f**) depict planned Le Fort I distraction in a child with Apert syndrome. Not the large magnitude of sagittal and vertical repositioning (Proplan, DuPuy Synthes Craniomaxillofacial, Paoli, PA, USA)

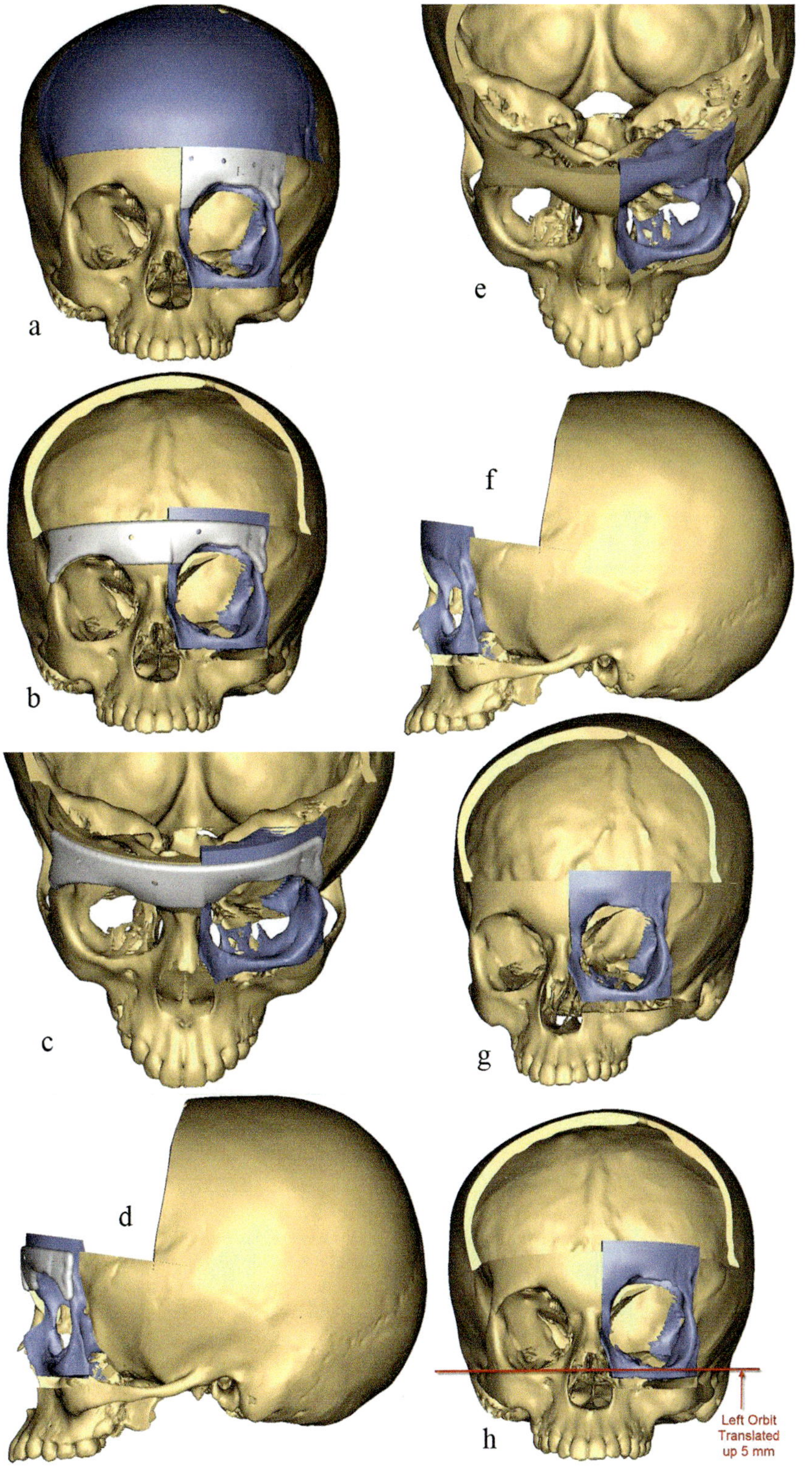

Fig. 12.10 Treatment plan for a patient with left-sided orbital dystopia (downward displacement 5 mm); (**a**) preoperative state with cutting jig in place; (**b**–**d**) left orbital upward translation using a specifically designed surgical guide; (**e**–**h**) projected postoperative position (Proplan, DuPuy Synthes Craniomaxillofacial, Paoli, PA, USA)

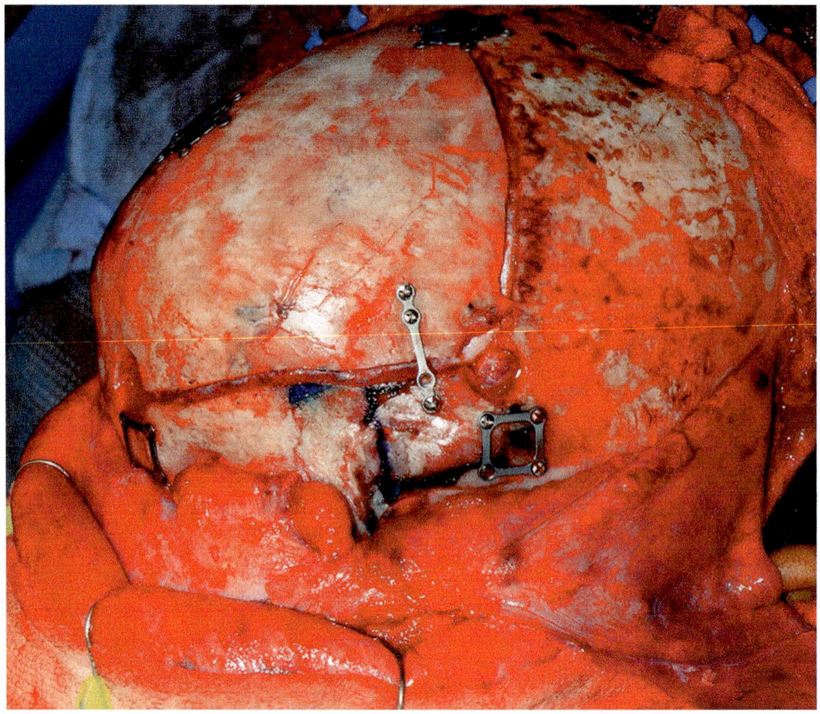

Fig. 12.11 Four-wall box orbital translocation: frontal bone flap and left orbit with plates and screws in place (DuPuy Synthes Craniomaxillofacial, Paoli, PA, USA)

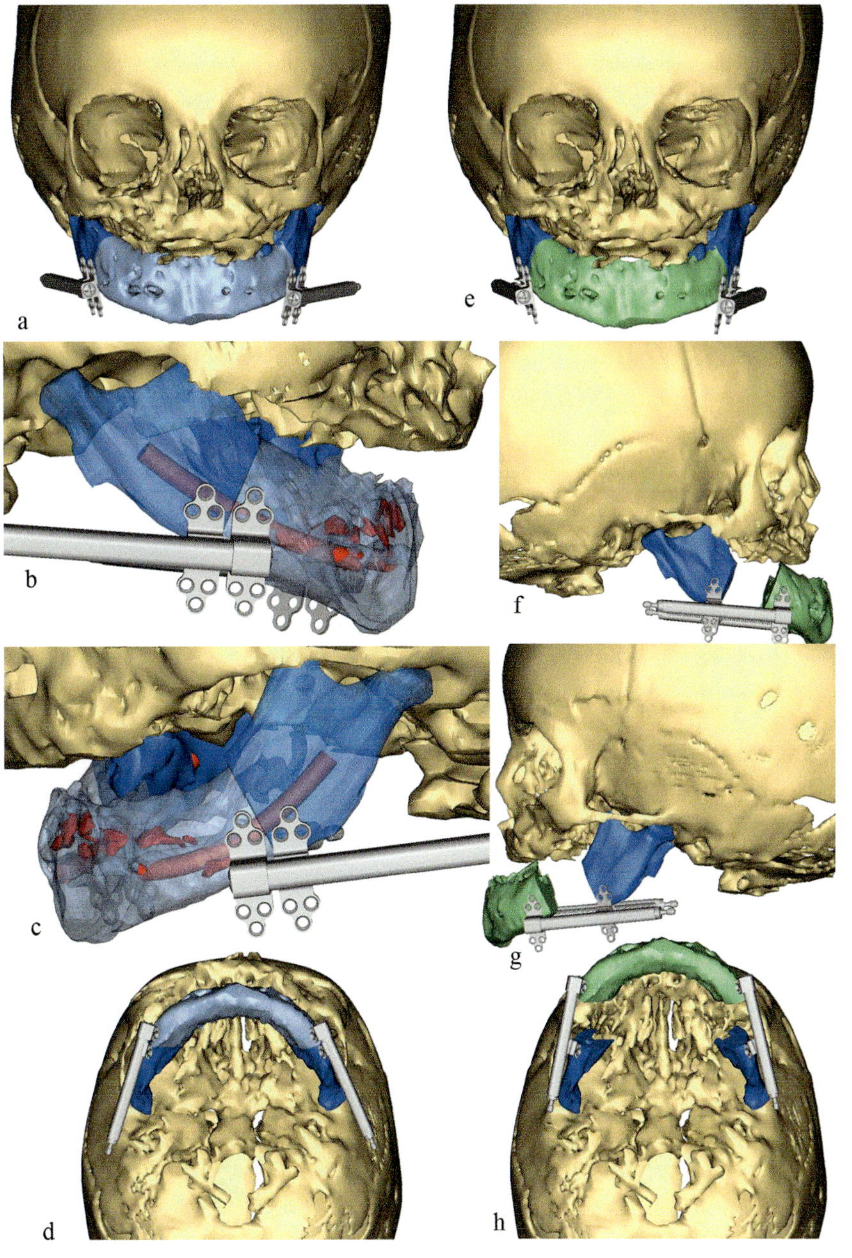

Fig. 12.12 Digital surgical planning for bilateral mandibular distractor placement procedure in a patient with tracheostomy-dependent neonatal micrognathia (Case 8). Graphic representation of the craniofacial complex before (**a**–**d**) and after (**e**–**h**) distraction is shown (Proplan, DuPuy Synthes Craniomaxillofacial, Paoli, PA, USA)

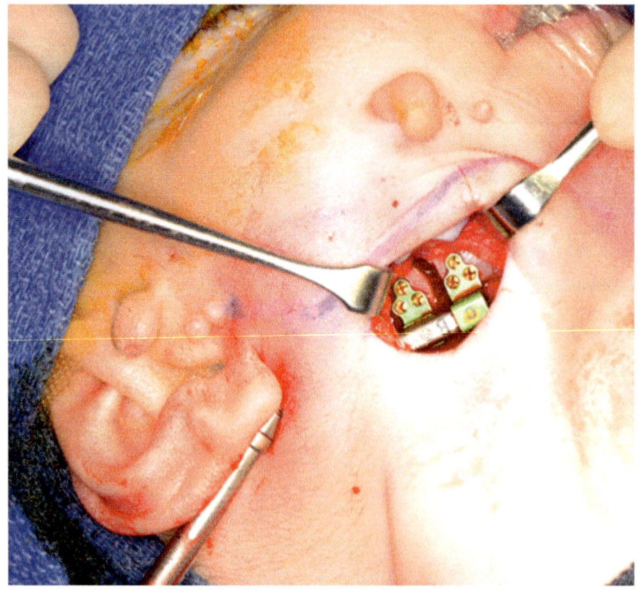

Fig. 12.13 Intraoperative photo of the distractor placed in situ according to the digital plan on the right hemimandible in the patient in Case 8 (DuPuy Synthes Craniomaxillofacial, Paoli, PA, USA)

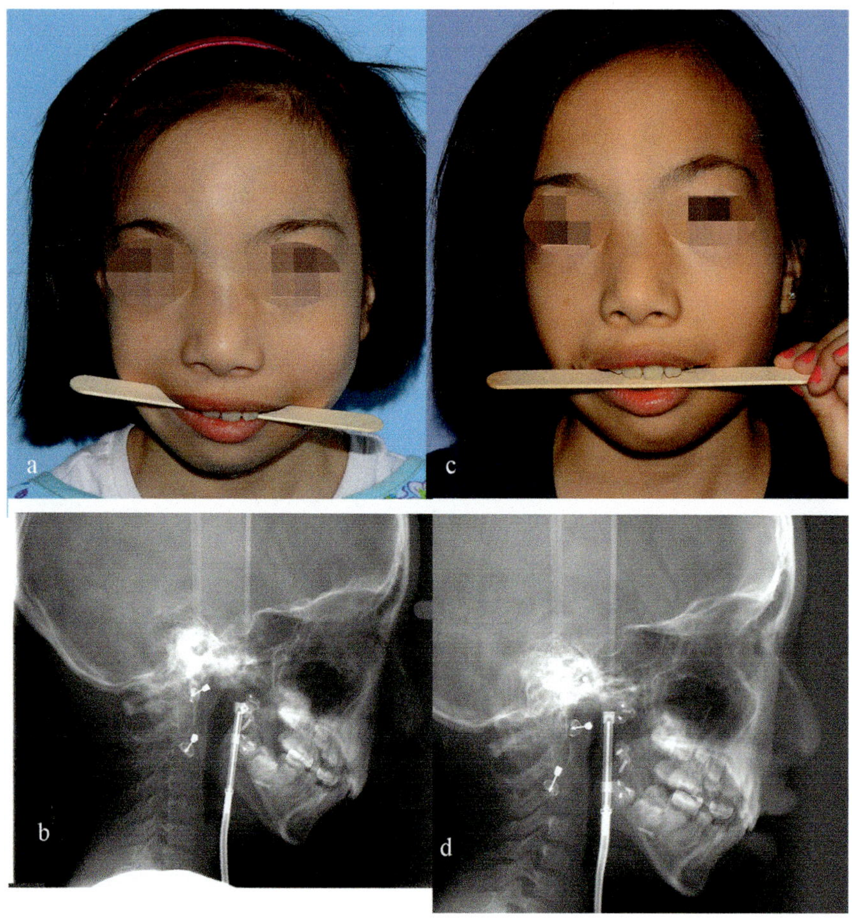

Fig. 12.14 (**a**) Patient with right-sided HFM (preoperative, Case 9). (**b**) Radiograph of the same patient with right-sided HFM with the mandibular distractor in place, before distraction (**c**, **d**) picture, and radiograph of the same patient after distraction

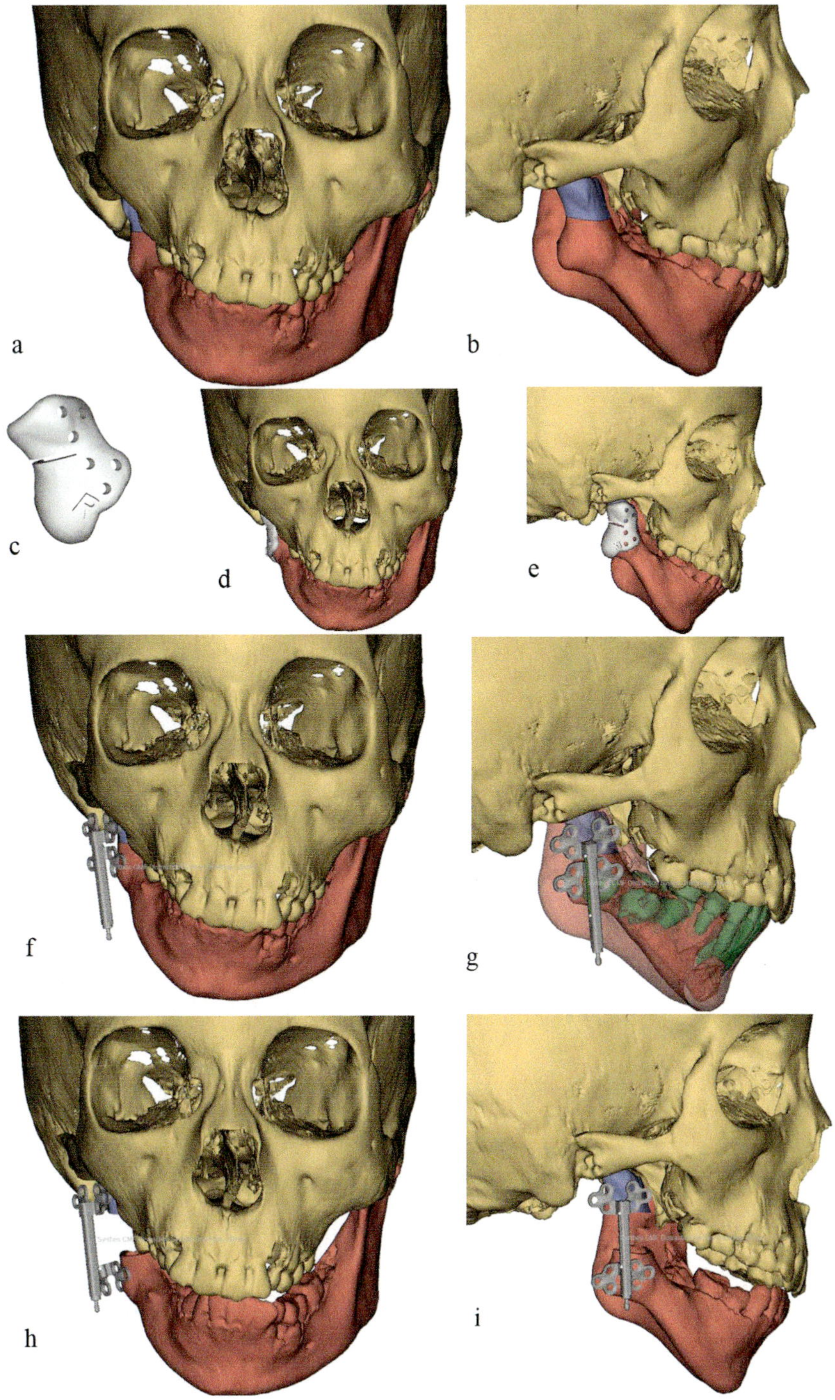

Fig. 12.15 3D planning for mandibular distractor placement in the same patient (Case 9) (Proplan, DuPuy Synthes Craniomaxillofacial, Paoli, PA, USA)

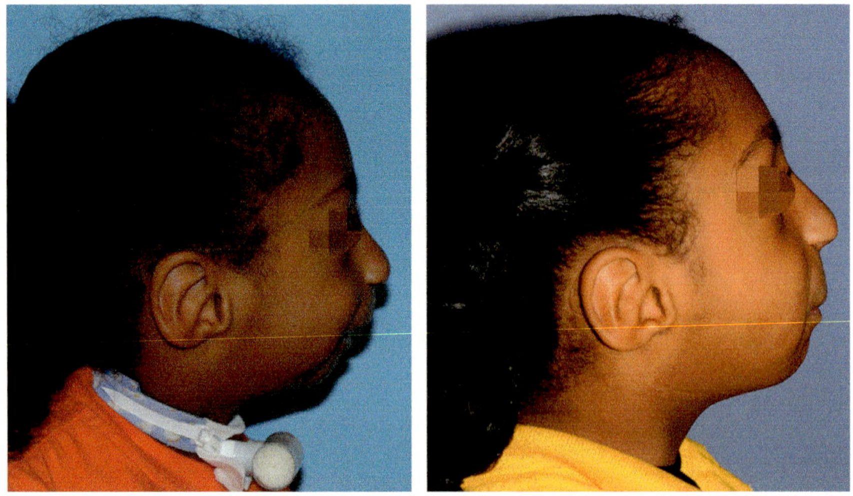

Fig. 12.16 Mandibular distraction for neonatal micrognathia in an older tracheostomy-dependent child: before surgery (*left*) and after distraction completion (*right*) (note the elimination of the tracheostomy cannula and the improvement in facial proportions on the profile view)

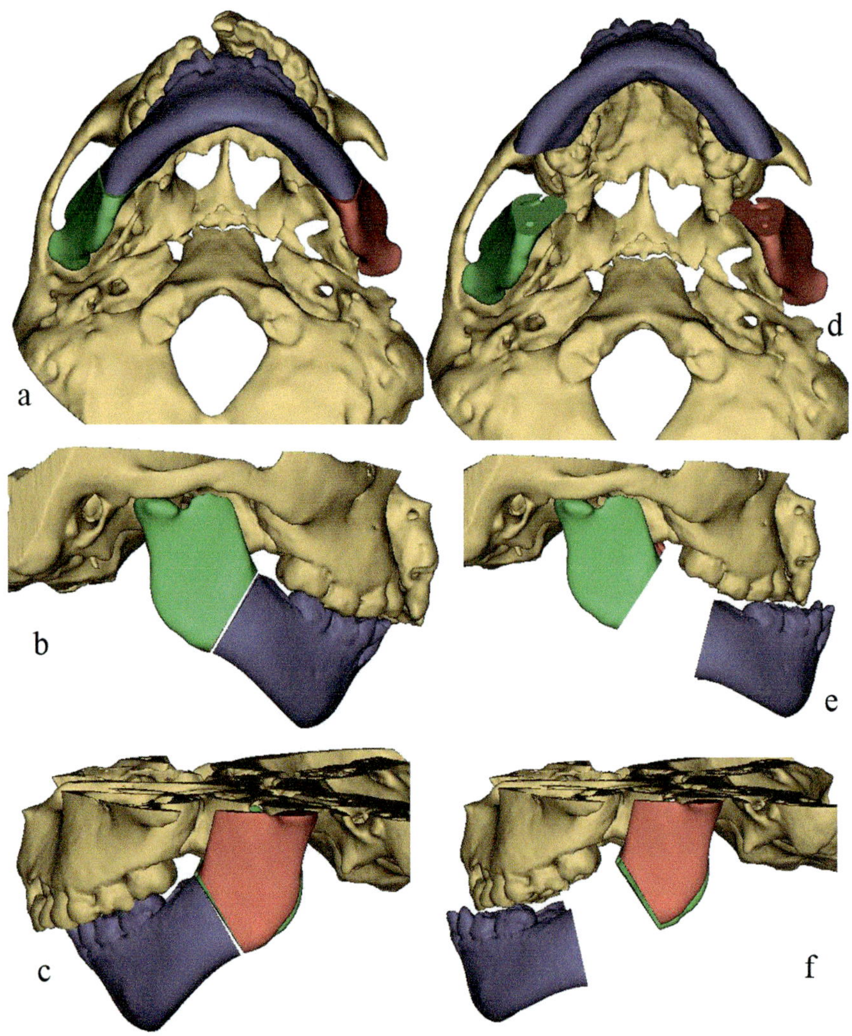

Fig. 12.17 Surgical planning for mandibular distractor placement in a tracheostomy-dependent child with micrognathia. 3D reconstruction of CT scan images before distraction (**a**–**c**) showing the osteotomy sites and the projected position after distraction (**d**–**f**) (Proplan, DuPuy Synthes Craniomaxillofacial, Paoli, PA, USA)

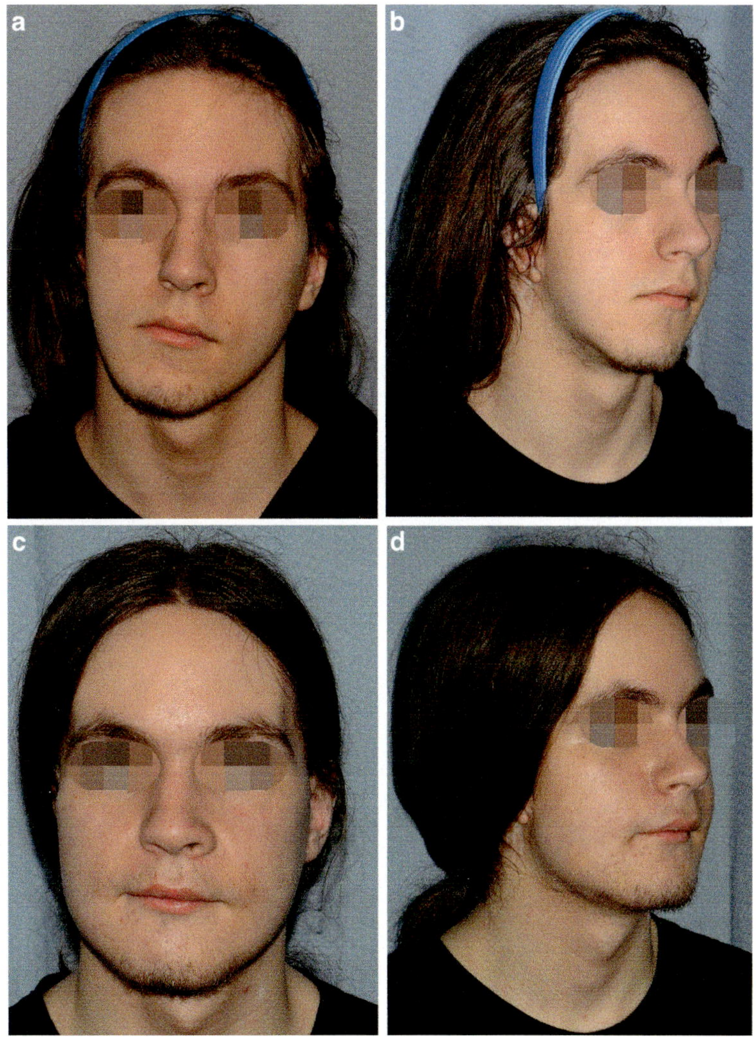

Fig. 12.18 Patient described in case 11. Preoperative (*first row* **a**, **b**) and postoperative (*second row* **c**, **d**) photographs were taken showing marked improvement in facial symmetry

Fig. 12.19 3D planning of the procedure in case 11. (**a**–**c**) Preoperative state: SNA = 83.6°, SNB = 80.1°, ANB = 8.7°; occlusal angle, 15.8°. (**d**) 4.0 mm maxillary advancement with 5.5 mm rotation to the left, with intermediate splint in position. (**e**) Final splint in position guiding mandibular repositioning – 5.0 mm advancement, 1.2 mm overbite reduction, left-sided rotation – after upper maxillary fixation in the new position. (**f**–**h**) Postoperative state, postoperative: SNA = 88.0°; SNB = 83.9°; ANB = 4.1°; occlusal angle = 10.7°. (**i**, **j**) Correction of the occlusal cant and symmetry (Proplan, DuPuy Synthes Craniomaxillofacial, Paoli, PA, USA)

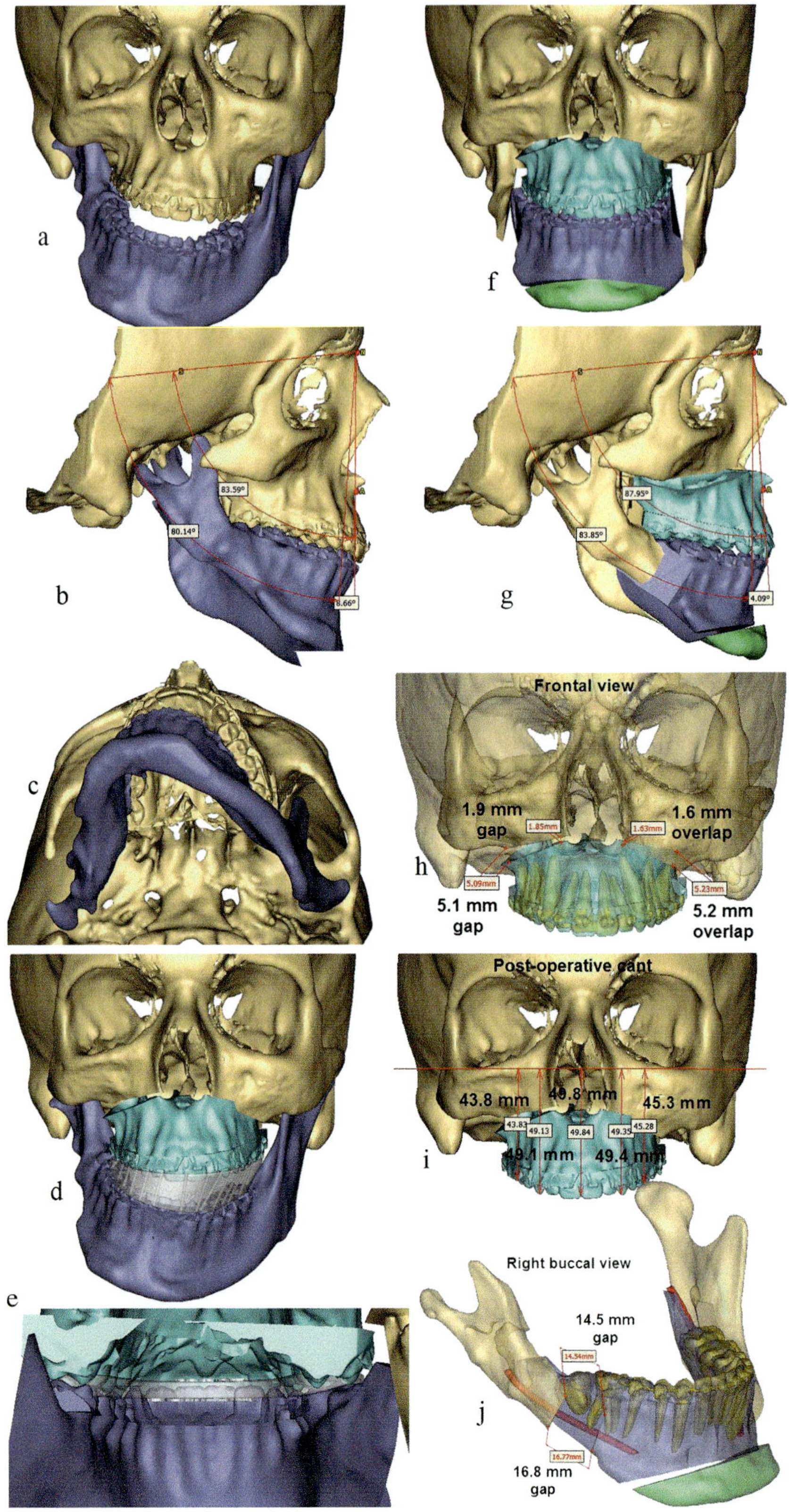

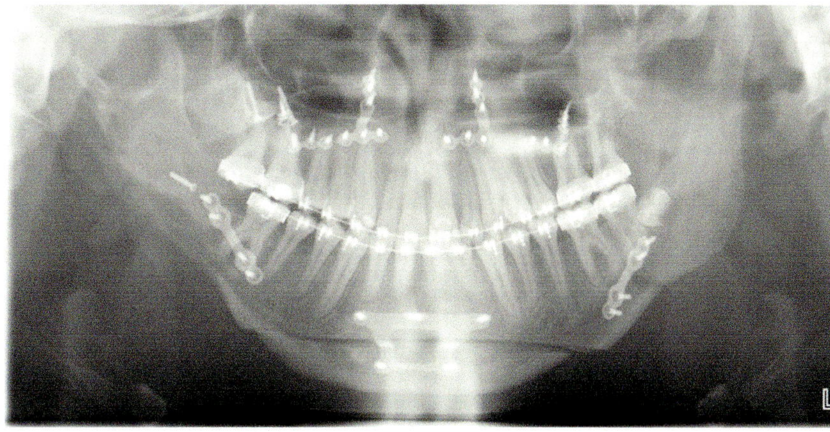

Fig. 12.20 Postoperative panoramic radiograph of the patient in Case 11 showing proper occlusion and correction of the occlusal cant

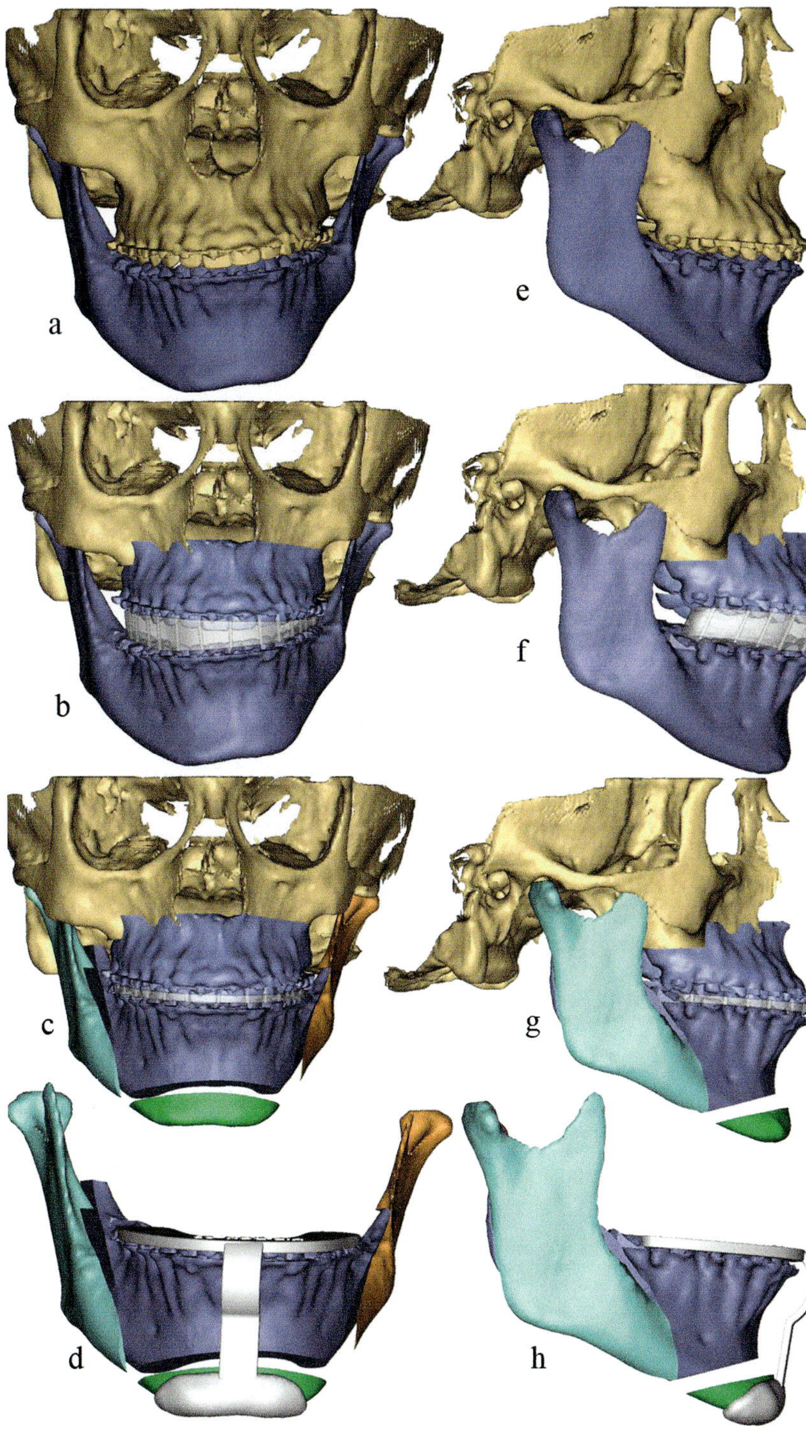

Fig. 12.21 This is the treatment plan for another orthognathic surgery case where a computer-generated intermediate splint and final splint were used to position the maxilla and the mandible, respectively (**a**–**c**). (**d**) The genioplasty plan was also translated into a surgical guide that accurately dictates the position of the genioplasty fragment (**e**–**h**) Note on lateral view the proposed bone movements and intermediate and final splints to achieve the desired result (Proplan, DuPuy Synthes Craniomaxillofacial, Paoli, PA, USA)

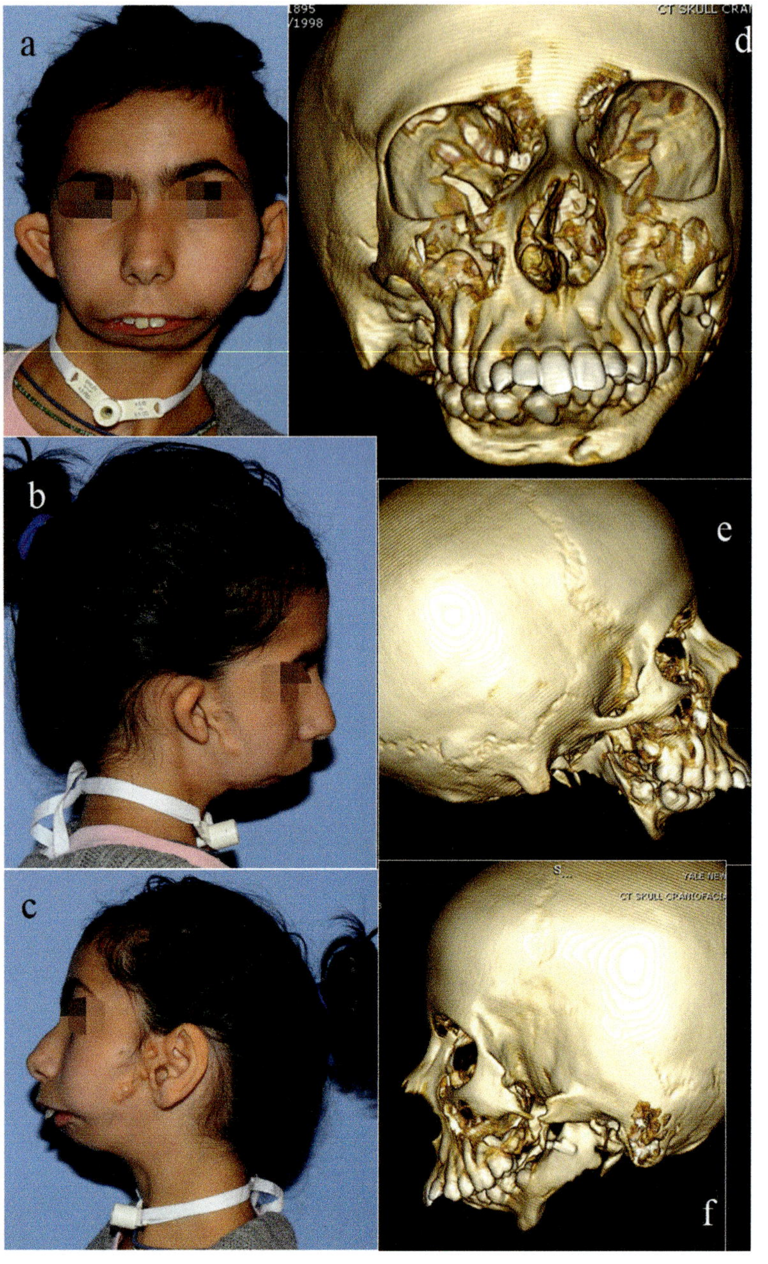

Fig. 12.22 Preoperative photographs of a tracheotomy-dependent child (Case 12) with severe mandibular deformity due to neonatal microsomia

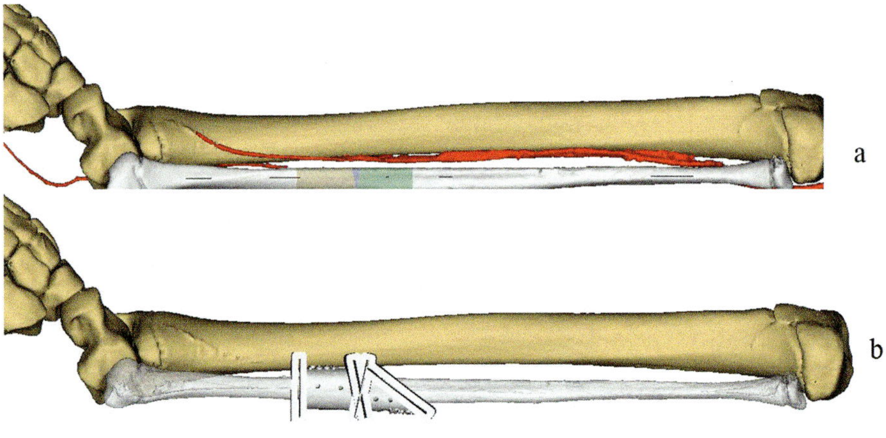

Fig. 12.23 3D planning and peroperative photos of the patient in Case 12. (**a**) Amount of fibula harvested. (**b**) Representation of the surgical cutting guide for fibula harvesting. (**c**, **d**) Projected 3D image for the planned reconstruction. (**e**, **f**) Preoperative surgical markings. (**g**) Fibular flap exposed. (**h**) Surgical template (cutting guide) for fibular flap osteotomies and remodeling. (**i**) Fibular flap after remodeling (note 3D plan jaw model). (**j**, **k**) Postoperative CT demonstrating the precision of preoperative plan (DuPuy Synthes Craniomaxillofacial, Paoli, PA, USA)

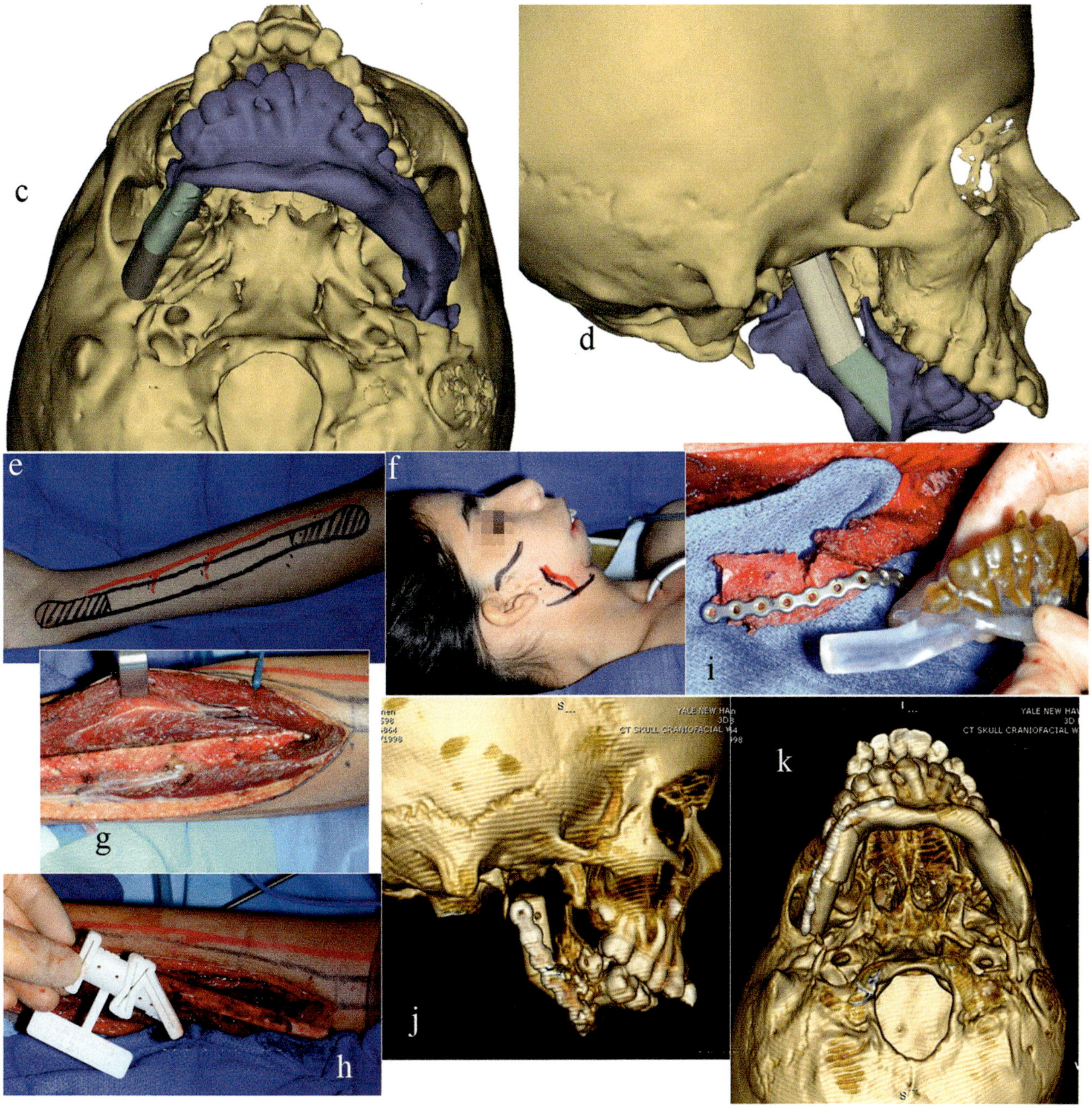

Fig. 12.23 (continued)

References

1. Robiony M, Salvo I, Costa F, Zerman N, Bandera C, Filippi S, et al. Accuracy of virtual reality and stereolithographic models in maxillofacial surgical planning. J Craniofac Surg. 2008;19(2):482–9.
2. Schendel SA, Hazan-Molina H, Rachmiel A, Aizenbud D. The future in craniofacial surgery: computer-assisted planning. Rambam Maimonides Med J. 2012;3(2):e0012.
3. Grauer D, Cevidanes LSH, Proffit WR. Working with DICOM craniofacial images. Am J Orthod Dentofac Orthop. 2009;136(3):460–70.
4. Flores RL, Deluccia N, Grayson BH, Oliker A, McCarthy JG. Creating a virtual surgical atlas of craniofacial procedures: Part I. Three-dimensional digital models of craniofacial deformities. Plast Reconstr Surg. 2010;126(6):2084–92.
5. Flores RL, Deluccia N, Oliker A, McCarthy JG. Creating a virtual surgical atlas of craniofacial procedures: Part II. Surgical animations. Plast Reconstr Surg. 2010;126(6):2093–101.
6. Meehan M, Teschner M, Girod S. Three-dimensional simulation and prediction of craniofacial surgery. Orthod Craniofac Res. 2003;6(Suppl 1):102–7.
7. Rudman K, Hoekzema C, Rhee J. Computer-assisted innovations in craniofacial surgery. Facial Plast Surg FPS. 2011;27(4):358–65.

8. Markiewicz MR, Bell RB. The use of 3D imaging tools in facial plastic surgery. Facial Plast Surg Clin North Am. 2011;19(4): 655–82.
9. Bell RB. Computer planning and intraoperative navigation in cranio-maxillofacial surgery. Oral Maxillofac Surg Clin North Am. 2010;22(1):135–56.
10. Marsh JL, Vannier MW. Surface imaging from computerized tomographic scans. Surgery. 1983;94(2):159–65.
11. Cutting C, Bookstein FL, Grayson B, Fellingham L, McCarthy JG. Three-dimensional computer-assisted design of craniofacial surgical procedures: optimization and interaction with cephalometric and CT-based models. Plast Reconstr Surg. 1986;77(6):877–87.
12. Cutting C, Grayson B, Bookstein F, Fellingham L, McCarthy JG. Computer-aided planning and evaluation of facial and orthognathic surgery. Clin Plast Surg. 1986;13(3):449–62.
13. Vannier MW, Conroy GC, Marsh JL, Knapp RH. Three-dimensional cranial surface reconstructions using high-resolution computed tomography. Am J Phys Anthropol. 1985;67(4):299–311.
14. Marsh JL, Vannier MW, Stevens WG, Warren JO, Gayou D, Dye DM. Computerized imaging for soft tissue and osseous reconstruction in the head and neck. Clin Plast Surg. 1985;12(2):279–91.
15. Vander Sloten J, Degryse K, Gobin R, Van der Perre G, Mommaerts MY. Interactive simulation of cranial surgery in a computer aided design environment. J Craniomaxillofac Surg. 1996;24(2):122–9.
16. Mommaerts MY, Jans G, Vander Sloten J, Staels PF, Van der Perre G, Gobin R. On the assets of CAD planning for craniosynostosis surgery. J Craniofac Surg. 2001;12(6):547–54.
17. Saber NR, Phillips J, Looi T, Usmani Z, Burge J, Drake J, et al. Generation of normative pediatric skull models for use in cranial vault remodeling procedures. Childs Nerv Syst. 2012;28(3):405–10.
18. Burge J, Saber NR, Looi T, French B, Usmani Z, Anooshiravani N, et al. Application of CAD/CAM prefabricated age-matched templates in cranio-orbital remodeling in craniosynostosis. J Craniofac Surg. 2011;22(5):1810–3.
19. Seruya M, Borsuk DE, Khalifian S, Carson BS, Dalesio NM, Dorafshar AH. Computer-aided design and manufacturing in craniosynostosis surgery. J Craniofac Surg. 2013;24(4):1100–5.
20. Mardini S, Alsubaie S, Cayci C, Chim H, Wetjen N. Three-dimensional preoperative virtual planning and template use for surgical correction of craniosynostosis. J Plast Reconstr Aesthet Surg. 2014;67(3):336–43.
21. Diluna ML, Steinbacher DM. Simulated fronto-orbital advancement achieves reproducible results in metopic synostosis. J Craniofac Surg. 2012;23(3):e231–4.
22. Shah A, Patel A, Steinbacher DM. Simulated frontoorbital advancement and intraoperative templates enhance reproducibility in craniosynostosis. Plast Reconstr Surg. 2012;129(6):1011e–2e.
23. Khechoyan DY, Saber NR, Burge J, Fattah A, Drake J, Forrest CR, et al. Surgical outcomes in craniosynostosis reconstruction: the use of prefabricated templates in cranial vault remodelling. J Plast Reconstr Aesthet Surg. 2014;67(1):9–16.
24. Ezaldein HH, Metzler P, Persing JA, Steinbacher DM. Three-dimensional orbital dysmorphology in metopic synostosis. J Plast Reconstr Aesthet Surg. 2014;67(7):900–5.
25. Metzler P, Ezaldein HH, Persing JA, Steinbacher DM. Comparing two fronto-orbital advancement strategies to treat trigonocephaly in metopic synostosis. J Craniomaxillofac Surg. 2014;42:1437–41.
26. Beckett JS, Persing JA, Steinbacher DM. Bilateral orbital dysmorphology in unicoronal synostosis. Plast Reconstr Surg. 2013;131(1):125–30.
27. Beckett JS, Chadha P, Persing JA, Steinbacher DM. Classification of trigonocephaly in metopic synostosis. Plast Reconstr Surg. 2012;130(3):442e–7e.
28. Pfaff MJ, Wong K, Persing JA, Steinbacher DM. Zygomatic dysmorphology in unicoronal synostosis. J Plast Reconstr Aesthet Surg. 2013;66(8):1096–102.
29. Steinbacher DM, Skirpan J, Puchała J, Bartlett SP. Expansion of the posterior cranial vault using distraction osteogenesis. Plast Reconstr Surg. 2011;127(2):792–801.
30. Taylor JA, Derderian CA, Bartlett SP, Fiadjoe JE, Sussman EM, Stricker PA. Perioperative morbidity in posterior cranial vault expansion: distraction osteogenesis versus conventional osteotomy. Plast Reconstr Surg. 2012;129(4):674e–80e.
31. Marchac A, Arnaud E. Cranium and midface distraction osteogenesis: current practices, controversies, and future applications. J Craniofac Surg. 2012;23(1):235–8.
32. Choi M, Flores RL, Havlik RJ. Volumetric analysis of anterior versus posterior cranial vault expansion in patients with syndromic craniosynostosis. J Craniofac Surg. 2012;23(2):455–8.
33. Nowinski D, Di Rocco F, Renier D, SainteRose C, Leikola J, Arnaud E. Posterior cranial vault expansion in the treatment of craniosynostosis. Comparison of current techniques. Childs Nerv Syst. 2012;28(9):1537–44.
34. Derderian CA, Bastidas N, Bartlett SP. Posterior cranial vault expansion using distraction osteogenesis. Childs Nerv Syst. 2012;28(9):1551–6.
35. Satoh K, Mitsukawa N. Suitable indication for the application of distraction osteogenesis: occipital enlargement for lambdoid synostosis. J Craniofac Surg. 2013;24(5):1530–4.
36. Ylikontiola LP, Sándor GK, Salokorpi N, Serlo WS. Experience with craniosynostosis treatment using posterior cranial vault distraction osteogenesis. Ann Maxillofac Surg. 2012;2(1):4–7.
37. White N, Evans M, Dover MS, Noons P, Solanki G, Nishikawa H. Posterior calvarial vault expansion using distraction osteogenesis. Childs Nerv Syst. 2009;25(2):231–6.
38. Nowinski D, Saiepour D, Leikola J, Messo E, Nilsson P, Enblad P. Posterior cranial vault expansion performed with rapid distraction and time-reduced consolidation in infants with syndromic craniosynostosis. Childs Nerv Syst. 2011;27(11):1999–2003.
39. De Jong T, van Veelen MLC, Mathijssen IMJ. Spring-assisted posterior vault expansion in multisuture craniosynostosis. Childs Nerv Syst. 2013;29(5):815–20.
40. Mulliken JB, Godwin SL, Pracharktam N, Altobelli DE. The concept of the sagittal orbital-globe relationship in craniofacial surgery. Plast Reconstr Surg. 1996;97(4):700–6.
41. Pai L, Kohout MP, Mulliken JB. Prospective anthropometric analysis of sagittal orbital-globe relationship following fronto-orbital advancement in childhood. Plast Reconstr Surg. 1999;103(5):1341–6.
42. Bender CA, Veneman W, Veenland JF, Mathijssen IMJ, Hop WCJ, Koudstaal MJ, et al. Orbital aspects following monobloc advancement in syndromic craniosynostosis. J Craniomaxillofac Surg. 2013;41(7):e146–53.
43. Jeelani NUO, Khan MA, Fitzgerald O'Connor EJ, Dunaway D, Hayward R. Frontofacial monobloc distraction using the StealthStation intraoperative navigation system: the ability to see where you are cutting. J Craniofac Surg. 2009;20(3):892–4.
44. Paige KT, Vega SJ, Kelly CP, Bartlett SP, Zakai E, Jawad AF, et al. Age-dependent closure of bony defects after frontal orbital advancement. Plast Reconstr Surg. 2006;118(4):977–84.
45. Dean D, Min K-J, Bond A. Computer aided design of large-format prefabricated cranial plates. J Craniofac Surg. 2003;14(6):819–32.
46. Winder J, Cooke RS, Gray J, Fannin T, Fegan T. Medical rapid prototyping and 3D CT in the manufacture of custom made cranial titanium plates. J Med Eng Technol. 1999;23(1):26–8.
47. Saringer W, Nöbauer-Huhmann I, Knosp E. Cranioplasty with individual carbon fibre reinforced polymer (CFRP) medical grade implants based on CAD/CAM technique. Acta Neurochir. 2002;144(11):1193–203.
48. Ono I, Tateshita T, Satou M, Sasaki T, Matsumoto M, Kodama N. Treatment of large complex cranial bone defects by

using hydroxyapatite ceramic implants. Plast Reconstr Surg. 1999;104(2):339–49.
49. Eufinger H, Wehmöller M. Individual prefabricated titanium implants in reconstructive craniofacial surgery: clinical and technical aspects of the first 22 cases. Plast Reconstr Surg. 1998;102(2):300–8.
50. Hanasono MM, Goel N, DeMonte F. Calvarial reconstruction with polyetheretherketone implants. Ann Plast Surg. 2009;62(6):653–5.
51. Bricolo A, Benati A, Bazzan A. Cranioplasty with acrylic resin, with heavy stainless steel mesh and with fragments of theca. Minerva Neurochir. 1967;11(3):208–11.
52. Cohen AJ, Dickerman RD, Schneider SJ. New method of pediatric cranioplasty for skull defect utilizing polylactic acid absorbable plates and carbonated apatite bone cement. J Craniofac Surg. 2004;15(3):469–72.
53. Biskup NI, Singh DJ, Beals S, Joganic EF, Manwaring K. Pediatric cranial vault defects: early experience with beta-tricalcium phosphate bone graft substitute. J Craniofac Surg. 2010;21(2):358–62.
54. Hutmacher DW. Scaffolds in tissue engineering bone and cartilage. Biomaterials. 2000;21(24):2529–43.
55. Chim H, Schantz J-T. New frontiers in calvarial reconstruction: integrating computer-assisted design and tissue engineering in cranioplasty. Plast Reconstr Surg. 2005;116(6):1726–41.
56. Jarrahy R. Controversies in the management of neonatal micrognathia: to distract or not to distract, that is the question. J Craniofac Surg. 2012;23(1):243–9.
57. D'Hauthuille C, Taha F, Devauchelle B, Testelin S. Comparison of two computer-assisted surgery techniques to guide a mandibular distraction osteogenesis procedure. Technical note. Int J Oral Maxillofac Surg. 2005;34(2):197–201.
58. Rachmiel A, Srouji S, Emodi O, Aizenbud D. Distraction osteogenesis for tracheostomy dependent children with severe micrognathia. J Craniofac Surg. 2012;23(2):459–63.
59. McCarthy JG, Schreiber J, Karp N, Thorne CH, Grayson BH. Lengthening the human mandible by gradual distraction. Plast Reconstr Surg. 1992;89(1):1–8. discussion 9–10.
60. Nagy K, Kuijpers-Jagtman AM, Mommaerts MY. No evidence for long-term effectiveness of early osteodistraction in hemifacial microsomia. Plast Reconstr Surg. 2009;124(6):2061–71.
61. Suh J, Choi TH, Baek S-H, Kim JC, Kim S. Mandibular distraction in unilateral craniofacial microsomia: longitudinal results until the completion of growth. Plast Reconstr Surg. 2013;132(5):1244–52.
62. Ascenço ASK, Balbinot P, Junior IM, D'Oro U, Busato L, da Silva Freitas R. Mandibular distraction in hemifacial microsomia is not a permanent treatment: a long-term evaluation. J Craniofac Surg. 2014;25(2):352–4.
63. Pluijmers BI, Caron CJJM, Dunaway DJ, Wolvius EB, Koudstaal MJ. Mandibular reconstruction in the growing patient with unilateral craniofacial microsomia: a systematic review. Int J Oral Maxillofac Surg. 2014;43(3):286–95.
64. Khetani MA, Collett BR, Speltz ML, Werler MM. Health-related quality of life in children with hemifacial microsomia: parent and child perspectives. J Dev Behav Pediatr. 2013;34(9):661–8.
65. Chen Y, Niu F, Yu B, Liu J, Wang M, Gui L. Three-dimensional preoperative design of distraction osteogenesis for hemifacial microsomia. J Craniofac Surg. 2014;25(1):184–8.
66. Paeng J-Y, Lee J-H, Lee J-H, Kim M-J. Condyle as the point of rotation for 3-D planning of distraction osteogenesis for hemifacial microsomia. J Craniomaxillofac Surg. 2007;35(2):91–102.
67. Sun H, Li B, Zhao Z, Zhang L, Shen SGF, Wang X. Error analysis of a CAD/CAM method for unidirectional mandibular distraction osteogenesis in the treatment of hemifacial microsomia. Br J Oral Maxillofac Surg. 2013;51(8):892–7.
68. Ducic Y, Young L. Improving aesthetic outcomes in pediatric free tissue oromandibular reconstruction. Arch Facial Plast Surg. 2011;13(3):180–4.
69. Stirling Craig E, Yuhasz M, Shah A, Blumberg J, Salomon J, Lowlicht R, et al. Simulated surgery and cutting guides enhance spatial positioning in free fibular mandibular reconstruction. Microsurgery. 2014;35:29–33.
70. Liu X, Gui L, Mao C, Peng X, Yu G. Applying computer techniques in maxillofacial reconstruction using a fibula flap: a messenger and an evaluation method. J Craniofac Surg. 2009;20(2):372–7.
71. Schepers RH, Raghoebar GM, Vissink A, Lahoda LU, Van der Meer WJ, Roodenburg JL, et al. Fully 3-dimensional digitally planned reconstruction of a mandible with a free vascularized fibula and immediate placement of an implant-supported prosthetic construction. Head Neck. 2013;35(4):E109–14.
72. Freudlsperger C, Bodem JP, Engel E, Hoffmann J. Mandibular reconstruction with a prefabricated free vascularized fibula and implant-supported prosthesis based on fully three-dimensional virtual planning. J Craniofac Surg. 2014;25(3):980–2.
73. Metzger MC, Hohlweg-Majert B, Schwarz U, Teschner M, Hammer B, Schmelzeisen R. Manufacturing splints for orthognathic surgery using a three-dimensional printer. Oral Surg Oral Med Oral Pathol Oral Radiol Endod. 2008;105(2):e1–7.
74. Choi J-Y, Song K-G, Baek S-H. Virtual model surgery and wafer fabrication for orthognathic surgery. Int J Oral Maxillofac Surg. 2009;38(12):1306–10.
75. Aboul-Hosn Centenero S, Hernández-Alfaro F. 3D planning in orthognathic surgery: CAD/CAM surgical splints and prediction of the soft and hard tissues results - our experience in 16 cases. J Craniomaxillofac Surg. 2012;40(2):162–8.
76. Sun Y, Luebbers H-T, Agbaje JO, Schepers S, Vrielinck L, Lambrichts I, et al. Accuracy of upper jaw positioning with intermediate splint fabrication after virtual planning in bimaxillary orthognathic surgery. J Craniofac Surg. 2013;24(6):1871–6.
77. Tsuji M, Noguchi N, Shigematsu M, Yamashita Y, Ihara K, Shikimori M, et al. A new navigation system based on cephalograms and dental casts for oral and maxillofacial surgery. Int J Oral Maxillofac Surg. 2006;35(9):828–36.

Craniomaxillofacial Free Flap Reconstruction Using Virtual Surgical Planning

13

James Leighton Mayo and Hugo St. Hilaire

Historical Perspectives

The concept of virtual surgical planning (VSP) has evolved significantly over the past 30 years. Developments in microsurgery, imaging techniques, and computer-assisted design and manufacture (CAD-CAM) technology have allowed VSP to become a routine tool for reconstructive microsurgeons.

Wei et al. (1986) [1] initially reported his experience on the use of the fibular free flap as a predictable composite flap in lower extremity reconstruction. These predominantly linear defects did not require complex osteotomies. Hidalgo (1989) [2], in his initial reports on the use of fibular free flaps for mandibular reconstruction, noted the relative ease with which the fibula can be contoured to reconstruct the more complex three-dimensional defects. While this can be said for a well-seasoned surgeon, creating a curvilinear neo-mandible while optimizing bony contacts in the absence of a stable construct creates a challenge. Efforts were initially made to fabricate guides using two-dimensional radiologic studies to facilitate planning and contouring of the osteotomy. Synchronously, Cutting and his group (1986) [3] were expanding the application of standard cephalometric studies and primitive computerized tomography (CT) data to assist in surgical planning for complex craniofacial cases.

Rose et al. (1993) [4] were the first to truly apply computerized surgical planning to design and produce replicates of reconstructed maxillofacial components to assist in the molding of bone-containing flaps. Computerized tomography data was used to create a three-dimensional model. The defect was virtually reconstructed, and an "analog reconstruction" was milled. This was applied to secondary reconstruction of the maxillofacial skeleton using the subscapular and the deep circumflex iliac system. The main drawback to this novel technology was the limited access to the appropriate technological support and the prohibitive cost.

The next decade allowed for an exponential growth in imaging technology, ability to manipulate data with more powerful computer systems, and more accessible CAD-CAM technology. Levine et al. (2009) [5] published their initial series of maxillofacial reconstructions using virtual surgical planning as we know it today. The ability to create virtual defects and reconstruct them with patient-specific bone-containing flaps was well illustrated and found to be predictably performed. The production of resection and shaping guides as well as pre-contoured plates streamlines complex maxillofacial reconstruction [6].

Simultaneous improvements in dental implantology and planning allowed for the implementation of a more prosthetically driven reconstruction with the immediate placement of implants and, in selected cases, immediate loading. The latter led to the development of the "Jaw in a Day" as reported by Levine et al. [7] where, in the setting of a benign osseous lesion, resection is performed with immediate reconstruction using a bone-containing flap and an immediate loaded implant-based prosthesis. Latest developments in virtual surgical planning and reconstruction include the patient-specific flap with a pre-bent plate fabricated to the special needs of a reconstruction.

Principles of Virtual Surgical Planning in Maxillofacial Reconstruction

Data Gathering

In order to allow appropriate rendering of the computerized tomography data, slice thickness of 1 mm or less is necessary. Imaging of the maxillofacial area as well as the donor site should be obtained. Of note, a library of "stock"

J.L. Mayo
Aesthetic and Reconstructive Surgery Institute, Orlando Health-University of Florida Cancer Center of Orlando, Orlando, FL, USA

H.S. Hilaire (✉)
Division of Plastic & Reconstructive Surgery, Department of Surgery, Louisiana State University, New Orleans, LA, USA
e-mail: hugost1@gmail.com; hsthil@lsuhsc.edu

A.M. Greenberg (ed.), *Digital Technologies in Craniomaxillofacial Surgery*, https://doi.org/10.1007/978-1-4939-1532-3_13

bone-containing flaps exists for use in situations in which a CT of the donor site cannot be obtained. This option may lead to less precise reconstruction, and the author recommends the use of patient-specific data. Appropriate understanding of the pathology and thorough discussion about resection margins need to be accomplished with the ablative surgeons when a two-team approach is used.

Planning Session

Through a web-based meeting, the operating surgeon and a team of biomedical engineers will virtually discuss and execute the surgical plan. The flexibility of a web-based meeting facilitates the participation of the ablative and reconstructive surgeon. In cases of primary reconstruction, the resection area along with the angulation of the osteotomies in all planes is defined. In cases of secondary reconstruction, the native skeletal structures can be manipulated and virtually repositioned. Once the defect to be reconstructed is adequately defined, the donor bone flap will be manipulated and positioned to reconstruct the defect. Close attention is given to the size of the segments and orientation of the osteotomies. Modification to the resection by creation of a more extensive defect may be required to ensure adequate length and vascularization of the bone flap segments. In the case of the fibula, the authors prefer keeping the segments larger than 2.0 cm in length.

When a patient-specific plate is fabricated, the plate specification, hole position, and angulation will be discussed. Following the completion of the meeting, a document summarizing the ablative and reconstructive plan will be produced for review by the operating surgeon.

Fabrication of Surgical Guides

Resection guides are then designed and fabricated using CAD-CAM technology. These guides should have ample surface contact area with the skeletal structure to ensure a unique position while being small enough to avoid encroachment on the soft tissue envelope or other important anatomical structures. Patient-specific plates, when utilized, will contain specific holes that correspond with one or more screw holes in the guide for securing the entire construct. Cutting guides, used to shape the bone-containing flap, are also created using similar technology. Again, in cases using patient-specific plates, screw holes will correspond to specific holes in the plate. The amount of musculature/periosteum left on the bone (typically 1–2 mm in fibula flaps) will be incorporated in the cutting guide. Three-dimensional stereolithic preop and post-op models can also be fabricated for intraoperative reference. Furthermore, shaping guides (e.g., condylar head) can be generated to ensure a close anatomic reconstruction.

Execution of the Surgery

A two-team approach allows more efficient surgery making the fibula a favorable donor site. Exposure of the maxillofacial defect, extirpation of the tumor, and dissection of the recipient vessels can be performed, while the fibula is harvested. The use of cutting guides allows the execution of the osteotomies in a more controlled and predictable fashion. Metal inserts can be placed in the cutting slot to ensure the reciprocating saw keeps the plan trajectory. The osteotomies and reassembly using a patient-specific plate can be performed, while the flap is still perfused at the donor site, thereby reducing ischemia time. Occasionally, minimal recontouring is required. This is likely the result of additive errors in positioning of the guides. The construct is harvested, and the microsurgical anastomosis is performed. The soft tissue elements are then inset, and the donor site is closed.

The application of VSP offers a more elegant and efficient execution of the surgical plan. In addition to providing resection and cutting guides, as well as a pre-contoured reconstruction plate, the planning session allows the surgeon to plan ahead and review the execution of the surgery to ensure an efficient and optimal outcome.

Common Flaps Used in Craniofacial Skeletal Reconstruction

Fibula

First introduced for reconstruction of lower extremity segmental bone defects by Taylor in 1975, the fibula free flap is now the workhorse for various head and neck bony reconstructions [8]. Hidalgo, in 1989, was the first to describe the use of the free fibula flap for mandibular reconstruction [2]. The straight hard cortical bone supplied by both endosteal and periosteal blood supply based on the peroneal artery offers a consistent, structurally sound yet easily and safely osteotomized construct for complex facial three-dimensional bony reconstruction. Early reports questioned the reliability of a septocutaneous component supplied by peroneal perforators through the posterior intermuscular septum. However, Wei and colleagues presented a series of patients who underwent reconstruction with the fibula osteoseptocutaneous flap predominantly for cancer reconstruction [9]. The favorable results demonstrated the true versatility of this flap as a reliable reconstruction modality. It is able to restore a bony framework capable of accepting osseointegrated dental implants, and provides a septocutaneous component capable of either intraoral or extraoral soft tissue coverage.

The fibula provides only 10% of lower leg support making it an acceptable donor site for vascularized bone. The fibula's blood supply is provided by the peroneal artery as periosteal blood flow and endosteal blood flow via a nutrient artery that enters the fibula 14–19 cm distal to the styloid process. The abundant periosteal blood supply obviates the need to include the nutrient source in flap harvest. The skin and soft tissue overlying the fibula laterally is supplied by septocutaneous perforators that branch from the peroneal artery traveling through the posterior intermuscular septum of the lateral compartment, and by musculocutaneous peroneal artery perforators traveling through the flexor hallucis longus and soleus muscles. The septocutaneous perforators alone are sufficient to provide blood flow to a septocutaneous component. Typically four to seven septocutaneous peroneal artery perforators ranging in size from 0.8 to 1.7 mm can be found at 3–6 cm intervals along the posterior fibula. This allows for numerous variations in skin paddle design with the most common location being mid-distal to preserve the proximal flap as the pedicle length component. The superficial peroneal nerve can be found in the skin island distribution making possible the construction of a sensate flap.

Preoperative CTA of the lower extremity is standard for our practice to exclude the 10% with peroneal artery dominant vascular architecture. The flap is harvested via a lateral approach with a tourniquet set to 350 mmHg. If a skin island is taken, typically this is designed with its anterior margin at or behind the anterior margin of the fibula to aid in closure of the defect. Up to a 5 cm width paddle can be harvested with an expectation for primary donor site closure. Those defects too wide to close primarily are closed with a split thickness skin graft. A 1–2 mm cuff of muscle is left on the bone, but it is important to refrain from leaving too much muscle, as this will impede plate fixation and formation of the bony construct after osteotomies. Osteotomies are made leaving at least 4 cm proximally and 6 cm distally to allow retained stability. Care must be taken to avoid the common peroneal nerve at the fibular head. Also, the peroneal artery takeoff from the tibioperoneal trunk is not far from its course along the posteromedial fibula representing another area requiring increased attention. The more distal fibula is used for reconstruction, and if the entire segment is not harvested, a section from the proximal aspect can be discarded. This will allow for additional pedicle length when shorter fibula segments are utilized.

The fibula free flap is quite versatile offering components of bone, muscle, and skin/soft tissue. The hard straight cortical bone allows the use of osteotomies to build a variety of three-dimensional facial constructs including frontal bone, orbit, maxilla, and mandible. The addition of the flexor hallucis longus muscle can be included to fill various defects from sinus obliteration to soft tissue defects created by cancer ablation. Finally, the skin paddle can be used for extraoral or intraoral coverage during mandible reconstruction. Its ability to be supplied by both proximal and distal perforators allows creativity in planning its position along the length of the fibula to be utilized for reconstruction. If necessary, two separate skin paddles can be harvested based on separate perforators. However, more commonly, a second free flap is utilized if both a lining and external flap are necessary. Common flaps for this purpose include ALT and forearm flaps. The second free flap can be anastomosed either to an additional neck recipient vessel or to the distal peroneal vessels. Donor site morbidity should be addressed, but only 4% suffer a decreased ambulatory status predominantly due to other factors [10] (Fig. 13.1).

Radial Artery Forearm Flap

Described by Yang et al. over 30 years ago, the radial fasciocutaneous flap holds a steadfast position within the armamentarium for head and neck reconstruction [11]. The radial forearm osteocutaneous flap, on the other hand, has been much less frequently utilized and is criticized for the donor site complications and poor bone stock [12]. The flap has the advantages of ease of harvest, long pedicle with good vessel caliber, consistent anatomy, and a thin/pliable skin paddle. However, the donor site aesthetics can be poor in such a highly visible and utilized functional body unit. As a composite flap, the risk of subsequent radius fracture has been reported in up to 43% of patients, 30% in larger series [13–15]. Still, the favorable qualities of the flap necessitate its consideration in head and neck reconstruction at the very least as a secondary option, if not as a primary construct in select cases [16, 17].

The radial artery is one of two end arteries to the forearm arising with the ulnar artery from the brachial artery at the proximal forearm. Perforators from the radial artery are plentiful in the exposed distal radial artery and travel through the lateral intermuscular septum. Venous drainage is abundant as the flap is drained by radial artery venae comitantes and through superficial veins via the cephalic vein [18]. Skin area can be quite variable from 4 to 30 cm in length and 4 to 15 cm in width. The section of radius available for harvest is the roughly 12 cm distally along the portion of the bone distal to the pronator teres insertion to the radial styloid. Up to 40% of the circumference of the radius can be taken without a significant increase in risk of fracture. The lateral antebrachial cutaneous nerve travels with the cephalic vein supplying the skin of the radial forearm. The medial antebrachial cutaneous nerve travels with the basilic vein.

The flap is harvested with the patient supine with the extremity under a tourniquet at 250 mmHG. After the distal skin paddle has been designed, dissection begins from ulnar side. Dissection is easiest in a subfascial plane ensuring that the paratenon is left intact over tendons distally. However, a suprafascial plane of dissection can be implemented in an effort to reduce the risk of wound healing difficulty over tendons. The lateral intermuscular septum to the radius is preserved as this includes key perforators. The radial border

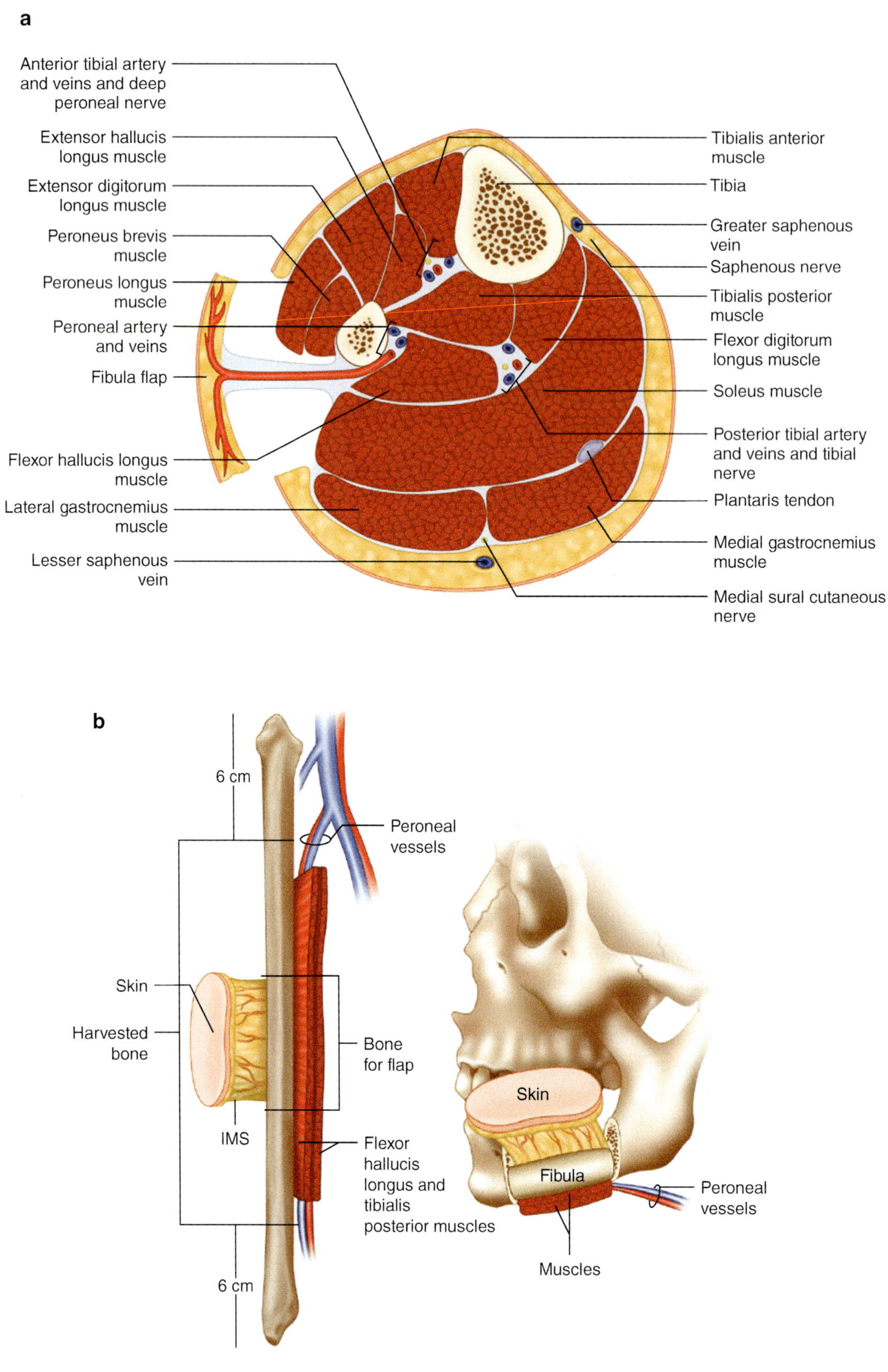

Fig. 13.1 (**a**) Peroneal artery perforators travel through the posterior intermuscular septum to supply the fasciocutaneous flap frequently harvested with the fibula flap. The vascular pedicle travels posteromedially to the fibula between the fibula and flexor hallucis longus. A variably sized cuff of this muscle can be included as necessary to add bulk to the flap. (**b**) The proximal fibula is discarded to increase pedicle length. The fasciocutaneous paddle is designed and harvested at a mid to distal fibula position where the most prominent perforators are located. 6 cm of proximal and distal fibula is left in situ in order to maintain stability. The fibula is then inset with the vascular pedicle traveling most often posteroinferiorly toward the recipient vessels in the ipsilateral neck

is then raised in a similar fashion. A boat-shaped section of the bone is then harvested including a small cuff of the flexor pollicis longus and pronator quadratus. The vascular pedicle is transected distally, and dissection proceeds proximally gaining pedicle length as necessary. Osteotomies can be performed in situ or after flap harvest. Risk of fracture is significantly reduced by prophylactically performing bicortical screw internal fixation of the radius [16].

Modifications and application of the flap are abundant. Small segment mandible defects can be reconstructed with the understanding that dental implants will not be placed. The skin paddle can be split to reconstruct more than one surface. The skin paddle can also be "sandwiched" around the vascularized radius for maxillary reconstruction [17]. The flap can be harvested as a sensate flap utilizing either the medial or lateral antebrachial cutaneous nerves as dictated by skin paddle design. Limitations are realized in the setting of large volume soft tissue defects. Ultimately, the versatile radial osteocutaneous free flap should be recognized as an option for head and neck reconstruction (Fig. 13.2).

Deep Circumflex Iliac Artery Flap

In 1979, Taylor et al. described the deep circumflex iliac vessels as the dominant blood supply to the iliac bone and surrounding tissues paving the way for the application of this versatile composite flap to a myriad of head and neck reconstructive challenges [19]. Favorable vessel size and pedicle length afford the ability to utilize the flap in various locations with the occasional need for a vein graft. Ample height and width are advantages in performing quality mandible reconstruction especially when osseointegrated dental implants are planned. In the setting of maxillary reconstruction, unlike purely soft tissue flaps such as latissimus or rectus abdominis free flaps, the DCIA composite flap offers a stable and very acceptable structure when combined with an internal oblique muscle component for intraoral lining. While being quite versatile, the DCIA flap also has the advantage of an acceptable donor site complication profile. In a review of 82 cases of iliac crest free flap head and neck reconstruction, Forest et al. found the most common complication to be persistent

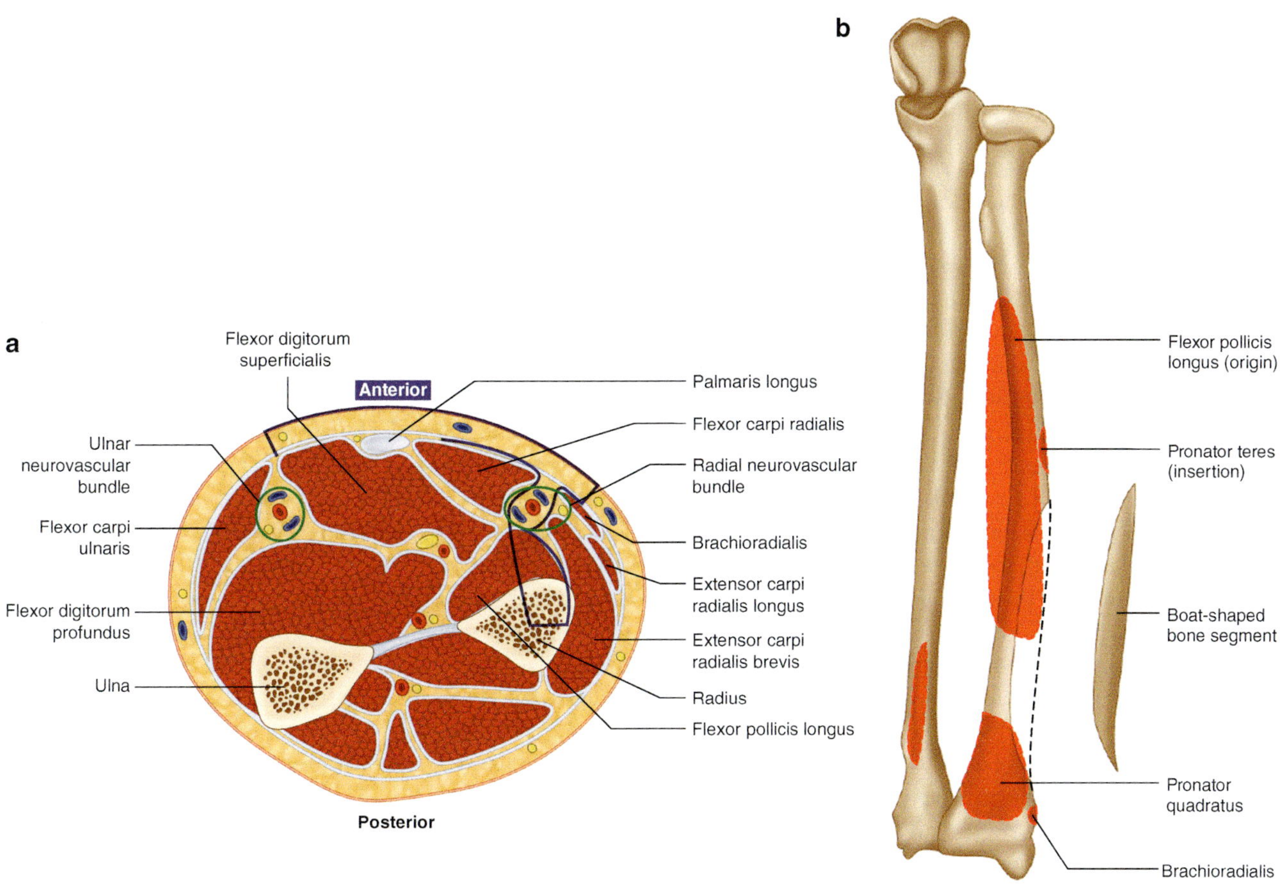

Fig. 13.2 (**a**) The radial forearm bone flap is harvested including the volar skin and fascia, the radial artery and vena commitantes and up to a 40% wedge of radius distally. Note the dual venous drainage via the superficial/cephalic system and the paired vena commitantes traveling with the radial artery. (**b**) The radial bone flap is harvested by removing up to a 40% wedge of bone from the insertion of the pronator teres distally to the radial styloid. The proximal and distal ends are tapered in a boat shape to help reduce the incidence of radial fracture after bone harvest

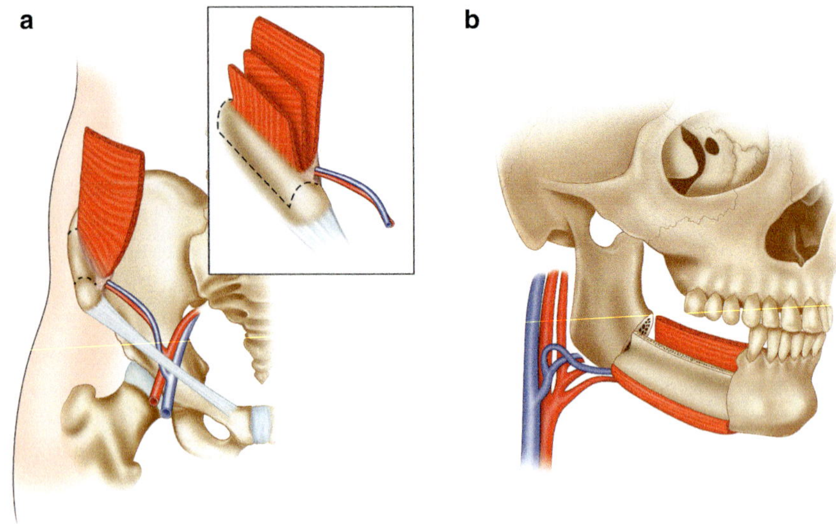

Fig. 13.3 (**a**) The dotted line represents the boundaries of the iliac bone flap based on the deep circumflex iliac vessels originating just proximal to the inguinal ligament from the external iliac vessels. Three muscle layers are encountered during dissection: the external oblique, internal oblique and transversus abdominis. Note that the anterior superior iliac spine is left intact to preserve the insertion of the inguinal ligament and reduce post-operative hernia. (**b**) The DCIA iliac bone flap is inset with the internal oblique muscle wrapping around to provide intraoral tissue that can mucosalize as necessary. The vascular pedicle travels in a posterior/inferior direction for ease of anastomosis to the recipient vessels in the neck. Not shown: plates are used to secure the vascularized bone construct to the existing stable mandible

anterolateral thigh paresthesias coinciding with the distribution of the lateral femoral cutaneous nerve [20]. Other less commonly seen complications include pain, hernia, and contour deformity when taken with a skin paddle. Overall functional loss is not significant, and the majority of the complications can be avoided with proper technique.

Muscular perforators from the deep circumflex iliac vessels supply the iliac crest. With a diameter of 2–2.5 mm, the deep circumflex iliac artery originates above the inguinal ligament from the external iliac artery. It travels from medial to lateral between the transversalis and iliacus fascia toward the anterior superior iliac spine (ASIS). Proximal to the ASIS, an ascending branch arises that supplies the internal oblique muscle offering a muscular component to the composite graft. Pedicle length averages 5–6 cm. The lateral femoral cutaneous nerve crosses deep to the deep circumflex vessels near the ASIS. The skin component can be up to 16 × 20 cm but is often included with the underlying muscles and iliac bone creating a bulky flap with limited mobility to the soft tissue component. In 30% of cases, a large deep circumflex iliac perforator to the skin can be identified.

Dissection of the flap proceeds from a medial to lateral direction. This helps prevent inadvertent clipping of the main pedicle due to the misidentification of the main pedicle for the ascending branch. Musculocutaneous perforators are included in the flap by way of inclusion of the external oblique, internal oblique, and transversus abdominis components. The main branch of the DICA/V is identified and dissected to its origin. Again, special attention is given to identifying and avoiding the lateral femoral cutaneous nerve as it crosses the vessels adjacent to the ASIS. Up to a 7 × 16 cm section of the iliac crest can be harvested. Osteotomies are performed either in situ, to reduce ischemia time, or after pedicle harvest on the back table.

Leaving the ASIS intact will aid in preventing hernia as well as meticulous closure of the transversus abdominis to the iliacus and the external oblique to the tensor fascia lata and gluteus muscles.

Numerous modifications to the DCIA composite flap have been reported. Including a deep circumflex iliac perforator, as found in 30%, will offer a more mobile skin paddle for intraoral resurfacing [21]. Alternatively, and more commonly, an internal oblique muscle component will be harvested based on the ascending branch. This muscular component will often be utilized for intraoral lining in maxillary defects that adds necessary bulk and will mucosalize in a timely manner [22]. For mandible reconstruction, the internal oblique can be wrapped around the intraoral section of the bone. This will provide a mucosalized and stable surface quite advantageous for the reception of dental implants. In an effort to retain structural integrity, only the inner table of the iliac crest can be harvested. However, functional morbidity is low in this procedure, and any contour abnormality is more related to soft tissue component harvest than the bone. Finally, the superficial circumflex iliac system can be included with the use of vein grafts to allow harvest of a larger skin component. With such varied components and relatively low donor site morbidity, the DCIA composite flap has numerous applications in head and neck reconstruction and should remain a strong arm of any experienced reconstructive surgeon's algorithm (Fig. 13.3).

Scapula

The scapular bone flap is most notable for the diversity of its soft tissue options as a composite flap. The blood supply to the lateral border of the scapula arises from the circumflex scapular artery, a branch of the subscapular system. The soft tissues supplied by the subscapular system are numerous and include both fasciocutaneous and muscle options based on either of the two main branches, the thoracodorsal and the circumflex scapular arteries. Swartz et al. presented an early review of 26 cases of maxillary and mandibular reconstruction highlighting the versatility of the flap, its ability to reconstruct complex three-dimensional structures, and its low donor site morbidity [23]. Urken et al. ultimately published the largest series of scapular bone flaps further touting the broad scope of reconstructive applications with flaps based off the subscapular system [24]. The need to harvest the flap with the patient in the lateral decubitus position is the flap's main disadvantage. The scapular bone flap is best applied in head and neck reconstruction for patients with peripheral vascular disease, elderly needing early return to function, and those requiring extensive, complex soft tissue defect repair [25].

The subscapular artery arises from the axillary artery. It divides into the thoracodorsal artery supplying both the latissimus dorsi and serratus muscles. The thoracodorsal artery also supplies a direct cutaneous perforator in up to 47% of patients [26]. The second branch of the subscapular artery is the circumflex scapular artery. This artery gives off a superficial branch which splits into a horizontal component and a vertical component supplying the scapula and parascapular fasciocutaneous flaps [27, 28]. The main trunk of the circumflex scapular artery continues to supply neighboring muscles, and a descending branch supplies the lateral border of the scapula providing the perfusion to the scapula bone flap commonly harvested. This branch will anastomose at the tip of the scapula with the angular artery from the thoracodorsal system. Of note, the thoracodorsal and circumflex scapular arteries can have individual origins from the axillary artery [26].

The pedicle to the circumflex scapular artery-based scapular bone flap is 5–6 cm. However, given the variability of composite flap components, pedicle length is quite variable. Numerous flap options exist, and dissection techniques will vary based on flap design. When harvesting the circumflex scapular artery, the patient is placed in the lateral decubitus position. Dissection proceeds proximally exposing vessels inferior to teres minor and superior to teres major. In general the pedicle is harvested at the origin of the thoracodorsal vessels. The lateral border of the scapula is harvested at 3–4 cm in width starting 2–3 cm below the glenoid fossa with a 12 mm cuff of transected teres major protecting the descending branch.

Modifications when included with various flap combinations based on the subscapular system are numerous. Should a longer pedicle be necessary, the bone segment can be based on the angular artery through the thoracodorsal system. The tip of the scapula itself can be harvested for mandibular angle and anterior maxillary defects. Fasciocutaneous segments which can be harvested include the scapula, parascapular, and thoracodorsal artery perforator flaps. An extended scapula flap can be harvested for large surface area defects [29]. Muscle flaps include the serratus and latissimus dorsi flaps. Any combination of these flaps can be harvested in existing arterial configuration or anastomosed to the main pedicle in a chimeric fashion. The abundance of modifications and options for flap components highlights the main indication for the application of the scapula bone flap to complex, three-dimensional defects with large soft tissue components. This coupled with a low donor site morbidity makes the scapular bone flap an integral component in bony head and neck reconstruction (Fig. 13.4).

Site-Specific Reconstruction

In order to fully appreciate the power of VSP, a defect-oriented approach will be used, focusing on mandibular, maxillary, and fronto-orbital defects.

Mandibular Defects

Condyle Reconstruction

The condyle represents a dynamic component of the mandible as it both rotates and translates. Adequate anatomical height and contour is important to ensure good occlusion and range of motion. Isolated condylar head and neck reconstruction lends itself to the use of a radial artery bone-containing flap. Fascia and skin can be included in the design in situations where the articular disk needs to be reconstructed. The long vascular pedicle provided by the radial artery will allow anastomosis in the neck (Fig. 13.5).

Condyle/Ramus Reconstruction

The condyle ramus unit is a relatively straight structure well reconstructed with a fibular free flap. Classically, the ipsilateral fibula will be used so that the distal fibula is used as a neo-condyle. The lateral aspect of the fibula will be oriented laterally in order to project the vascular pedicle medially. This will bring the vascular pedicle anteriorly, in a more favorable location for microvascular anastomosis. Height of the neo-condyle/ramus is obtained from the preoperative studies or from mirror imaging when the native anatomy is distorted. Shaping guides can be fabricated to ensure adequate anatomical contour. In cases of benign disease in which the articular disk of the temporomandibular joint can be preserved, the neo-condyle will be inserted along its inferior surface and suspended using an absorbable suture

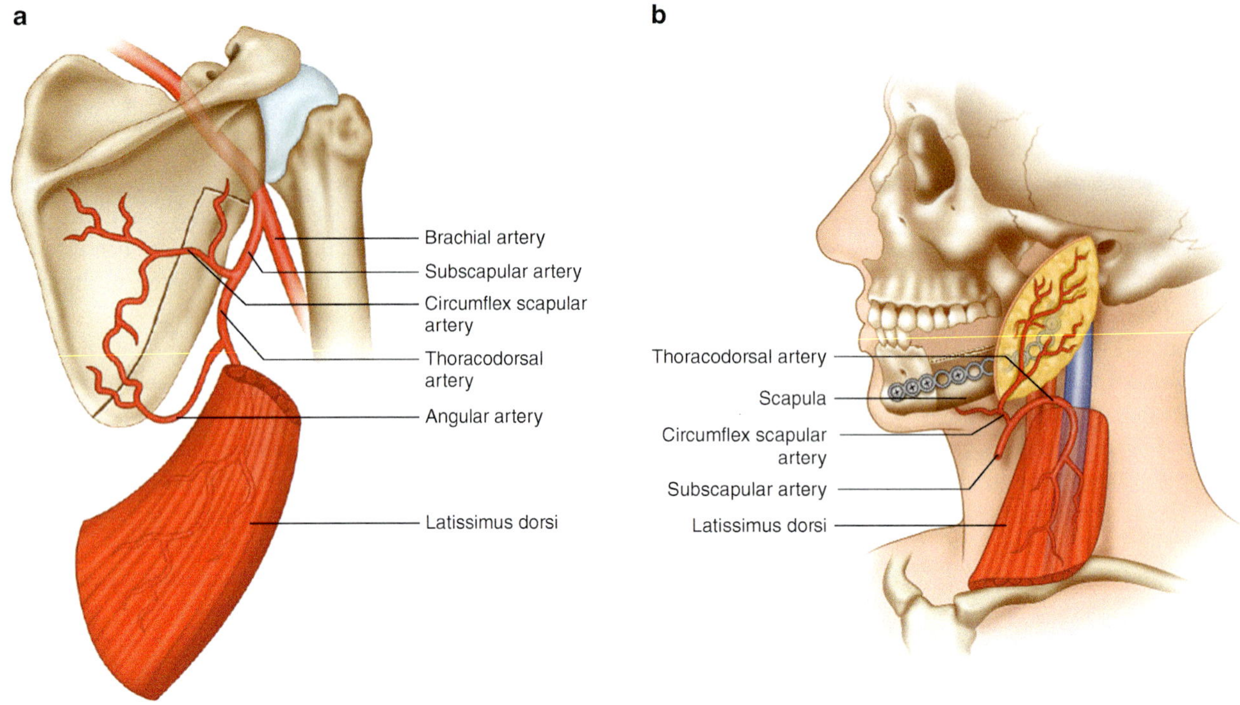

Fig. 13.4 (**a**) The consistent, complex subscapular arterial system provides blood flow to a variety of tissue components including skin, muscle and bone. The scapula has dual blood supply with the lateral scapular bone receiving blood supply from the circumflex scapular artery and the scapular tip from the angular artery via the thoracodorsal system. (**b**) The scapula bone flap is inset for mandible reconstruction using a fasciocutaneous flap based on the superficial circumflex vessels for intra- or extraoral coverage, as well as a latissimus muscle flap which can provide tissue bulk to the neck following a neck dissection and/or radiation therapy. Soft tissue options include the scapula, parascapula, and thoracodorsal artery perforator flaps

(PDS) through a drill hole in the lateral lip of the glenoid fossa. This requires a separate preauricular approach to the temporomandibular joint. In order to optimize functional outcome, the masseter can be resuspended to the lateral aspect of the reconstruction. Should the occlusion need to be corrected, dental splints can be fabricated as well (Fig. 13.6).

Body/Symphysis

The mandibular body extends from the mandibular angle to the mental foramen and, as such, is a relatively linear segment. In situations where the fibula is selected for reconstruction, care needs to be taken to evaluate the available recipient vessels as well as the requirement for the location of the skin paddles. The curvilinear nature of the parasymphyseal area is typically reconstructed with two segments. Recontouring of the neo-symphysis is sometimes necessary to avoid an excessively projected chin. A defect involving the bilateral parasymphyseal area lends itself well to performing the osteotomies at the donor site and assembling the construct to the reconstruction plate, prior to microvascular transfer, as the construct can be inserted in appropriate position. The use of patient-specific plates will ensure appropriate reconstruction so that the mandibular plane angle is adequately reconstructed avoiding over or under projection of the mentum (Fig. 13.7).

Maxillary Reconstruction

The maxilla represents a "U"-shaped structure, and anatomical reconstruction is favorable, especially when the ultimate goal involves a dentate reconstruction with osseointegrated dental implants. In order to fully appreciate the power of VSP in maxillary reconstruction, defects will be subdivided into: segmental, total, and orbito-maxillary. Unique to maxillary reconstruction is the proximity to the paranasal sinuses and nasal cavity. Preoperative presence of an oronasal or oroantral fistula needs to be evaluated and addressed through the utilization of soft tissue in addition to the bony component.

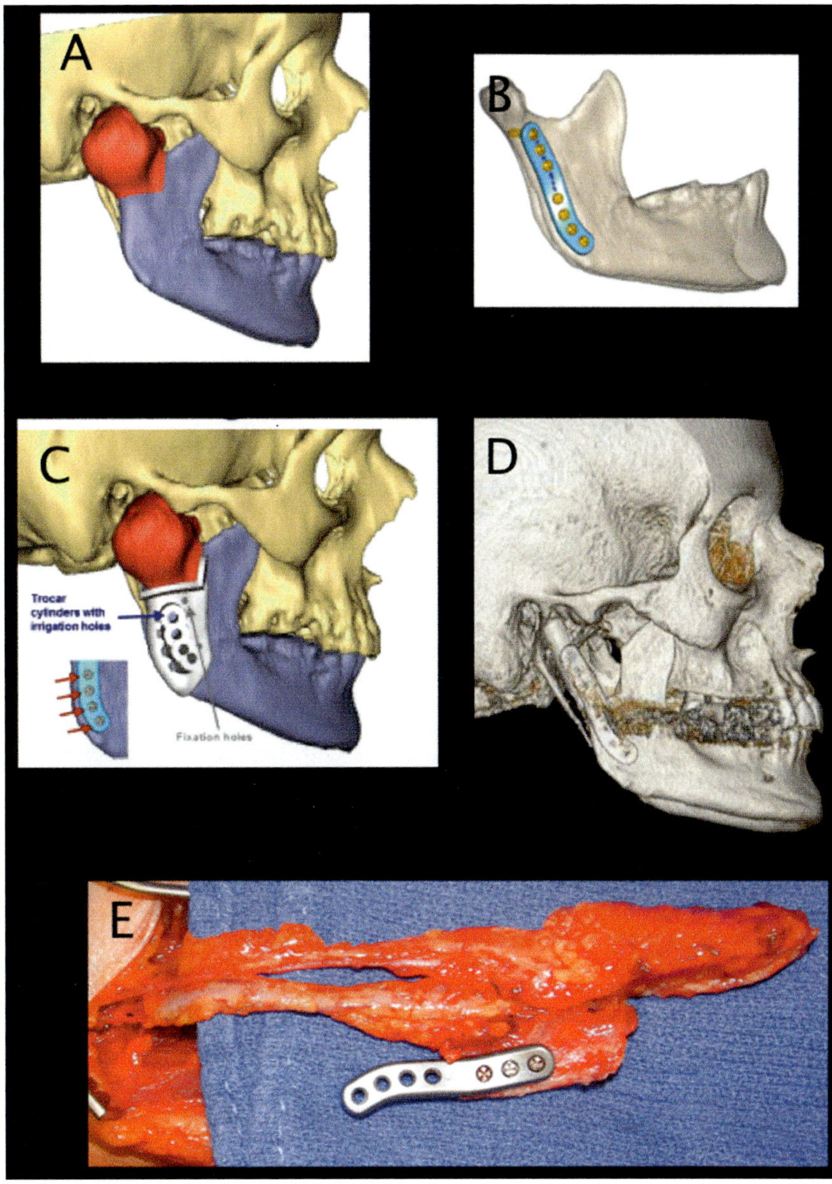

Fig. 13.5 (**a**) 3D CT scan of a 54-year-old with an osteochondroma of the right mandibular condyle. The *red* outlines the planned resection. (**b**) Using mirror-imaging technique, the normal anatomy is restored, and a patient-specific plate is virtually created. (**c**) Using the previous information, a resection guide including drilling guides for the screws is fabricated. (**d**) 3D CT of the final reconstruction with a radial artery osteocutaneous flap. (**e**) Radial artery osteocutaneous flap elevated with patient-specific reconstruction plate prior to transfer (Courtesy of Dr. Daniel Petrisor, MD, DDS) (DuPuy Synthes Craniomaxillofacial, Paoli, PA, USA)

Segmental Defects

The maxilla can be broken down into four segments spanning from the pterygoid plate to the ipsilateral canine, to midline. This subdivision of the maxilla allows easy reproduction of its curvilinear nature when dealing with a linear bone-containing flap such as the fibula or the lateral aspect of the scapula. The ipsilateral facial artery and vein are the favored recipient vessels. If the facial vessels are not available, vein grafts may be necessary to reach other vessels lower in the neck (Fig. 13.8).

Total Maxillary Reconstruction

Either as the result of oncologic resection or of trauma, total maxillary defects are a reconstructive challenge. Typically, the only stable structures that remain are the pterygoid plates. It is therefore difficult to appropriately control the position of the anterior neo-maxilla. Intraoperative navigation has been used, but requires significant resources that may not be readily available. The use of virtually created positioning guides and pre-bent plates using a stereolithic model of the reconstructed maxilla will circumvent this problem. The fibula

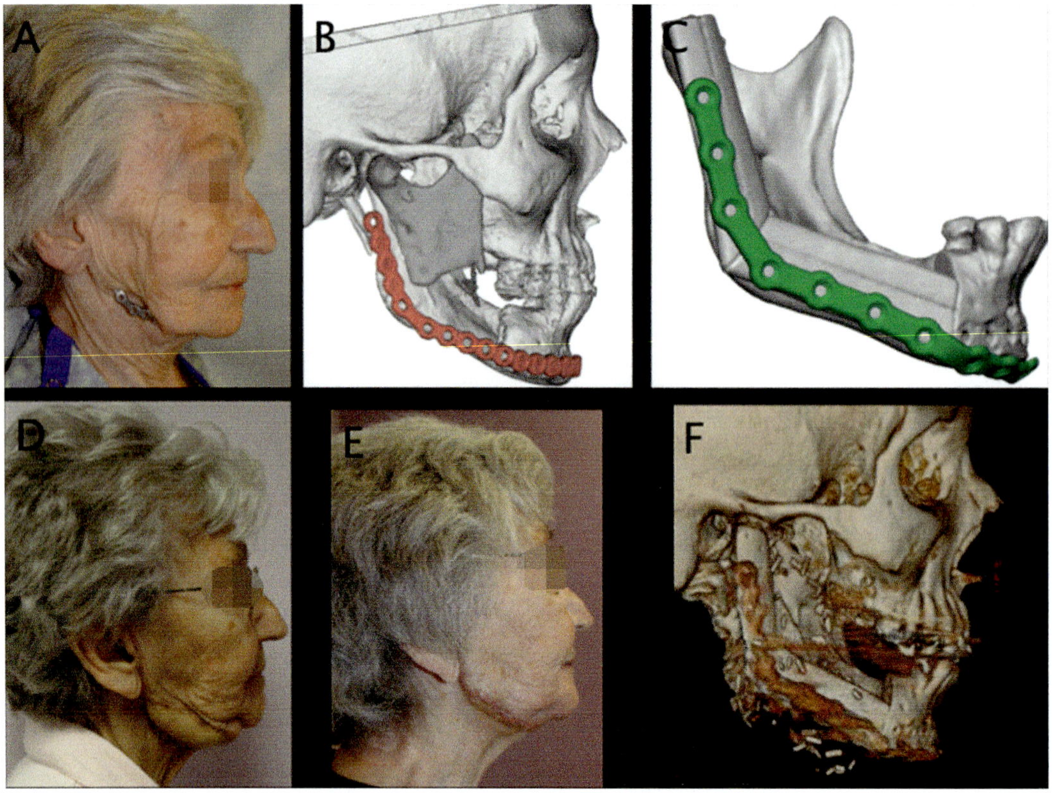

Fig. 13.6 (**a**) 72-year-old female with a long history of osteomyelitis of the right mandible who underwent a mandibular resection and now presents with exposed hardware. (**b**) 3D CT scan shows migration of the hardware. Extension of the osteolytic process was noted in the native proximal segment. It was decided to resect the proximal segment and reconstruct the condyle/ramus unit and body with the ipsilateral fibula to allow anterior projection of the vascular pedicle. (**c**) A patient-specific plate was fabricated. Care was taken to avoid the screw holes from the previous reconstruction plate. (**d**) Early clinical picture showing the external position of the skin paddle. (**e**) At 6 weeks, the skin paddle is de-epithelialized, and the area is resurfaced with native skin. (**f**) Postoperative 3D CT showing adequate condylar position and restoration of the mandible (3D Systems Healthcare, Rock Hill, SC, USA)

provides adequate bone stock to reliably reconstruct a total maxillary defect. Furthermore, a generous skin paddle is available as well as vascularized muscle to obliterate the maxillary sinus. The optimal recipient vessels are the facial artery and vein, and the proximal fibula will abut the ipsilateral pterygoid plates (Figs. 13.9 and 13.10).

Orbito-Maxillary Defect

Either as a result of a supra-structure maxillectomy as an oncologic resection or from trauma, orbito-maxillary defect reconstruction can be complex. The fibula remains a very powerful donor site as it can be predictably osteotomized. The distal fibula will typically lie at the medial orbital rim, and a segmental removal of the fibula of 4–5 cm will ensure adequate freedom from the vascular pedicle to inset the maxillary component. The skin paddle can be used to provide intraoral lining. In the case of a hemimaxillectomy, a two-segment reconstruction spanning from the pterygoid plate to the midline is commonly utilized. The vascular pedicle needs to be oriented laterally, as the facial artery and vein are the usual recipient vessels (Fig. 13.11).

Fronto-Orbital Defect

Rodriguez et al. [30] initially reported the use of the fibular free flap for fronto-orbital bar reconstruction in the treatment of mucocele. The fibula offers adequate bone stock, a long vascular pedicle capable of reaching the superficial temporal system, and recruitment of muscle (flexor hallucis longus) to seal off the anterior cranial fossa. The lateral aspect of the fibula will typically be oriented externally, and a midline osteotomy is necessary to ensure adequate contour restoration. Care must be taken to avoid undue pressure on the vascular pedicle as it exits the cranium (Fig. 13.12).

Conclusion

It is clear that the development of VSP has created a paradigm shift in complex composite maxillofacial reconstruction. The technology is now relatively easily accessible, and has allowed the busy reconstructive microsurgeon to be more efficient when managing complex cases. The future of VSP lays in the incorporation of the soft tissue component vascular pedicle and perforators to optimize the designs of the flaps. In the future, developments that incorporate tissue engineering will allow improved anatomic skeletal reconstruction.

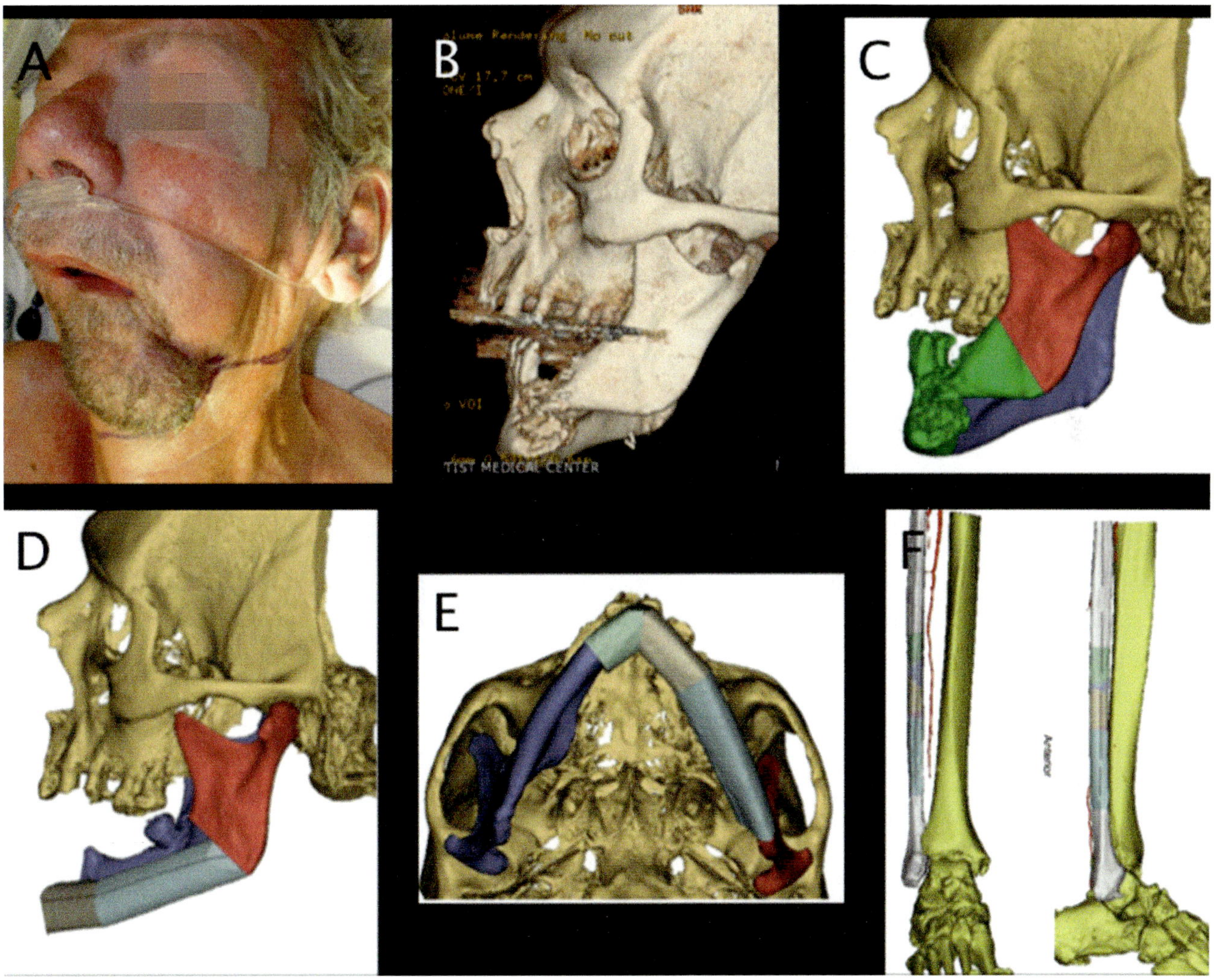

Fig. 13.7 (**a**) 67-year-old male with stage III osteoradionecrosis of the left mandible with oro-cutaneous fistula present. (**b**) 3D CT scan illustrating pathological fracture of the left mandible and rotation of the proximal segment. (**c**) The area of resection is defined according to the CT findings with generous margins. The resection extends from the left mandibular angle to the right parasymphyseal area. (**d**) The native anatomy is manipulated to restore adequate anatomy, and the contralateral fibula is used to reconstruct the defect with three segments. (**e**) Planned reconstruction with restoration of mandibular width. (**f**) Patient-specific CT data from the fibula is used to design the osteotomies and fabricate cutting guides. (**g**) Following adequate exposure, the resection guides are secured in position. (**h**) A stereolithic model of the reconstructed mandible is used as a template to pre-bend a reconstruction plate (**i**) Fibular free flap with the cutting guide in position. Because of the extensive radiation damage, the fibular skin is inset intraorally, and the ipsilateral anterolateral thigh flap (ATF) will be used to reconstruct the external skin. (**j**) Early postoperative clinical picture showing restoration of mandibular projection with stable soft tissue. (**k**) Postoperative 3D CT showing adequate mandibular reconstruction. (**l**) Intraoral photograph illustrating adequate intraoral lining with good vestibular depth (DuPuy Synthes Craniomaxillofacial, Paoli, PA, USA)

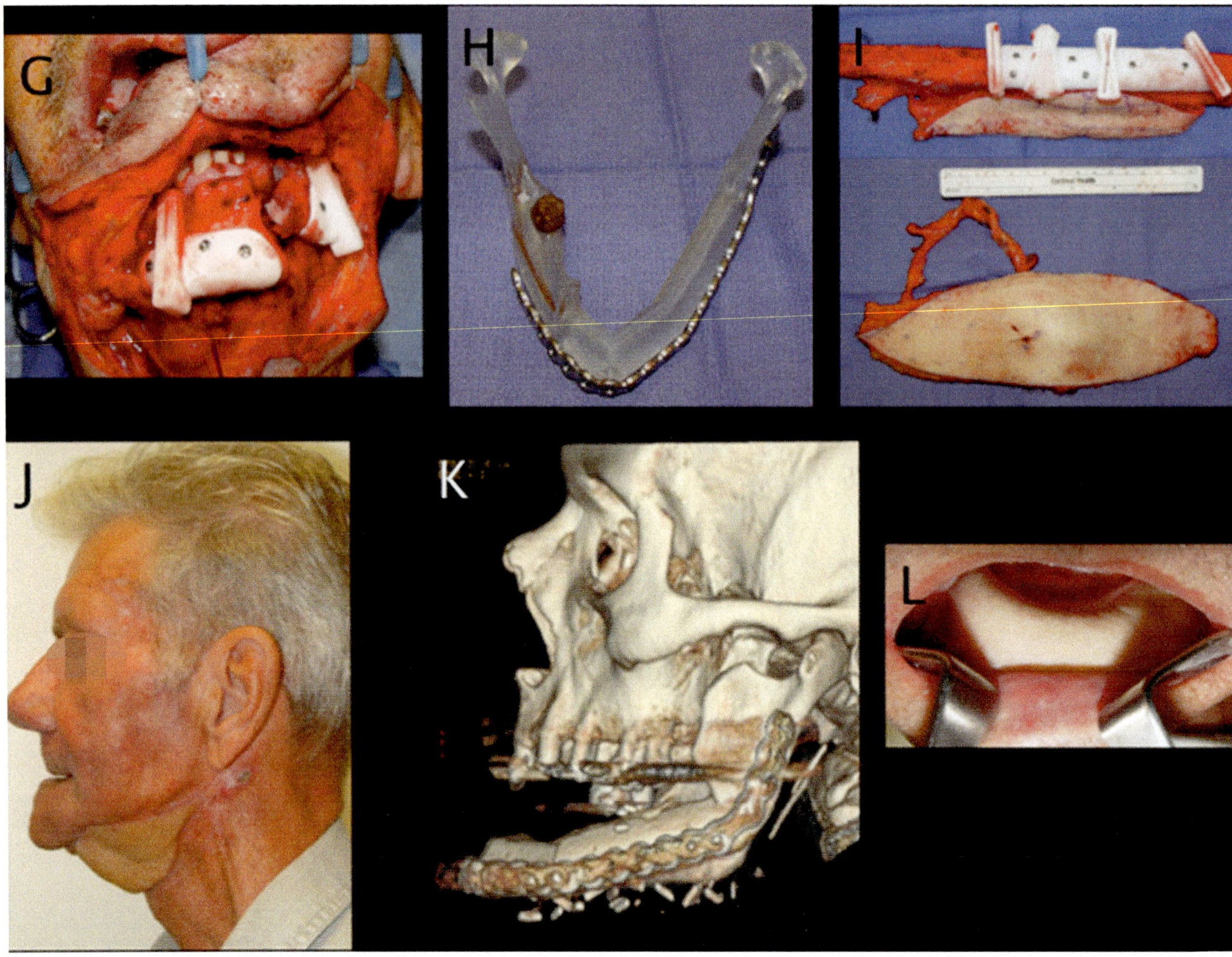

Fig. 13.7 (continued)

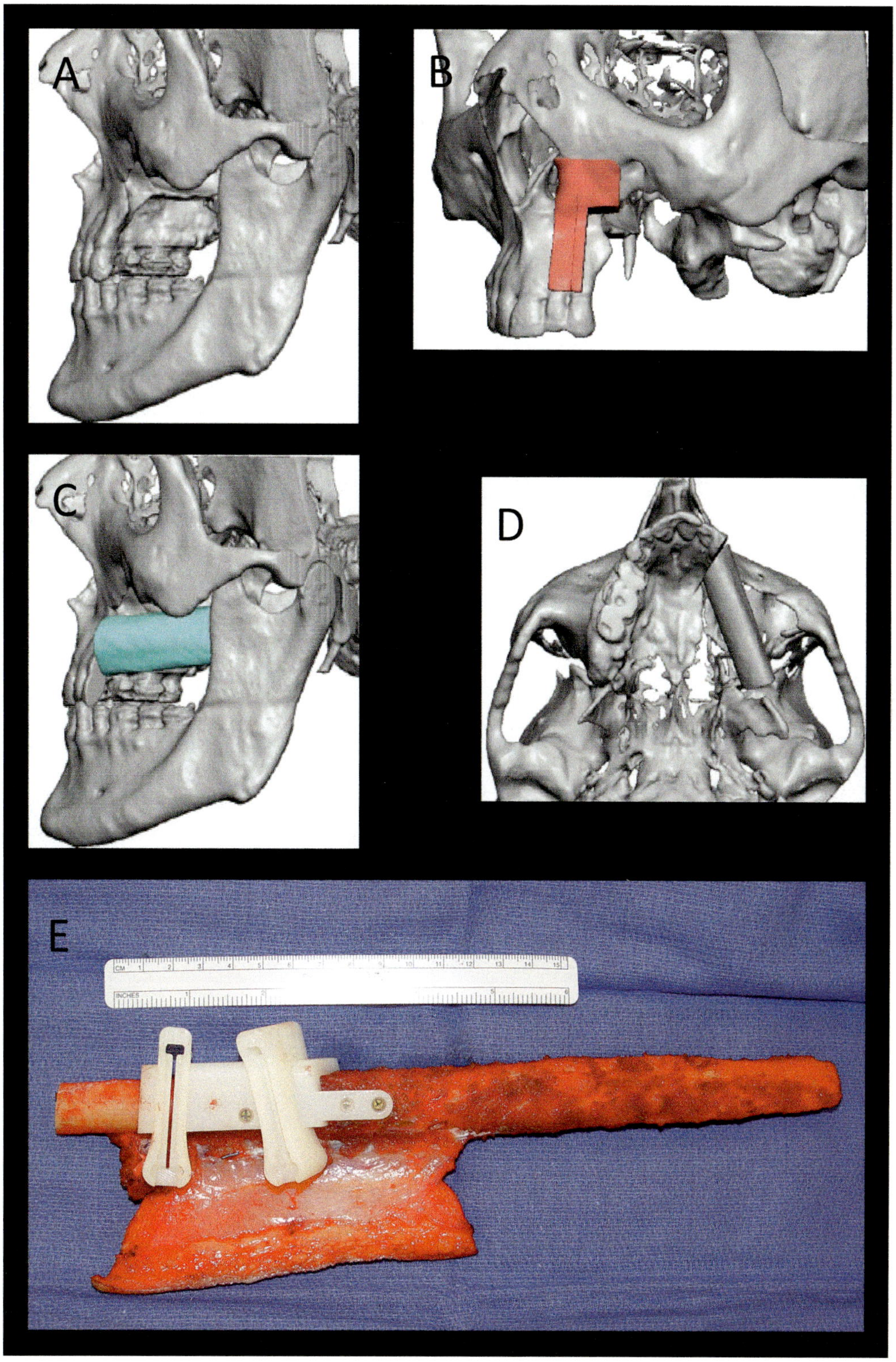

Fig. 13.8 (**a**) 3D CT of a 42-year-old male post excision of a benign odontogenic tumor who presents for skeletal reconstruction to allow placement of dental implants. The left maxillary defect extended from the canine to the pterygoid plate. Furthermore, a large oroantral communication was present. (**b**) Because of the exposed root of the canine, a resection guide was fabricated to ensure adequate bony contact anteriorly. (**c** and **d**) The planned reconstruction used the ipsilateral fibula and will extend from the pterygoid plates to the canine area. (**e**) The harvested fibula with the cutting guide in position. (**f**) A stereolithic model of the reconstructed neo-maxilla is fabricated to allow pre-contouring of the plates. (**g**) The resection guide in appropriate position. (**h** and **i**) Early postoperative 3D CT showing the fibula in appropriate, planned, position (3D Systems Healthcare, Rock Hill, SC, USA)

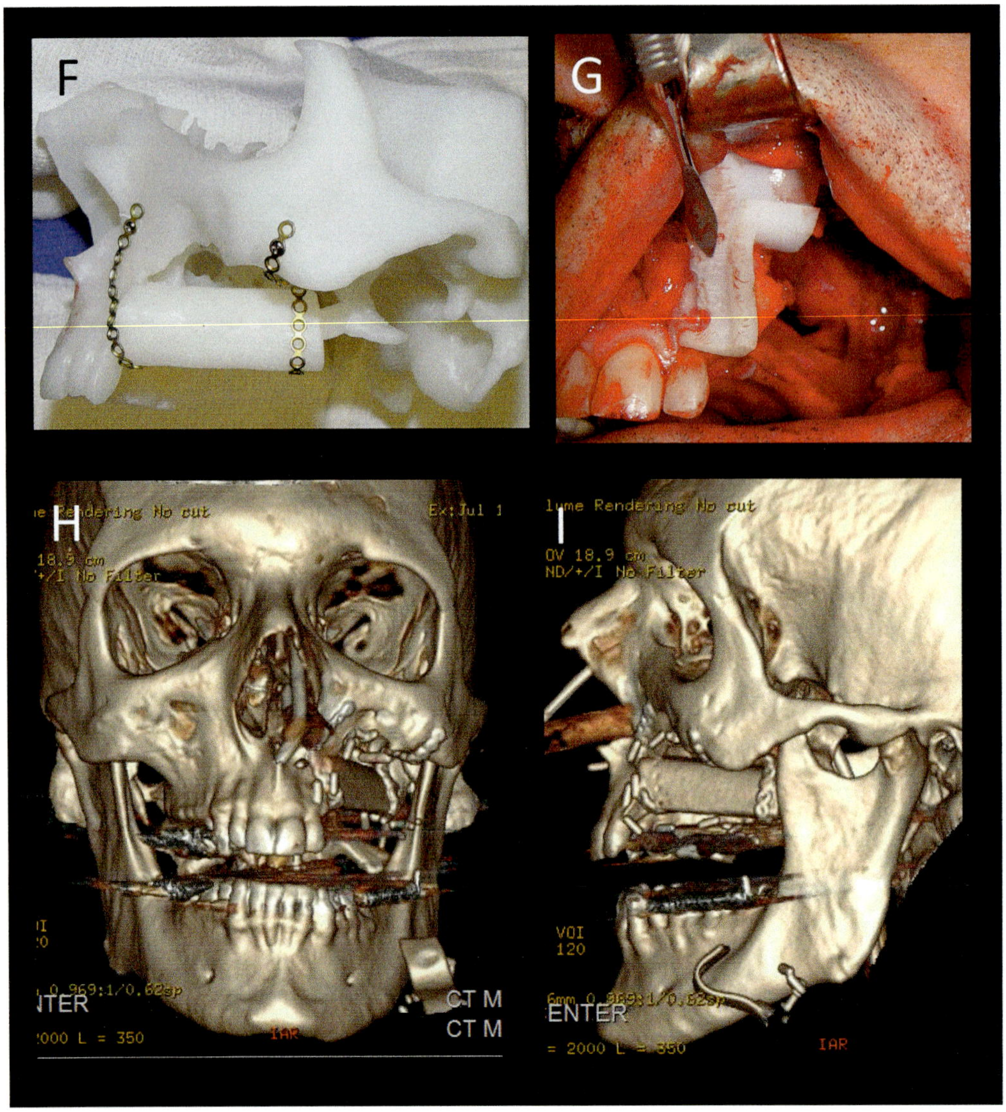

Fig. 13.8 (continued)

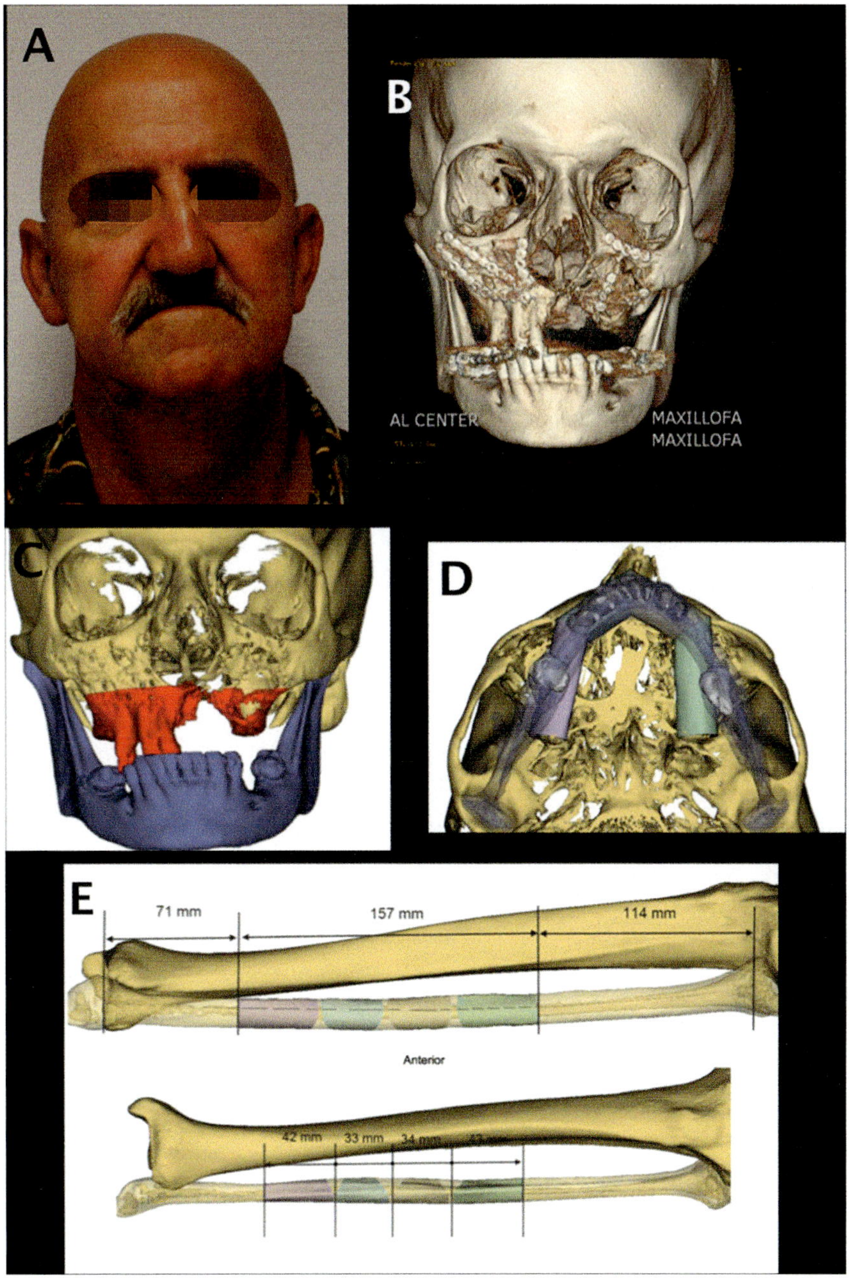

Fig. 13.9 (**a** and **b**) 64-year-old male s/p motor vehicle accident where he sustained multiple facial fractures which were complicated by avascular necrosis of the maxilla nonresponsive to hyperbaric oxygen treatment and local debridement. (**c**) The area to be resected was defined. (**d**) A four-piece fibular free flap reconstruction was planned. (**e**) Patient-specific CT data was use to define the fibular reconstruction. (**f**) Following harvest of the left fibula, the cutting guide is applied, and appropriate osteotomies are performed. (**g**) The neo-maxilla is assembled using pre-contoured plates bend from a reconstructed stereolithic model. (**h** and **i**) CT scan at 6 months following the fibular free flap reconstruction after removal of hardware and placement of six osseointegrated implants. (**j**) Six months following placement of the fixtures, the second stage is performed with removal of the skin paddle and vestibuloplasty. (**k**) Clinical photograph following the prosthetic restoration (performed by Dr. Sammy Tom, DDS) (DuPuy Synthes Craniomaxillofacial, Paoli, PA, USA)

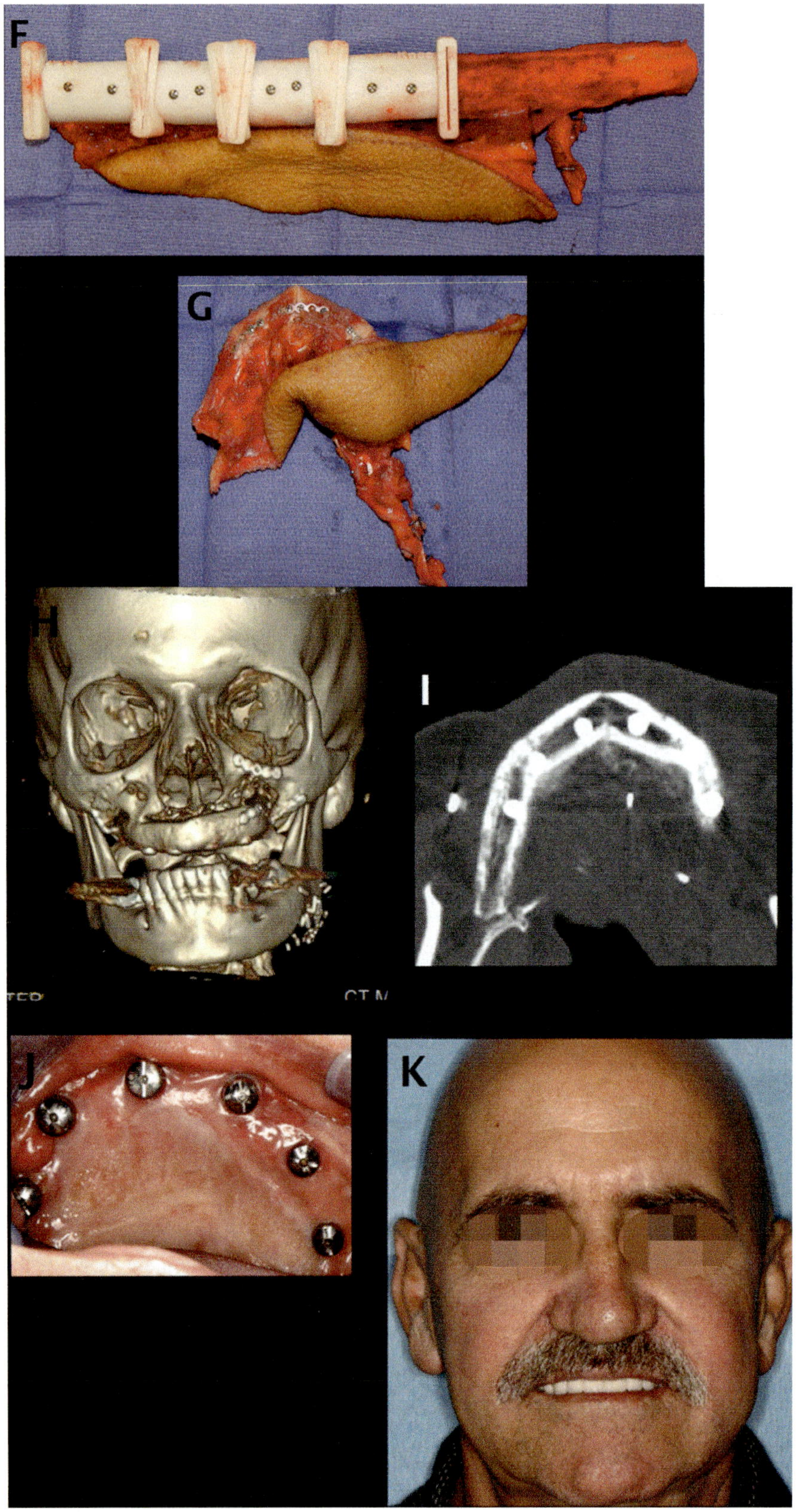

Fig. 13.9 (continued)

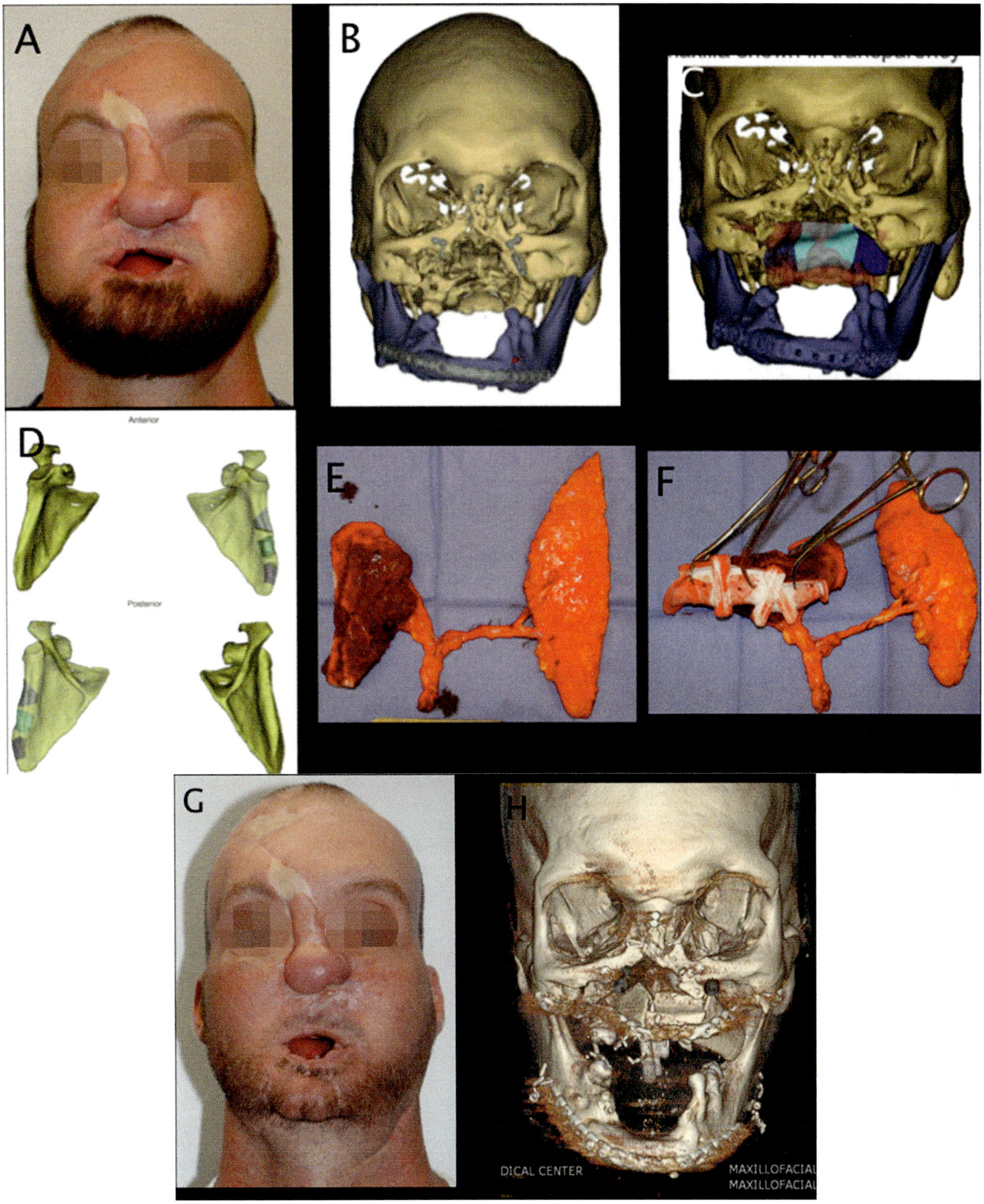

Fig. 13.10 (**a**) 43-year-old male status post-accidental gunshot wound to the face who underwent multiple previous reconstructions presented with near absence of his maxilla and large oronasal fistula. (**b**) Preoperative CT imaging showing a maxillary defect extending from the second molar on the right to the first molar on the left. (**c**) Virtual surgical planned maxillary reconstruction using the right scapula using a superimposed "stock" maxilla. (**d**) 3D CT of the patient scapula with the reconstructed segment in position from which the cutting guides will be created. (**e**) Harvested chimeric scapular flap with thoracodorsal artery perforator flap skin component that will be used to resurface the oronasal fistula. (**f**) Cutting guides in position prior to performing the osteotomies. (**g**) Early postoperative pictures and (**h**) Postoperative 3D CT (DuPuy Synthes Craniomaxillofacial, Paoli, PA, USA)

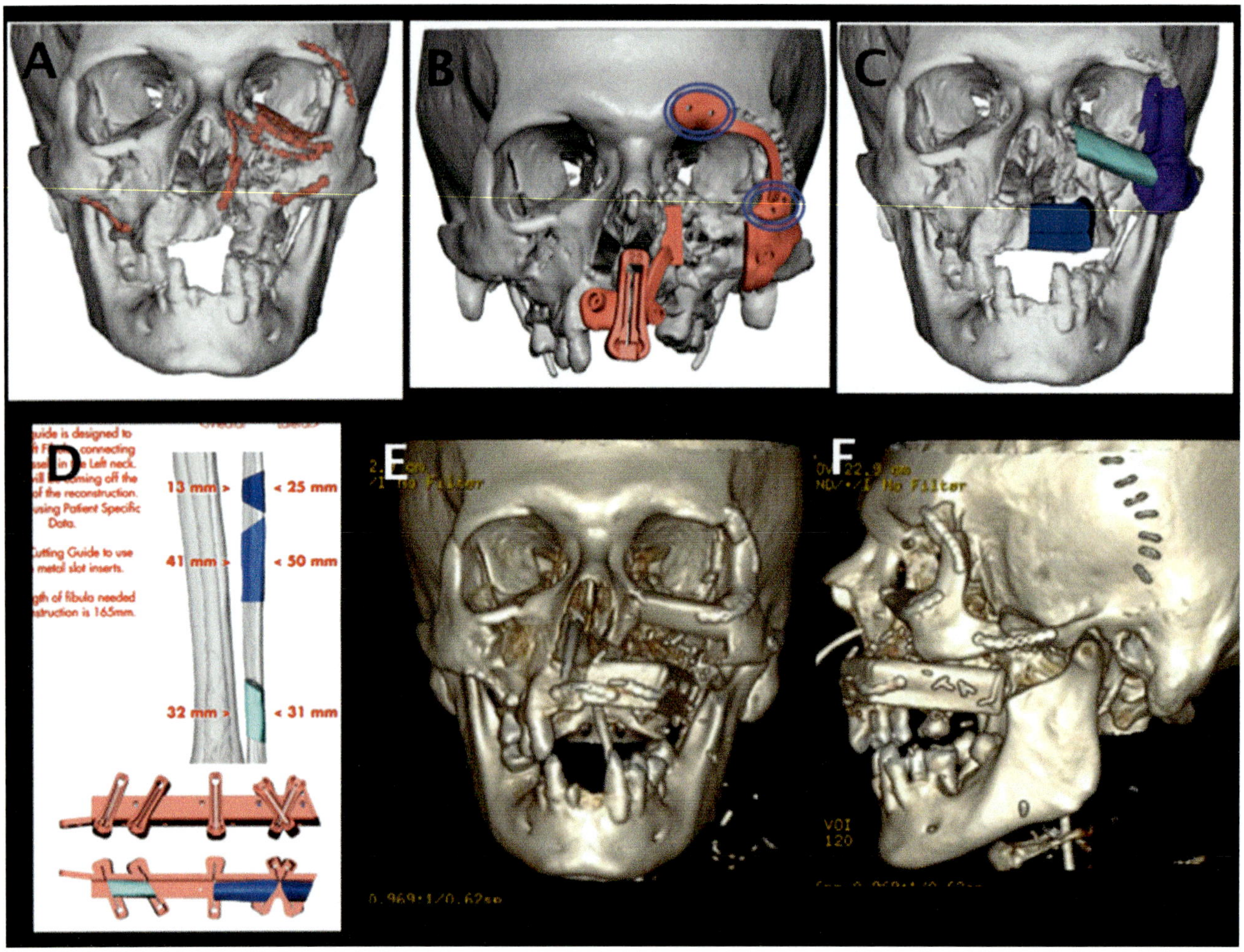

Fig. 13.11 (**a**) 63-year-old male who sustained a high velocity midfacial injury presented with malunion of left maxillary and orbitozygomatic fractures. (**b**) The surgical plan included left hemimaxillectomy and repositioning of the left zygoma. (**c**) The reconstructive plan used the fibula to reconstruct the orbital rim and hemimaxilla following repositioning of the zygoma. (**d**) This information was transferred to the patient-specific CT data to generate fibular cutting guides. (**e** and **f**) Postoperative 3D CT showing adequate position of the zygoma, orbital rim, and neo-hemimaxilla (3D Systems Healthcare, Rock Hill, SC, USA)

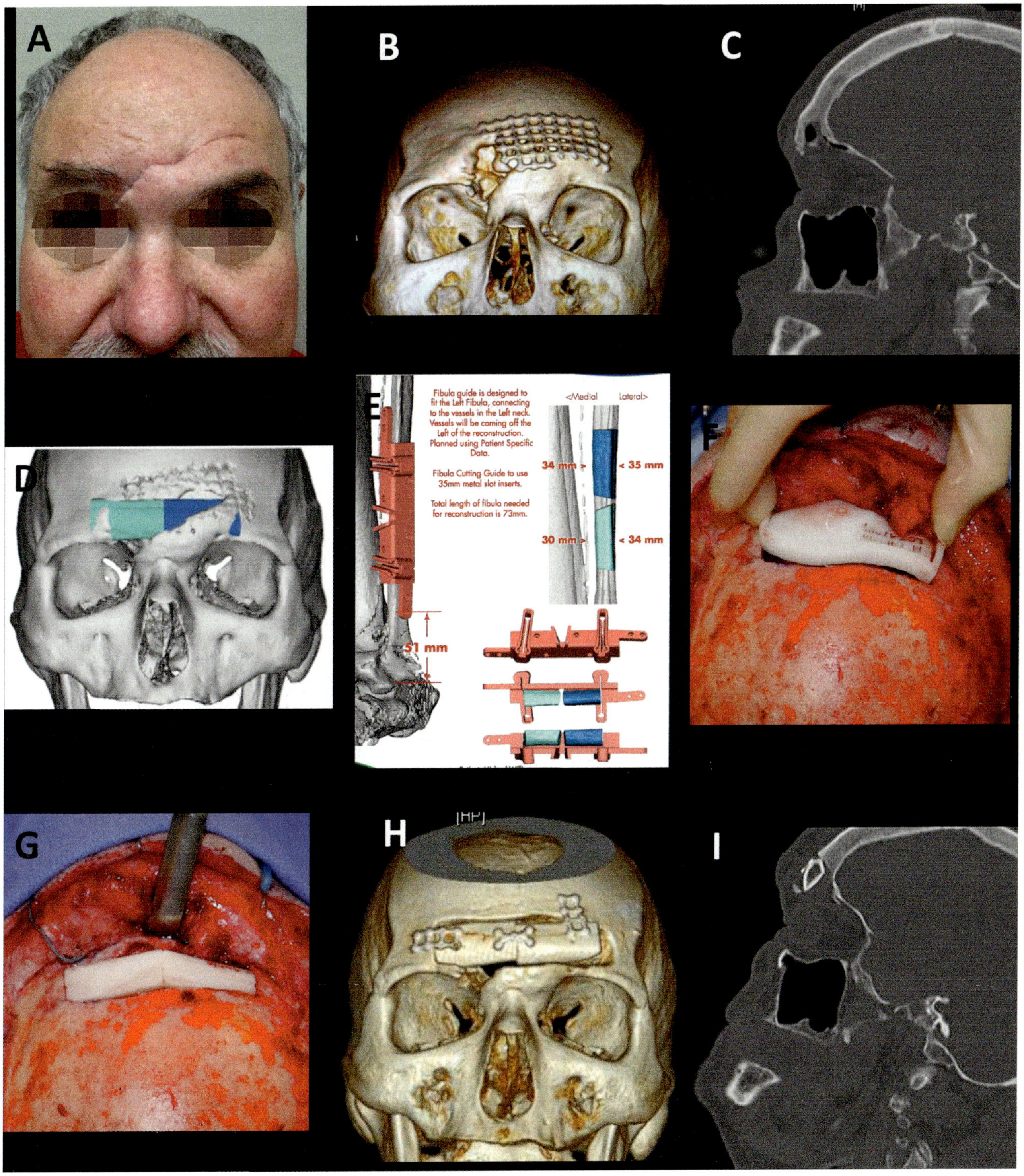

Fig. 13.12 (**a**) 63-year-old male s/p anterior table frontal fracture, repaired 1 year prior with obliteration now presents with chronic fronto-orbital pain and clear soft tissue injury. (**b**) 3D CT showing hardware in position. (**c**) Sagittal CT showing air within the frontal sinus confirming inadequate obliteration. (**d**) Planned fronto-orbital reconstruction using the left fibular free flap along with a segment of flexor hallucis longus to allow for adequate seal of the anterior cranial fossa. (**e**) Cutting guides are created using patient-specific CT data from the left fibula. (**f**) Resection guides in position. (**g**) A plastic reconstruction analog was also created to ensure adequate contouring of the anterior table of the frontal sinus. (**h**) 3D CT showing the fibula in appropriate position. (**i**) Sagittal CT illustrating adequate seal of the anterior cranial fossa. The patient is now symptom free (3D Systems Healthcare, Rock Hill, SC, USA)

References

1. Wei F-C, Chen H-C, Chuang C-C, Noordhoff MS. Fibular osteoseptocutaneous flap: anatomic study and clinical application. Plast Reconstr Surg. 1986;78(2):191–9.
2. Hidalgo DA. Fibular free flap: a new method of mandible reconstruction. Plast Reconstr Surg. 1989;84(1):71–9.
3. Cutting C, Bookstein FL, Grayson B, Fellingham L, McCarthy JG. Three-dimensional computer-assisted design of craniofacial surgical procedures: optimization and interaction with cephalometric and CT-based models. Plast Reconstr Surg. 1986;77(6):877–85.
4. Rose EH, Norris MS, Rosen JM. Application of high-tech three-dimensional imaging and computer-generated models in complex facial reconstructions with vascularized bone grafts. Plast Reconstr Surg. 1993;91(2):252–64.
5. Hirsch DL, Garfein ES, Christensen AM, Weimer KA, Saddeh PB, Levine JP. Use of computer-aided design and computer-aided manufacturing to produce orthognathically ideal surgical outcomes: a paradigm shift in head and neck reconstruction. J Oral Maxillofac Surg. 2009;67:2115–22.
6. Saad A, Winters R, Wise MW, Dupin CL, St-Hilaire H. Virtual surgical planning in complex composite maxillofacial reconstruction. Plast Reconstr Surg. 2013;132(3):626–31.
7. Levine JP, Bae JS, Soares M, Brecht LE, Saadeh PB, Ceradini DJ, Hirsch DL. Jaw in a day: total maxillofacial reconstruction using digital technology. Plast Reconstr Surg. 2013;131(6):1386–91.
8. Taylor GI, Miller GD, Ham FJ. The free vascularized bone graft. A clinical extension of microvascular techniques. Plast Reconstr Surg. 1975;55(5):533–44.
9. Wei FC, Seah CS, Tsai YC, Liu SJ, Tsai MS. Fibula osteoseptocutaneous flap for reconstruction of composite mandibular defects. Plast Reconstr Surg. 1994;93(2):294–304.
10. Momoh AO, Yu P, Skoracki RJ, Liu S, Feng L, Hanasono MM. A prospective cohort study of fibula free flap donor-site morbidity in 157 consecutive patients. Plast Reconstr Surg. 2011;128(3):714–20.
11. Yang GF, Chen PJ, Gao YZ, Liu XY, Li J, Jiang SX, et al. Forearm free skin flap transplantation: a report of 56 cases. 1981. Br J Plast Surg. 1997;50(3):162–5.
12. Zenn MR, Hidalgo DA, Cordeiro PG, Shah JP, Strong EW, Kraus DH. Current role of the radial forearm free flap in mandibular reconstruction. Plast Reconstr Surg. 1997;99(4):1012–7.
13. Timmons MJ, Missotten FE, Poole MD, Davies DM. Complications of radial forearm flap donor sites. Br J Plast Surg. 1986;39(2):176–8.
14. Bardsley AF, Soutar DS, Elliot D, Batchelor AG. Reducing morbidity in the radial forearm flap donor site. Plast Reconstr Surg. 1990;86(2):287–92.
15. Vaughan ED. The radial forearm free flap in orofacial reconstruction. Personal experience in 120 consecutive cases. J Craniomaxillofac Surg. 1990;18(1):2–7.
16. Avery CME. Review of the radial free flap: still evolving or facing extinction? Part two: osteocutaneous radial free flap. Br J Oral Maxillofac Surg. 2010;48(4):253–60.
17. Cordeiro PG, Santamaria E. A classification system and algorithm for reconstruction of maxillectomy and midfacial defects. Plast Reconstr Surg. 2000;105(7):2331–46.
18. Timmons MJ. The vascular basis of the radial forearm flap. Plast Reconstr Surg. 1986;77(1):80–92.
19. Taylor GI, Townsend P, Corlett R. Superiority of the deep circumflex iliac vessels as the supply for free groin flaps. Plast Reconstr Surg. 1979;64(6):1745–59.
20. Forrest C, Boyd B, Manktelow R, Zuker R, Bowen V. The free vascularised iliac crest tissue transfer: donor site complications associated with eighty-two cases. Br J Plast Surg. 1992;45(2):89–93.
21. Kimata Y, Uchiyama K, Sakuraba M, Ebihara S, Hayashi R, Asakage T, Nakatsuka T, Harii K. Deep circumflex iliac perforator flap with iliac crest for mandibular reconstruction. Br J Plast Surg. 2001;54(6):487–90.
22. Brown JS, Jones DC, Summerwill A, Rogers SN, Howell RA, Cawood JI, Vaughan ED. Vascularized iliac crest with internal oblique muscle for immediate reconstruction after maxillectomy. Br J Oral Maxillofac Surg. 2002;40(3):183–90.
23. Swartz WM, Banis JC, Newton ED, Ramasastry SS, Jones NF, Acland R. The osteocutaneous scapular flap for mandibular and maxillary reconstruction. Plast Reconstr Surg. 1986;77(4):530–45.
24. Gibber MJ, Clain JB, Jacobson AS, et al. Subscapular system of flaps: an 8-year experience with 105 patients. Head Neck. 2015;37(8):1200–6.
25. Dowthwaite SA, Theurer J, Belzile M, Fung K, Franklin J, Nichols A, et al. Comparison of fibular and scapular osseous free flaps for oromandibular reconstruction: a patient-centered approach to flap selection. JAMA Otolaryngol Head Neck Surg. 2013;139(3):285–92.
26. Rowsell AR, Davies DM, Eisenberg N, Taylor GI. The anatomy of the subscapular-thoracodorsal arterial system: study of 100 cadaver dissections. Br J Plast Surg. 1984;37(4):574–6.
27. Dos Santos LF. The vascular anatomy and dissection of the free scapular flap. Plast Reconstr Surg. 1984;73(4):599–603.
28. Nassif TM, Vidal L, Bovet JL, Baudet J. The parascapular flap: a new cutaneous microsurgical free flap. Plast Reconstr Surg. 1982;69(4):591–600.
29. Thoma A, Heddle S. The extended free scapular flap. Br J Plast Surg. 1990;43(6):709–12.
30. Rodriguez ED, Stanwix MG, Nam AJ, St-Hilaire H, Simmons OP, Manson PN. Definitive treatment of persistent frontal sinus infection: elimination of dead space and sinonasal communication. Plast Reconstr Surg. 2009;123(3):957–67.

Navigation and Computer-Assisted Craniomaxillofacial Surgery

14

Nils-Claudius Gellrich and Majeed Rana

Procedures for Computer-Assisted Surgery

Imaging Modalities

The success of a surgical procedure using computer-assisted surgery (CAS) depends largely on the quality of imaging modalities. The more accurate the relevant anatomical bony and soft tissue information is presented, the more precise and detailed the operation can be planned preoperatively. The surgeon has access to a wide range of imaging techniques; all of them are associated with certain advantages and disadvantages. The perfect method does not exist because each method is based on a measurement of physical properties of the body and possibly also means a radiation exposure for the patient. The chosen imaging modality depends on surgeon choice and the specific requirements of each case. Table 14.1 shows the various imaging procedures in oral and maxillofacial surgery, which plays a role in CAS and provides each compared with their advantages and disadvantages.

Computed tomography (CT) is now one of the most important methods of investigation. The CT can be used both for diagnostics and for intraoperative navigation, reconstruction and follow-up. Although CT scans are associated with relatively high radiation doses of about 3–10 mSv, this risk must be weighed in an individual case versus the benefits. Given the short duration of the investigation and the superimposition-free, three-dimensional and accurate representation, especially of bony structures, the CT is a very useful imaging technique.

Cone beam CT (CBCT) is associated with less radiation exposure and similar information density as the conventional CT produces [1–3], and it is now preferred [4] in the dental and oral and maxillofacial surgical field. In a direct comparison of the two methods, the image quality of CBCT in an area with metallic dental restoration, mandibular CT is partially superior [5]. The CBCT is particularly suitable for the pre- and postoperative hard tissue-based imaging, as it demonstrates the reconstruction result and no image artefacts such as from functionally stable reconstruction plates. For intraoperative navigation, the CT data set could be merged with a subvolume CBCT data set. This technique can enhance the larger field of view of the initial non-referenced CT data with the subvolume data set containing registration markers that allows for a complete workflow in computer-assisted planning and surgery.

Magnetic resonance imaging (MRI) shows greater detail especially for tumours and soft tissue changes compared to CT because of the increased blood flow and the associated increase in water content, so that an accurate localization and assessment of the spread of the tumour or changes of muscular structures are possible. However, bony structures cannot be adequately reflected, as they contain little water and little fat. The main application of diffusion-weighted MRI (DWMRI) is the tracking of fibre tracts in the brain, but it now also plays a role in tumour staging, because it allows a fast diagnosis without contrast injection. It may help to detect tumours and to differentiate cystic or oedematous structures of tumours [6–9]. Perfusion MRI is a technique based on the stated principles of MR imaging technique that provides the magnetic resonance perfusion imaging through which a representation of the blood flow to organs and tissues is possible and thus the blood supply to tumours can be visualized.

The PET is the most sensitive technique for restaging procedures but cannot visualize the physiological nature of tumours when compared to MRI, for example, slime-forming tumours [10]. The single-photon emission computed tomography (SPECT) is compared to PET, although much cheaper and less time-consuming, but this comes at the expense of a lower spatial resolution due to a reduced-resolution camera (Fig. 14.1). Stereophotogrammetry (3D face scan) scanner uses an optical sensor across the face and

N.-C. Gellrich (✉) • M. Rana
Department of Oral & Craniomaxillofacial Surgery, Hannover Medical School, Hanover, Germany
e-mail: MKG-Chirurgie@mh-hannover.de

A.M. Greenberg (ed.), *Digital Technologies in Craniomaxillofacial Surgery*, https://doi.org/10.1007/978-1-4939-1532-3_14

Table 14.1 Advantages and disadvantages of anatomical, functional and optical imaging techniques

Classification	Methods	Advantages and disadvantages
Anatomical imaging	CT	+ Short examination time + Representation of bony structures + Representation of foreign bodies + Superposition-free representation + Three-dimensional images + Low cost
		– Radiation exposure – Undifferentiated representation of soft tissue – Contrast agent – Artefacts of dental restorations
	CBCT	+ Bone-high spatial resolution + Low radiation exposure + Superposition-free representation + Three-dimensional images
		– Blurring – Undifferentiated representation of soft tissue – Artefacts – Small layer thickness (≤0.5 mm)
Functional imaging	MRI	+ Highly detailed images of soft tissue + No radiation exposure + Three-dimensional images
		– Representation of bony structures – Time-consuming – Artefacts – Distortions/inaccuracies
	Diffusion-weighted MRI	+ High sensitivity in the diagnosis of bone metastases + Differentiation of cancerous non-cancerous changes
		– Motion artefacts – Image distortion
	Perfusion MRI	Representation of the blood flow to organs and tissues
	PET	+ Low radiation exposure + Good restaging procedures
		– High cost – Poor interpretation of physiologically active tissue – No reliable detection of slime-forming tumours
	SPECT	+ Low radiation exposure + Low effort + Low cost
		– Lower spatial resolution – Lower sensitivity of the cameras
Optical imaging	3D face scan	Representation of the soft tissue surface

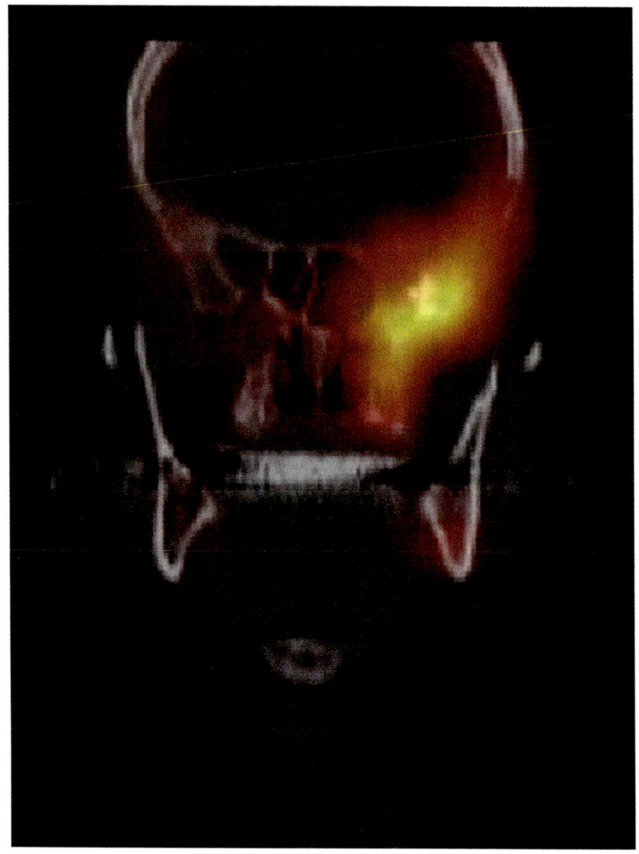

Fig. 14.1 Single-photon emission computed tomography (SPECT) examination of the left orbit, a metastasis of a breast carcinoma is shown in a 2D coronal view

provides spatial data on the soft tissue surface. The sensor operates on the principle of phase-measuring triangulation and offers the advantage of contactless data acquisition, which is free of ionizing radiation to the patient [11]. This process plays a role primarily in the review of the necessary reconstruction and success of the reconstruction after ablative surgery is involved. Precisely because of the specific advantages and disadvantages of each method, as shown in Table 14.1, it is natural to combine different techniques to achieve maximum sensitivity and specificity (Fig. 14.2).

Computer-Assisted Preoperative Planning

In craniomaxillofacial surgery, computer-assisted preoperative planning (CAPP) and computer-assisted surgery (CAS) could improve the treatment especially for acquired or congenital midfacial deformities. The major part of using navigation is the computer-assisted preoperative planning (CAPP) (Fig. 14.3). Comprehensive software tools are available to visualize the worldwide accepted standard for

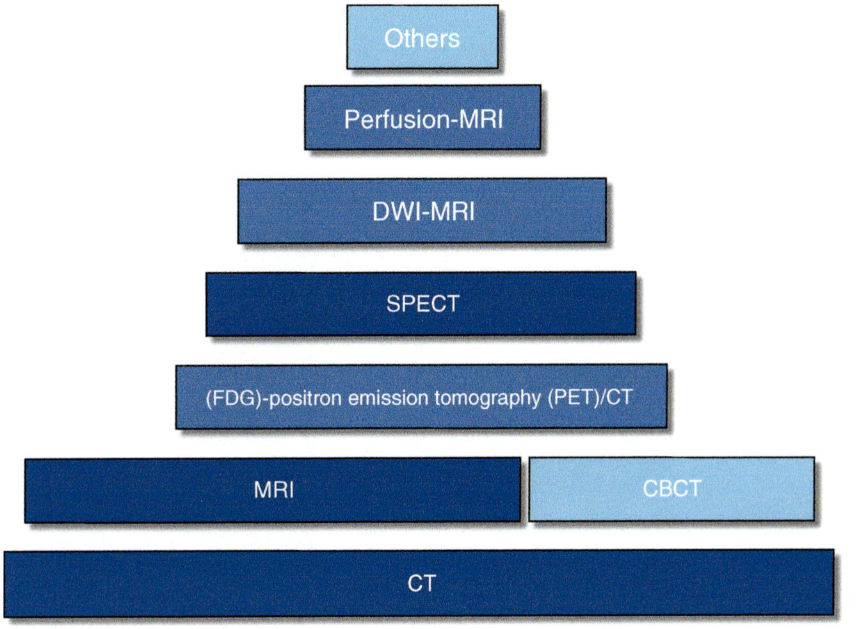

Fig. 14.2 Demonstrates the required imaging modalities in ablative head and neck surgery for tumour treatment and diagnosis

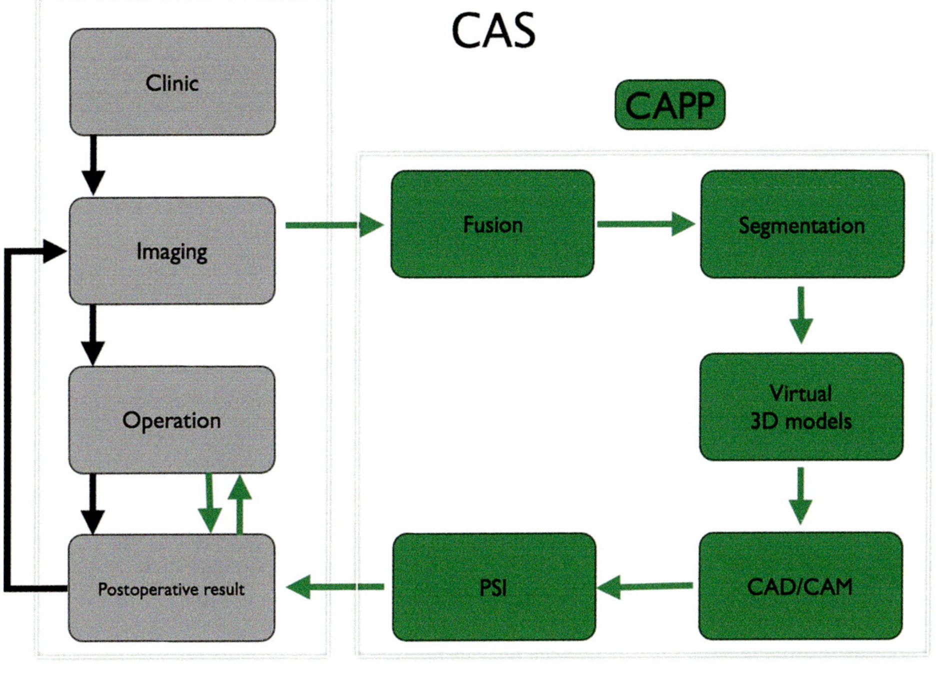

Fig. 14.3 Workflow of CAS: in *grey* the normal clinical workflow is demonstrated; the *green boxes* show the several items of CAPP

exchanging medical digital information (DICOM data; Digital Imaging and Communication in Medicine). Therefore, the surgeon is not dependent anymore on the preselection done by the radiologist in the era of two-dimensional hard copies of CT scans. The complete data set should be used for the preoperative computer-assisted planning, computer-assisted design and, if requested, manufacturing of individual implants (CAD/CAM) and computer-assisted surgery (CAS) using navigation devices. The first step is to import DICOM data of the patient's anatomy into the planning application (iPlan 3.0.5, Brainlab®, Feldkirchen, Germany) (Fig. 14.4). To analyse the clinical situation, a symmetric view of the data and its 3D volume reconstruction is necessary for further planning; therefore,

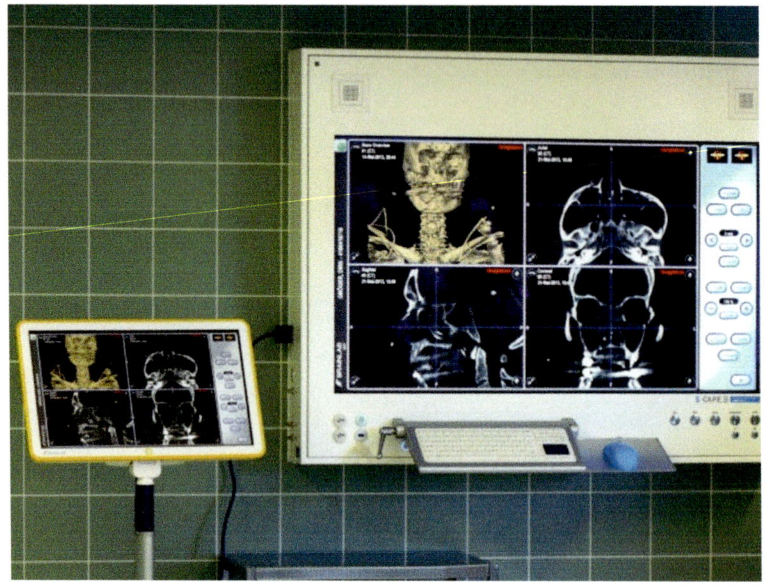

Fig. 14.4 Kick®-Navigation system is connected with a monitor in the operation room (Escape®) (Brainlab®, Feldkirchen, Germany)

the CT slice is oriented according to the Frankfurt Horizontal Mid-Sagittal (FHMS) planes in all dimensions (axial, coronal and sagittal).

After that alignment, several image data sets (CT, MRI, CBCT) can be co-registered by a so-called image fusion, a surface and voxel-based matching method, to have the whole multimodal information available within the previously adjusted alignment. This method of multimodal rigid image registration is based on mutual information, using features like multi-resolution, intensity rebinding and parameter space scaling.

Similar to this co-registration of data sets, a registration of the real-world patient with its virtual data is required during the surgery. For that registration, reference points like anatomical landmarks could be defined during the planning procedure, in which the CT or CBCT data is preferred to set such landmarks. Registration points are then planned virtually on the screw heads within a dental splint. A method like this provides unobtrusive, rigid and exact landmarks, which are clearly visible on virtual data sets (CT images) as well as during a navigation procedure, as no surgical preparation is needed to reach those screws. During the acquisition of the CT or CBCT data, either four surgically inserted navigation landmarks (bony landmarks, 2.0 cross-drive titanium mini screws (DuPuy Synthes Craniomaxillofacial, Paoli, PA, USA) or an individual dental splint with additional titanium screws (Fig. 14.5) is used for registration of the individual patient. These screws are used as registration points during planning and surgery, instead of using anatomical reference points. A dental splint with additional titanium screws should be used to increase registration accuracy.

After all necessary pre-planning steps have been finalized, the anatomical structures and the target template are segmented out of the image sets. For the anatomical structures, an automatic atlas-based algorithm is used. The central task of such an algorithm is to find the one-to-one correspondence between a patient's data set and an atlas data set that defines correct and verified anatomical templates. The structures are segmented automatically by an elastic deformation of the templates to match the patient's anatomy. Using this algorithm, not only bone structures, but anatomical regions like the orbit could be segmented and used for further surgical reconstruction planning. As a result of that procedure, all necessary anatomical structures at the area of interest for further treatment are now available as 3D segmented objects (Fig. 14.6). For the treatment of unilateral deformities or traumatic bony defects, easy tools (mirroring, interpolation and Smartbrush) are available to virtually reconstruct the desired result. These tools are difficult to use for bilateral complex deformities; therefore, it is necessary to have an archive of different templates of the facial region available.

For the treatment of tumour lesions, the tumour shape is outlined manually, or by using different tools for brushing, as a tumour is not a general structure within a patient's anatomy, and thus not automatically segmented with an atlas. Segmentation of the tumour lesion with the new Smartbrush algorithm is started by marking some points inside the desired area. Within an automatically determined region of interest (ROI) around these points, a region-growing algorithm is performed which computes the final 2D segmentation. After that, segmentation of the desired structure in a plane perpendicular to the segmented slice has to be performed. For final segmentation of the tumour, smoothing is applied to the created object. If necessary, the result of the 3D interpolation can quickly be adjusted manually. The change to one slide is then interpolated to the complete object to improve the result of the whole segmented structure. According to this planning step, clearly defined anatomical representations of patient's anatomy together with a

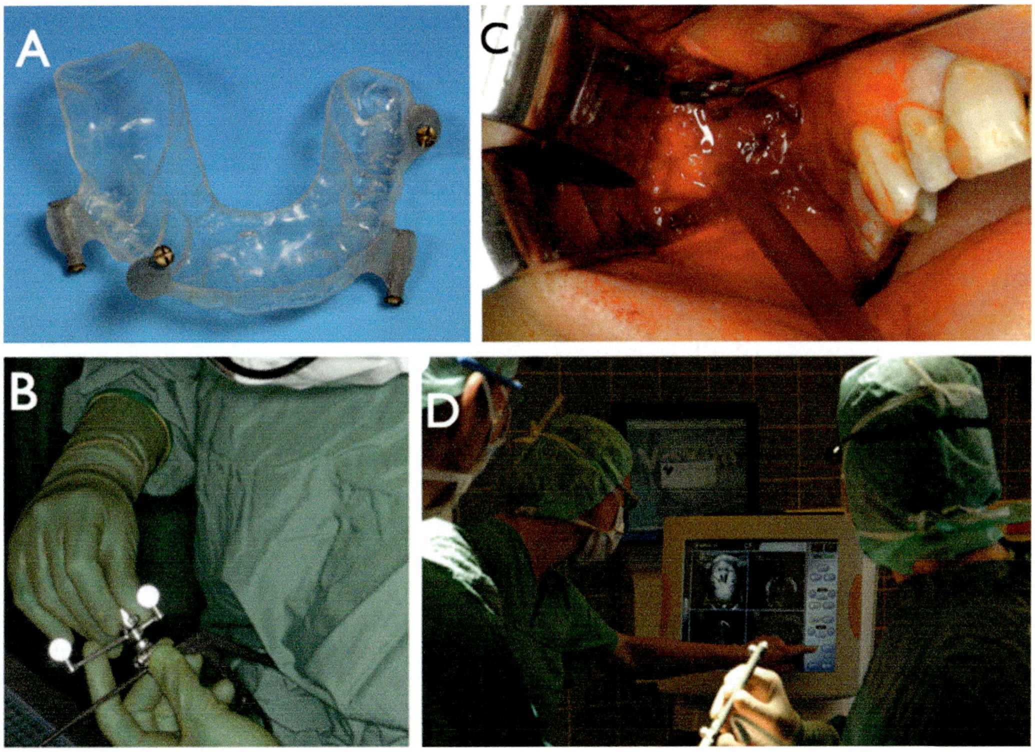

Fig. 14.5 Individual laboratory-made vacuum-formed splint for the upper jaw (navigational splint) with titanium mini 2.0 screws (DuPuy Synthes Craniomaxillofacial, Paoli, PA, USA) (**a**), positioning a holder with three sphere markers to a biopsy clamp (**b**), intraoperative biopsy with a calibrated clamp (**c**), screenshots are acquired during intraoperative navigation (**d**) (Brainlab®, Feldkirchen, Germany)

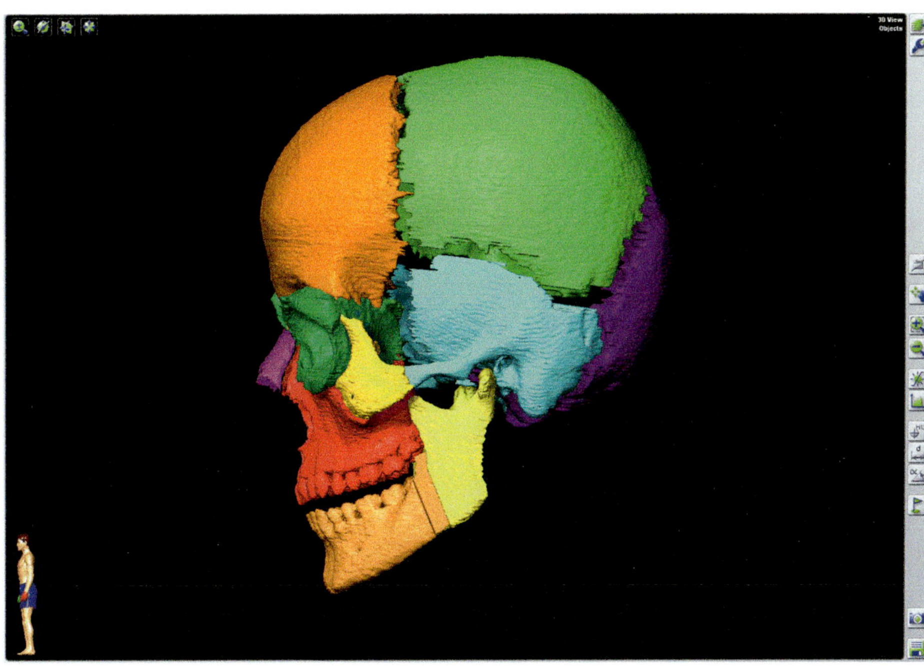

Fig. 14.6 Atlas-based 3D segments available using iPlan 3.0.5 (Brainlab®, Feldkirchen, Germany)

target region at the tumour position for resection or taking the biopsies are received. To ensure to reach the exact positions for the target, additional trajectories are planned starting at the exit point of anatomical landmarks or screws and defining a path along the midface or orbital roof directly to the tumour region. Those trajectories could be referenced and used for navigation during surgery as well. All preplanned virtual patient data, objects and trajectories are transferred to an image-guided surgery system ("navigation system"). As a basis for trauma treatment, the desired template is virtually positioned at the demanded position. For tumour treatment planning, CT and MR images of a patient are recorded, whereas the MRI data set is used to identify the tumour tissue and the CT data set to define and visualize the patient's bony anatomy.

Today, a variety of assistance systems in the sense of interactive image analysis platforms exist for the CAPP. In oral and maxillofacial surgery, the platforms of Brainlab (iPlan®, Feldkirchen, Germany) [12], IVS Solutions (VoXim, Chemnitz, Germany) [13] and StealthStation® (Medtronic, Minneapolis, Minnesota, USA)[14] are proven systems.

Intraoperative Infrared-Based Navigation

The intraoperative navigation can be compared with the navigation systems in motor vehicles. The satellite receiver emitted by the vehicle GPS signals to locate and determine its position. In the case of intraoperative navigation, the position is determined by an optical or magnetic system for the collection of the coordinates of the patient and the instruments used. The maps correspond to the custom reference points on the patient before the operation and records the CT or magnetic resonance imaging and information from the preoperative intervention planning. To calibrate this system, a starting position is set so that the virtual patient on the screen corresponds to the real patient on the operating table. According to the "local rigid body concept" (LRBC) in which at least three stationary reference elements must span a coordinate system of the object [15], this process is carried out by four reference points that must be clearly identifiable on the patient and must be found also in the record. Under-referencing is thus understood as the process in which there is a registration of the image data previously collected with the coordinate system of the patient in the operating room. The intraoperative accuracy mainly depends on the resolution of the imaging and referencing accuracy from the registration [16, 17].

Before surgery the patient is fixed in the Mayfield clamp or a mini tripod "Skull Reference Base" with three trackable spheres, fixed with a single mini titanium screw on the patient's skull, to identify the exact position and orientation of the patient [18] (Fig. 14.7). Intraoperative accuracy is checked using at least four precise "navigation landmarks". Infrared-based navigation system (Kick-Brainlab®) is used intraoperatively.

By using a stereoscopic infrared camera, such a system is able to reference a "real-world patient's" position with its planned virtual data and to further track and display instrument positions in real time. For that, the patient as well as any instrument needs to be equipped with passive infrared markers, which could be captured by the camera. This specific technique also enables the surgeon to guide the tip of any tracked surgical tool (forceps, drill, chisel and endoscope) or to localize the focus of a surgical microscope. The patient position and anatomy are registered to the planned data by equipping the patient with navigation landmarks, like the above-mentioned dental splint, and by pointing the screw heads according to their planned positions. During surgery the position of the tip can be monitored in real time to ensure the desired position and depth within the patient's skull. Additionally intraoperative landmarks can be recorded (acquired), and a "screenshot" is done to document the result. The virtual plan can be transferred after surgery to compare it with the postoperative imaging data set (Fig. 14.8).

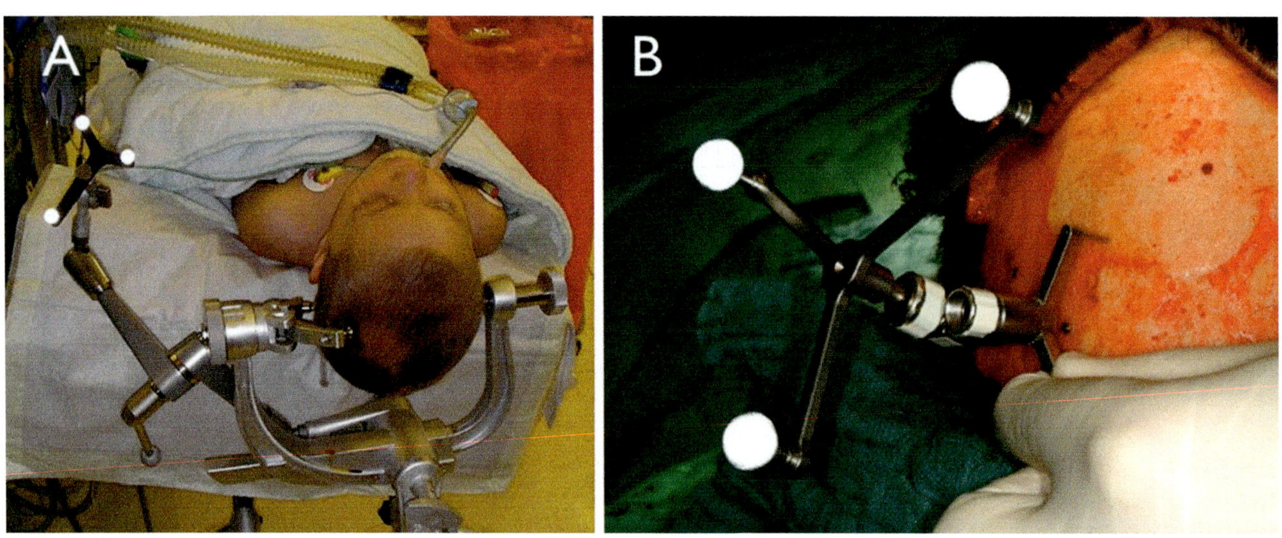

Fig. 14.7 "Mayfield Clamp" (**a**) and a mini tripod "Skull Reference Base" (**b**) with three trackable spheres, fixed with a single mini titanium screw on the patient's skull, to identify the exact position and orientation of the patient

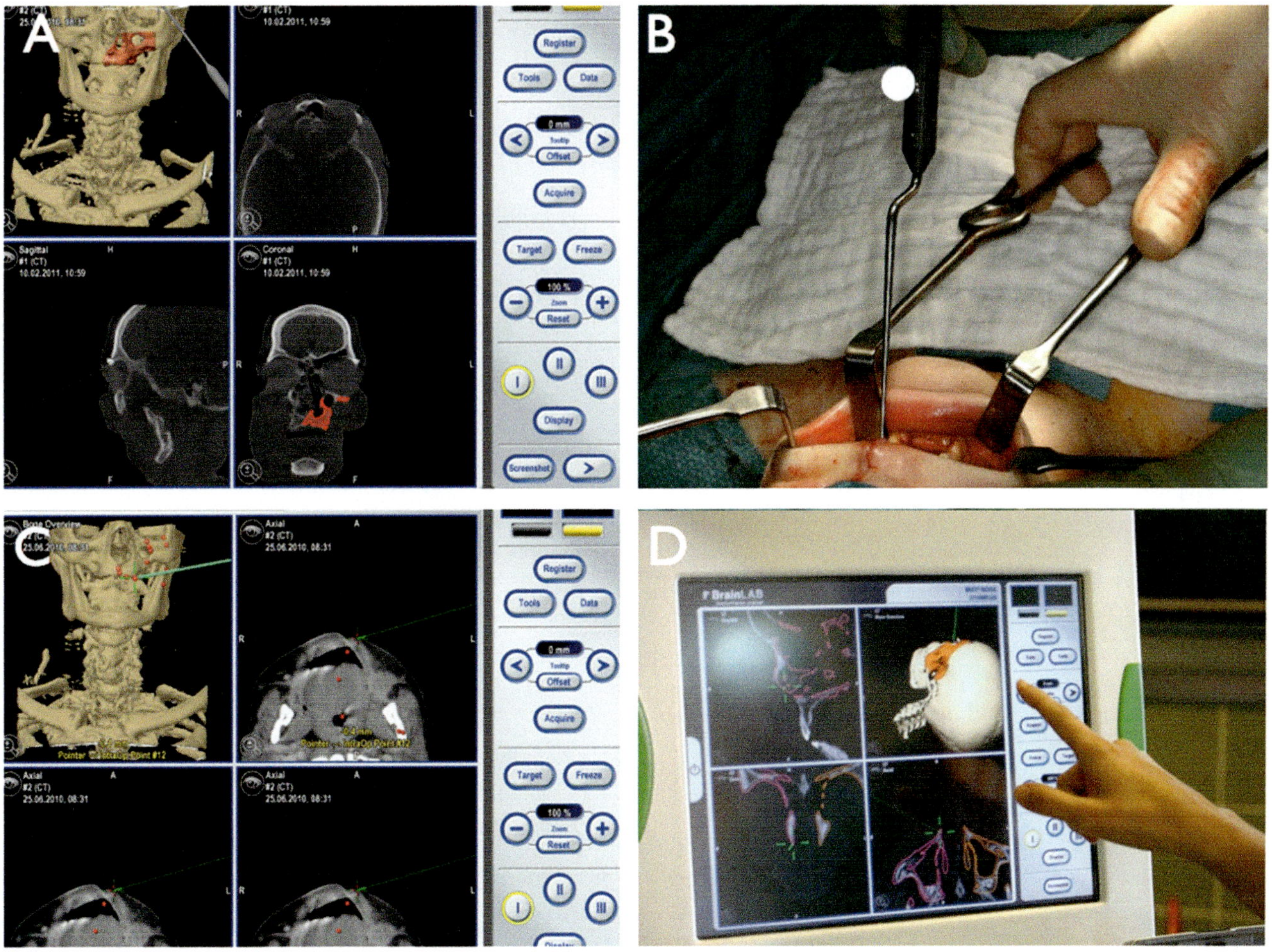

Fig. 14.8 Intraoperative navigation is used for the resection of a maxillary tumour. Intraoperative landmarks are recorded (acquired), and a "screenshot" is done to document the result (**a**–**c**). The virtual plan is transferred after surgery to compare it with the postoperative imaging data set (**d**) (Brainlab®, Feldkirchen, Germany)

Intraoperative imaging increases the accuracy and safety of surgery because it allows real-time control of the individual operation steps by accurate navigation. When using intraoperative imaging, various aspects play a role, and the safety of the staff and the patient has to be taken into account (Fig. 14.9). Intraoperative radiation exposure using intraoperative CT or CBCT should be minimized as far as possible. The costs must be estimated with respect to the expected benefits [19, 20]. In principle, different imaging procedures such as CT, MRI and 3D C-arm, and ultrasonography are used intraoperatively [21]. Intraoperative CT additionally means a high radiation dose to the patient. In oral and maxillofacial surgery, intraoperative imaging has proved that the application of the CBCT as practical, with the main advantage of CBCT being that artefacts (scatters) of the metallic dental restorations do not overlap the necessary form for reporting structures.

Postoperative Control

Postoperative three-dimensional imaging is used for postoperative documentation of successful repositioned fractures, ideally positioned patient-specific implants (PSI) (Fig. 14.10) or sufficient therapy for tumour follow-up or restaging use. The postoperative data thus allows a precise comparison in later recurrence control, and targeted use of radiation therapy by the three-dimensional data which is sent to the radiotherapists, so that they can set up according to the information an individualized treatment plan. Comparing the pre- and postoperative records may also aid in the success of the procedure, and the radiotherapy or chemotherapy will be evaluated qualitatively and quantitatively, so that the work of the surgeon and radiation therapists becomes more transparent and thus more controllable. Upon receipt of the histological findings, the sampling points of the tumour according to its origin can be colour coded, so that later there is a three-dimensional image of any residual tumour tissue.

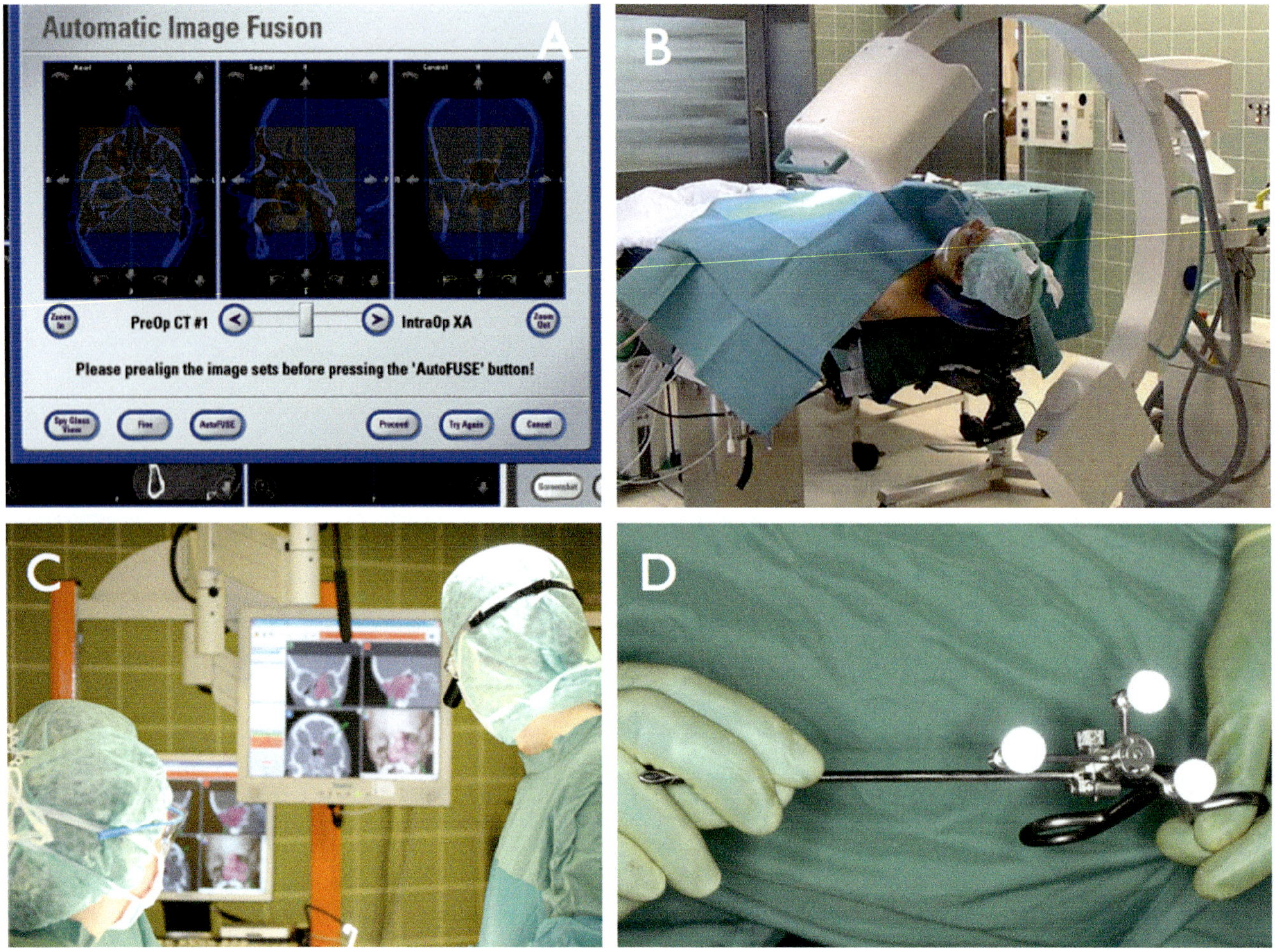

Fig. 14.9 Automatic image fusion in navigation system KICK® (**a**). Intraoperative 3D C-arm (Ziehm® Imaging, Orlando, FI, USA) for intraoperative imaging (**b**). Navigation system IVS Solutions (VoXim, Chemnitz, Germany) (**c**). Calibrated clamp (**d**)

Navigation Systems

In principle, optical, electromechanical, electromagnetic and ultrasound-based systems can be distinguished (Table 14.2). Together, these systems have in common that a multiplanar view is used, in the axial, sagittal, and coronal planes. In addition, in many cases, a virtual 3D model of the data set is created.

The most commonly used systems in CAS represent the optical systems, as they are very precise and are hardly affected by the environmental conditions in the operating room. In these systems, the surgical instruments and probes to be detected intraoperatively with passive markers. The camera-infrared cameras are integrated, which emit light. This light is reflected by the spherical markers, which are attached to the instrument. The reflected light from CCD cameras (charge-coupled device) is detected, and the position of each marker is then determined by triangulation in three-dimensional space. In these systems, an accuracy of about 1 mm is achieved, which is assessed in comparison to other systems as high [22, 23].

Electromechanical systems operate on a multi-joint sensor arm through which it calculates the position of a probe that is attached to the arm and can be displayed on the CT data set. In clinical studies, intraoperative accuracy of 1–3 mm is reported [24–26]. The advantage of these systems is that they are independent of the environmental conditions in the operating room, but at the same time, they can be cumbersome due to their shape and size during surgery.

Electromagnetic systems operate with a magnetic field source and transmitter, which is attached to a head mount. A sensor mounted on the surgical instrument sensor detects changes in the electromagnetic field and thus calculates its position. The problem with this system is that all metal objects in the operating room affect the magnetic field and therefore must be removed [27]. An attempt is made to counteract this, by using sequentially activated coils [28]. The accuracy of these systems is reported in various studies

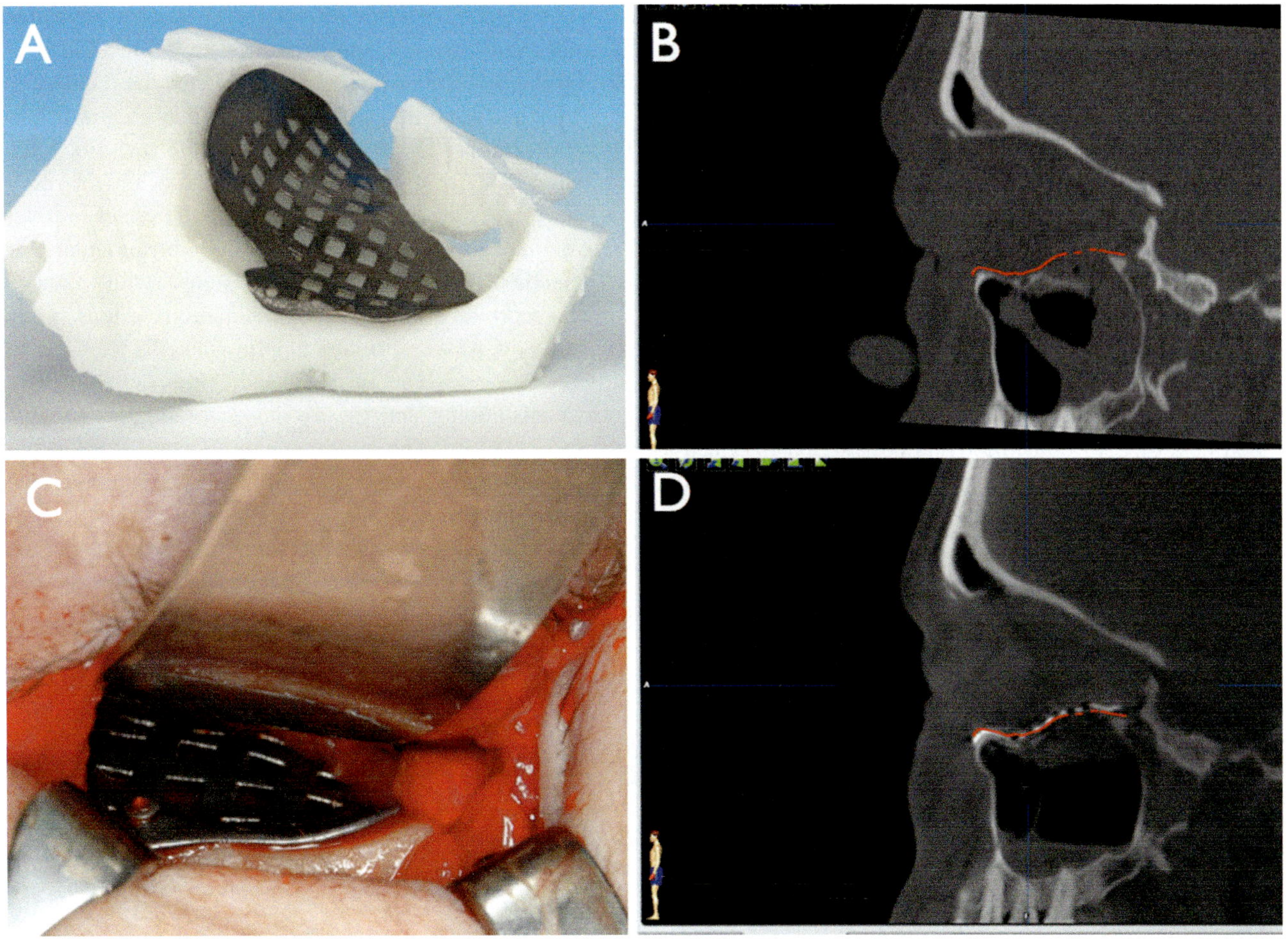

Fig. 14.10 PSI of the left orbit with a polyamide model (KLS-Martin®, Tuttlingen, Germany) (**a**), preoperative three-dimensional image (sagittal view) and the ideal position of the implant (*red*) (**b**), successful reconstructed orbital fracture and ideally positioned patient-specific implant (PSI) (**c**), postoperative three-dimensional image (sagittal view) and (**d**), the ideal position of the implant (*red*) and the inserted implant (*grey*) (iPlan, Brainlab, Munich, Germany)

Table 14.2 Examples of optical, electromechanical, electromagnetic and ultrasound-based navigation systems

Technology	Company	Navigation system
Optical	Medtronic	StealthStation®
	IVS Technology	VoXim®
	Stryker	eNlite
		NavSuite
	Scopis medical	Scopis®
	Brainlab	Curve, VectorVision, Kick®, Kolibri™
	XION medical	MATRIX POLAR
	Collin	DigiPointeur®
Electromechanical	ISG Technologies	Viewing Wand
Electromagnetic	Medtronic	StealthStation® Fusion
	Brainlab	Kick® EM
	Fiagon	Fiagon Smart
Ultrasound based	SonoWand	Invite™

with about 2 mm [29–31]. Ultrasound-based systems use acoustic signals emitted by a surgical microphone. The microphone position can be calculated by a computer using three radiopaque beads, which are attached to the patient's head, and three microphones installed in the room and is superimposed with CT images [32]. The problem with this system is the dependence of the acoustic signals from the temperature and airflow as extra noise affecting the measurement accuracy [33].

Use of Computer-Assisted Surgery and Intraoperative Navigation in Oral and Maxillofacial Surgery

The range of applications of CAS in oral and maxillofacial surgery is today widely diversified and used routinely in many areas. CAS in oral and maxillofacial surgery is mainly used in the context of virtual planning, intraoperative navigation and postoperative quality control. The major part of this is CAPP. Other than in neurosurgery where the goal is to visualize a lesion which is present, (e.g. navigation-guided biopsy), in craniomaxillofacial surgery navigation is used to achieve reconstructive goals (ideal maxillary, orbital or mandibular reconstruction) as well as to guide ablative surgery.

Minimally Invasive Surgery and Biopsies

Navigation-assisted biopsies were introduced as the first application field of CAS in the head and neck region [34], and a typical application is frameless stereotaxy [13]. Minimally invasive procedures are distinguished in that they provide the least traumatizing technique, thus reducing the mortality while sparing adjacent structures. As a result, the patient has less postoperative pain symptoms, and aesthetics are maintained.

In the field of oral and maxillofacial surgery, navigated biopsies such as in approaches to retromaxillary or intraorbital area are desirable, as well as for the removal of small benign or malignant processes. When approaches in the retromaxillary or intraorbital regions are performed, the advantage of CAS is that the transoral approach to the retromaxillary space can be achieved through the use of intraoperative navigation, instead of the preauricular or retromandibular transcutaneous incisions, with reduced surgical morbidity. Even in post-traumatic revisions in the sinuses, the CAS is especially helpful since the localization of the endoscopes can be navigated intraoperatively with correct positioning and the avoidance of injuries to vital structures [13, 35]. The most common indication of CAS in this area is to provide biopsies preoperatively in which the trajectory is planned. Guidelines for the selection of approaches are: localization, tumour entity, and extent of the tumour, which are defined in the context of preoperative planning (Fig. 14.11).

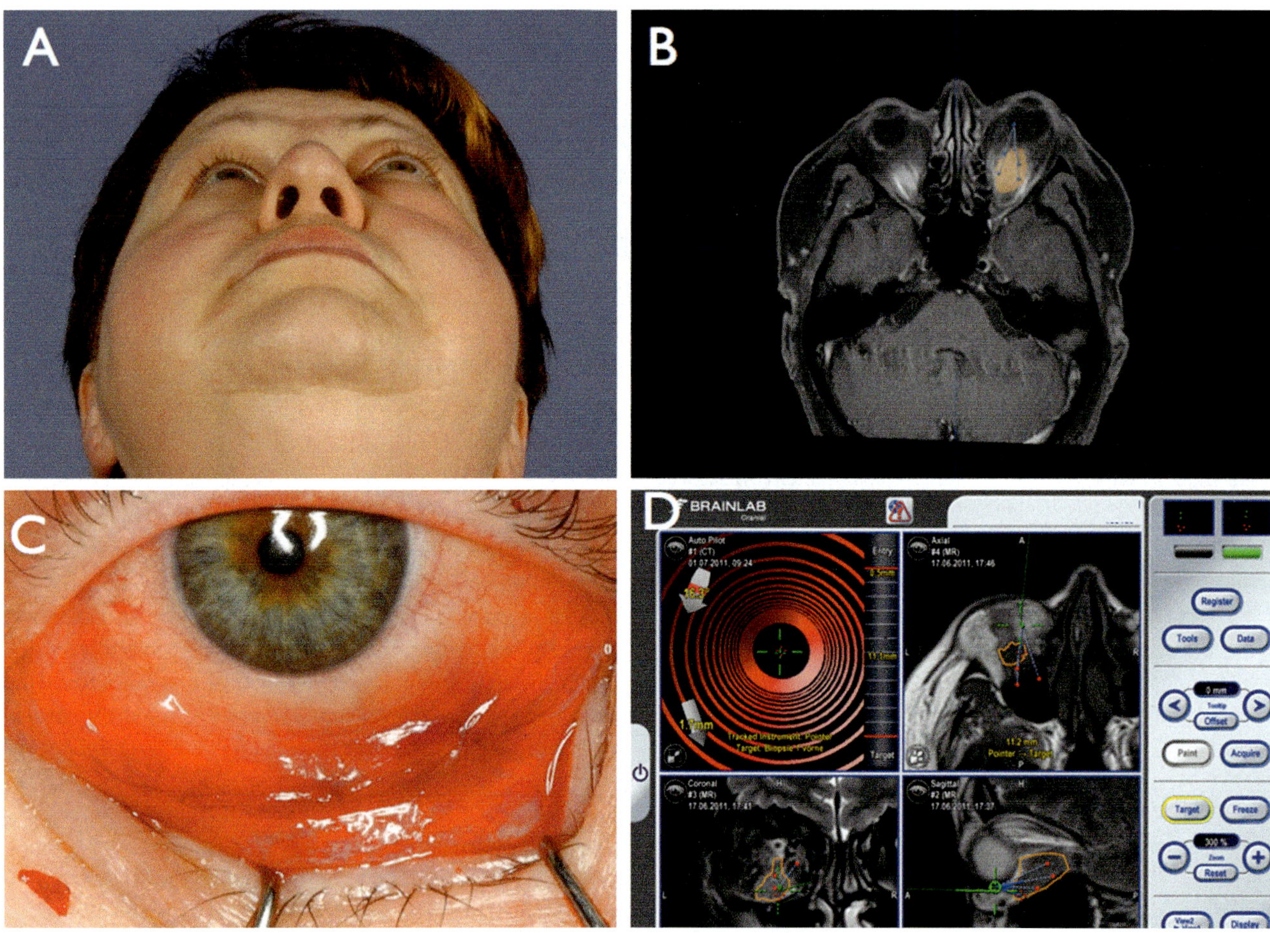

Fig. 14.11 (**a**) Front view of a 53-year-old female with an unknown orbital tumour. (**b**) Display of the MRI data set in the axial view. The area to be biopsied was marked preoperatively (*brown*) and can be identified intraoperatively in the multiplanar display of the MRI data set, four pre-planned trajectories are marked (*blue*). (**c**) Transconjunctival approach. (**d**) Navigation-assisted exploration of the orbital cavity. The tip is pointing to the tumour (*green*), which is displayed in the multiplanar mode (axial, sagittal and coronal). Autopilot feature displays the deviation from a desired path in all spatial directions to ensure to follow a planned track (Brainlab®, Feldkirchen, Germany)

Traumatology

The acute treatment of facial fractures as a result of injuries caused by interpersonal violence or accidents, when indicated primarily consists of open reduction and internal fixation with the aim of restoring the facial skeleton and the overlying soft tissues. Secondarily, a functional recovery of the affected structures is sought [35]. Owing to the short data acquisition time, imaging is based on the intraoperative volume tomography (3D C-arm) obtained in the ideal case, with the minimum average of 2–3 min. The results of the repositioned fracture segments can now be controlled intraoperatively by navigation, and screenshots of crucial anatomical structures can be saved for documentation [36].

With regard to aesthetic and functional fracture reconstruction, CAS has proven to be very helpful, as the result can be accurately predicted by the detailed planning with the help of imaging techniques. The intraoperative navigation also allows continuous control of the reconstruction steps, so that positioning errors can be prevented and thus the need for further correction is minimized [37, 38].

The reliable reconstruction of the face by virtual planning for unilateral fractures is now routinely achieved by mirroring the unaffected side, so that prior to surgery, patient-specific implants (PSI) can be fabricated [39] (Fig. 14.12).

Possible workflows of CAS in traumatology are the data acquisition across different imaging modalities (CT, CBCT). Subsequently, the planning and simulation for fracture treatment are done. With the help of CAPP, three paths can also be used independently or jointly run for the preparation of PSI, intraoperative navigation and intraoperative CBCT. After repositioning the fractures, intraoperative imaging is used. In complex fractures, it could be possible for additional control through the use of the navigation. For insertion of PSI, the situation is monitored by intraoperative navigation and finally documented with intraoperative imaging (if available).

For primary orbital reconstruction using titanium implants, two different methods are now used for the reconstruction of large bony defects. The first method is to use a pre-bent titanium mesh (PBTM) based on a 3D polyamide model of the ideal orbit form based on the virtual

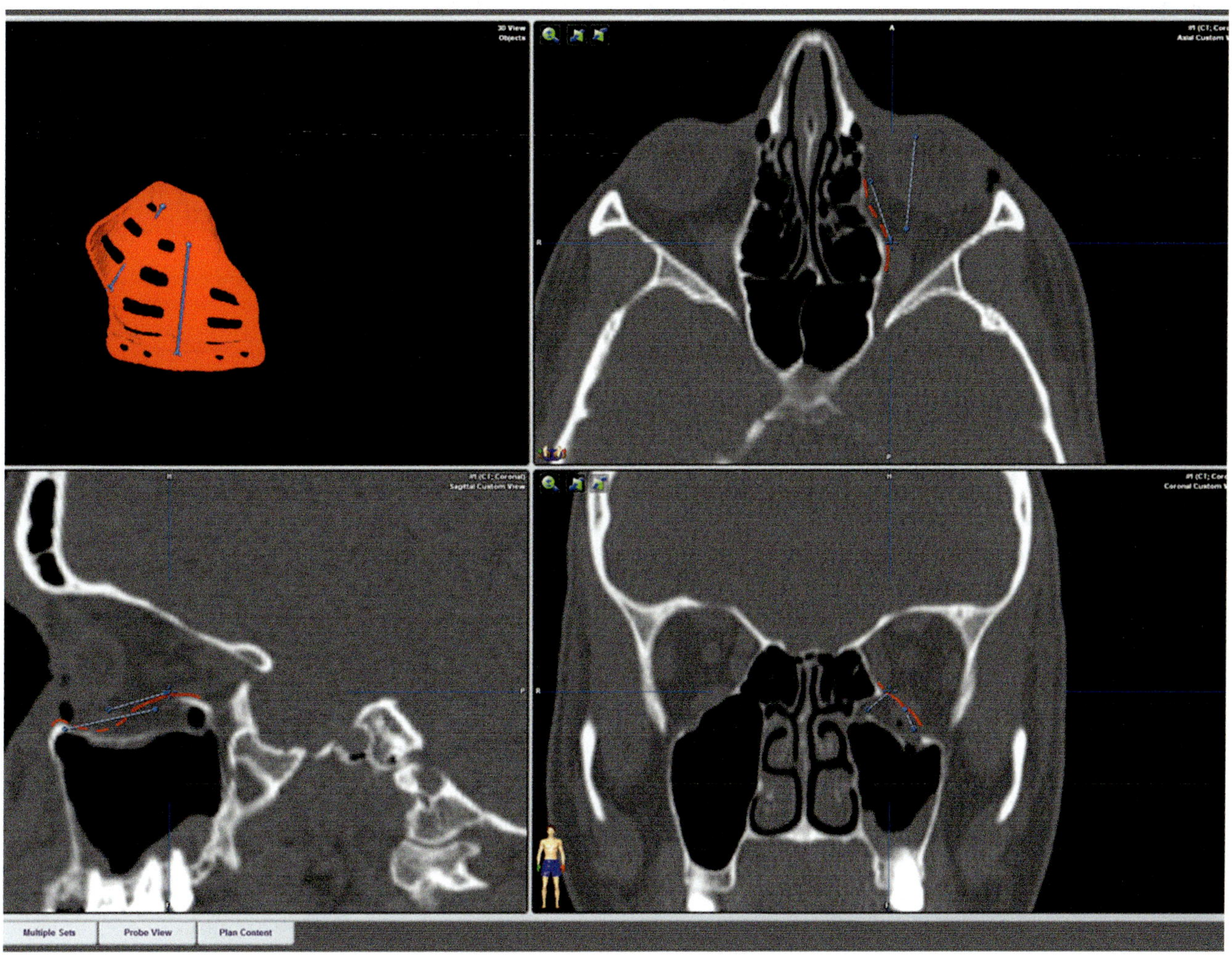

Fig. 14.12 Preoperative view of a left orbital fracture. PSI is coloured (*red*) (KLS-Martin®, Tuttlingen, Germany) (iPlan, Brainlab, Munich, Germany)

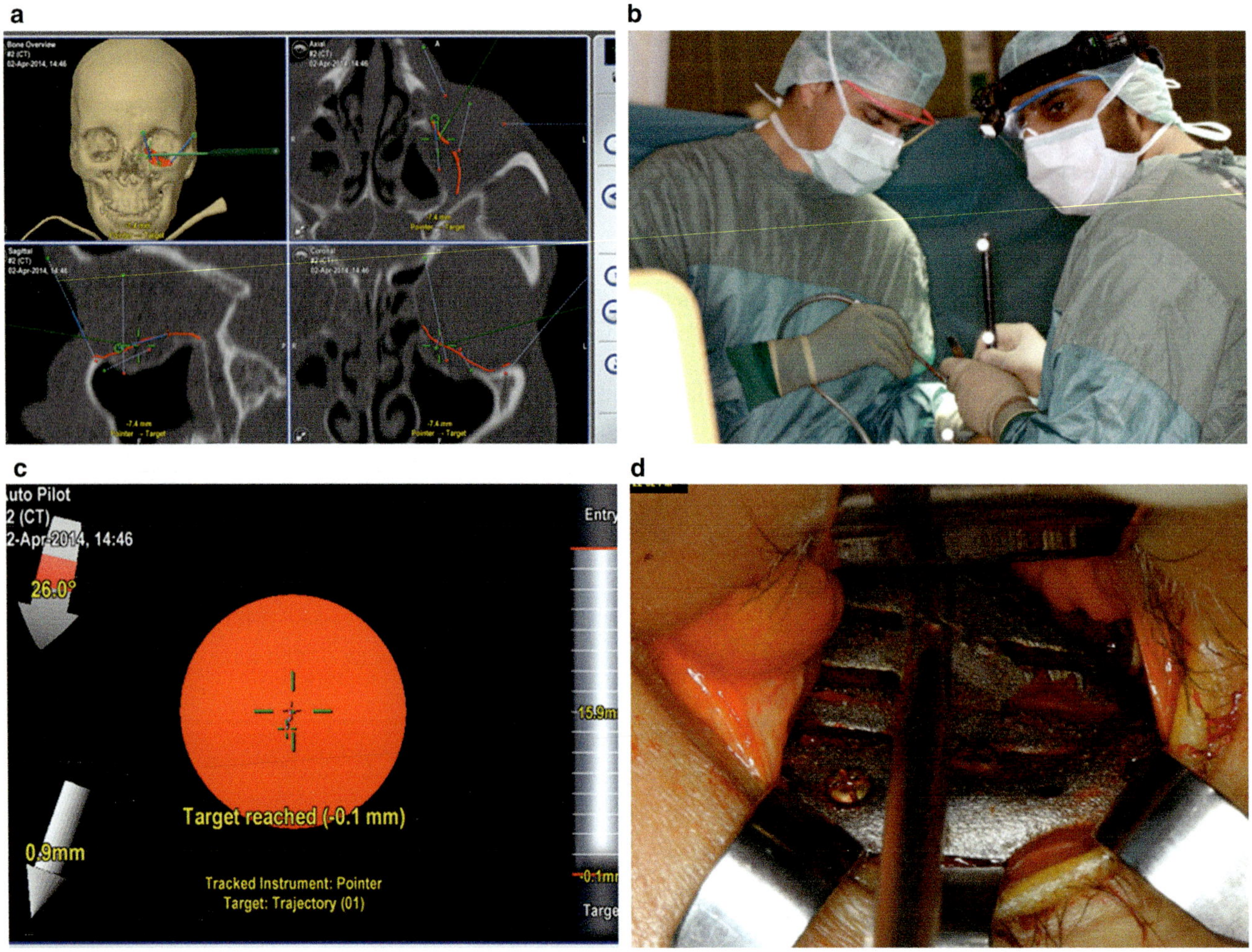

Fig. 14.13 (**a**) *Upper left*: screenshot of 3D image with the pointer resting on a navigational landmark of the PSI. *Lower right* and *left*, and *Upper left*: screenshots showing position of pointer in sagittal and coronal views, and axial view (tip of pointer is represented by the centre of the green crosshairs) (Brainlab®, Feldkirchen, Germany). (**b**) intraoperative navigation used to confirm correct implant position. (**c**) screenshot showing pointer has reached the navigation landmark. (**d**) intraoperative view of PSI in position with pointer resting on it for navigational control (KLS-Martin®, Tuttlingen, Germany)

plan produced by Phacon® (Leipzig, Germany). Titanium mesh (DuPuy Synthes Craniomaxillofacial, Paoli, PA, USA) can then be manually bent preoperatively to the desired contour as previously described [40]. The second method is to use patient-specific implants (PSI) (Fig. 14.13). The virtual model of the reconstructed ideal orbit is exported as a stereolithographical (STL) file to the program Geomagic-Freeform® Plus (Morrisville, NC, USA) to design the desired titanium implant needed to reconstruct the bony defects. Key elements of the design include a rounded edge for easier insertion and, to prevent restriction of orbital contents, a drainage system, navigational guides, rulers and drill holes (Fig. 14.14). Once the design is finalized, the implant was produced via additive manufacturing (selective laser sintering) by KLS-Martin® (Tuttlingen, Germany).

The planning for secondary reconstructions is more challenging due to the soft tissue loss and scarring [35]. Here, the displaced bones are also visualized, and ideal approaches are planned in the preoperative planning. The reconstruction of bilateral trauma and complex midfacial fractures or panfacial fractures is difficult, since there is no reference for the plan-

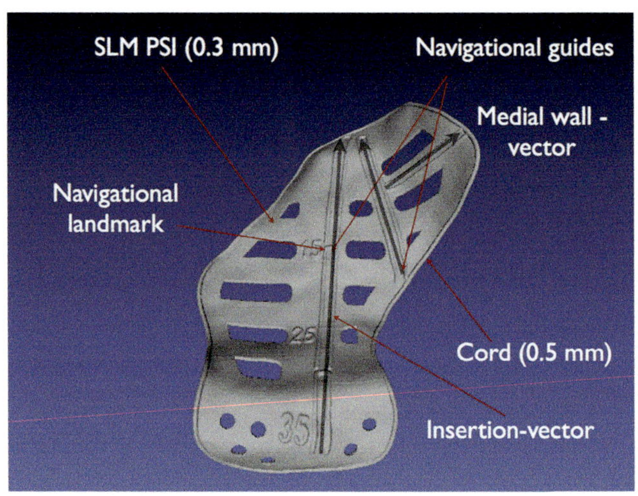

Fig. 14.14 A selective laser melted (sintered) patient-specific implant designed for the right orbit, 0.3 mm thick. An atraumatic cord with a thickness of 0.5 mm runs around the border. A horizontal drainage system is incorporated throughout. Navigational landmarks and guides are provided to facilitate implant placement with intraoperative navigation. Screw holes are placed anteriorly for fixation to the inferior orbital rim (KLS-Martin®, Tuttlingen, Germany)

ning of the reconstruction results based on the presence of unaffected structures. But even in this field, algorithms are now being developed that use a system based on standard model skulls of rigid and elastic deformation to allow a virtual reconstruction.

Another challenge with orbital wall or orbital floor defects is the limited visibility in the intraorbital surgical field. This may cause incorrect positioning of the implants, which in turn leads to unintended secondary reconstructions. Here, intraoperative navigation brings a decisive advantage because it can check the positioning of the implant placement and compare it with the preoperative specified goals [36].

A further advantage that CAS provides in traumatology is that, by the verification of the correct placement of the prefabricated patient-specific implants, the operation time can be reduced [36, 39]. Therefore, a higher precision can be achieved by the use of the PSI by means of intraoperative navigation.

Orthognathic Surgery and Congenital Deformities

For the treatment of acquired or congenital facial deformities, skeletal malocclusion is an especially important field for the application CAPP and CAS in oral and maxillofacial surgery. Although the objectives in orthognathic surgery have changed considerably since the 1980s, the surgical techniques have hardly changed since the introduction of the intraoral surgical approaches developed by Obwegeser and Bell [41, 42]. Today, the focus on high-quality results is desirable. Achieving this requires careful planning and subsequent counselling of patients, consistent treatment, and the application of appropriate techniques. Computer-assisted planning of malocclusion may be superior to conventional planning [43, 44]. Treating facial aesthetics provides another element of importance, in addition to the functional improvement of the malocclusion and mastication associated with these disorders.

The main starting point for the implementation of CAPP and CAS is the desired congruence between the coordinate system of planning procedures and real patients. This objective is not reached by existing conventional planning methods, where the registration has clear weaknesses through so-called facebow recordings, and a lack of reproducibility within an articulator system [42]. In this method, the amount of intraoperative displacement of the maxillary and mandibular repositioning is determined by simulating the surgical movements of the jaw segments on the articulator. This is the least reproducible step in the surgical planning, because of the wide variety of nonstandardized techniques that are utilized. Instead, a fusion of 3D data sets provides the unique opportunity that the registration of real patients is standardized with the data on the computer. To increase accuracy, it is better to have a positioning plate to keep the mandibular condyles in their habitual position [45].

Conventional techniques attempt to set the original condylar position by hand through the use of an interocclusal splint. This can be an especially difficult with the LeFort I Maxillary Osteotomy in which malpositioning of the segment occurs because of a retruded position of the condyle [46, 47]. The Göttingen concept employs interocclusal centric splints, which are intraoperatively attached to a facebow in centric condylar position, which is considered the therapeutic condylar position [48, 49].

At the start of the virtual planning, the desired position of the maxilla and mandible must be specified. Then with the help of an optical collision detection, it is possible to calculate an appropriate dental occlusion of the upper and lower jaw. Finally, a Boolean operation is performed to obtain a preliminary virtual splint from which a physical splint is then printed using a 3D printer. Osteotomies can be planned in detail with the help of CAPP, and the displacements of the maxillary and mandibular segments are virtually simulated until a satisfactory treatment plan is realized. It is in the especially anatomically difficult to reach areas, such as the Le Fort III level, that the intersegmental distances and positioning of the bone segments and osteotomies can be planned preoperatively. After creating the three-dimensional image data using CT or CBCT, an auto-segmentation algorithm is used to prepare the virtual Le Fort I, II, or III Maxillary Osteotomy, Bilateral Mandibular Sagittal Split or Vertical Ramus Osteotomies, and Genioplasty as indicted. In the next step, plaster models of the arch of the upper and lower jaw of the patient are scanned by a three-dimensional dental surface scanner and imported into the initial CT or CBCT data sets, so that the visual depiction of the teeth is improved. This step is crucial for the occlusion and the creation of the interdental splints (Fig. 14.15).

Further, a photorealistic 3D surface scanner may be used to acquire the facial soft tissue of the patient and for fusion with the preoperative anatomical data, whereby the expected outcomes can be better visualized. The preoperatively planned position of the maxilla and mandible is then navigated by the system during operation. An example of the possible operations of the CAS during orthognathic surgery is presented in (Fig. 14.16).

Dental Implantology

The objectives of CAPP and CAS in dental implant surgery are the preservation of vital structures and reduction of postoperative complications. In addition, the functional and aesthetic results are improved. The use of the CAS and CAPP can prevent the erroneous positioning of the implant

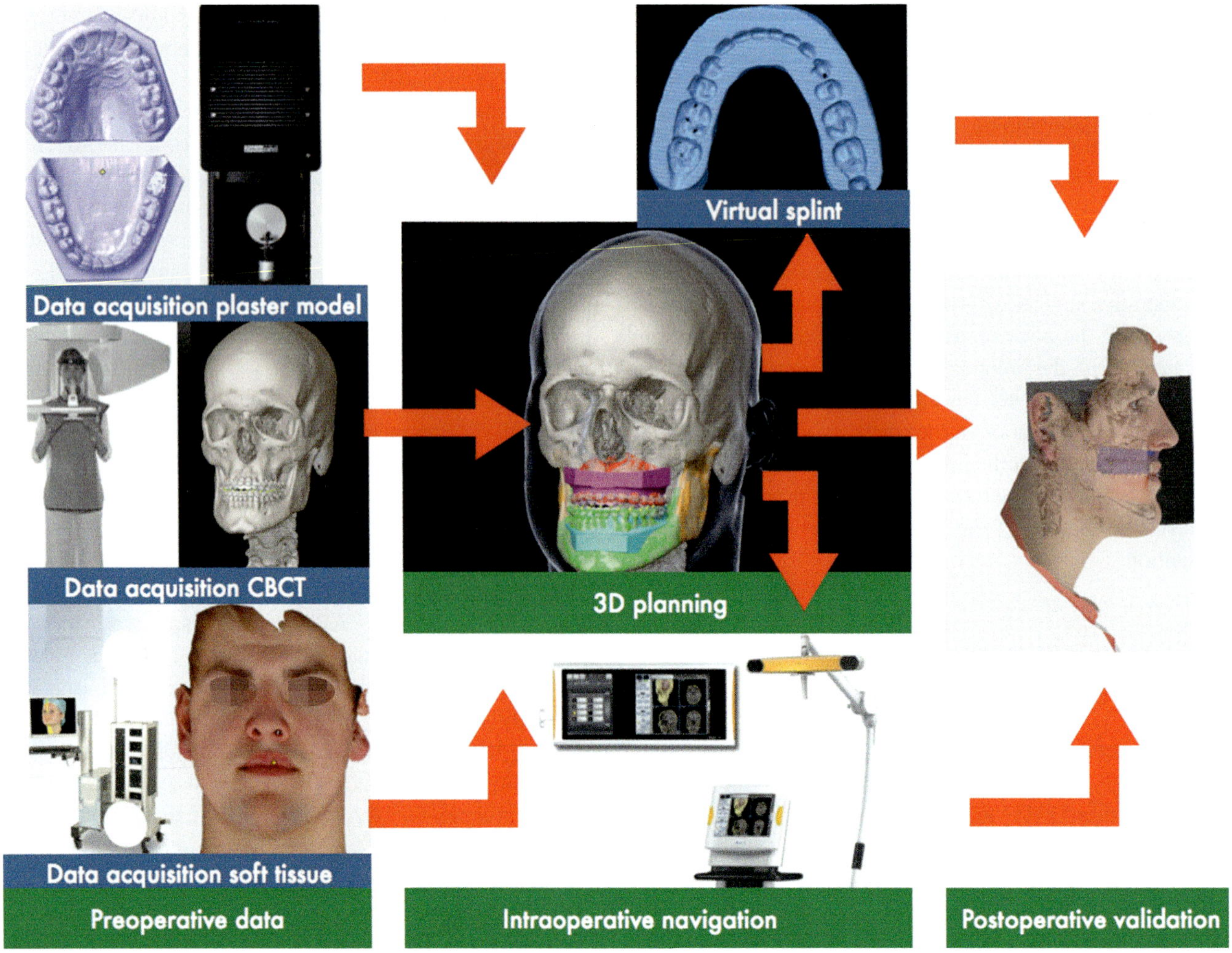

Fig. 14.15 Workflow of virtual planning in orthognathic surgery based on the preoperative data to the postoperative evaluation. First, the merging of all preoperative data (STL export of gypsum models, DICOM export of CBCT's and OBJ export of face scans) is achieved with the planning software iPlan 3.0.5. (Brainlab®, Feldkirchen, Germany). After completion of planning, the production of the physical splint based on the principle of rapid prototyping is performed. Planning is controlled intraoperatively by the use of navigation in addition to the physical splint. Postoperatively, it is monitored by the superimposition of the pre- and postoperative data set with the planning

and the violation of critical structures [50, 51]. Typical indications are the insertion of zygoma implants after ablative tumour surgery in the upper jaw and implant placement after extensive bone grafting [52] (Fig. 14.17).

The success of an implant-supported rehabilitation depends on precise preoperative planning of implant position and prosthetic treatment options. In this area, the so-called backwards planning plays a crucial role, since during the preoperative planning, the desired end result is the starting point of the design. Starting from this treatment goal, the CAS supports the surgeon through the collected image data not only in the planning, but also in the implementation and documentation of the procedure.

In order to ensure successful treatment, the following steps are generally used. Based on the data from a planned prosthesis and imaging, the implant position can be determined by backwards planning (prosthetically-driven implant planning). When planning the prosthesis, the detailed intra- and extra-oral examination should be at the forefront of assessing the needs of the patient.

For successful implementation of the planning, the data quality of the imaging methods is crucial. Three-dimensional data sets are collected favourably with CT and CBCT, as they allow a layered representation without superimposition of the structures. In addition, bone quality and quantity can be determined in advance by the grey values [53]. The CT when compared with the two-dimensional process has a

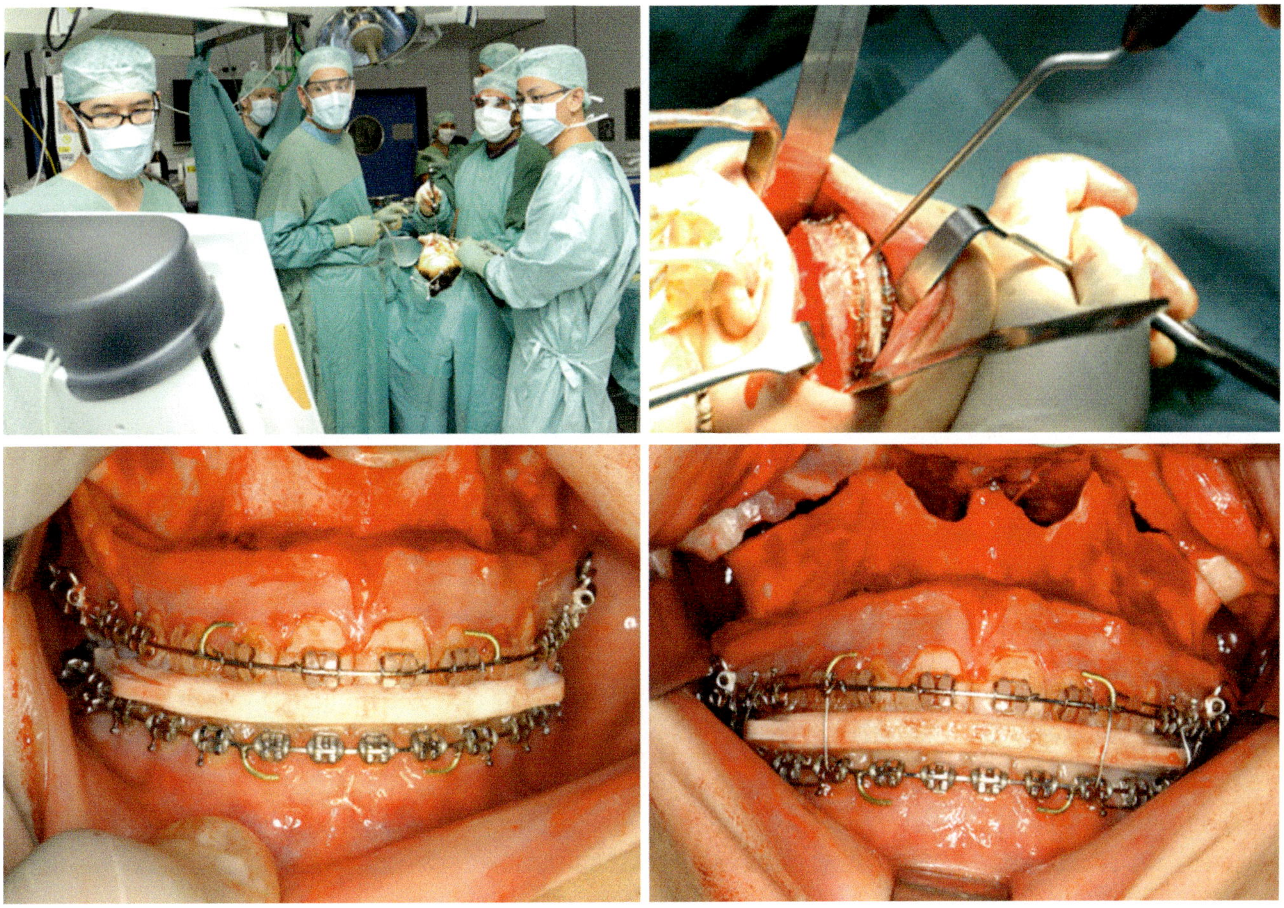

Fig. 14.16 Rapid printed virtual dental splint used with intraoperative navigation for the position of a LeFort I Osteotomy of the upper jaw

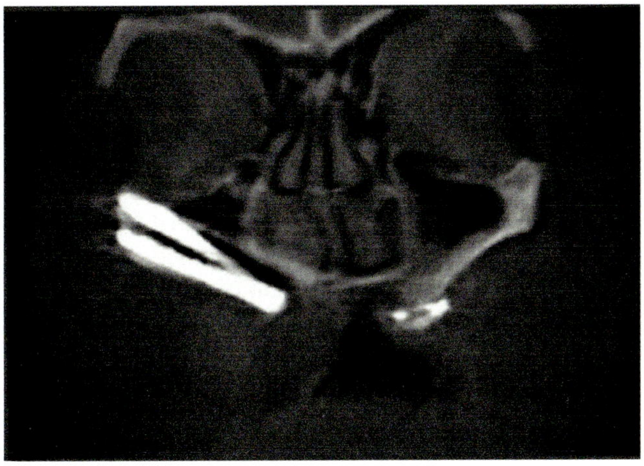

Fig. 14.17 Coronal view after the insertion of two right zygoma implants

range of 0.33–0.5 mm precision [54, 55]. However, a CBCT has advantages over CT in that it allows an accurate representation of the anatomy and geometry, with less artefacts by metallic restorations and brackets, such as gold and chromium-cobalt-molybdenum alloys [56, 57]. The CBCT study in the field of oral and maxillofacial surgery is a type of CT examination which is based on the principle of the conical beam, and is of superior quality to the fan-shaped beam. However, the selection of the imaging method is to be taken only after careful consideration, since the CBCT cannot display a high resolution of the soft tissue.

In planning the implant position, various possibilities are available, such as the planning on a radiograph or a model. However, when compared to the CAPP, 2D images have the distinct disadvantage in that there is no information on bone mineral density and anatomic at risk structures. This is in contrast to CAPP, where a three-dimensional model can be created, with the data obtained from the CT or CBCT. The 3D model allows for looking at different views and to highlight important structures. In addition, the implant can be virtually planned, and based on the data, drilling templates for implant placement can be fabricated. Dental navigation systems can assist the surgeon in the process of implementing the plan (Fig. 14.18).

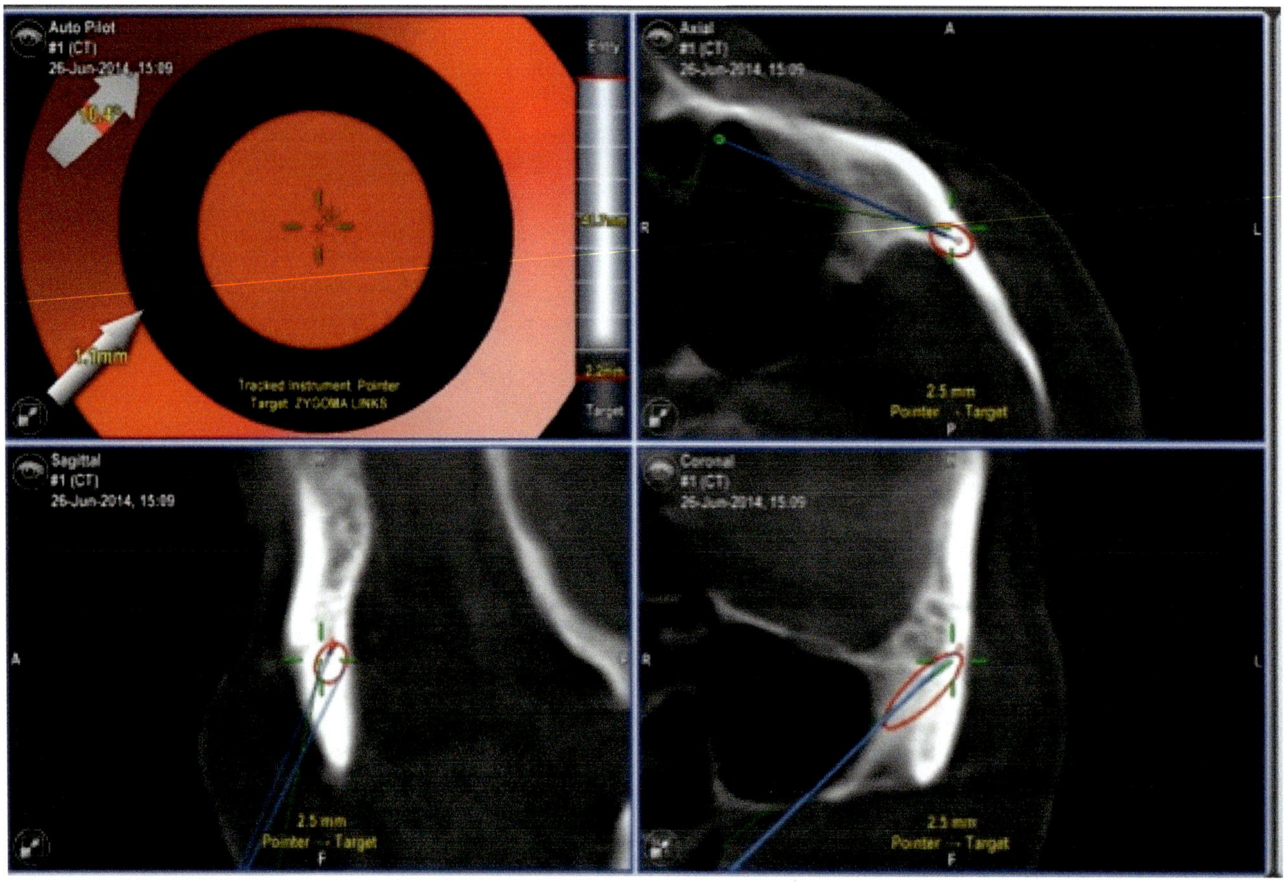

Fig. 14.18 Navigated-assisted insertion of a zygoma implant in the left zygomatic buttress (iPlan 3.0.5, Brainlab®, Feldkirchen, Germany)

Tumour Surgery

Tumour surgery is another main area for the application of CAPP and CAS. Head and neck oncologic treatment benefits greatly from the interdisciplinary exchange of information and conferences. However, when it comes to therapy, mainly the views of single disciplines are applied to the given information: the oncologic surgeon resects the tumour, the reconstructive surgeon repairs the defect, the radiotherapist plans and performs the radiotherapy, and, if required, the oncologist plans and controls the chemotherapy. Using CAS, the resection margins can now be better defined, and a complete tumour resection can be performed without the violation of vital structures [18]. As part of the diagnosis, CT is still the gold standard for imaging. With suitable software (VoXim® 6.2, IVS Technology, Chemnitz, Germany), it is also possible to represent the tumour in multimodal view and a 3D volume reconstruction (Fig. 14.19).

In head and neck oncologic surgery, complete resection and analysis of resection margins are fundamental. Navigation techniques define resection margins more accurately and facilitate complete tumour removal by preserving vital structures [12]. CAS has the advantage that the marginal resections are marked and named virtually (Fig. 14.20). As a result, the assignment of histological results is greatly simplified. If in the long term, a restaging is necessary, previously stored data can be used and merged with the newly collected data sets and compared. In the late 1990s, the group of Gellrich, Schramm and Schmelzeisen used navigation to achieve an unambiguous assignment of voxels in the space between real patients and 3D data [58]. However, even with this combined imaging modality, the intraoperative evaluation of the distance between the resection margins and the tumour margin remains a challenge in oncologic surgery. Preoperatively the tumour shape and margins can be outlined manually after using different software tools, such as brushing. A major problem during tumour resection (without navigation) is to name and exactly allocate the anatomical 3D position of specimens. Advantages of intraoperative navigation is not only to plan tumour resection margins, but also the

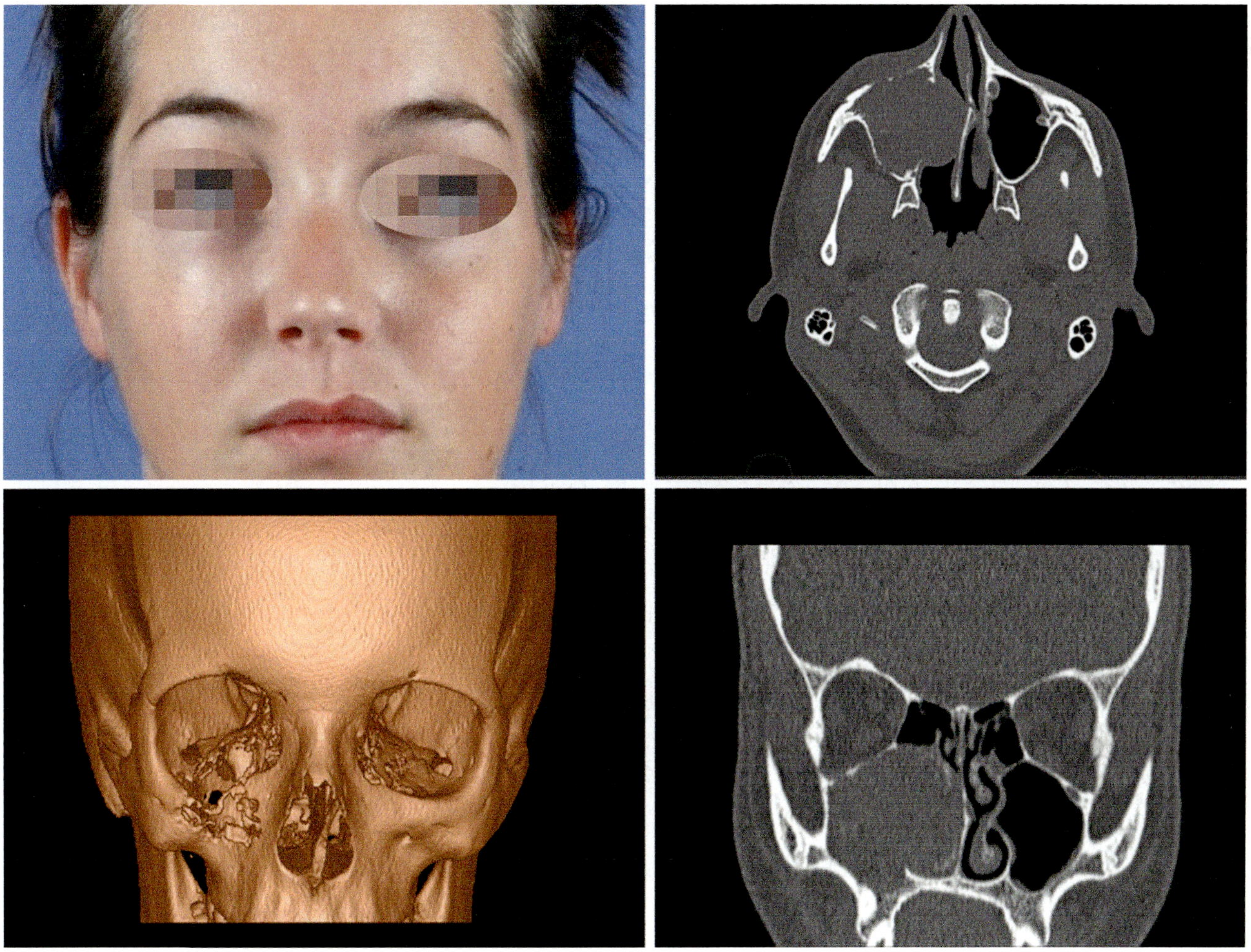

Fig. 14.19 21-year-old female patient with sino-nasal carcinoma of the right maxillary sinus in the multimodal view (axial, coronal, three-dimensional) (VoXim® 6.2, IVS Technology, Chemnitz, Germany)

definitive marking and mapping of frozen sections. These data could be stored and transferred in DICOM format to communicate the patient's specific tumour information (invasion of vessels, nerves, skull base, non-resectable tumour) to the oncologist, radiotherapist and pathologist for further oncologic treatment (Fig. 14.21).

In the field of ablative surgery, CAS has many advantages over surgery without navigation. Careful planning, and taking into account all relevant information, can greatly facilitate intraoperative interventions and optimize the result obtained due to the precision that CAS offers. Perhaps the greatest advantage of the CAS lies in the possibility of designing patient-specific implants. As a result, not only is the function and organ preservation secured, but also greatly improved aesthetic outcomes can be achieved. A time-sparing, possibly simultaneous, so-called "true-to-original" reconstruction can be implemented using CAS. In summary, histopathological findings should be three-dimensionally mapped, information should be without loss, and ideally language-independent digitally stored so as to improve the interdisciplinary interface for the benefit of the patient.

Mandibular Reconstruction

Partial mandibulectomy may be necessary [59] in oral tumours, osteoradionecrosis, osteomyelitis, or bisphosphonate-associated osteonecrosis of the mandible. Following surgery, the mandibular discontinuity defect must be reconstructed to restore its original contours. The mandible can be reconstructed with a vascularized soft tissue graft combined with an alloplastic reconstruction plate [60]. Reconstruction

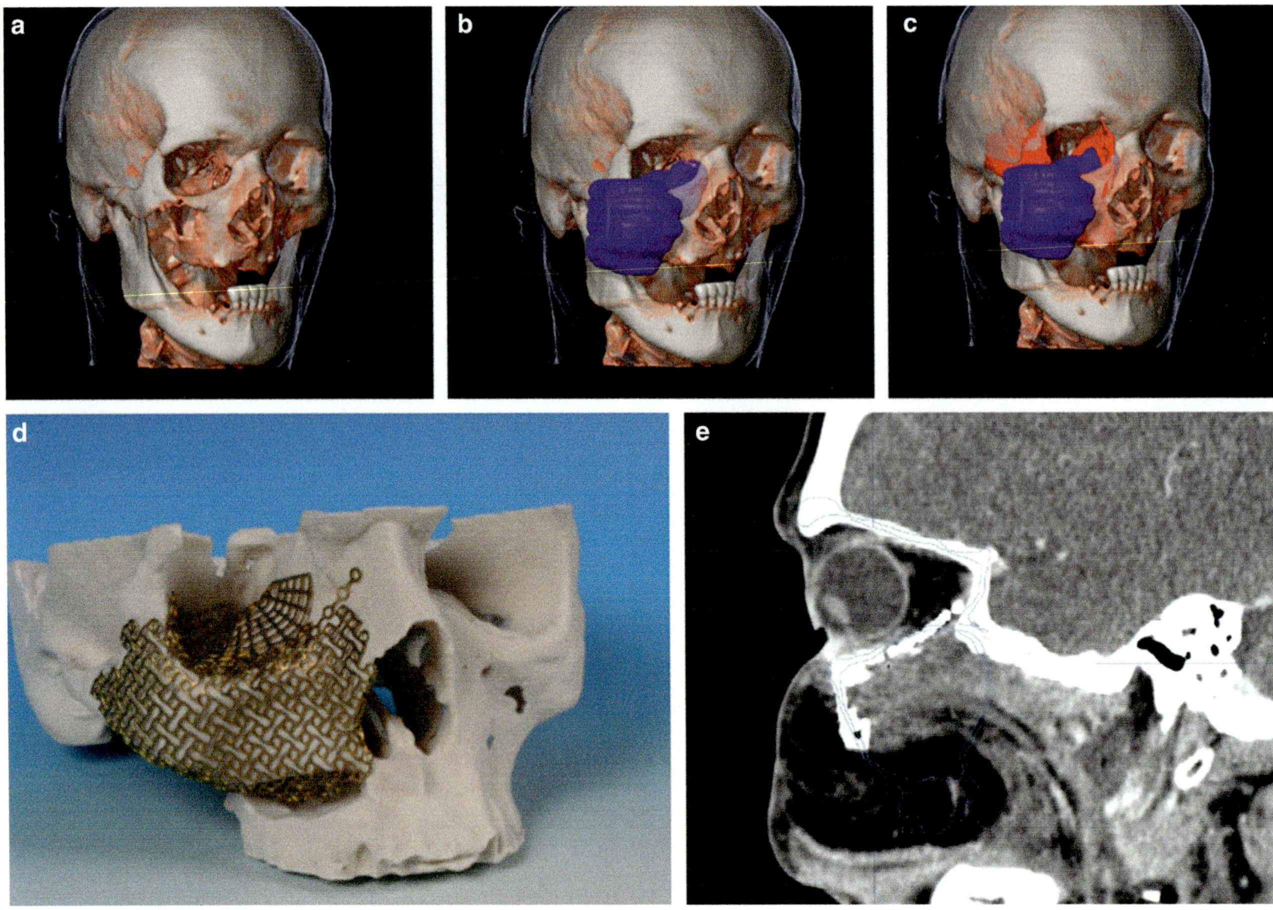

Fig. 14.20 (**a**, **b**, and **c**) Segmented tumour on the upper jaw and the planned resection (*red*). Intraoperative edge sections surrounding the tumour. (**d**) Three-dimensional mesh (DuPuy Synthes Craniomaxillofacial, Paoli, PA, USA) is molded on a stereolithographic (STL) midfacial skull model, produced via rapid prototype modeling. (**e**) Postoperative result (iPlan 3.0.5, Brainlab®, Feldkirchen, Germany)

plates for functionally stable internal fixation are conventionally bent along the outer contour of the mandible to recreate the original form. Simultaneously, or in a secondary procedure that is required for masticatory rehabilitation, autogenous bone (vascularized or non-vascularized), is fixed into position with the reconstruction plate [61].

The disadvantage of this approach is that because these bone grafts (fibular and iliac crest grafts) are aligned with the usual outer anatomic contour of the original mandible, it becomes difficult to achieve optimal prosthetically driven dental implant placement. As a result, the dental implants have been inserted into the available mandibular bone, and not in the correct alignment to the maxilla, with a compromised occlusion and masticatory function.

The biological requirement of proper dental rehabilitation defines the shape, volume, and the position of the autogenous bone graft, and thereby also the inner and outer contour of the patient-specific reconstruction plate. With conventional methods, however, these requirements are often impossible to meet. In the past, this often resulted in bone graft reconstructions that were located too far lateral for correct dental implant placement. Such a discrepancy between the desired and actual position of the bone graft in a vertical or transverse plane complicates the dental implant prosthetic rehabilitation.

With the help of preoperative planning in three dimensions, the shape of the PSI to reconstruct the mandibular contour can now be planned virtually. Through the automatic

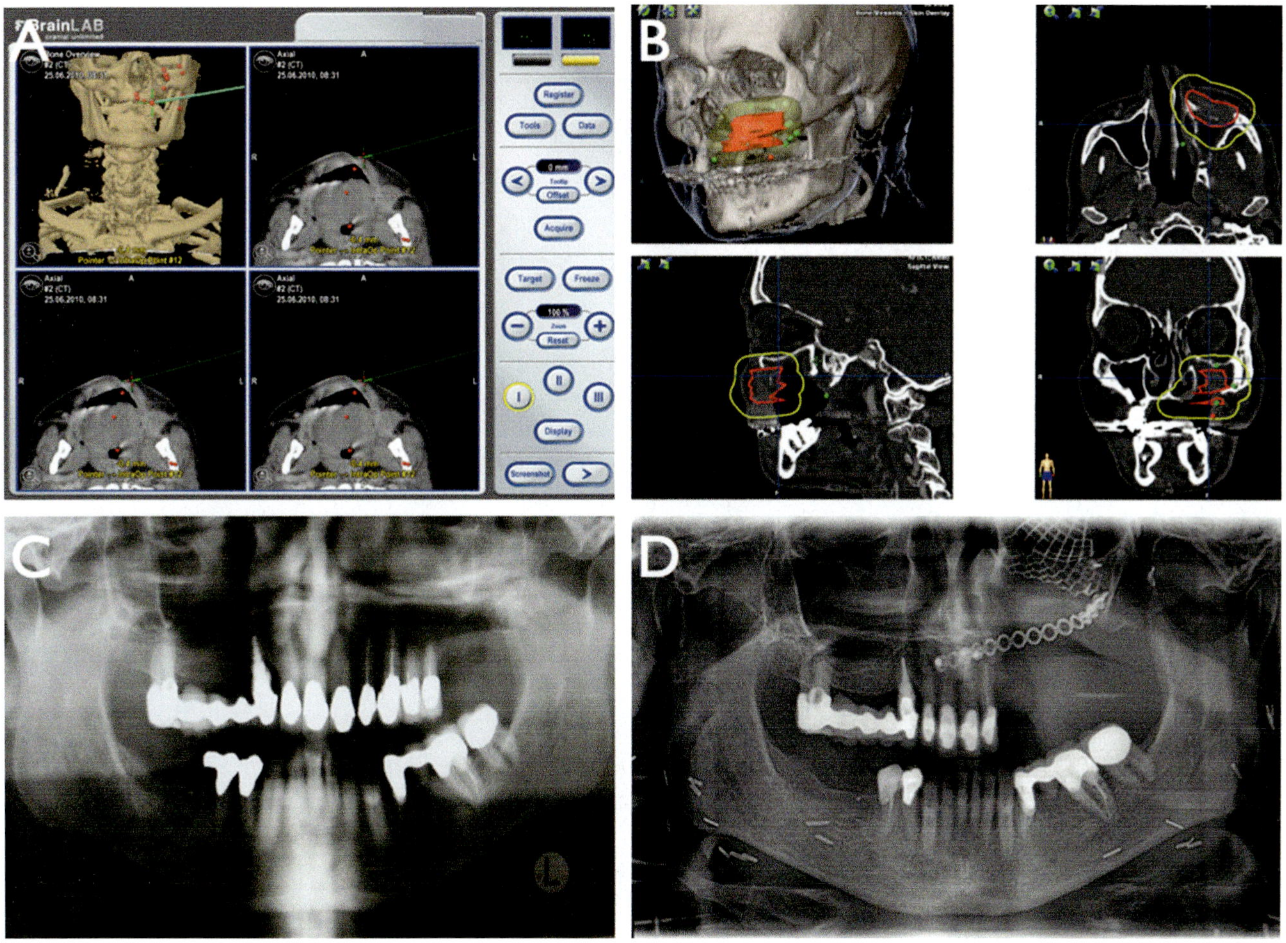

Fig. 14.21 (**a**) Screenshots of a primary T4a squamous cell carcinoma (SCC). (**b**) Resected tumour (SCC) of the left maxilla with invasion of pterygoid plates. (**c**) Panoramic view preoperative. (**d**) Panoramic view postoperative (Brainlab®, Feldkirchen, German)

segmentation, and the ability to manipulate the three-dimensional structures with appropriate tools, preoperative planning is facilitated. At the same time, the export of STL data allows the production of PSI through the pre-bending of three-dimensional models; thus, a reliable accuracy of implant fit can be achieved (Fig. 14.22).

The superimposition of pre- and postoperative records by planning systems allows quality control [60]. By this method, both the operation time is shortened and the reconstruction result can be predicted at the hard tissue level [58].

The benefit of computer-assisted planning of PSI in mandible reconstruction has been extensively documented over the last decade. These systems are have proven to offer a more predictable surgical procedure, some of which allow the virtual planning of dental implant placement. However, the precise reconstruction of an accurate segmented mandible continues to remain a challenge. Since these systems do not represent a complete 3D planning software, they have to be supplemented by additional software tools and hardware devices. As a consequence, the handling of these systems is of a collaborative and sometimes experimental nature, and web meetings with an engineer are required. At the present time, using CAS in primary alloplastic mandible reconstruction, allows for the PSI, as well as the resection and drilling guides to be fabricated prior to surgery. High levels of consistency between the fused preoperative plan and the intraoperative as well as postoperative CT data set can be achieved.

Modern treatment strategies for mandibular reconstruction and the backwards planning workflow could help to improve oral rehabilitation (Fig. 14.23).

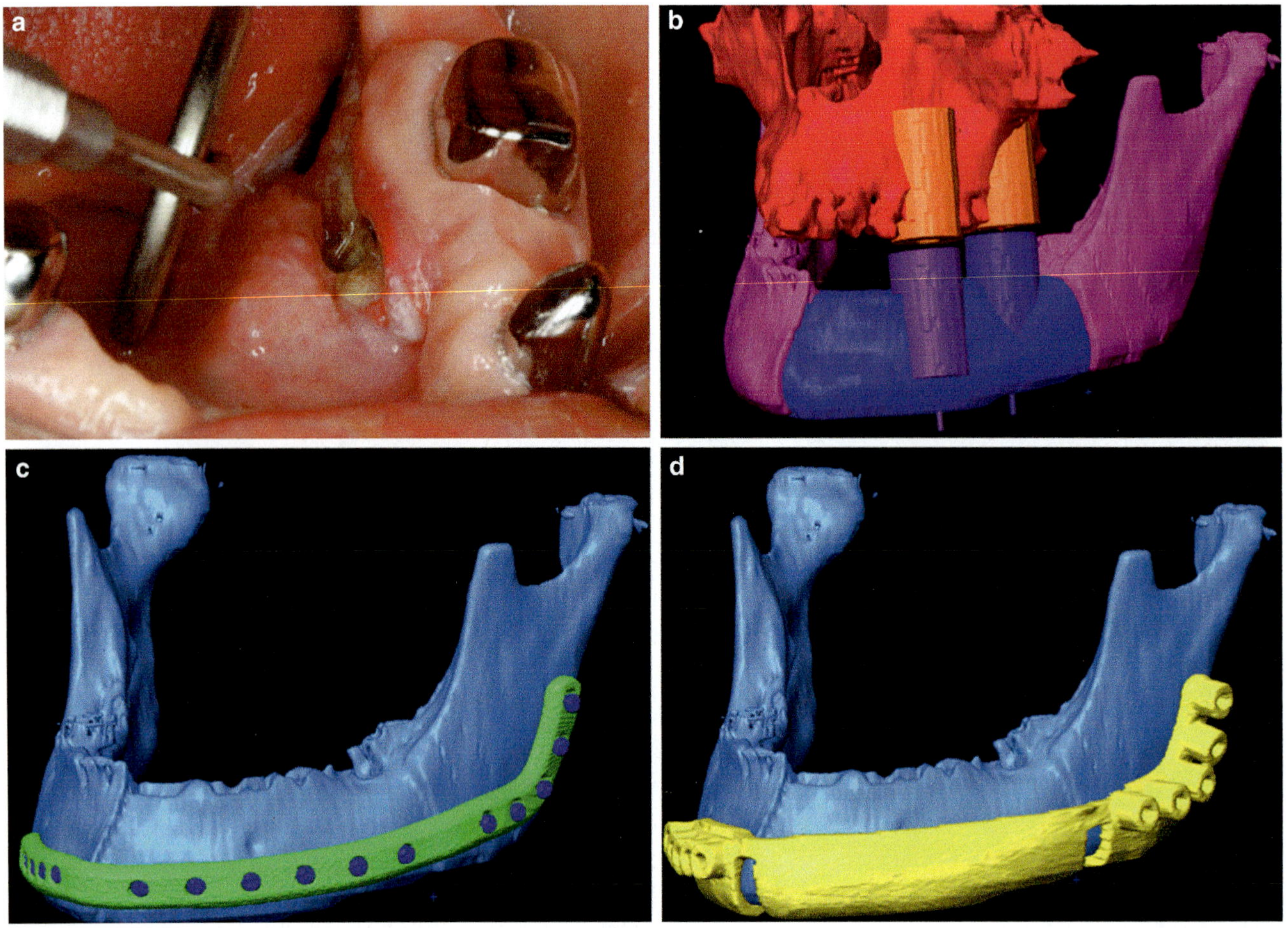

Fig. 14.22 (**a**) Intraoral view of a SCC of the left mandible. (**b**) Frontal view of a 3D skull with new anatomical structures of the mandible (*blue*) using automatic atlas-based algorithm and desired implant position (*multicolour*). (**c**) Reconstruction plate (*green*) (**d**) Cutting guide (*yellow*) (iPlan 3.0.5, Brainlab®, Feldkirchen, Germany)

Summary

Computer-assisted preoperative and postoperative planning (CAPP), and computer-assisted surgery (CAS) including navigation allow for the optimized use of 3D medical imaging data sets based on the DICOM standard. Without harm to the patient, a virtual surgical plan can be visualized and defined, and then followed, allowing greater precision during surgery. Based on the language independence of visualization, multiple ways of intraspecialty and interspecialty communication can be improved. Furthermore, the preoperative fabrication of patient-specific implants (PSI) is possible based on virtual planning with STL export. Modern digital workflows permit the reinsertion of the STL info of the actual patient-specific implant (PSI) into the data set for intraoperative navigation use, so that the positioning of the implant can be closely monitored for precise placement. These digital surgical workflows add a new transparency to CMF surgery that can be easily transferred to all surgical specialties, and represents a huge commitment towards quality control of the preoperative, intraoperative, and postoperative treatment pathways.

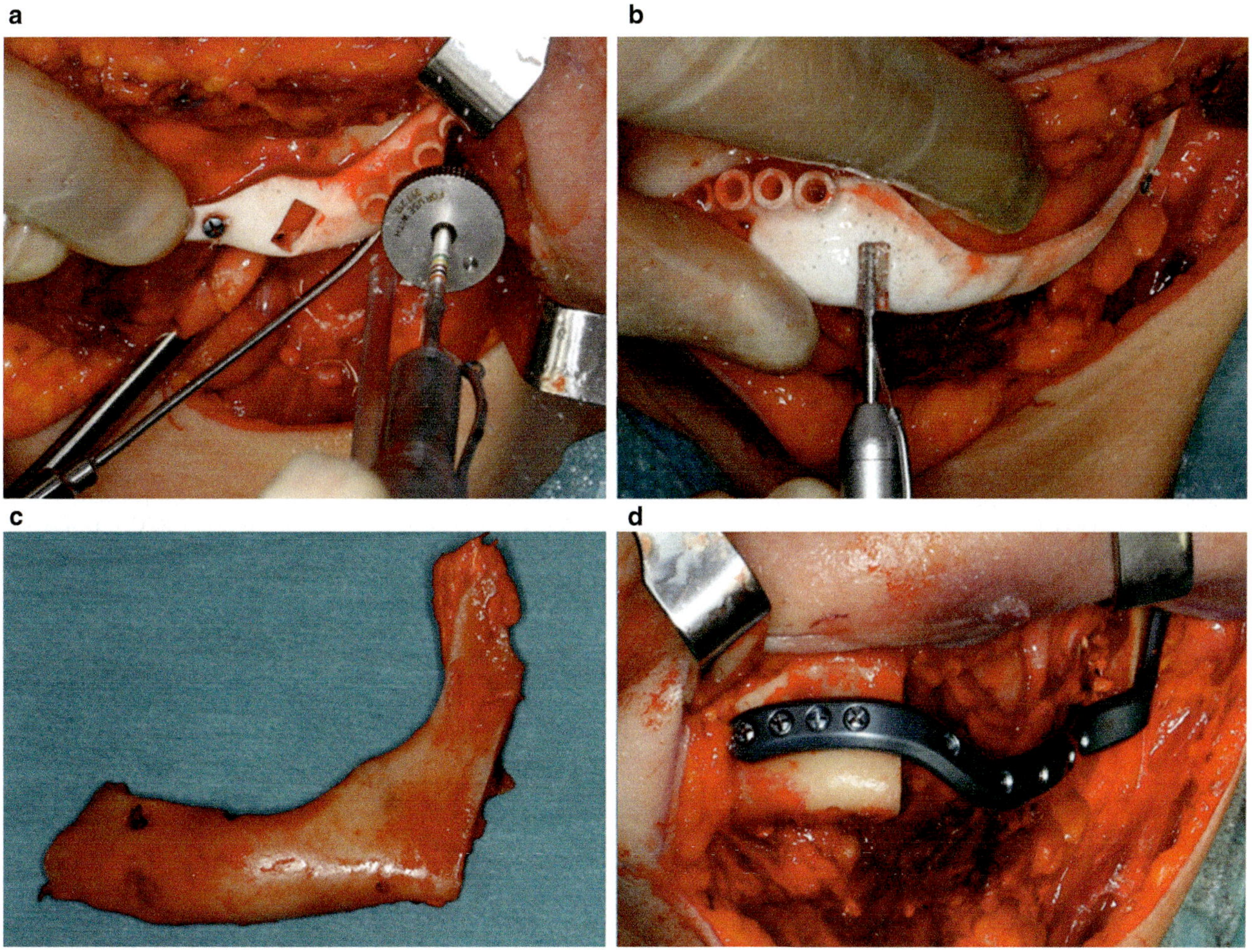

Fig. 14.23 (**a**), (**b**), and (**c**) Intraoperative view performing a mandible resection, using drilling guides and cutting guides. (**d**) PSI for the mandible is used to perform the reconstruction (DuPuy Synthes Craniomaxillofacial, Paoli, PA, USA)

References

1. Hassfeld S, Streib S, Sahl H, Stratmann U, Fehrentz D, Zoller J. Low-dose computerized tomography of the jaw bone in pre-implantation diagnosis. Limits of dose reduction and accuracy of distance measurements. Mund Kiefer Gesichtschir. 1998;2(4):188–93.
2. Schnelle C. Vergleich der Strahlenexposition bei der Digitalen-Volumen-Tomographie, der Panoramaschichtaufnahme und der Computertomographie [dissertation]. Düsseldorf: Heinrich-Heine-Universität; 2001.
3. Schulze D, Heiland M, Thurmann H, Adam G. Radiation exposure during midfacial imaging using 4- and 16-slice computed tomography, cone beam computed tomography systems and conventional radiography. Dentomaxillofac Radiol. 2004;33(2):83–6.
4. Zizelmann C, Gellrich NC, Metzger MC, Schoen R, Schmelzeisen R, Schramm A. Computer-assisted reconstruction of orbital floor based on cone beam tomography. Br J Oral Maxillofac Surg. 2007;45(1):79–80.
5. Liang X, Jacobs R, Hassan B, Li L, Pauwels R, Corpas L, et al. A comparative evaluation of cone beam computed tomography (CBCT) and multi-slice CT (MSCT): part I. On subjective image quality. Eur J Radiol. 2010;75(2):265–9.
6. Namimoto T, Yamashita Y, Sumi S, Tang Y, Takahashi M. Focal liver masses: characterization with diffusion-weighted echo-planar MR imaging. Radiology. 1997;204(3):739–44.

7. Hein PA, Kremser C, Judmaier W, Griebel J, Rudisch A, Pfeiffer KP, et al. Diffusion-weighted MRI—a new parameter for advanced rectal carcinoma? Rofo. 2003;175(3):381–6.
8. Herneth AM, Guccione S, Bednarski M. Apparent diffusion coefficient: a quantitative parameter for in vivo tumor characterization. Eur J Radiol. 2003;45(3):208–13.
9. Kamel IR, Bluemke DA, Ramsey D, Abusedera M, Torbenson M, Eng J, et al. Role of diffusion-weighted imaging in estimating tumor necrosis after chemoembolization of hepatocellular carcinoma. AJR Am J Roentgenol. 2003;181(3):708–10.
10. Barrington SF, Maisey MN, Wahl RL. Atlas of clinical positron emission tomography. London: Hodder Arnold; 2006.
11. Rana M, Gellrich NC, Joos U, Piffko J, Kater W. 3D evaluation of postoperative swelling using two different cooling methods following orthognathic surgery: a randomised observer blind prospective pilot study. Int J Oral Maxillofac Surg. 2011;40(7):690–6.
12. Rana M, Essig H, Eckardt AM, Tavassol F, Ruecker M, Schramm A, et al. Advances and innovations in computer-assisted head and neck oncologic surgery. J Craniofac Surg. 2012;23(1):272–8.
13. Schramm A, Gellrich NC, Schmelzeisen R. Navigational Surgery of the Facial Skeleton. Berlin/Heidelberg/New York: Springer; 2006.
14. Pirris SM, Nottmeier EW. A case series on the technical use of three-dimensional image guidance in subaxial anterior cervical surgery. Int J Med Robot. 2015;11(1):44–51.
15. Zamorano LJ, Nolte L, Kadi AM, Jiang Z. Interactive intraoperative localization using an infrared-based system. Neurol Res. 1993;15(5):290–8.
16. Heermann R, Schwab B, Issing PR, Haupt C, Hempel C, Lenarz T. Image-guided surgery of the anterior skull base. Acta Otolaryngol. 2001;121(8):973–8.
17. Bartling SH, Leinung M, Graute J, Rodt T, Dullin C, Becker H, et al. Increase of accuracy in intraoperative navigation through high-resolution flat-panel volume computed tomography: experimental comparison with multislice computed tomography-based navigation. Otol Neurotol. 2007;28(1):129–34.
18. Schramm A, Gellrich NC, Naumann S, Bühner U, Schön R, Schmelzeisen R. Non-invasive referencing in computer assisted surgery. Med Biol Eng Comput. 1999;37:644–5.
19. Heiland M, Pohlenz P, Blessmann M, Werle H, Fraederich M, Schmelzle R, et al. Navigated implantation after microsurgical bone transfer using intraoperatively acquired cone-beam computed tomography data sets. Int J Oral Maxillofac Surg. 2008;37(1):70–5.
20. Heiland M, Schulze D, Blake F, Schmelzle R. Intraoperative imaging of zygomaticomaxillary complex fractures using a 3D C-arm system. Int J Oral Maxillofac Surg. 2005;34(4):369–75.
21. Eggers G, Kress B, Rohde S, Muhling J. Intraoperative computed tomography and automated registration for image-guided cranial surgery. Dentomaxillofac Radiol. 2009;38(1):28–33.
22. Stelter K, Ledderose G, Hempel JM, Morhard DF, Flatz W, Krause E, et al. Image guided navigation by intraoperative CT scan for cochlear implantation. Comput Aided Surg. 2012;17(3):153–60.
23. Chu ST. Endoscopic sinus surgery under navigation system—analysis report of 79 cases. J Chin Med Assoc. 2006;69(11):529–33.
24. Anon JB, Lipman SP, Oppenheim D, Halt RA. Computer-assisted endoscopic sinus surgery. Laryngoscope. 1994;104(7):901–5.
25. Sipos EP, Tebo SA, Zinreich SJ, Long DM, Brem H. In vivo accuracy testing and clinical experience with the ISG viewing wand. Neurosurgery. 1996;39(1):194–202. discussion -4
26. Olivier A, Germano IM, Cukiert A, Peters T. Frameless stereotaxy for surgery of the epilepsies: preliminary experience. Technical note. J Neurosurg. 1994;81(4):629–33.
27. Klimek L, Mosges R. Computer-assisted surgery in the ENT specialty. Developments and experiences from the first decade. Laryngorhinootologie. 1998;77(5):275–82.
28. Anon JB, Klimek L, Mosges R, Zinreich SJ. Computer-assisted endoscopic sinus surgery. An international review. Otolaryngol Clin N Am. 1997;30(3):389–401.
29. Zaaroor M, Bejerano Y, Weinfeld Z, Ben-Haim S. Novel magnetic technology for intraoperative intracranial frameless navigation: in vivo and in vitro results. Neurosurgery. 2001;48(5):1100–7. discussion 7-8
30. Frantz DD, Wiles AD, Leis SE, Kirsch SR. Accuracy assessment protocols for electromagnetic tracking systems. Phys Med Biol. 2003;48(14):2241–51.
31. Mascott CR. Comparison of magnetic tracking and optical tracking by simultaneous use of two independent frameless stereotactic systems. Neurosurgery. 2005;57(4 Suppl):295–301. discussion 295–301.
32. Reinhardt HF, Horstmann GA, Gratzl O. Microsurgical removal of deep vascular malformations using sonar-stereometry. Ultraschall Med. 1991;12(2):80–3.
33. Nitsche N, Hubert M, Strasser G, Schuiz H, Wunderlich A, Arnold W. Einsatz eines berührungsfreien computergestützten Orientierungssystems bei Nasennebenhöhlenoperationen. Oto-Rhino-Laryngologia Nova. 1993;3(4):173–9.
34. Watanabe E, Mayanagi Y, Kosugi Y, Manaka S, Takakura K. Open surgery assisted by the neuronavigator, a stereotactic, articulated, sensitive arm. Neurosurgery. 1991;28(6):792–9. discussion 9-800
35. Gellrich NC, Schramm A, Hammer B, Rojas S, Cufi D, Lagreze W, et al. Computer-assisted secondary reconstruction of unilateral posttraumatic orbital deformity. Plast Reconstr Surg. 2002;110(6):1417–29.
36. Schramm A, Wilde F. Die computergestützte Gesichtsschädelrekonstruktion. HNO. 2011;59(8):800–6.
37. Kokemuller H, von See C, Essig H, Tavassol F, Rucker M, Schramm A, et al. Reconstruction of complex midfacial defects with individualized titanium implants. HNO. 2011;59(4):319–26.
38. Schmelzeisen R, Schramm A. Computer-assisted reconstruction of the facial skeleton. Arch Facial Plast Surg. 2003;5(5):437.
39. Essig H, Dressel L, Rana M, Rana M, Kokemueller H, Ruecker M, et al. Precision of posttraumatic primary orbital reconstruction using individually bent titanium mesh with and without navigation: a retrospective study. Head Face Med. 2013;9(1):18.
40. Rana M, Modrow D, Keuchel J, Chui C, Rana M, Wagner M, et al. Development and evaluation of an automatic tumor segmentation tool: a comparison between automatic, semi-automatic and manual segmentation of mandibular odontogenic cysts and tumors. J Craniomaxillofac Surg. 2014;43:355–9.
41. Bell WH. Le Forte I osteotomy for correction of maxillary deformities. J Oral Surg. 1975;33(6):412–26.
42. Obwegeser H. The indications for surgical correction of mandibular deformity by the sagittal splitting technique. Br J Oral Surg. 1964;1:157–71.
43. Zizelmann C, Hammer B, Gellrich NC, Schwestka-Polly R, Rana M, Bucher P. An evaluation of face-bow transfer for the planning of orthognathic surgery. J Oral Maxillofac Surg. 2012;70(8):1944–50.
44. Xia JJ, Shevchenko L, Gateno J, Teichgraeber JF, Taylor TD, Lasky RE, et al. Outcome study of computer-aided surgical simulation in the treatment of patients with craniomaxillofacial deformities. J Oral Maxillofac Surg. 2011;69(7):2014–24.
45. Schwestka-Polly R, Kubein-Meesenburg D, Luhr HG. Techniques for achieving three-dimensional positioning of the maxilla applied in conjunction with the Gottingen concept. Int J Adult Orthodon Orthognath Surg. 1998;13(3):248–58.
46. Helm G, Stepke MT. Maintenance of the preoperative condyle position in orthognathic surgery. J Craniomaxillofac Surg. 1997;25(1):34–8.
47. Saka B, Petsch I, Hingst V, Härtel J. The influence of pre- and intraoperative positioning of the condyle in the centre of the articular fossa on the position of the disc in orthognathic surgery. A magnetic resonance study. Br J Oral Maxillofac Surg. 2004;42(2):120–6.
48. Schwestka-Polly R, Kubein-Meesenburg D, Luhr HG. Results of the application of the Goettingen concept for three-dimensional repositioning of the maxilla in orthognathic surgery. Mund Kiefer Gesichtschir. 1999;3(3):123–30.

49. Schwestka-Polly R. Fortschritte in der gelenkbezüglichen kieferorthopädisch-kieferchirurgischen Therapie. Inf Orthod Kieferorthop. 2004;36(04):205–18.
50. Miller RJ, Bier J. Surgical navigation in oral implantology. Implant Dent. 2006;15(1):41–7.
51. Miller RJ. Navigated surgery in oral implantology: a case study. Int J Med Robot. 2007;3(3):229–34.
52. Hohlweg-Majert B, Schon R, Schmelzeisen R, Gellrich NC, Schramm A. Navigational maxillofacial surgery using virtual models. World J Surg. 2005;29(12):1530–8.
53. Schneider U, Pedroni E, Lomax A. The calibration of CT Hounsfield units for radiotherapy treatment planning. Phys Med Biol. 1996;41(1):111–24.
54. Gaggl A, Schultes G, Karcher H. Navigational precision of drilling tools preventing damage to the mandibular canal. J Craniomaxillofac Surg. 2001;29(5):271–5.
55. Nickenig HJ, Spiekermann H. CT/DVT-basierte implantatprothetische Führungsschablonen vs. traditionelle Orientierungsschablonen. Z Zahnärztl Implantol. 2006;22:272–80.
56. Cohnen M, Kemper J, Mobes O, Pawelzik J, Modder U. Radiation dose in dental radiology. Eur Radiol. 2002;12(3):634–7.
57. Möbes O, Becker J, Schnelle C, Ewen K, Kemper J, Cohnen M. Strahlenexposition bei der digitalen Volumentomographiem, Panoramaschichtaufnahme und Computertomographie. Dtsch Zahnarztl Z. 2000;55:336–9.
58. Kokemüller H, See C, Essig H, Tavassol F, Rücker M, Schramm A, et al. Rekonstruktion komplexer Mittelgesichtsdefekte durch individualisierte Titanimplantate. HNO. 2011;59(4):319–26.
59. Schramm A, Gellrich NC. Intraoperative Navigation und computerassistierte Chirurgie. In: Schwenzer N, editor. Mund-Kiefer-Gesichtschirurgie. Georg Thieme Verlag; Stuttgart, Germany. 2011.
60. Eckardt A, Swennen GR. Virtual planning of composite mandibular reconstruction with free fibula bone graft. J Craniofac Surg. 2005;16(6):1137–40.
61. Rana M, Warraich R, Kokemuller H, Lemound J, Essig H, Tavassol F, et al. Reconstruction of mandibular defects – clinical retrospective research over a 10-year period. Head Neck Oncol. 2011;3:23.

Digital Planning of Craniomaxillofacial Radiation Therapy

15

Gido Bittermann, Marc C. Metzger, and Rainer Schmelzeisen

Introduction

Cancer of the head and neck requires a multidisciplinary approach in order to obtain optimal balance between tumour control and quality of life. Locally advanced oral squamous cell carcinoma (SCC) is commonly treated by a combination of surgical resection, reconstruction and radiotherapy or radiochemotherapy. Given the involvement of multiple disciplines, precise communication is indispensable and a challenge. Optimization of patient management has been promoted by the setting up of tumour boards or multidisciplinary teams (MDT) that discuss various options and drawbacks.

The anatomy of the head and neck offers a further challenge in the management of these patients. The balance between complete resection and organ preservation with good postoperative function and quality of life is often difficult to achieve.

Once a decision for surgery is made, the next important step is precise communication between the surgeon, pathologist and radiation oncologists regarding specimen orientation and location of any additional biopsies or tumour bed delineation. An interdisciplinary interface enables a workflow of preoperative 3D imaging, intraoperative navigation and postoperative processing to produce a precise delineation of the tumour margins to aid in communication with the pathologist and to help the radiation oncologist in the planning and delivery of adjuvant radiotherapy. The aim is a standardised interdisciplinary communication to allow precise mapping of any frozen sections and a focused delivery of adjuvant irradiation at the tumour bed. Figure 15.1. depicts how image-guided navigation procedures and an interdisciplinary interface could improve the communication between surgeons, pathologists and radiation oncologists.

G. Bittermann (✉) • M.C. Metzger • R. Schmelzeisen
Department of Craniomaxillofacial Surgery, University of Freiburg, Freiburg, Germany
e-mail: gido.bittermann@uniklinik-freiburg.de; marc.metzger@uniklinik-freiburg.de; rainer.schmelzeisen@uniklinik-freiburg.de

Preoperative Planning

3D data sets acquired from preoperative imaging (e.g. computed tomography (CT) or magnetic resonance imaging (MRI)) are fused and have been shown to be a helpful tool in examining hard and soft tissues together [1]. Sometimes information gathered from positron emission tomography (PET) is added to preoperative data [2, 3]. In this way the tumour and its associated destruction are delineated in three dimensions [4]. The different tissues can then be marked by simulated segmentation to plan the resection, as well as the bony and soft tissue reconstruction. This allows three-dimensional surgical planning with visualisation of tumour extent and possible resection margins (Fig. 15.2).

Surgical Resection

Modern head and neck cancer therapy strives for complete resection of the tumour. In this surgical treatment, the analyses of tumour and resection margins are fundamental. The desired goal in cancer surgery is cure for which a R0 resection of the malignant neoplasm is a starting point [5, 6]. The status of resection margins has an influence on the outcome with respect to recurrence and mortality [5]. Patients with positive (R1 or R2 resection) or close surgical margins show a significantly less favorable outcome [7].

It is becoming more common to send frozen section biopsies intraoperatively to the processing pathologist. Precise collection and mapping of frozen sections will aid in achieving complete resection at the microscopic level.

A.M. Greenberg (ed.), *Digital Technologies in Craniomaxillofacial Surgery*, https://doi.org/10.1007/978-1-4939-1532-3_15

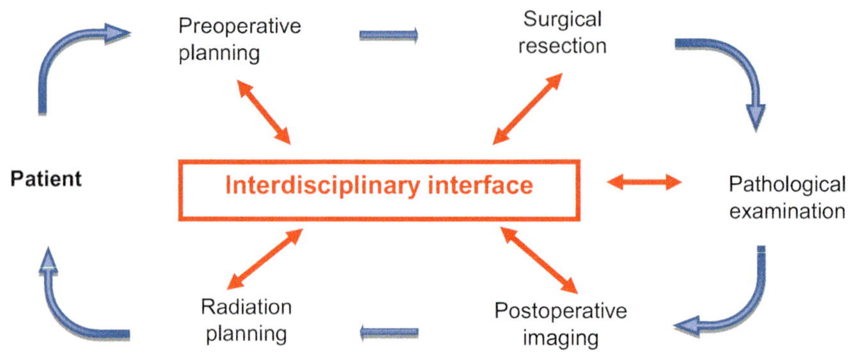

Fig. 15.1 Image-guided navigation procedures and an interdisciplinary interface could improve the communication between surgeons, pathologists and radiation oncologists

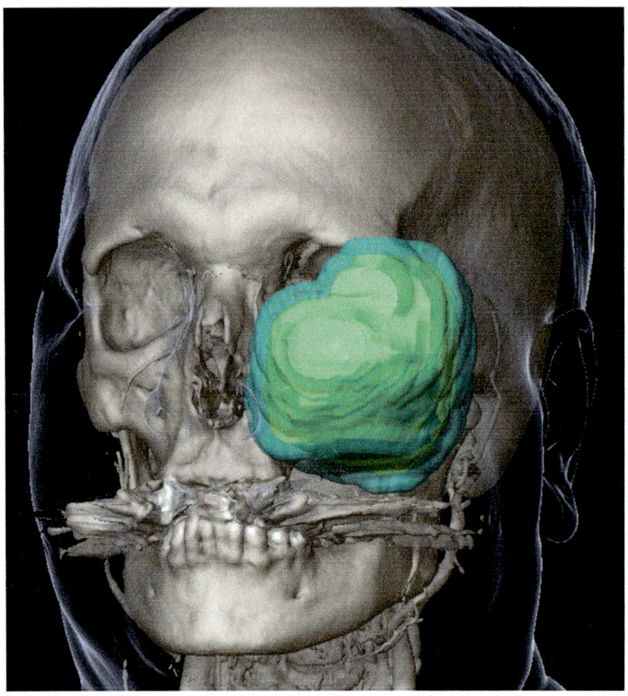

Fig. 15.2 Representation of preoperative planning: segmentation of an advanced tumour (*yellow*) of the left maxillary sinus and the left orbital cavity. A virtual resection margin (*blue*) was added around the tumour volume (iPlan, Brainlab, Munich, Germany)

Traditionally, the method of labeling is relegated to the surgeon's memory of where the sample was taken from, so that additional targeted resection may be performed. The pathologist receives a specimen and a label with a minimal idea of its orientation. From this a response of positive or negative is sought. If positive (tumour cells could be detected in the sample), it falls upon the memory of the surgeon to localise where the sample was precisely taken which will ultimately affect the final resection margin. Various refinements in the field of computer-aided surgery (CAS) have been implemented in order to improve marking of resection margins and the tumour bed by intraoperative navigation [8–11]. Surgical navigation has become an established technique in the field of head and neck surgery [8].

Intraoperative Navigation

CAS systems require a headset transmitter to be secured to the patient with an additional transmitter on a pointer. Based on preoperative imaging and the identification of fiducial markers on the CAS monitor, the optical detector allows the computer to integrate spatial information from the actual patient with a virtual treatment plan. This allows precise localisation of the patient and surgical instrument on/in the patient [12]. The navigation pointer is then used to map and label the frozen section specimen and to control the boundaries of the resection by comparing the preoperative 3D plan with the intraoperative findings.

Marking of Resection Margins

When collecting frozen sections, the site of the biopsy is marked and mapped by the navigation probe, and this precise localisation data is stored at the interdisciplinary interface. The labeled frozen sections and the data set with coordinates are then transmitted to the pathologist who can colour code the positive and negative results on the virtual image. The data coordinates provide the pathologist with accurate localisation and positional relationship of the samples. The CAS allows clear marking of frozen sections in space and labeling by digital data coordinates, rendering them accurate and repeatable to mark corresponding points where sections are returned positive. Intraoperatively, CAS procedures enable fairly precise three-dimensional anatomical orientation with more defined localisation of skull base and midface resection boundaries (Fig. 15.3a, b) [9, 10].

After complete tumour ablation, the resection margins are marked with the navigation pointer if the margin lies on bone or close to it. Although the accuracy and reliability of the navigation workflow is generally accepted for midface and cranial vault operations, intraoperative navigation of the mandible and adjacent soft tissue structures, e.g. the tongue or the floor of the mouth, is still challenging [9, 13].

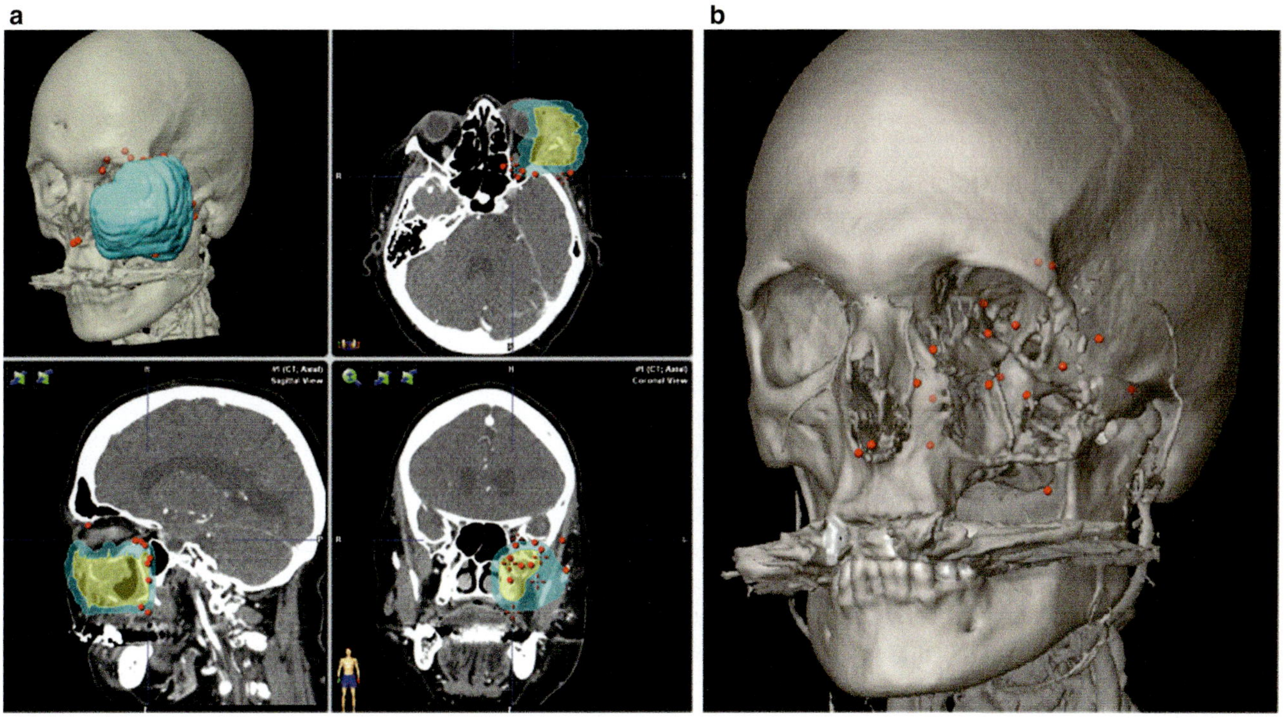

Fig. 15.3 3D reconstruction of CT data set after complete tumour excision of an advanced maxillary sinus carcinoma and after intraoperative labelling of frozen sections. (**a**) Intraoperative CAS marking in relationship to the preoperative resection planning. (**b**) The pathologist receives a specimen and a label with precise intraoperative orientation. This data also serves to communicate (interdisciplinary interface) to the oncologist the exact extent of the resection and the areas where additional focus may be needed based on positive frozen sections (iPlan, Brainlab, Munich, Germany)

This is either because of the mandible's independent movement from the rest of the cranium or soft tissue shifts as the result of gravity and swelling. If the margin lies on soft tissue, marking is made with titanium ligature clips, so they are radio-opaque and biocompatible and do not interfere with radiation [14].

Markers, regardless whether titanium, gold seeds or virtually aided, placed in surgical cavity walls provide additional localisation information compared to CT imaging alone [9, 15, 16]. The cavity walls will be referred to as the tumour bed. The markers are placed at the deep, superficial, medial, lateral, inferior and superior boundary of the resection margin. Immediate microvascular free tissue reconstruction is an established method in cases of insufficient adjacent tissue and has gained acceptance as standard practice [17]. The type and extent of reconstruction is an additional challenge for radiation delivery, especially when using tissue transfer. In the course of tumour resections, defects are often reconstructed with free vascularised tissue. When there is neck lymph node involvement, R1–Rx tumour resection or close tumour margins, comprehensive treatment of advanced head and neck cancers frequently mandates the use of adjuvant external beam radiotherapy, but it is challenging for the oncologist to plan radiotherapy focused on the resection margins and the underlying tissue while sparing the tumour free vascularised graft [17, 18]. It is well known that wound healing after tissue reconstruction is reduced by postoperative radiation [19, 20]. On the other side, an increase of the irradiation dose correlates with an increase of the tumour control. The radiation oncologist requires as much information as possible from the surgeon in order to accurately plan radiation dosages to the affected tissue and minimise unnecessary radiation of adjacent tissues as well as vital structures. Traditionally, radiation therapy protocols are based on printed pathology reports, pre- and postoperative imaging as well as surgical operative notes which are notoriously indecipherable [10]. An essential prerequisite of external beam irradiation is accurate localisation of tumour bed, for which many oncologists are using CT images [21]. Delineation of reconstructed tissue from resection margins on postoperative CT scans is often difficult. Precise orientation of the boundaries between resection margin and free flap reconstruction therefore becomes important. In this situation marking of resection margins could be helpful [9]. Planning radiotherapy is further complicated by variation between the virtual resection margin and the true postsurgical one. Additionally soft tissue distortions occur as the result of gravity and swelling which alter the appearance of the resection margins. In order to avoid this, the margins are marked with titanium ligature clips. Recent investigations could demonstrate that image-guided navigation procedures and an interdisciplinary interface improves the communication between surgeons, pathologists and radiation oncologists [9–11].

Postoperative Processing

An additional 3D imaging (CT or cone beam CT (CBCT)) is performed postoperatively, and the titanium clips are identified. Preoperative and postoperative images could be fused, and all landmarks and clips were highlighted when viewed axially. Tumour resection margins are then outlined manually using the brushing tool on the software (Fig. 15.4). When final histology of the resected specimen is received, this is incorporated with the localisation of the frozen sections. This provides a three-dimensional representation of the histological findings in relation to the resection margins on the virtual patient.

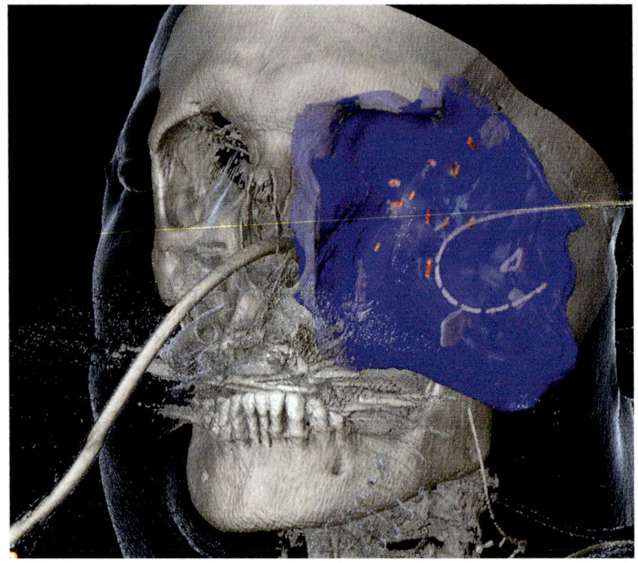

Fig. 15.4 3D reconstruction and precise delineation of the former tumour bed after complete tumour excision, marking of the tumour resection margin and free flap reconstruction. The titanium clips are highlighted (*red*) and a virtual blanket (*blue*) represents the former tumour bed (iPlan, Brainlab, Munich, Germany)

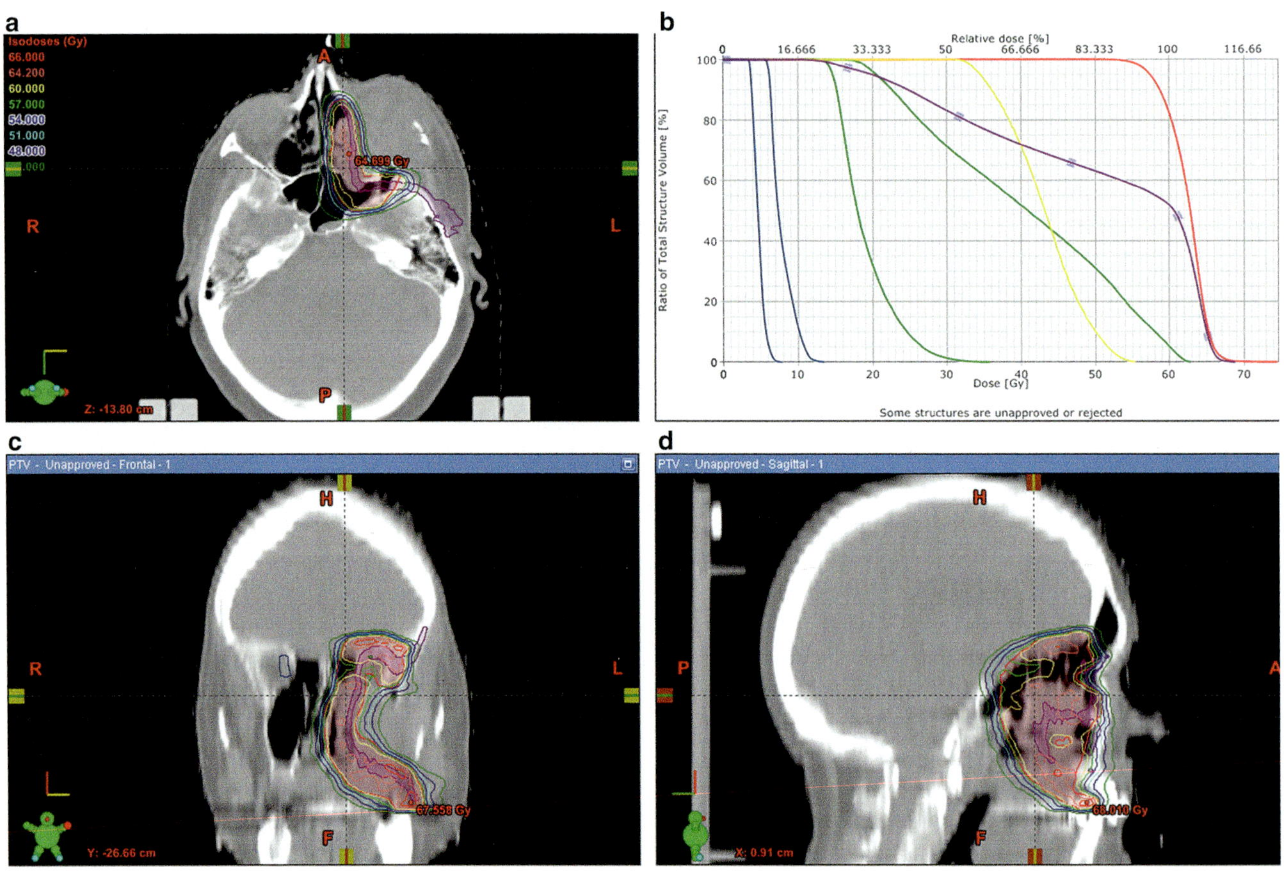

Fig. 15.5 Advances in radiotherapy such as intensity-modulated radiation therapy (IMRT) aim to increase the dose within the tumour bed, while reducing the dose to the surrounding healthy tissue and the free flap reconstruction. (**a–d**) Virtual planning of radiation treatment of an advanced left maxillary sinus tumour as volume-modulated arc therapy (VMAT) using Eclipse Software Version 10.1 (Varian Medical Solutions, Palo Alto, USA)

Planning Adjuvant Irradiation

Locally advanced oral squamous cell carcinoma (SCC) is commonly treated by a combination of surgical resection immediate reconstruction, and adjuvant radio- or radiochemotherapy. Adjuvant radiotherapy for the treatment of advanced head and neck squamous cell carcinoma improves local control and survival but is associated with increased radiation-related side effects due to irradiation of non-target tissue. As radiation morbidity is directly related to irradiated volume, limiting radiotherapy treatment volume can expectedly decrease late toxicity [22]. It is well known that wound healing after tissue reconstruction is reduced by postoperative radiation [23–25].

In the field of head and neck surgery, advanced tissue replacement for defect coverage is often necessary by means of free tissue transfer after expanded tumour resections. Accurate delineation of the tumour bed is a prerequisite of radiotherapy and is critical to achieving long-term local control for adjuvant radiotherapy. CAS labeling of tumour margin localisation can modify the radiotherapy field borders to focus irradiation on the former tumour bed. However, CAS alone is insufficient in delineating tumour margins away from hard tissue in the soft tissue and, the delineation of reconstructed tissue from resection margins on postoperative scans is often difficult [9, 10]. Additionally, soft tissue distortions, as the result of gravity and swelling, will alter the appearance of the resection margins. In such a situation, marking of tissue margins by titanium clips is useful [21, 26]. Data coordinates generated by the navigation procedure or by conventional clipping provide the pathologist with accurate localisation and the positional relationship of the samples, and the radiation oncologist with the exact extent of the resection and delineation of the tissue reconstruction. By incorporating the navigation and clips together, this provides a very accurate delineation of the target tissue margins on postoperative 3D imaging for the radiation therapist to focus the adjuvant radiation and thus reduce the exposure of the free vascular flap reconstruction (Fig. 15.5). Subsequently, the communication between the surgeon, pathologist and radiation oncologist is complemented by a visual orientation aid.

References

1. Messmer P, Gross T, Suhm N, Regazzoni P, Jacob AL, Huegli RW. Modality-based navigation. Injury. 2004;35(Suppl 1):S-A24–9.
2. Caldwell CB, Mah K, Skinner M, Danjoux CE. Can PET provide the 3D extent of tumor motion for individualized internal target volumes? A phantom study of the limitations of CT and the promise of PET. Int J Radiat Oncol Biol Phys. 2003;55(5):1381–93.
3. Beyer T, Townsend DW, Brun T, Kinahan PE, Charron M, Roddy R, et al. A combined PET/CT scanner for clinical oncology. J Nucl Med. 2000;41(8):1369–79.
4. Feichtinger M, Pau M, Zemann W, Aigner RM, Karcher H. Intraoperative control of resection margins in advanced head and neck cancer using a 3D-navigation system based on PET/CT image fusion. J Craniomaxillofac Surg. 2010;38(8):589–94.
5. Binahmed A, Nason RW, Abdoh AA. The clinical significance of the positive surgical margin in oral cancer. Oral Oncol. 2007;43(8):780–4.
6. Liao CT, Chang JT, Wang HM, Ng SH, Hsueh C, Lee LY, et al. Surgical outcome of T4a and resected T4b oral cavity cancer. Cancer. 2006;107(2):337–44.
7. Loree TR, Strong EW. Significance of positive margins in oral cavity squamous carcinoma. Am J Surg. 1990;160(4):410–4.
8. Schramm A, Suarez-Cunqueiro MM, Barth EL, Essig H, Bormann KH, Kokemueller H, et al. Computer-assisted navigation in craniomaxillofacial tumors. J Craniofac Surg. 2008;19(4):1067–74.
9. Bittermann G, Scheifele C, Prokic V, Bhatt V, Henke M, Grosu AL, et al. Description of a method: computer generated virtual model for accurate localisation of tumour margins, standardised resection, and planning of radiation treatment in head & neck cancer surgery. J Craniomaxillofac Surg. 2012;41:279–81.
10. Essig H, Rana M, Meyer A, Eckardt AM, Kokemueller H, von See C, et al. Virtual 3D tumor marking-exact intraoperative coordinate mapping improve post-operative radiotherapy. Radiat Oncol. 2011;6:159.
11. Guijarro-Martinez R, Gellrich NC, Witte J, Tapioles D, von Briel C, Kolotas C, et al. Optimization of the interface between radiology, surgery, radiotherapy, and pathology in head and neck tumor surgery: a navigation-assisted multidisciplinary network. Int J Oral Maxillofac Surg. 2013;43:156–62.
12. Metzger MC, Rafii A, Holhweg-Majert B, Pham AM, Strong B. Comparison of 4 registration strategies for computer-aided maxillofacial surgery. Otolaryngol Head Neck Surg. 2007;137(1):93–9.
13. Lubbers HT, Jacobsen C, Matthews F, Gratz KW, Kruse A, Obwegeser JA. Surgical navigation in craniomaxillofacial surgery: expensive toy or useful tool? A classification of different indications. J Oral Maxillofac Surg. 2011;69(1):300–8.
14. Oh JL, Nguyen G, Whitman GJ, Hunt KK, Yu TK, Woodward WA, et al. Placement of radiopaque clips for tumor localization in patients undergoing neoadjuvant chemotherapy and breast conservation therapy. Cancer. 2007;110(11):2420–7.
15. Kirby AM, Evans PM, Nerurkar AY, Desai SS, Krupa J, Devalia H, et al. How does knowledge of three-dimensional excision margins following breast conservation surgery impact upon clinical target volume definition for partial-breast radiotherapy? Radiother Oncol. 2010;94(3):292–9.
16. Kirova YM, Castro Pena P, Hijal T, Fournier-Bidoz N, Laki F, Sigal-Zafrani B, et al. Improving the definition of tumor bed boost with the use of surgical clips and image registration in breast cancer patients. Int J Radiat Oncol Biol Phys. 2010;78(5):1352–5.
17. Choi S, Schwartz DL, Farwell DG, Austin-Seymour M, Futran N. Radiation therapy does not impact local complication rates after free flap reconstruction for head and neck cancer. Arch Otolaryngol Head Neck Surg. 2004;130(11):1308–12.
18. Chen TC, Wang CP, Ko JY, Yang TL, Lou PJ. The impact of pathologic close margin on the survival of patients with early stage oral squamous cell carcinoma. Oral Oncol. 2012;48(7):623–8.
19. Nemeth Z, Somogyi A, Takacsi-Nagy Z, Barabas J, Nemeth G, Szabo G. Possibilities of preventing osteoradionecrosis during complex therapy of tumors of the oral cavity. Pathol Oncol Res. 2000;6(1):53–8.
20. Wang Z, Qiu W, Huang G. Influence of radiotherapy on reconstruction flaps in oral and maxillofacial regions. Zhonghua Er Bi Yan Hou Ke Za Zhi. 1999;34(3):177–9.

21. Kirby AN, Jena R, Harris EJ, Evans PM, Crowley C, Gregory DL, et al. Tumour bed delineation for partial breast/breast boost radiotherapy: what is the optimal number of implanted markers? Radiother Oncol. 2013;106(2):231–5.
22. Yang TJ, Tao R, Elkhuizen PH, van Vliet-Vroegindeweij C, Li G, Powell SN. Tumor bed delineation for external beam accelerated partial breast irradiation: a systematic review. Radiother Oncol. 2013;108(2):181–9.
23. Chao AH, Chang DW, Shuaib SW, Hanasono MM. The effect of neoadjuvant versus adjuvant irradiation on microvascular free flap reconstruction in sarcoma patients. Plast Reconstr Surg. 2012;129(3):675–82.
24. Baker SR, Krause CJ, Panje WR. Radiation effects on microvascular anastomosis. Arch Otolaryngol. 1978;104(2):103–7.
25. Zafereo ME, Weber RS, Lewin JS, Roberts DB, Hanasono MM. Complications and functional outcomes following complex oropharyngeal reconstruction. Head Neck. 2009;32(8):1003–11.
26. Ohdaira T, Nagai H. Intraoperative localization of early-stage upper gastrointestinal tumors using a magnetic marking clip-detecting system. Surg Endosc. 2007;21(5):810–5.

Index

A.M. Greenberg (ed.), *Digital Technologies in Craniomaxillofacial Surgery*, https://doi.org/10.1007/978-1-4939-1532-3